# THIS BOOK IS THE PROPERTY OF:

STATE _____

PROVINCE _____

COUNTY _____

PARISH _____

SCHOOL DISTRICT _____

OTHER _____

Book No. _____

Enter information
in spaces
to the left as
instructed

| ISSUED TO | Year Used | CONDITION | |
|---|---|---|---|
| | | ISSUED | RETURNED |
| | | | |
| | | | |
| | | | |
| | | | |
| | | | |
| | | | |
| | | | |
| | | | |

**PUPILS to whom this textbook is issued must not write on any page or mark any part of it in any way, consumable textbooks excepted.**

1. Teachers should see that the pupil's name is clearly written in ink in the spaces above in every book issued.

2. The following terms should be used in recording the condition of the book: New; Good; Fair; Poor; Bad.

# Fitness for Life

## SIXTH EDITION

**Charles B. Corbin**
Arizona State University

**Guy C. Le Masurier**
Vancouver Island University

Contributing author:

**Karen E. McConnell**
Pacific Lutheran University

Human Kinetics

**Library of Congress Cataloging-in-Publication Data**

Corbin, Charles B.
  Fitness for life / Charles B. Corbin, Arizona State University, Guy C. Le Masurier,  Vancouver Island University, Karen E. McConnell, Pacific Lutheran University. -- Sixth edition.
      pages cm
  Includes index.
  1.  Physical fitness.  I. Title.
  RA781.C584 20104
  613.7--dc23

                              2013032671
  ISBN-13: 978-1-4504-0022-0 (hard cover)       ISBN-13: 978-1-4504-9753-4 (soft cover)

The web addresses cited in this text were current as of October 28, 2013, unless otherwise noted.

**Acquisitions Editor:** Scott Wikgren; **Developmental Editor:** Ray Vallese; **Assistant Editor:** Derek Campbell; **Copyeditor:** Tom Tiller; **Indexer:** Nancy Ball; **Permissions Manager:** Dalene Reeder; **Graphic Designer:** Nancy Rasmus; **Cover Designer:** Keith Blomberg; **Photographs (cover):** © Human Kinetics, © Photodisc, © Andres Rodriguez, © Michael Svoboda, **Photographs (interior):** © Human Kinetics, unless otherwise noted; **Photo Asset Manager:** Laura Fitch; **Visual Production Assistant:** Joyce Brumfield; **Photo Production Manager:** Jason Allen; **Art Manager:** Kelly Hendren; **Associate Art Manager:** Alan L. Wilborn; **Art Style Development:** Joanne Brummett; **Illustrations:** © Human Kinetics; **Printer:** Courier Companies, Inc.

We thank Truly Fit in Urbana, Illinois, for assistance in providing one of the locations for the photo shoot for this book.

We also wish to thank the *Fitness for Life* editorial board. **Content Advisors:** Stephen D. Ball, PhD; and Hans van der Mars; **Research Advisors:** Phil Abbadessa, MEd; Pamela Hodges Kulinna, PhD; and Jennifer Reeves, MEd; **Adapted Physical Education Advisors:** Phil Abbadessa, MEd; David LaCilento, BAE; and Janet A. Seaman, PED; **Editorial Review Board:** Stephen D. Ball, PhD; Robyn Bretzing; Don Cain, PhD; Brian Culp, EdD; Luis Columna,PhD; Valerie Harville; Marilyn Laidlaw, NBCT; Scot Talbot, MA; and Mark Watt.

Printed in the United States of America    10 9 8 7 6 5 4 3 2

The paper in this book was manufactured using responsible forestry methods.

**Human Kinetics**
Website: www.HumanKinetics.com

*United States:* Human Kinetics
P.O. Box 5076
Champaign, IL 61825-5076
800-747-4457
e-mail: humank@hkusa.com

*Canada:* Human Kinetics
475 Devonshire Road Unit 100
Windsor, ON N8Y 2L5
800-465-7301 (in Canada only)
e-mail: info@hkcanada.com

*Europe:* Human Kinetics
107 Bradford Road
Stanningley
Leeds LS28 6AT, United Kingdom
+44 (0) 113 255 5665
e-mail: hk@hkeurope.com

*Australia:* Human Kinetics
57A Price Avenue
Lower Mitcham, South Australia 5062
08 8372 0999
e-mail: info@hkaustralia.com

*New Zealand:* Human Kinetics
P.O. Box 80
Torrens Park, South Australia 5062
0800 222 062
e-mail: info@hknewzealand.com

E6361

# Contents

## UNIT V  Healthy Choices

## UNIT VI  Wellness Perspective

# Touring *Fitness for Life*

**Do** you want to be healthy and fit? Do you want to look your best and feel good?

*Fitness for Life* is based on the proven HELP philosophy: **H**ealth for **E**veryone for a **L**ifetime in a very **P**ersonal way.

**H** = Health

**E** = Everyone

**L** = Lifetime

**P** = Personal

The HELP philosophy allows you to take personal control of your future fitness, health, and wellness.

*Fitness for Life* helps you become a physically literate person so that you can

- understand and apply important concepts and principles of fitness, health, and wellness;

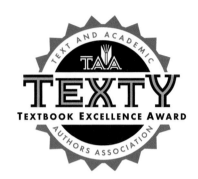

- understand and use self-management skills that promote healthy lifestyles for a lifetime;
- be an informed consumer and critical user of fitness, health, and wellness information; and
- adopt healthy lifestyles now and later in life.

*Fitness for Life* is the winner of the Texty Award for textbook excellence.

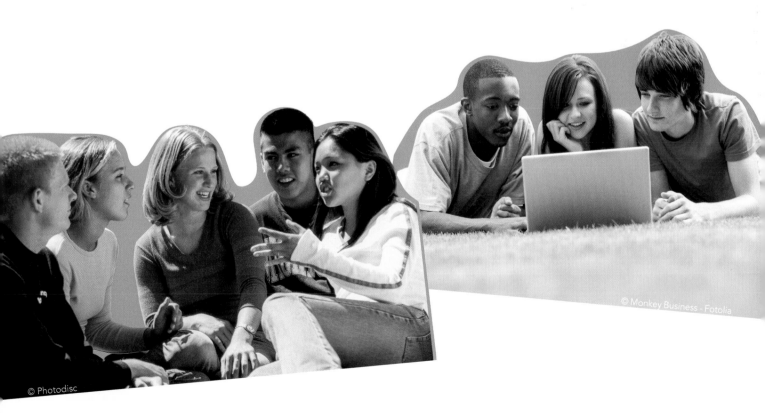

© Photodisc

© Monkey Business - Fotolia

*Fitness for Life* will help you meet your fitness and physical activity goals. Take this guided tour to learn about all of the features of this textbook. Two lessons are included in each chapter to help you learn key concepts relating to fitness, health, and wellness.

**UNIT OPENER:** Provides a brief overview of the content in each unit.

**HEALTHY PEOPLE 2020 GOALS:** Lists national health goals covered in each unit.

**FEATURES:** Lists the Self-Assessment, Taking Charge, Self-Management, and Taking Action features in each unit.

**STUDENT WEB RESOURCES:** Provides the web address for finding additional information in each lesson.

**CHAPTER OPENER:** Provides a brief overview of the content of the chapter.

**IN THIS CHAPTER:** Lists the main elements of each chapter.

# UNIT III
## Moderate and Vigorous Physical Activity

**Healthy People 2020 Goals**
- Increase the percentage of teens who meet aerobic activity guidelines.
- Increase overall cardiovascular health.
- Reduce the risk of heart disease and other chronic diseases.
- Increase education to promote health-enhancing behaviors and reduce health risks.
- Reduce the percentage of teens with high blood pressure and other health risks.
- Improve teens' understanding of health promotion and disease prevention.
- Reduce overweight and obesity among teens.
- Reduce sport and recreation injuries.
- Improve community facilities (s_____ environment (such as sidewalks).
- Increase physical education in _____
- Increase the percentage of tee_____
- Improve health literacy and in_____

**Self-Assessment Features in This**
- Walking Test
- Step Test and One-Mile Run
- Assessing Jogging Technique

**Taking Charge Features in This**
- Learning to Manage Time
- Self-Confidence
- Activity Participation

**Self-Management Features in**
- Skills for Managing Time
- Skills for Building Self-Con_____
- Skills for Choosing Good A_____

**Taking Action Features in Thi**
- Your Moderate Physical A_____
- Target Heart Rate Workou_____
- Your Vigorous Physical A_____

## 2
## Adopting a Healthy Lifestyle and Self-Management Skills

**www Student Web Resources**
www.fitnessforlife.org/student

**In This Chapter**

LESSON 2.1
Adopting Healthy Lifestyles

SELF-ASSESSMENT
Practicing Physical Fitness Tests

LESSON 2.2
Learning Self-Management Skills

TAKING CHARGE
Building Knowledge and Understanding

SELF-MANAGEMENT
Skills for Building Knowledge and Understanding

TAKING ACTION
Fitness Trails

**LESSON OBJECTIVES:** Describes what you will learn in each lesson.

**LESSON VOCABULARY:** Lists key terms in each lesson, which are defined in the glossary and on the student website.

**CONSUMER CORNER:** Provides information to help you become a good consumer and avoid quackery.

**WEB ICONS:** Indicate that additional information is available on the student website.

**FIT FACT:** Offers interesting information about key topics.

**FITNESS TECHNOLOGY:** Helps you become aware of new technological information related to fitness, health, and wellness and helps you try out and use new technology.

---

## Lesson 13.2

# Energy Balance

**Lesson Objectives**

After reading this lesson, you should be able to
1. explain how to use the FIT formula for fat control,
2. describe how many calories are expended in doing various physical activities,
3. explain how physical activity helps a person maintain a healthy body fat level, and
4. describe some common myths about fat control.

**Lesson Vocabulary**

calorie, calorie expenditure, calorie intake, energy ba[...]

**Do** you know how many calories you expend in a typical day? Do you know how many calories you consume in a typical day? One major health goal is to achieve and maintain an acceptable level of body fat throughout your life. To do this, you must balance the calories you consume and the calories you expend. In this lesson, you'll learn the FIT formula for fat control and appropriate activities for gaining weight and losing body fat.

### Balancing Calories

The term *calorie* is commonly used to describe the amount of energy in a food. The true term is *kilocalorie* (a unit of energy or heat), but when talking about diet and nutrition, *calorie* is typically used. Energy balance refers to balancing calorie [...] and calorie expenditure [...]

**FIT FACT**

One pound of fa[...]
Therefore, you ca[...]
kilogram) of fat [...]
fewer than you no[...]
or by burning 3,[...]
normal in physical [...]
provides more calo[...]
will cause you to g[...]
you can gain a poun[...]
calories more than y[...]
given time or by exp[...]
fewer than usual in p[...]
a given time.

---

## CONSUMER CORNER: TV Tactics—Creating Needs

You've now learned about developing a strategy and using tactics to achieve a goal. Companies also develop strategies and tactics. Sometimes their strategies help them but are not good for you. For example, a company's strategy may be to get you to buy something you don't really want or need. To help them carry out their strategies, companies buy advertising in various medi[...] such as television, the web (pop-[...] zines, radio, and newspap[...] companies pay f[...] media [...]

every day. Of course, not all advertisements are deceptive, but many are. It takes a very critical eye to detect the messages being conveyed in ads and to distinguish bet[...] good and bad information.

As you[...] advertisement, [...] tactics being [...] What is this [...] duct they're [...] he product [...] apter, you [...] identify [...] can use [...] keting [...] mer.

Lesson 19.2

---

## FITNESS TECHNOLOGY: Motion Analysis Systems

Many technological advances have helped people become more skilled at a variety of sport activities. One of the most noteworthy is the use of motion analysis systems, which can be as simple as a basic video camera and playback system or as complicated as a high-speed video camera and software that helps analyze whether a performer's movements (biomechanics) are efficient and effective. Whether simple or complex, a motion analysis system video-records a person performing a sport or activity. Next, a skill-learning expert, such as a sport pedagogist or coach, views the video and analyzes the performer's movements. For example, football players and coaches routinely review game footage together to look at defensive and offensive formations, as well as opponents' tactics. High-powered systems

allow users to analyze the action in very slow motion and generate computer analysis to provide information that helps the performer make corrections. Motion analysis systems can be used for many kinds of activity (such as softball pitching and tennis) but are especially popular among golfers, who use the biomechanical feedback to improve their swings.

### Using Technology

Make a video of your performance of a motor skill. Analyze the performance using information you've learned from an instructor or from information gained in the Science in Action student activity.

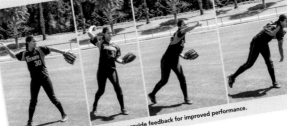

Movement sequences can be studied to provide feedback for improved performance.

ability that includes both eye–hand coordination (the ability to use your hands and eyes together, as in hitting a ball) and eye–foot coordination (the ability to use your eyes and feet together, as in kicking a ball). You may be good in one area but not as good in another. In addition to working on the areas that need improvement, you should consider selecting activities for your program that match your strengths.

Once you've assessed your skill-related fitness abilities, you can develop a profile of your results to help you select lifetime sports and other activities.

In this lesson, you'll learn both how to do that and how to make plans for becoming proficient in your chosen activities.

### Building a Skill-Related Fitness Profile

One student, Sue, did all of the skill-related physical fitness assessments presented in this chapter, then developed a profile for her skill-related fitness (see

Lesson 6.1

*Skill Learning and Injury Prevention* **113**

**EXERCISES:** Provide instructions and pictures to teach you correct technique for exercises.

**SELF-ASSESSMENT:** Helps you learn more about your fitness and behaviors that affect your health and wellness and helps you prepare a personal plan for improvement.

### HEEL RAISE

1. Place a board that is 2 inches (5 centimeters) thick on the floor. Stand with the balls of your feet on the board and the handles even with your shoulders.
2. Grasp the handles with your palms facing away from your body. Keep your hands and arms stationary during the lift.
3. Rise onto the balls of your feet, then lower to the starting position.

Gastrocnemius

Soleus

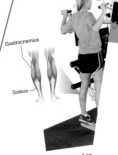

This exercise uses your han...

### LAT PULL-DOWN

1. Sit on the bench (or floor, depending on the machine). Adjust the seat height so that your arms are fully extended when you grab the bar.
2. Grab the bar with your palms facing away from you. Your arms should be at least shoulder-width apart.
3. Pull the bar down...
4. Return to the star...

Lesson 3.1

### ✓ SELF-ASSESSMENT: Walking Test

Many of the self-assessments you perform in this course require very intense physical activity. If you're a very active person and are quite fit, the mile run or PACER may be the best way to estimate your cardiorespiratory endurance, but the walking test is also a good one. The test is especially good for people who are beginners, who haven't done a lot of recent activity, or who are regular walkers but do not regularly get more vigorous activity. The walk test is also good for older people and for those who cannot do running tests due to joint or muscle problems. As directed by your teacher, record your scores and fitness ratings for the walking test. You can then use the information in preparing your personal physical activity plan. If you're working with a partner, remember that self-assessment information is personal and considered confidential. It shouldn't be shared with others without the permission of the person being tested.

1. Walk a mile at a fast pace (as fast as yo... can go while keeping...

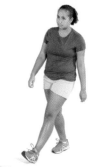

The walking test is a good assessment for beginners or people who do... o a lot of vigorous activity.

...priate chart to determine ...rating. Locate your heart ...column of the chart and ...e along the bottom row. ...here the row and column ...ermine your rating.

### ✦ SCIENCE IN ACTION: Optimal Challenge

Scientists in many fields have collaborated to find ways to help people stay active, eat well, and stick with other healthy lifestyle behaviors. They have discovered that in order to be successful, you must set goals that provide "optimal challenge." The key is giving effort (trying hard). If a challenge is too easy, there's no need to try hard—it's not really a challenge. On the other hand, if a goal is too hard, we fail, which may lead us to give up or quit because our effort seems hopeless (see figure 3.2).

An optimal challenge requires *reasonable* effort. Meeting an optimal challenge provides us with success and makes us want to try again. In fact, providing optimal challenge is one reason that video games are so popular. They challenge you by making the task more difficult as you improve, and this optimal challenge makes you want to play again and again. You can use optimal challenge when setting your own goals to help yourself succeed.

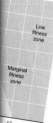

Success

Boredom

Failure

Too easy   Optimal   Too hard

**Figure 3.2** Some challenges can lead to boredom or failure, but optimal challenges can lead to success.

#### Student Activity

Imagine that you want to help a friend learn a skill—for example, hitting a tennis ball or a golf ball. How could you use optimal challenge to help your friend learn the skill?

Low fitness zone

Marginal fitness zone

17    18    19 or more

...r males). ...ission of author James

...l Activity    **143**

**SCIENCE IN ACTION:** Helps you understand how new information is generated using the scientific method.

day (figure 3.1*b*). Process goals make good short-term goals because you can easily monitor your progress and, with effort, succeed. In contrast, *product* goals do not make especially good short-term goals, because they can be discouraging, especially for a person who is just beginning to change. For example, if you chose a product goal of performing, say, 25 push-ups, it might (depending on your current fitness level) take you so long to meet the goal that you would give up. But a short-term process goal—such as performing 5 to 10 push-ups each day for two weeks—would be possible for you to achieve with effort. Thus, as you meet a series of short-term process goals, you work toward meeting long-term product goals.

The Taking Charge and Self-Management features in this chapter focus on setting goals for physical activity and building physical fitness. Elsewhere in the book, you'll get the chance to set long-term goals for fitness, health, and wellness (product goals) and for making healthy lifestyle changes (process goals) that lead to good fitness, health, and wellness. You'll also get the chance to set short-term goals that help you move toward achieving your long-term goals.

> ❝ If you want to live a happy life, tie it to a goal, not to people or things. ❞
>
> —Albert Einstein, Nobel Prize–winning physicist

**FITNESS QUOTES:** Provide quotes from famous people about fitness, health, and wellness.

**LESSON REVIEW:** Helps you review and remember the information you learned in the lesson.

#### Lesson Review

1. How does the SMART formula help you set goals?
2. How can you use long-term and short-term goals to plan your program? In your answer, use fitness and physical activity examples.
3. What is the difference between a process goal and a product goal? In your answer, use fitness and physical activity examples.

56

## ⚡ TAKING CHARGE: Improving Physical Self-Perception

Each person has a mental picture of himself or herself. If you think you do well in a certain activity, you'll probably take part in that type of activity. If you feel embarrassed about your appearance or ability level while doing an activity, you'll probably avoid that activity. Here are two very different examples of physical self-perception.

Michael was not sure that he wanted to go back to school after the summer break. It seemed as if all of his friends had grown taller in the last few months, but he had stayed the same height. Michael felt embarrassed and a little jealous, even though none of his friends seemed to notice. His height certainly did not alter his ability to play tennis. In fact, his friends still called him "King of the Court" because he usually won.

Raul was one of the shortest people in his class, but his height did not stop him from being involved in activities. He realized that he had never been a great basketball player, but he still liked to play with his friends from school. He also discovered that height had nothing to do with his ability to go hiking, nor did it prevent him from being a good wrestler.

### For Discussion

Michael had a negative self-perception because of his height. What can he do to change his negative perception? How does Raul keep a positive self-perception? What else can a person do to develop a positive self-perception? Consider the guidelines presented in the Self-Management feature as you answer the discussion questions.

## ➡ SELF-MANAGEMENT: Skills for Self-Perception

A self-perception is an idea you have about your own thoughts, actions, or appearance. It is influenced by how you think other people view you. Some of the many kinds of self-perception are academic, social, and artistic. In this book, the focus is on physical self-perceptions—the way you view your physical self.

Four aspects of physical self-perception are strength, fitness, skill, and physical attractiveness. People with good physical self-perceptions are happy with their current strength and fitness levels; they also feel that their skills are adequate to meet their needs, and they like the way they look. We know that people who have positive physical self-perceptions are more likely to be physically active than those who do not. The following list provides guidelines you can use to maintain or improve your physical self-perceptions.

- **Assess your physical self-perceptions.** You may use the worksheet provided by your teacher.

- **Consider your self-assessment results.** Use the self-assessment worksheet to determine whether you have any areas in which your physical self-perceptions are especially low (strength, fitness, skill, or physical ...

- **Perform ... improve ... tice regu... skills.** Re... you look... can help...

- **Consid... yourse...** standa... ing lik... or in ... life t... they... app... cial... You...

... star has an eating disorder or practices healthy habits. Consider your heredity and set realistic standards for yourself.

- **Think positively.** Almost all people have a physical characteristic that they would like to change. But studies show that the things people don't like about themselves are rarely seen as problems by other people. You're often your own worst critic, and thinking positively can help you present yourself in a positive way.

- **Do not let the actions of a few insensitive people cause you to feel negatively about yourself.** There will always be some people who are insensitive to others' feelings. These people often have low self-perceptions and try to build themselves up by tearing other people down. Recognize that criticism from these people is their problem, not yours.

- **Consider how your behavior and actions influence the way other people view you.** Acting cheerful and friendly has as much to do with how others perceive you as your physical characteristics.

- **Realize that all people have some imperfections.** Try to build on your strengths and improve your areas of weakness.

- **Find a realistic role model and be a role model for others.** Instead of trying to be like someone who is totally unlike you, find someone you admire who has characteristics you can realistically achieve. And, just as you look to others for models, remember that others may look to you as a model. Providing a positive model for others can help you think positively about yourself.

### 🧩 Academic Connection: Quartiles

Various statistics can be used to describe scores for a group of people. The term *quartile* is used to describe the scores for each quarter of a distribution. In the following example, each number represents a score (in inches) on the waist girth test for 36 15-year-old females. The distribution is divided into quartiles (25 percent of scores per quartile, listed in different colors).

A good fitness rating for waist girth for 15-year-old females is 32 inches or less. Which color of quartile includes scores for the good fitness range? What percentage of girls were in the good fitness zone for waist girth? What percentage of girls had scores that did not qualify them to be in the good fitness zone?

#### Distribution of Waist Girth Scores (Inches) for 15-Year-Old Females

|    |    |    |    | 34 |    |    |    |    |    |    |    |    |    |    |    |
|----|----|----|----|----|----|----|----|----|----|----|----|----|----|----|----|
|    |    |    |    | 33 | 34 |    |    |    |    |    |    |    |    |    |    |
|    |    |    | 32 | 33 | 34 | 35 |    |    |    |    |    |    |    |    |    |
|    | 28 |    | 30 | 32 | 33 | 34 | 35 | 36 |    |    |    |    |    |    |    |
| 27 | 28 | 29 | 30 | 32 | 33 | 34 | 35 | 36 | 37 | 38 | 39 | 40 |    |    |    |
|    | 28 |    | 30 | 32 | 33 | 34 | 35 | 36 | 37 | 38 | 39 | 40 | 41 | 42 | 43 |

#### Check Your Answers

The red quartile includes scores in the good fitness range, so 25 percent of the girls were in the good fitness zone. That also means that 75 percent, or three quartiles, of the girls were not in the good fitness zone.

---

**TAKING CHARGE AND SELF-MANAGEMENT:** Provide guidelines for learning self-management skills that help you adopt healthy behaviors.

**FOR DISCUSSION:** Helps you take charge by making good decisions.

**ACADEMIC CONNECTION:** Relates concepts from other academic subject areas to fitness, health, and wellness.

**TAKING ACTION:** Lets you try out teacher-directed activities that can help you become fit and active for a lifetime.

**CHAPTER REVIEW:** Helps you reinforce what you've learned in the chapter's two lessons.

## TAKING ACTION: Target Heart Rate Workouts

Cardiorespiratory endurance is important for living a long and healthy life. It's also essential for competing, participating in your favorite physical activities, and maintaining a healthy body weight. As you've learned in this chapter, you must do vigorous physical activity above your threshold of training and in your target zone to build cardiorespiratory endurance. **Take action** by doing vigorous activity that fulfills the FIT formula: at least three days each week (addressing F for frequency in the FIT formula), in your target heart rate zone (addressing I for intensity), and for at least 20 minutes each session (addressing T for time). Consider the following tips as you take action by performing a target heart rate workout.

- Determine your target heart rate by using either the percent of heart rate reserve method or the percent of maximal heart ra...
- Before ch... consider y...
- Before do... a 5-minu... warm-up...
- Check y... ceived e... you're r... workou...
- After y... cool-d...

Take action by doing a workout that elevates your heart r...

**CHAPTER REVIEW**

### Reviewing Concepts and Vocabulary

As directed by your teacher, answer items 1 through 5 by correctly completing each sentence with a word or phrase.

1. Factors that affect your fitness, health, and wellness are called _____.
2. Factors influencing fitness, health, and wellness over which you have little control are called _____.
3. Factors influencing fitness, health, and wellness over which you have the most control are called _____.
4. The steps that lead you from dependence to independence are referred to together as the _____.
5. The fitness test used to assess cardiorespiratory endurance by running when signaled by a beep is called the _____.

For items 6 through 10, as directed by your teacher, match each term in column 1 with the appropriate phrase in column 2.

6. sedentary person
7. inactive thinker
8. planner
9. activator
10. active exerciser

a. just bought exercise equipment
b. is active most days of the week
c. is sometimes active
d. is considering becoming active
e. is inactive

For items 11 through 15, as directed by your teacher, respond to each statement or question.

11. Explain what a self-management skill is and why it can be useful.
12. What are some of the fitness test items used in major fitness test batteries such as Fitnessgram, and what do they measure?
13. Describe the five stages of change.
14. What are fitness trails, and how can they be useful in staying active?
15. What are some guidelines for building knowledge and understanding?

### Thinking Critically

Write a paragraph to answer the following question. Of all the self-management skills described in lesson 2, which one would most help you be more active or eat better? Give the reasons for your answer.

### Project

Assume that you are the head of a marketing company assigned to create an ad campaign promoting healthier eating and more active living. Prepare a script for a television commercial for the promotion. If resources are available, create a video of the commercial.

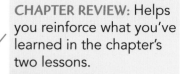

51

**THINKING CRITICALLY:** Requires the use of critical-thinking skills to apply chapter information.

**PROJECT:** Provides an enrichment activity for use outside the classroom.

In addition to all the textbook features, the Fitness for Life program includes several other components:

- **Student Web Resource:** You have access to a wide variety of resources at www.fitnessforlife.org/student. These resources will aid your understanding of the textbook content and include video clips that demonstrate how to do the self-assessment exercises in each chapter, worksheets, interactive review questions, and expanded discussions of topics that are marked by web icons throughout this book.
- **Teacher Web Resource:** Your teacher has access to a special web resource with lessons and activities that you can do to better learn and understand the information in this textbook.

Now read on, and enjoy *Fitness for Life*!

# UNIT I
# Building a Foundation

• • • • • • • • • • • • • • • • • • • • • •

**Healthy People 2020 Goals**

- Live high-quality, longer lives.
- Reduce preventable disease, injury, and early death.
- Increase awareness and understanding of what determines good health.
- Encourage all people to adopt healthy lifestyles that promote lifetime health, fitness, and wellness.
- Create environments that promote health, fitness, and wellness for all.

**Self-Assessment Features in This Unit**

- Physical Fitness Challenges
- Practicing Physical Fitness Tests
- Assessing Muscle Fitness

**Taking Charge Features in This Unit**

- Learning to Self-Assess
- Building Knowledge and Understanding
- Setting Goals

**Self-Management Features in This Unit**

- Skills for Learning to Self-Assess
- Skills for Building Knowledge and Understanding
- Skills for Setting Goals

**Taking Action Features in This Unit**

- The Warm-Up
- Fitness Trails
- Exercise Circuits

# 1

# Fitness, Health, and Wellness for All

## In This Chapter

 **Student Web Resources**
www.fitnessforlife.org/student

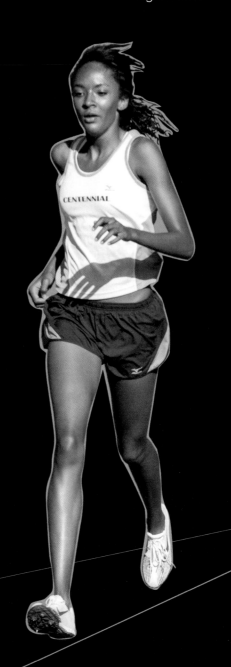

# Lesson 1.1
## Scientific Foundations

**Lesson Objectives**

After reading this lesson, you should be able to

1. describe the scientific method;
2. define *health and medical science* and *nutrition science*;
3. define *kinesiology* and list the seven types of science it encompasses; and
4. describe and differentiate the warm-up, the workout, and the cool-down.

 **Lesson Vocabulary**

biomechanics, calisthenics, cool-down, dietitian, dynamic warm-up, exercise anatomy, exercise physiology, exercise psychology, exercise sociology, health and medical science, kinesiology, motor learning, motor skill, nutrition science, sport pedagogy, stretching warm-up, warm-up, workout

**Science** is the study of knowledge based on observation and experimentation. In school, you study various sciences, such as natural science (focused on nature), social science (focused on individual and social behavior), and mathematics (focused on numbers and their operations). Examples of natural science include biology, chemistry, and physics; examples of social science include psychology, sociology, and geography; and examples of mathematics include algebra, geometry, and calculus.

### FIT FACT

Many of the names of sciences end with "-ology," which means "the study of."

## The Scientific Method

Scientists of all types use the scientific method to discover new knowledge and establish principles that help us make good decisions and solve problems. A simplified form of the scientific method is presented here. The steps—identifying a problem, establishing a hypothesis, collecting information, and interpreting information—are shown in figure 1.1.

The information presented in this book is based on studies that use the scientific method as described in figure 1.1, and each chapter includes a special feature called Science in Action. This feature helps you see how research in **health and medical science, kinesiology** (exercise science), and **nutrition science** can help us make good decisions about fitness, health, and wellness.

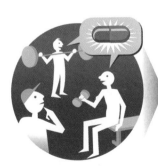 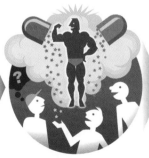 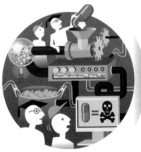 

**Problem**
Friends are considering taking a dietary supplement. Should I take one?

**Hypothesis**
They think a supplement might help them get fit faster.

**Collect information**
Conduct a search for information about benefits and risks associated with the supplement.

**Interpret information**
Analysis and conclusion: the risks are greater than the benefits. Don't take the supplement.

**FIGURE 1.1** A simplified form of the scientific method.

You've probably used the scientific method yourself when conducting experiments in science classes. You've also read studies that used the scientific method. But you may not have thought about using the scientific method in your personal life. As you work your way through the Fitness for Life program, you'll learn to use the scientific method to help you solve problems and make healthy lifestyle decisions. You'll also use the scientific method to plan programs for building your fitness, health, and wellness.

## Health and Medical Science

Medicine is the art and science of healing. Historically, the practice of medicine has been focused on diagnosing and treating disease. In prehistoric times, people often associated illness with demons and evil influences. But as early as 2000 BC, Egyptians performed surgery and began to build a more scientific base for medicine. Modern medical practitioners use evidence-based approaches, and research studies are required before medical procedures and medicines are approved.

Because of advances in health and medical science, life expectancy in the United States has increased dramatically over the last century. In 1900, the life expectancy for Americans was 47 years. Over the next century, it almost doubled, reaching nearly 80 years. Health and medical scientists have developed medicines that treat bacterial infections, and as a result infectious diseases such as typhoid fever and smallpox, which used to be among the leading causes of death, have been conquered. Before 1900, fewer than 100 medicines were available to doctors. Now there are more than 10,000, and in the United States they must be tested before the government's Food and Drug Administration (FDA) approves them. With infectious illness reduced, the main causes of early death in developed countries today are heart disease, cancer, diabetes, and other chronic diseases related to unhealthy lifestyles.

Health science focuses on preventing disease and promoting wellness and high quality of life. Some health scientists study personal health issues in order to help individuals prevent disease and promote wellness. Public health scientists, on the other hand, study patterns of health and illness among populations in order to help prevent epidemics of illness; thus they are sometimes called epidemiologists.

> " Physical fitness is not only one of the most important keys to a healthy body; it is the basis of dynamic and creative intellectual activity. "
>
> —John F. Kennedy, U.S. president

© REmy MASSEGLIA

## Kinesiology (Exercise Science)

The past two centuries have sometimes been called the golden age of medicine because they have seen many of the most significant advances in health and medical science. Toward the end of the 20th century, a relatively new science called kinesiology emerged as more and more evidence accumulated showing the health and wellness benefits of physical activity and exercise. The U.S. National Research Council now recognizes kinesiology as a major area of science along with other major branches such as those listed at the beginning of this chapter.

Put simply, kinesiology is the study of human movement. There are, of course, many types of human movement. Some involve small muscle movements, such as the movement of your eyes when reading, the movement of your fingers when typing, and the movement of your hands when playing a musical instrument. Kinesiology is the study of all human movement, but it focuses on large-muscle physical activity; in fact, the phrase "physical activity" is a very general term for large muscle movement. There are many types of physical activity, including moderate activities such as walking, vigorous activities such as aerobics, sport and recreational activities, and exercise for muscle fitness and flexibility. These activity types are included in the Physical Activity Pyramid, which is described in more detail throughout this book.

## FIT FACT

One national health goal established by the U.S. Department of Health and Human Services (USDHHS) is to eliminate disparities in fitness, health, and wellness. People who study kinesiology look for ways of helping *all* people be active, fit, healthy, and well—regardless of race, ethnicity, social or economic class, disability, age, sex, or gender identity.

The general category of kinesiology includes seven sciences. The most prominent are featured in this chapter and in special features that appear throughout this book. They include **exercise physiology, exercise anatomy, biomechanics, exercise psychology, exercise sociology, motor learning,** and **sport pedagogy**. These sciences provide the foundation for our current understanding of the health benefits of physical activity and exercise. Exercise professionals, including physical education teachers, study all of the sciences in kinesiology as part of their training. You don't need to know as much about kinesiology as your teachers, but an understanding of the sciences of kinesiology will help you to understand the information in this book.

## Exercise Physiology

Physiology is a branch of biology focused on the study of body systems. More specifically, exercise physiology is a branch of kinesiology that explores how physical activity affects body systems. For example, exercise physiologists study the cardiovascular, respiratory, skeletal, muscular, and other body systems to see how they are affected by exercise. Understanding the basic principles of exercise physiology is essential for planning physical activity programs for promoting lifelong fitness, health, and wellness.

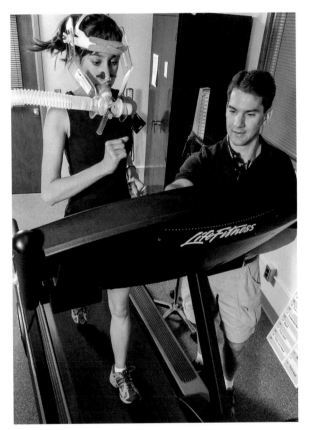

Exercise physiology is the branch of kinesiology that explores how physical activity affects body systems.

## Exercise Anatomy

Human anatomy is a branch of biology focused on studying the structure of the human organism. Scientists who study human anatomy focus on the tissues that make up the body (muscle, bone, tendon, ligament, skin, organ). Scientists who study exercise anatomy are especially interested in understanding how we use our muscles—and how our muscles work together with our bones, ligaments, and tendons—to produce movement. Understanding exercise anatomy can help you choose good exercises for building your personal fitness program.

## Biomechanics

The human body is much like a machine. It uses a complex system of levers (bones) that are moved by the force produced when you contract your muscles. Biomechanics is the branch of kinesiology that seeks to understand the human machine in motion through the principles of physics. Knowing the basic principles of biomechanics can help you move efficiently and avoid injury.

## Exercise Psychology

Psychology is commonly referred to as the science of mind and behavior. More specifically, exercise psychology focuses on the study of human behavior in all types of physical activity, including sport and exercise for fitness. Exercise psychology, including sport psychology, can help motivate people to be active, set realistic goals, and perform better in sports.

## Exercise Sociology

Sociology is the study of society and social relationships. Within this broad field, exercise sociology focuses on social relationships and interactions in physical activity, including sports. Exercise sociology has helped people understand teamwork and

cooperation; social responsibility; and cultural and ethnic differences in physical activity. Understanding key principles of exercise and sport sociology will help you experience positive social interactions in your physical activity.

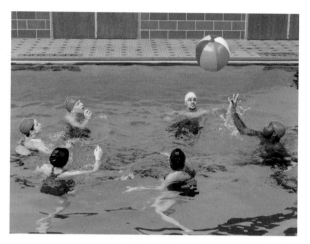

Exercise sociology is the branch of kinesiology that focuses on social relationships and interactions in physical activity, including sports.

## Motor Learning

When you see the word *motor*, you may think of an automobile engine, but the term *motor learning* in this book refers to skill learning. When you perform a movement skill (also called a **motor skill**), your brain sends a signal through a nerve that tells the relevant muscles to contract. Nerves and muscle fibers that work together to produce movement are

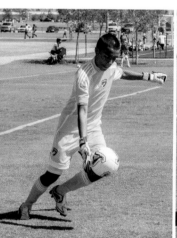
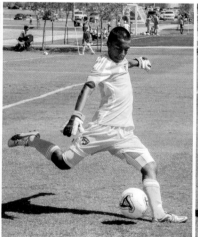
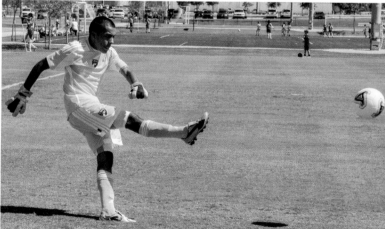

Biomechanics is the branch of kinesiology that seeks to understand the human body in motion through the principles of physics.

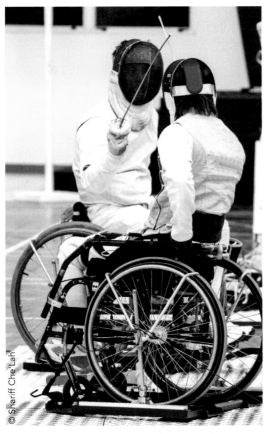

Motor learning is the branch of kinesiology that involves the study of nerves and muscles to see how they work together to perform motor skills.

called a motor unit. Performing a motor skill, such as throwing a ball, requires action by many motor units (nerves and muscles). People who study motor learning have developed rules and principles that help us learn motor skills and control movements. In this book, you'll learn the best ways to develop and practice the skills used in all of the activities presented in the Physical Activity Pyramid.

## Physical Education and Sport Pedagogy

Pedagogy is the art and science of teaching. People who study pedagogy as a science focus on discovering the best ways to teach. Sport pedagogy is the study of teaching and learning in many different physical activity settings, including school physical education, on sports teams, and in fitness clubs. The word *sport* is used broadly to include more than just traditional American sports. In other regions of the world, *sport* is used similarly to the term *physical activity*. So sports, or sporting activities, include activities such as riding a bike, taking a hike, performing muscle fitness exercises, and performing traditional sports such as basketball, volleyball, or tennis. People who study pedagogy as a science focus on developing a better understanding of the most appropriate approaches to teaching and the many factors that influence learning. They apply learning principles to help students meet important educational objectives. Examples include applying motor learning principles to help students improve their skills, applying management principles to increase physical activity during classes, and using motivational principles to encourage full participation and optimal learning.

## FITNESS TECHNOLOGY: World Wide Web

The World Wide Web has given many people immediate access to all kinds of health and fitness information. As you'll learn elsewhere in this book, some of the information available on the web is good. However, much of it is inaccurate, especially health information. In each chapter of this book, you'll find a web address that leads you to sound information about fitness, health, and wellness. Look for special web symbols included throughout the book; just type in the address from the first page of the chapter, and you'll find good, reliable information. These web pages will also give you links to other good sources of fitness and health information.

### Using Technology

Access the web address provided at the beginning of each chapter in this book. You will find additional information related to topics in each lesson. Explore the topics to learn more. Explore some of the websites provided to find good fitness and health information.

## SCIENCE IN ACTION: Guidelines for Warming Up and Cooling Down

The time you spend doing physical activity each day is your physical activity session. The activity session has three phases: warm-up, workout, and cool-down. The **warm-up** is the activity you perform before your workout in order to get ready for it. The **workout** is the main part of your activity session. It can involve exercise to build fitness, participation in a competitive event, or activity done just for fun. The **cool-down** is the activity you perform after your workout to help you recover. You can use the information presented here about warming up and cooling down to prepare yourself for the various workouts described in this book.

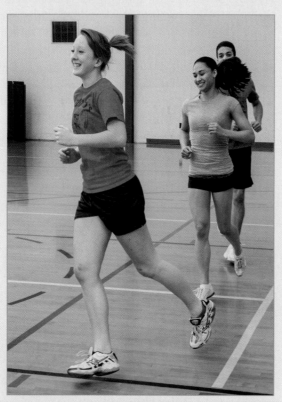

The general warm-up helps your heart and other body systems get ready for more vigorous physical activity.

### The Warm-Up

Experts have studied the warm-up for nearly 100 years. For many years, exercise physiologists thought that a **stretching warm-up** was the preferred method of getting ready for a workout. For this reason, the most common type of warm-up includes static stretching (slowly stretching a muscle beyond its normal length and holding the stretch for several seconds). The American College of Sports Medicine (ACSM) notes that a warm-up improves range of motion and may reduce the risk of injury. But some recent research has raised questions about whether the traditional stretching warm-up really prevents injury. Additionally, questions have been raised about the effects of a stretching warm-up on certain types of performance. The best evidence now suggests that your warm-up can vary depending on the workout you plan to perform. Here are some warm-up guidelines:

**You don't need to perform a warm-up prior to a workout of low to moderate intensity (such as walking or slow jogging).** Low to moderate physical activity is used as a general warm-up as recommended by ACSM, so a workout consisting of low- to moderate-intensity exercise doesn't require a special warm-up.

**ACSM recommends 5 to 10 minutes of general warm-up involving low- to moderate-intensity physical activity prior to a vigorous workout or competition.** The goal is to increase your body and muscle temperature. This general warm-up helps your heart and other body systems get ready for more vigorous exercise. The general warm-up can include walking, jogging, and **calisthenics**, such as those included in a **dynamic warm-up** (see the Taking Action feature near the end of the chapter).

**The National Strength and Conditioning Association (NSCA) recommends a series of dynamic exercises prior to a workout or competition that requires strength, speed, and power.** Examples of dynamic exercises include jogging, skipping, hopping, jumping, and calisthenics using your arms, legs, shoulders, and hips (see this chapter's Taking Action feature). You can also perform sport-related movements that use your body parts similarly to how you'll use them in sport competition. Examples include jumping and shooting drills for basketball and swinging a club or bat with gradually increasing intensity. Dynamic warm-up exercises are good for increasing your body temperature and for getting your muscles ready for more vigorous exercise. They can serve as all or part of the general warm-up recommended by ACSM.

**A stretching warm-up may be performed prior to a workout or competition, including activities that require strength, speed, and power, if the stretch is not held too long.** The NSCA recommends dynamic movement exercises as the preferred warm-up before activities requiring strength, speed, and power. For this reason, some may choose not to perform a stretching warm-up before these activities. However, for those who enjoy a stretching warm-up, stretching exercises can be included as long as each stretch is not held for more than 60 seconds, even prior to a strength, speed, and power workout. Recent research indicates that as long as the stretches don't exceed 60 seconds, they don't inhibit performance. Research also indicates that abruptly stopping a stretching warm-up after regularly performing one increases risk of injury. If you choose a stretching warm-up you should use a variety of stretching exercises to address all of your major muscle groups and joints (see this chapter's Taking Action feature). Stretches should be held for 15 to 30 seconds. Stretching is more effective when your muscles are warm, so you should stretch only after performing a general warm-up.

**Stretching exercises used to build flexibility, rather than for warming up, are best performed as a separate part of your workout.** The stretching warm-up and the stretching workout are not the same thing. A stretching warm-up is used to prepare you for physical activity. The stretching workout includes exercises to build flexibility, a health-related component of physical fitness. ACSM recommends that stretching for flexibility be done after the general warm-up as part of the workout or as a separate workout session after the cool-down. The flexibility workout is typically much more comprehensive than a warm-up. You will have the opportunity to study flexibility and the flexibility workout later in this book.

## The Cool-Down

After a workout, your body needs to recover from the demands of physical activity; to aid this process, ACSM recommends a cool-down of 5 to 10 minutes after a vigorous workout. The cool-down usually consists of slow to moderate activity, such as walking or slow jogging, that allows your heart and muscles to gradually recover. The cool-down helps prevent dizziness and fainting. Hard exercise increases the flow of blood to your muscles; for example, running causes more blood to be pumped to your arms and legs than to your head. If you suddenly stop running, the blood can pool in your legs. This leaves your heart with less blood to pump to your brain, which may cause you to feel dizzy or faint. But if you continue moving after a hard run, your muscles will squeeze the veins of your legs. This helps return the blood to your heart, which can then pump more blood to your brain, making you less likely to feel dizzy or faint. The following list provides some more cool-down guidelines.

- Do not lie down or sit down immediately after vigorous activity.
- Gradually reduce the intensity of activity during the cool-down (for example, if you were running, slow to a jog, then a walk, and then consider gentle stretching).
- Walk or do other moderate total body movements.
- You may choose to do some of the stretching exercises presented in the chapter titled Flexibility after your general cool-down while your muscles are still warm.

---

### Student Activity

How does the information in this feature change the way you would warm up before, and cool down after, a workout?

---

9

# Nutrition Science

Nutrition science is the study of how plants and animals use food to grow and sustain life. This book, of course, focuses on human nutrition. Nutrition scientists study nutrients (carbohydrate, protein, fat, vitamin, and mineral) to better understand which ones contribute to healthy growth and development. One type of nutrition science—food science—is the study of the chemical makeup of food. Another type—food technology—focuses on food processing, packaging, preservation, and safety. **Dietitians** are experts who help people apply principles of nutrition in daily life.

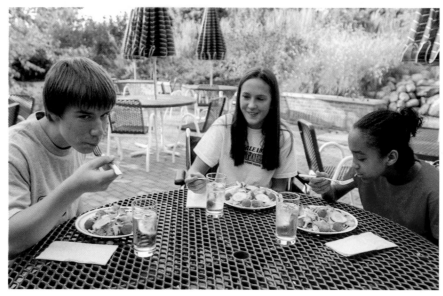

For healthy growth and development, apply the principles of nutrition in daily life.

## Lesson Review

1. What is the scientific method and what are its four steps?
2. What are the *health and medical* and *nutrition sciences*, and how do they relate to fitness, health, and wellness?
3. What is *kinesiology*, and what are the seven types of science it encompasses?
4. What are the warm-up and the cool-down, and how are they best performed?

Each chapter of this book includes a feature titled Self-Assessment. In most chapters, the self-assessment is designed to help you determine your personal fitness level. You'll record and analyze your assessment results. In this self-assessment, you'll try 11 challenges. They're called challenges rather than tests because *they are not meant to be tests of fitness; nor are they meant to be exercises that you do to get fit.* Instead, trying these challenges is a fun way to better understand the differences between the various parts of physical fitness. Please do not draw conclusions about your fitness based on your performance in these challenges. As you work your way through this book, you'll learn many self-assessments to help you determine your true fitness level.

The cardiorespiratory endurance and flexibility challenges will help you warm up before performing the other challenges. You may also want to consider additional warm-up exercises recommended by your teacher.

# PART 1: Health-Related Physical Fitness Challenges

## Running in Place (cardiorespiratory endurance)

1. Determine your resting heart rate for one minute. To do this, use your fingers to feel your pulse at your wrist or neck, then count your pulse (heartbeats) for one minute.

2. Run 120 steps in place for one minute. Count one step every time a foot hits the floor.

3. Rest for 30 seconds, then count your pulse (heart rate) for one minute. People with good cardiorespiratory endurance recover quickly after exercise. Is your heart rate after this exercise within 15 beats per minute of your resting heart rate before running in place?

**This challenge focuses on cardiorespiratory endurance.**

## Two-Hand Ankle Grip (flexibility)

1. Squat with your heels together. Lean the upper body forward and reach with your hands between your legs and behind your ankles.

2. Clasp your hands in front of your ankles.

3. Interlock your hands for the full length of your fingers. Keep your feet still.

4. Hold the position for five seconds.

**This challenge focuses on flexibility.**

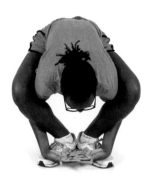

## Single-Leg Raise (muscular endurance)

1. Bend forward at your waist so that your upper body rests on a table and your feet are on the floor.

2. Raise one leg so that it is extended straight out behind you. Complete several such raises with each leg. Performing multiple repetitions (8 or more) requires muscular endurance. Stop if you reach 25 with each leg.

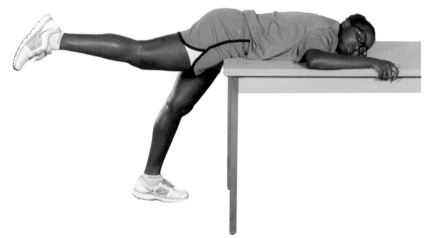

This challenge focuses on muscular endurance.

## Arm Skinfold (body fat level)

1. Let your right arm hang relaxed at your side. Have a partner gently pinch the skin and the fat under the skin on the back of your arm halfway between your elbow and shoulder. Together the skin and fat under the skin is called a skinfold.

2. Several skinfolds in different body locations can be used to determine the total amount of fat in the body. At this point there is no need to measure the skinfold. The skinfold on the arm is used only to illustrate the concept of body composition.

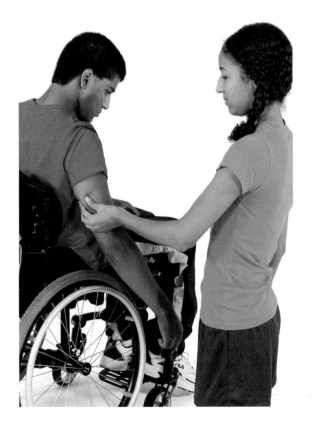

This challenge focuses on body composition.

## 90-Degree Push-Up (strength)

1. Lie facedown on a mat or carpet with your hands under your shoulders, your fingers spread, and your legs straight. Your legs should be slightly apart and your toes should be tucked under.

2. Push up until your arms are straight. Keep your legs and back straight—your body should form a straight line.

3. Lower your body by bending your elbows until your upper arms are parallel to the floor (elbows at a 90-degree angle), then push up until your arms are fully extended. Do one push-up every three seconds. You may want to have a partner say "up-down" every three seconds to help you. Performing up to 5 push-ups requires muscular strength.

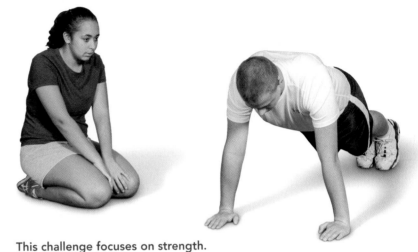

This challenge focuses on strength.

## Knees-to-Feet (power)

1. Kneel so that your shins and knees are on a mat. Hold your arms back. Point your toes straight backward.

2. Without curling your toes under you or rocking your body backward, swing your arms upward and spring to your feet.

3. Hold your position for three seconds after you land.

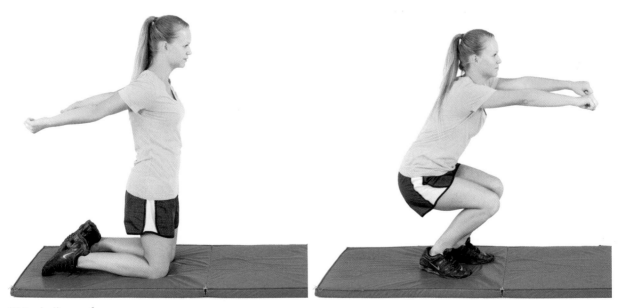

This challenge focuses on power.

# PART 2: Skill-Related Physical Fitness Challenges

## Line Jump (agility)

1. Balance on your right foot on a line on the floor.
2. Leap onto your left foot so that it lands to the right of the line.
3. Leap across the line onto your right foot; land to the left of the line.
4. Leap onto your left foot, landing on the line.

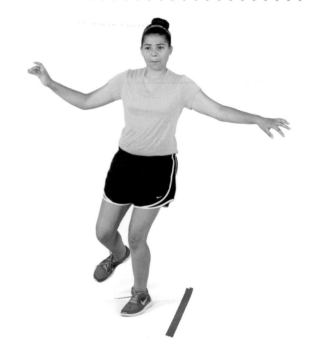

This challenge focuses on agility.

## Double Heel Click (speed)

1. Jump into the air and click your heels together twice before you land.
2. Your feet should be at least three inches (eight centimeters) apart when you land.

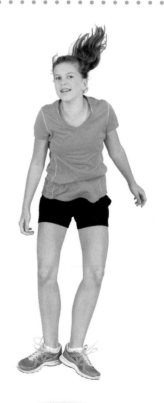

This challenge focuses on speed.

## Backward Hop (balance)

1. With your eyes closed, hop backward on one foot five times.
2. After the last hop, hold your balance for three seconds.

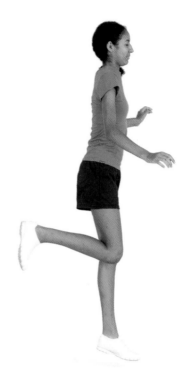

This challenge focuses on balance.

## Double-Ball Bounce (coordination)

1. Hold a volleyball in each hand. Beginning at the same time with each hand, bounce both balls at the same time, at least knee high.
2. Bounce both balls three times in a row without losing control of them.

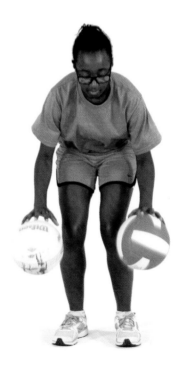

This challenge focuses on coordination.

## Coin Catch (reaction time)

1. Point your right elbow outward in front of you. Your right hand, palm up, should be beside your right ear. If you're left-handed, do this activity with your left hand.

2. Place a coin as close to the end of your elbow as possible.

3. Quickly lower your elbow and grab the coin in the air with the hand of the same arm.

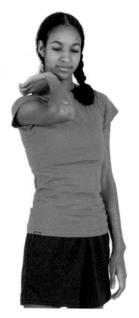

**This challenge focuses on reaction time.**

# Lesson 1.2

# Lifelong Fitness, Health, and Wellness

## Lesson Objectives

After reading this lesson, you should be able to

1. define *physical fitness*, *health*, and *wellness* and describe how they are interrelated;
2. describe the five components of health and wellness;
3. describe the six parts of health-related physical fitness and the five parts of skill-related physical fitness; and
4. define *self-assessment* and explain how it is important to good fitness, health, and wellness.

## Lesson Vocabulary

agility, balance, body composition, body fat level, cardiorespiratory endurance, coordination, flexibility, functional fitness, health, health-related physical fitness, hypokinetic condition, muscular endurance, physical fitness, power, public health scientist, reaction time, skill-related physical fitness, speed, strength, wellness

**If** you could have one wish come true, what would it be? Some people would wish for material things, such as money, a new car, or a new house. But after thinking about it, most people indicate that they would wish for good fitness, health, and wellness for themselves and their family. If you possess health, fitness, and wellness, you can enjoy life to its fullest. Without them, no amount of money will allow you to do all of the things you would like to do. More than 90 percent of all people, including teens, agree that good health is important because it helps you feel good, look good, and enjoy life with the people you care about most.

As you read this book, you'll learn more about healthy lifestyle choices that can help you be fit, healthy, and well. You'll learn how to prepare a healthy personal lifestyle plan and how to use self-management skills to stick with your plan. The goal of this book is to help you become an informed consumer who makes effective decisions about your lifelong fitness, health, and wellness.

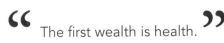
**"** The first wealth is health. **"**
—Ralph Waldo Emerson, poet

Before you can start developing a plan, you need some basic information. In this lesson, you'll learn definitions for some key words used throughout this course. You'll better understand the meaning of the words *fitness*, *health*, and *wellness*, and you'll learn about their components.

## What Is Health? What Is Wellness?

Early definitions of **health** focused on illness. The first medical doctors concentrated on helping sick people overcome their health problems; in other words, their main job was treating people who were ill.

But in 1947, the World Health Organization (WHO), which now includes representatives from 194 countries, issued a statement indicating that health meant more than freedom from disease or illness. This recognition led people to develop a more comprehensive definition of health, which now includes **wellness**. According to the WHO statement, the sheer fact of not being sick doesn't mean you are well. Wellness is the positive component of health that includes having a good quality of life and a good sense of well-being exhibited by a positive outlook on life.

Figure 1.2 shows that a healthy person both is not ill (the blue circle) and has a strong wellness component (the green circle). Illness is the negative component of health that we want to treat or prevent, whereas wellness is the positive component of health that we want to promote.

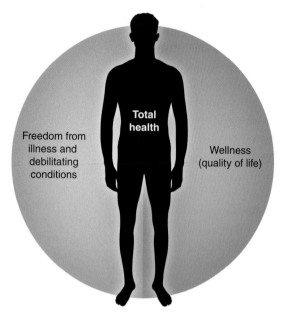

**FIGURE 1.2** Being healthy means having wellness in addition to not being ill.

Health and wellness have many components, and a chain is often used to show how the components are linked (figure 1.3). For a chain to be strong, each link must be strong. Likewise, to have good health and wellness, you must have all of the health and wellness components, not just one or two. The goal is to promote the positive while avoiding the negative in each component, as shown in figure 1.3. If you're happy, informed, involved, fit, and fulfilled, then you have incorporated the positive aspects of

the health components into your life. You possess wellness, and your risk of illness is reduced. The bottom line is this: Health is freedom from disease and debilitating conditions as well as optimal wellness in all five components (physical, emotional-mental, social, intellectual, and spiritual).

# Personal Health and Community Health

One major goal of this book is to help each reader achieve good personal health, including wellness. Another important goal is to promote community health, which refers to the health of a group rather than an individual—from small groups such as families and networks of friends, to larger groups such as towns and cities, and on to very large groups such as states and countries. Just as each person sets health goals, communities do so as well. Your school is a community, and many schools have a coordinated school health program (CSHP). A CSHP program has many components including physical education, health education, wellness programs, and other programs designed to improve the personal health of students and the health of the school community.

One example of a large-scale program designed to promote health in a large community is the Healthy People 2020 project, in which the U.S. Department of Health and Human Services has set national health goals to be accomplished by

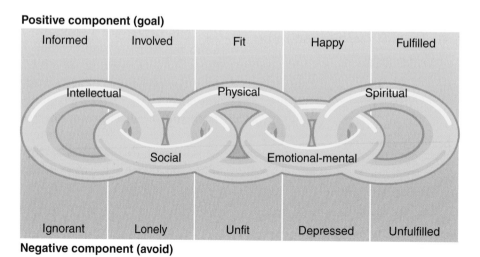

**FIGURE 1.3** The total health and wellness chain.
Based on Corbin et al. 2011.

the year 2020. The project is part of an ongoing program. Every 10 years, experts from more than 400 groups nationwide work together to develop health goals for the nation. **Public health scientists** and other experts from every state and many federal and private agencies develop the goals. Many of the Healthy People 2020 objectives are described on the unit opening pages of this book.

## What Is Physical Fitness?

**Physical fitness** refers to the ability of your body systems to work together efficiently to allow you to be healthy and perform activities of daily living. Being efficient means doing daily activities with the least effort possible. A fit person is able to perform schoolwork, meet home responsibilities, and still have enough energy to enjoy sport and other leisure activities. A fit person can respond effectively to normal life situations, such as raking leaves at home, stocking shelves at a part-time job, and marching in the band at school. A fit person can also respond to emergency situations—for example, by running to get help or aiding a friend in distress.

### FIT FACT

Studies indicate that fitness scores in the United States have declined in recent years for recruits in physically demanding lines of work, such as policing, fire fighting, and the military.

## The Parts of Physical Fitness

Physical fitness is made up of 11 parts—6 of them health related and 5 skill related. All of the parts are important to good performance in physical activity, including sports. But the 6 are referred to as contributing to **health-related physical fitness** because scientists in kinesiology have shown that they can reduce your risk of chronic disease and promote good health and wellness. These parts of fitness are **body composition, cardiorespiratory endurance, flexibility, muscular endurance,** **power,** and **strength.** They also help you function effectively in daily activities.

As the name implies, **skill-related physical fitness** components help you perform well in sports and other activities that require motor skills. For example, **speed** helps you in sports such as track and field. These 5 parts of physical fitness are also linked to health but less so than the health-related components. For example, among older adults, **balance, agility,** and **coordination** are very important for preventing falls (a major health concern), and **reaction time** relates to risk for automobile accidents. Each part of physical fitness is described in more detail in the two following features: The Six Parts of Health-Related Fitness and The Five Parts of Skill-Related Fitness.

### FIT FACT

Cardiorespiratory endurance is also referred to as cardiovascular fitness and aerobic fitness. The Institute of Medicine, an independent U.S. nonprofit organization, reviewed names for this fitness component and chose cardiorespiratory endurance, especially for use with youth. They chose the name because this type of fitness requires the cardiovascular and respiratory systems to work well together (cardiorespiratory) to allow your entire body to function for a long time without fatigue (endurance).

## Health-Related Physical Fitness

Think about a runner. She can probably run a long distance without tiring; thus she has good fitness in at least one area of health-related physical fitness. But does she have good fitness in all six parts? Running is an excellent form of physical activity, but being a runner doesn't guarantee fitness in all parts of health-related physical fitness. Like the runner, you may be more fit in some parts of fitness than in others. The feature named The Six Parts of Health-Related Fitness describes each part and shows an example. As you read about each part, ask yourself how fit you think you are in that area.

## The Six Parts of Health-Related Fitness

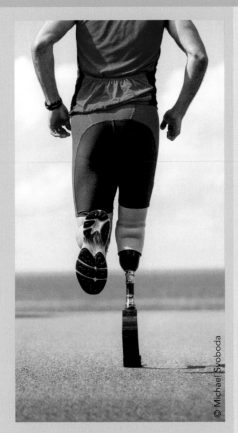

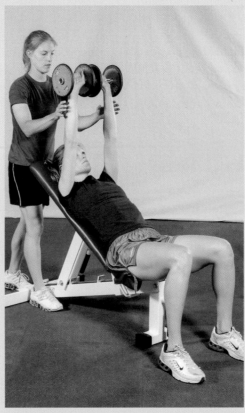

© Michael Svoboda

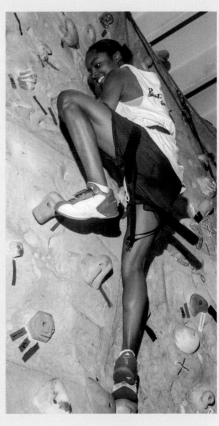

**Cardiorespiratory endurance** is the ability to exercise your entire body for a long time without stopping. It requires a strong heart, healthy lungs, and clear blood vessels to supply your large muscles with oxygen. Examples of activities that require good cardiorespiratory endurance are distance running, swimming, and cross-country skiing.

**Strength** is the amount of force your muscles can produce. It is often measured by how much weight you can lift or how much resistance you can overcome. Examples of activities that require good strength are lifting a heavy weight and pushing a heavy box.

**Muscular endurance** is the ability to use your muscles many times without tiring—for example, doing many push-ups or curl-ups (crunches) or climbing a rock wall.

How do you think you rate in each of the six health-related parts of fitness? To be healthy, you should be fit for each of the six parts. Totally fit people are less likely to develop a **hypokinetic condition**—a health problem caused partly by lack of physical activity—such as heart disease, high blood pressure, diabetes, osteoporosis, colon cancer, or a high **body fat level**. You'll learn more about hypokinetic conditions in other chapters of this book. People who are physically fit also enjoy better wellness. They feel better, look better, and

have more energy. You don't have to be a great athlete in order to enjoy good health and wellness and be physically fit. Regular physical activity can improve anyone's health-related physical fitness.

### Skill-Related Physical Fitness

Just as the runner in our example may not achieve a high rating in all parts of health-related physical fitness, she also may not rate the same in all parts of skill-related physical fitness. Though most sports

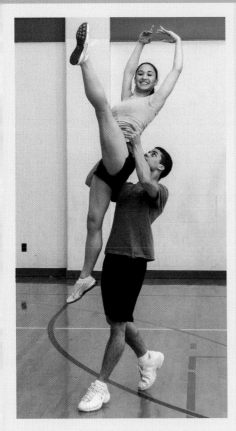

**Flexibility** is the ability to use your joints fully through a wide range of motion without injury. You are flexible when your muscles are long enough and your joints are free enough to allow adequate movement. Examples of people with good flexibility include dancers and gymnasts.

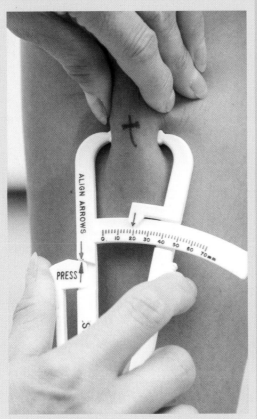

**Body composition** refers to the different types of tissues that make up your body, including fat, muscle, bone, and organ. Your level of body fat is often used to assess the component of body composition related to health. Body composition measures commonly used in schools include body mass index (based on height and weight), skinfold measures (which estimate body fatness), and body measurements such as waist and hip circumferences.

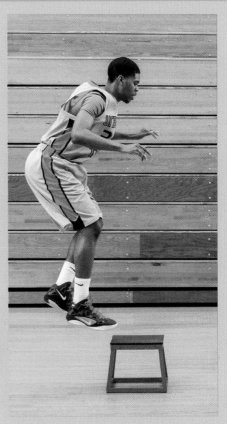

**Power** is the ability to use strength quickly; thus it involves both strength and speed. It is sometimes referred to as explosive strength. People with good power can, for example, jump far or high, put the shot, and speed-swim.

require several parts of skill-related fitness, different sports can require different parts. For example, a skater might have good agility but lack good reaction time. Some people have more natural ability in some areas than in others. No matter how you score on the skill-related parts of physical fitness, you can enjoy some type of physical activity.

Remember, too, that good health doesn't come from being good in skill-related physical fitness. It comes from doing activities designed to improve your health-related physical fitness, and it can be enjoyed both by great athletes and by people who consider themselves poor athletes.

As noted earlier, health-related fitness offers a double benefit. It not only helps you stay healthy but also helps you perform well in sport and other activities. For example, cardiorespiratory endurance helps you resist heart disease and helps you perform well in sports such as swimming and cross-country running. Similarly, strength helps you perform well in sports such as football and wrestling, muscular endurance is important in soccer and tennis,

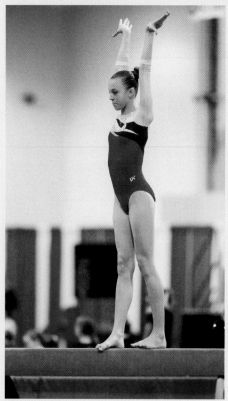

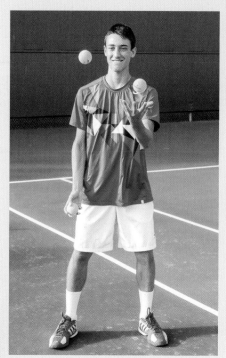

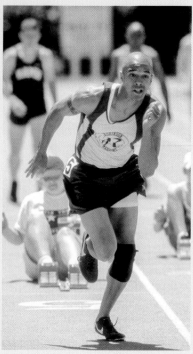

**Balance** is the ability to keep an upright posture while standing still or moving. People with good balance are likely to be good, for example, at gymnastics and ice skating.

**Coordination** is the ability to use your senses together with your body parts or to use two or more body parts together. People with good eye–hand or eye–foot coordination are good at juggling and at hitting and kicking games, such as soccer, baseball, volleyball, tennis, and golf.

**Speed** is the ability to perform a movement or cover a distance in a short time. For example, people with good leg speed can run fast, and people with good arm speed can throw fast or hit a ball that is thrown fast.

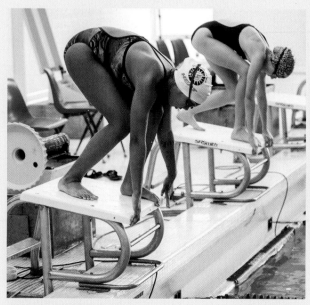

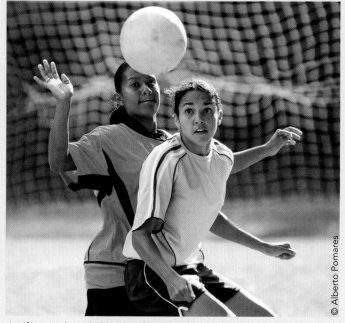

© Alberto Pomares

**Reaction time** is the amount of time it takes you to move once you recognize the need to act. People with good reaction time can make fast starts in track and swimming and can dodge fast attacks in fencing and karate.

**Agility** is the ability to change the position of your body quickly and control your body's movements. People with good agility are likely to be good, for example, at wrestling, diving, soccer, and ice skating.

## FIT FACT

Power, formerly classified as a skill-related part of fitness, is now classified as a health-related part of fitness. A report by the independent Institute of Medicine provides evidence of the link between physical power and health. The report indicates that power is associated with wellness, higher quality of life, reduced risk of chronic disease and early death, and better bone health. Power, and activities that improve power, have also been found to be important for healthy bones in children and teens.

flexibility helps in sports such as gymnastics and diving, power helps in track activities such as the discus throw and the long jump, and having a healthy amount of body fat makes your body more efficient in many activities.

### Functional Fitness

**Functional fitness** refers to the ability to function effectively when performing normal daily tasks. You have functional fitness if you can do your schoolwork, get to and from school, participate in leisure activities without fatigue, respond to emergency situations, and perform other daily tasks safely and without fatigue (for example, driving a car or doing housework and yardwork). From this point of view, health-related fitness not only helps you stay healthy but also helps you function; for example, it helps you avoid fatigue when working or playing. Similarly, skill-related fitness not only helps you perform well in sports but also can help you function in life, such as when you need to stop quickly while driving a car. As you work your way through this book, you'll learn how each part of health- and skill-related fitness contributes to your functional fitness.

# Fitness, Health, and Wellness Are Interrelated

Fitness, health, and wellness are all states of being, and you can maximize all three by living a healthy lifestyle. The interrelationship of fitness, health, and wellness is shown in figure 1.4 by the overlapping circles. For example, if you're active on a regular basis, your fitness improves. That reduces your risk of disease, which improves your health. Your wellness and quality of life are also improved because you feel better and can better enjoy the activities of daily life.

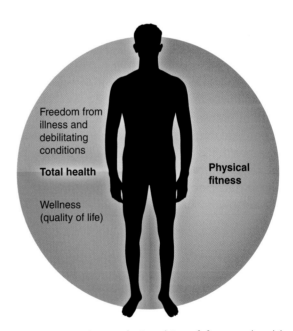

**FIGURE 1.4** Interrelationship of fitness, health, and wellness.

### Lesson Review

1. What is meant by the terms *physical fitness*, *health*, and *wellness*, and how they are interrelated?
2. What are the five components of health and wellness, and how are they defined?
3. What are the six parts of health-related physical fitness and the five parts of skill-related physical fitness, and how are they defined?
4. What is self-assessment, and how it is important to good fitness, health, and wellness?

23

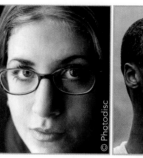
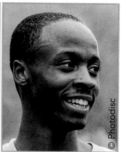

© Photodisc

© Photodisc

Self-management skills help you adopt a healthy lifestyle both now and throughout life. Self-assessment is a type of self-management skill that enables you to test yourself to see what you can do. You can perform many kinds of self-assessment. For example, you can assess your physical fitness, eating patterns, stress level, health risks, knowledge, and ability to perform in a sport. This book includes many self-assessments focused on physical fitness, as well as some that address health, wellness, and healthy lifestyle choices. The following example focuses on health-related physical fitness.

Julia and Troy were friends who wanted to know more about their health-related physical fitness. They had taken fitness tests in school but had learned little about why they were doing the tests or how to test themselves. They wanted to learn how to assess their own fitness.

Julia remembered some of the tests she had taken in elementary school, such as running a 50-yard (about 46-meter) dash and performing something called a "shuttle run." Troy had not taken a fitness test in physical education, but he had been tested for his baseball team to see how far he could throw a ball and how

fast he could run to first base.

Julia and Troy thought about doing a self-assessment that included all of the tests Julia had been given in school and all of the tests Troy had done for his baseball team. But they weren't sure how to do the tests in the correct way, and they weren't sure that these were the best tests. What they really wanted to learn was how to do a self-assessment for health-related physical fitness.

## For Discussion

Discuss a plan of self-assessment that Julia and Troy could follow to determine their health-related physical fitness. Did the tests Julia performed in elementary school assess health-related physical fitness? Did the tests Troy performed for his baseball team measure health-related physical fitness? What do you think the tests they performed really measured?

The guidelines in the following Self-Management feature will help you as you answer the discussion questions above and will be useful as you try the various self-assessments included in this book.

# SELF-MANAGEMENT: Skills for Learning to Self-Assess

Before you go on a trip, you use a map to make plans. The map helps you decide where you want to go. Assessing your own fitness is much like using a map. You can assess your current fitness and physical activity in order to help you learn where you need to improve and make your plans for doing so. You can also use the assessment information to develop strategies and tactics to commit to your plan. Use the following guidelines as you learn to do personal fitness and activity self-assessments.

- **Try a wide variety of tests.** Fitness and physical activity include many parts, and performing a variety of self-assessments enables you to get a total picture of your

fitness and activity needs. You will learn various self-assessment techniques in this class.

- **Choose self-assessments that work best for you.** You'll try all the self-assessments you learn in this book, but ultimately you won't need to use them all. You should choose at least one assessment for each type of health-related physical fitness and one assessment to determine your current activity level. After you've tried many self-assessments, you'll be prepared to select the ones that work best for you.

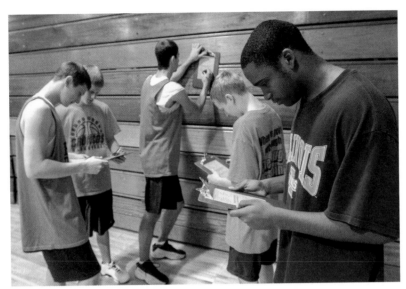

Learning to assess your own fitness is an important life skill.

- **Practice.** When you first drive a car, it's not easy, but your skill improves with practice. Similarly, the first time you do self-assessments, you'll make mistakes, but the more you practice, the better you'll get. So, once you decide which assessments to use on a regular basis, practice using them!

- **Use self-assessments for personal improvement.** Once you've learned to use self-assessments, repeat them from time to time to monitor your progress. Avoid making assessments too often, but check yourself periodically to see how you're doing. It takes several weeks to see improvement in health-related physical fitness after starting a new activity program. Avoid daily or even weekly self-assessments in favor of self-assessing after several weeks when improvement is more likely.

- **Use health standards rather than comparing yourself with others.** Sometimes people are discouraged when they get test results, often because they had unrealistic expectations. Rather than comparing yourself with others, evaluate yourself in relation to health standards and to your own previous performances. This type of comparison helps you stay realistic. *The standards used in this book are based on the level of fitness needed for good health and wellness—not on comparisons of one person with another.*

- **Information from self-assessments is personal.** Self-assessments are done to gain information that will help you build an accurate personal profile and plan for healthy active living. In many assessments you will work with a partner. Partners must agree to keep test results private. Information may be submitted to an instructor, parent, or guardian— again with the expectation that information is kept private. Information should not be shared with others without the permission of the person being tested. Think of doing a self-assessment like hiring a personal trainer. A personal trainer would have you do a series of tests to determine your strengths and weaknesses and then work with you to come up with a plan to meet your goals. The personal trainer would keep your information totally confidential.

As noted in the Science in Action feature in lesson 1, your warm-up should vary depending on the workout you plan to perform. Because *Fitness for Life* includes many types of activity, the type of warm-up you perform will vary from day to day. Before engaging in low- to moderate-intensity activity, no warm-up is typically necessary, though you may choose to do one if you wish. The activities in the warm-up you use prior to vigorous activity will vary depending on the nature of your workout activity. For vigorous activities that involve strength, speed, and power, you may choose a dynamic warm-up. If you prefer a stretching warm-up prior to vigorous activities, the stretches should last 15 to 30 seconds. Be sure not to stretch longer than 60 seconds, because that can result in reduced performance in some activities. You will **take action** here by trying both a stretching warm-up and a dynamic warm-up. After you've tried them, you can work with your teacher and use the guidelines in the Science in Action feature to create warm-up activities for each type of workout you're planning to do.

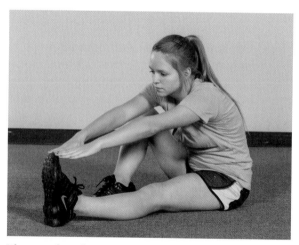

Those who choose a stretching warm-up before vigorous exercise should hold stretches for 15 to 30 seconds.

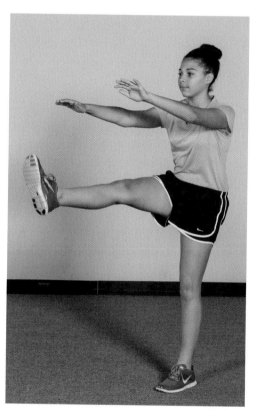

For vigorous activities that do involve strength, speed, and power, you can use a dynamic warm-up.

## Reviewing Concepts and Vocabulary

As directed by your teacher, answer items 1 through 5 by correctly completing each sentence with a word or phrase.

1. The study of human movement is called _____.
2. The _____ is a series of steps that can help you make good decisions and solve problems.
3. The science that uses principles of physics to understand the human machine is called _____.
4. A hypokinetic condition is a health problem caused by _____.
5. The part of fitness that refers to the types of body tissue is called _____.

For items 6 through 10, as directed by your teacher, match each term in column 1 with the appropriate phrase in column 2.

6. muscular endurance
7. agility
8. pedagogy
9. physical activity
10. wellness

a. movement of the body using larger muscles
b. positive component of health
c. ability to change body position quickly
d. art and science of teaching
e. ability to use muscles continuously without tiring

For items 11 through 15, as directed by your teacher, respond to each statement or question.

11. What is physical fitness?
12. How do health-related physical fitness and skill-related physical fitness differ?
13. Explain how the understanding of health has changed over time.
14. What are some important factors to consider when choosing a warm-up before your workout?
15. What are some guidelines for using self-assessments?

## Thinking Critically

Write a paragraph to answer the following question.

You are asked to make an important decision about your fitness, health, or wellness. How would you use the scientific method to make that decision?

## Project

Interview several healthy older adults about their fitness, health, and wellness. Ask questions such as these: How would you rate your health? How would you rate your wellness? How would you rate your health-related physical fitness? (Ask the person to use ratings such as good fitness, marginal fitness, and poor fitness.) How do you think teens rate their fitness, health, and wellness compared to people your age? Present the information to a group such as your class or family members.

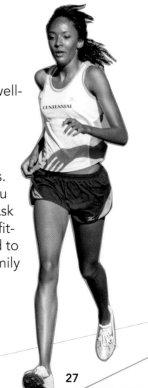

# 2

# Adopting a Healthy Lifestyle and Self-Management Skills

(www) **Student Web Resources**
www.fitnessforlife.org/student

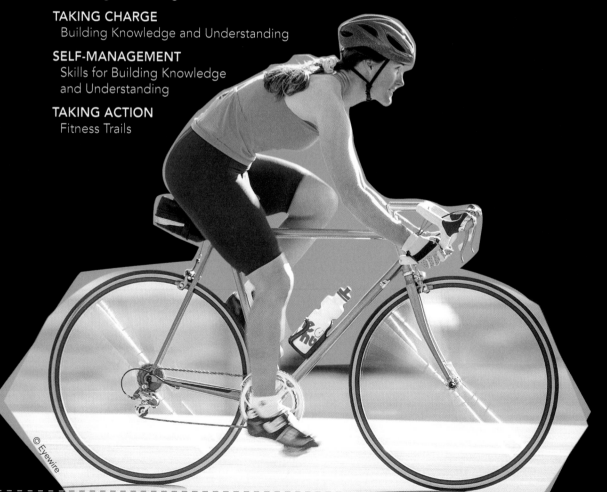

© Eyewire

# Lesson 2.1
# Adopting Healthy Lifestyles

**Let's** take a moment to consider the nature of fitness, health, and wellness. Each is a **state of being** that an individual person can possess to his or her benefit. If you possess fitness, you can work and play efficiently. If you possess health and wellness, you are free from disease and can enjoy a good quality of life. These states are interrelated, so if you do something to change one, you affect the others. Your fitness, health, and wellness are also affected by many other factors. Medical and scientific experts refer to these factors as **determinants**, and the U.S. government's Healthy People 2020 project suggests that all people learn about them in order to stay fit, healthy, and well.

> " One who has health has hope; and one who has hope has everything. "
>
> —Ancient proverb

## Determinants of Fitness, Health, and Wellness

As shown in figure 2.1, your fitness, health, and wellness are affected by five types of determinants: personal, environmental, health care, social and individual, and healthy lifestyle choices. Some are more within your control than others. The figure shows the determinant types in varying shades of orange—the lighter the color, the less control you have; the darker the color, the more control.

### Personal Determinants

You have relatively little control, or none at all, over personal determinants, such as heredity, age,

sex, and disability; thus they are shaded in light orange in the figure. Nonetheless, these factors can greatly affect your fitness, health, and wellness. For example, a person might inherit genes that put him or her at risk for certain diseases, and disease risk also increases with age. Sex is also a factor. For example, males, especially after the teen years, tend to have more muscle than females do. As for age, up to a certain point in life, muscles grow, and some parts of fitness improve just because of normal changes in the body. We also know that women have a longer life expectancy than men. Another potential factor is disability, which can affect a person's capacity to perform certain tasks but does not necessarily affect his or her health or quality of life.

You'll learn more about personal determinants and their effects on fitness, health, and wellness in other chapters of this book. Although you cannot control personal determinants, you can be aware of them. Being aware can help you decide to alter other determinants over which you do have control.

### FIT FACT

A disability is an objective condition (impairment), while a handicap is the inability to do something you would like to do. A disabled person is not necessarily handicapped. We are all physically different, and various personal determinants affect what you can and cannot do. Understanding your own strengths and limitations helps you be the best you can be and allows you to help others be the best they can be.

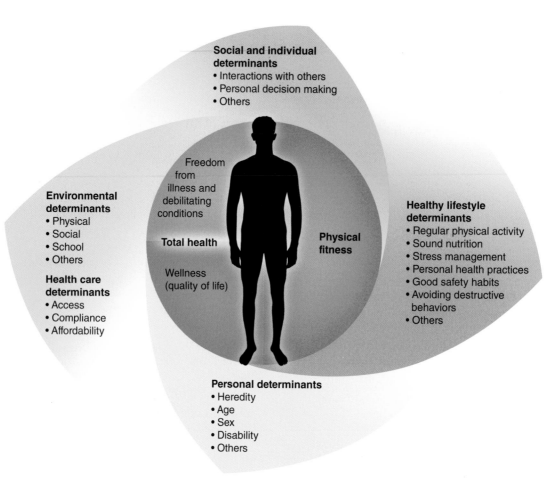

**FIGURE 2.1** The five determinants of fitness, health, and wellness.

Adapted, by permission, from C. Corbin et al., 2013, *Concepts of fitness and wellness: A comprehensive lifestyle approach,* 10th ed. (St. Louis, MO: McGraw-Hill). © The McGraw-Hill Companies

## Environmental and Health Care Determinants

Fitness, health, and wellness are also affected by environmental and health care determinants. In figure 2.1, they are colored in a darker shade of orange than the personal determinants because you have more control over them. For example, as an adult, you can choose to live or work in a healthy environment; you can also recycle in order to help protect the environment. There are other ways you can take action to improve the environment but, of course, there are limits on your control. For example, you cannot directly control the quality of the air in your neighborhood. Environmental determinants are discussed throughout this book.

Health care refers to being able to see a doctor or other health-care professional as needed and having access to health-care facilities and medicine. Health

care also includes opportunities to learn about prevention of illness and promotion of wellness. People who receive good health care live longer and have higher-quality lives compared to those who don't. This factor is shown in a darker shade of orange because you have some control over it. Having access to good health care, seeking it when needed, and complying with health care recommendations are all important to your health and wellness.

## Social and Individual Determinants

As an individual in a free society, you have the freedom to make choices and decisions that affect your fitness, health, and wellness. For example, you choose your friends and make decisions about how you interact with them, and these social choices make a difference. Teens who choose friends who avoid destructive habits and practice healthy ones

## ⚛ SCIENCE IN ACTION: Heredity and Fitness, Health, and Wellness

Exercise physiologists have studied human genes to determine whether heredity plays a role in fitness, health, and wellness. Their studies show that the genes we inherit from our parents do make a difference. For example, some people inherit genes that make them more likely to have a specific disease; other genes make it more likely that a person will be able to build muscle mass. And of course genes make a difference in how tall you are and how much you weigh. Recently, scientists have also discovered that, because of genetics, people respond differently to exercise. They learned this by studying groups of people who all did the same exercise. People who got big benefits are called responders, and those who benefited less are called nonresponders.

Even though heredity surely makes a difference in your fitness, health, and wellness, scientists also emphasize that making healthy lifestyle choices can help counteract heredity. Early in life, heredity plays a major role in your health, fitness, and wellness. However, people who practice a healthy lifestyle throughout life are among the healthiest people regardless of their heredity. What you inherit matters, but over the long haul what you do can be even more important.

---

### Student Activity

Choose one part of health-related fitness and describe how your own heredity influences it.

---

are more likely to be fit, healthy, and well themselves. Individual determinants are also important. Being a good consumer—for example, by using good information to choose healthy foods—is a way each individual can contribute to good fitness, health, and wellness. In figure 2.1, social and individual determinants are colored in a relatively dark shade of orange because you can exercise a lot of control over the choices you make, both as an individual and with your friends and other people. Personal decision making and peer interaction are discussed in special features throughout this book.

### Healthy Lifestyle Choices

By far the most important determinants of your fitness, health, and wellness are your lifestyle choices. A healthy lifestyle is made up of behaviors that you adopt to improve your fitness, health, and wellness. Because you generally have a lot of control over these determinants, they are colored in dark orange in figure 2.1. With good information and good <u>self-management skills</u>, you can adopt each of the healthy lifestyle behaviors illustrated in the figure. Self-management skills help you become more active and eat better; they also help you adapt

well in stressful situations. You'll learn more about self-management skills in lesson 2.

Adopting a healthy lifestyle gives you many benefits. First, it reduces your risk of disease and early death. In fact, nearly 60 percent of early deaths result from unhealthy lifestyle choices. Healthy choices, on the other hand, can help you prevent and treat various illnesses. For example, eating well and being active can help prevent heart disease and manage diabetes. You might assume that because illness and disease are more common in later life, you don't have to worry about them now. You might even share an attitude that is common among teenagers: "I'm young and healthy; it can't happen to me." But evidence indicates that the disease process begins early in life. Therefore, choosing and adopting a healthy lifestyle early in your life can do a lot to prevent disease and illness later on.

### FIT FACT

Healthy living pays off. For example, Oakland County, Michigan, cut health insurance costs by 15 percent after starting a program to promote healthy lifestyle choices.

# Benefits of a Healthy Lifestyle for Teens

Living a healthy lifestyle helps you not only later in life—you can also enjoy many benefits now. Examples include looking and feeling good, learning better, enjoying daily life, and effectively handling emergencies.

## Looking Good

Do you care about how you look? Experts agree that regular physical activity is one healthy lifestyle choice that can help you look your best. Others are proper nutrition, good posture, and good body mechanics.

## Feeling Good

People who do regular physical activity also feel better. If you're active and therefore physically fit, you can resist fatigue, you're less likely to be injured, and you're capable of working more efficiently. National surveys indicate that active people sleep better, do better in school, and experience less depression than people who are less active. Research indicates that regular activity can increase brain chemicals called endorphins that give you a sensation of feeling great after exercise such as a run. You can also help yourself feel your best by eating well and managing stress wisely (for diet and stress management strategies, see the separate chapters on nutrition and stress).

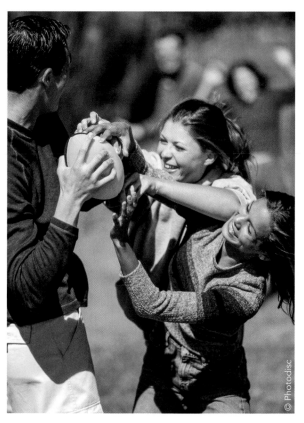

Regular physical activity can help you feel good and look your best.

## Learning Better

In recent years, scientists have found that you learn better if you are active, eat well, get enough sleep, and manage stress effectively. More specifically, studies show that teens who are active and fit score

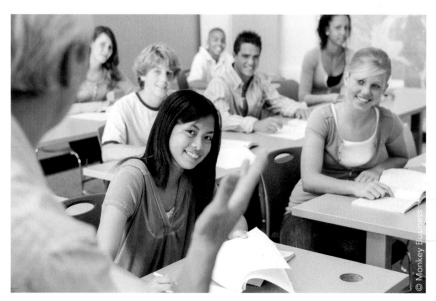

Physical activity and other healthy lifestyle choices can help you learn better.

better on tests and are less likely to be absent from school. In addition, teens who are active and eat regular healthy meals, especially breakfast, are more alert at school and less likely to be tired in the classroom. And recent studies show that regular exercise and good fitness are associated with high function in the parts of the brain that promote learning.

## Enjoying Life

Everyone wants to enjoy life. But what if you're too tired on most days to participate in the activities you really like? Regular physical activity increases your physical fitness, which is the key to being able to do more of the things you want to do. People who are fit, healthy, and well are able to enjoy life to the fullest.

## Meeting Emergencies

Sometimes challenging situations arise suddenly in life. You can prepare yourself to meet emergencies, as well as day-to-day demanding situations, by engaging in regular physical activity and making

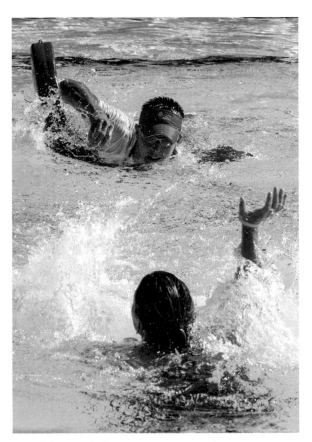

Good fitness helps you to respond in emergency situations.

other healthy lifestyle choices. For example, if you're physically fit and active, you'll be able to run for help, change a flat tire, and offer various kinds of assistance to others as needed.

## Program Overview

Throughout this book, you'll learn how determinants influence your fitness, health, and wellness. We focus especially on three **priority healthy lifestyle choices** that are very important in helping you prevent disease, get and remain fit, and enjoy a good quality of life. These three choices are regular physical activity, sound nutrition, and effective stress management. The fact that these are choices means, of course, that they are largely in *your* control.

## Stairway to Lifetime Fitness, Health, and Wellness

Do you live a healthy lifestyle? Do you eat well? If you eat meals at home, then you probably do eat well, but will you continue doing so when you're on your own? Are you physically active? Many teens are. But will you remain active as you grow older? Will you do the same kinds of activity you do now? If you answered no to any of these questions, you need to begin developing a lifetime plan for practicing a healthy lifestyle. One way to accomplish this goal is to climb what is called the Stairway to Lifetime Fitness, Health, and Wellness. As you can see in figure 2.2, when you climb this stairway, you move from a level of dependence to a level of independence. You move from having others make decisions for you to making good decisions on your own.

### Step 1: Making Healthy Lifestyle Choices—Directed by Others

Think about the way you eat, the various physical activities you're involved in, and your other lifestyle practices—even simple things such as brushing your teeth. When you were a kid, other people made most decisions about your lifestyle at home, at school, and in the community. As you've grown older, you've started making more decisions for yourself. As an adult, you'll be almost totally responsible for making your own decisions. School programs will no longer serve as your incentive to

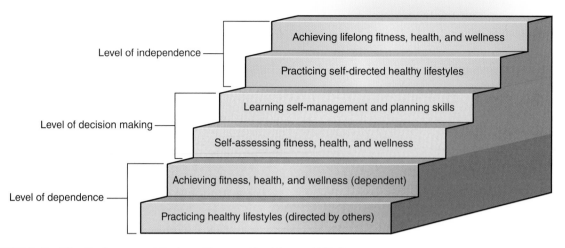

**FIGURE 2.2** The Stairway to Lifetime Fitness, Health, and Wellness.

exercise, and other opportunities for physical activity will probably decrease. You'll also choose your own food. Living out the healthy lifestyle choices made for you (or facilitated) by other people is a good first step, but it's up to you to keep climbing the stairway.

## Step 2: Achieving Fitness, Health, and Wellness—Dependent

The first step is about taking action based on what others expect. If you stick with the healthy living practices described in step 1, you will improve your fitness, health, and wellness (step 2). The resulting fitness, health, and wellness that you enjoy are dependent on others. In other words, you are not primarily responsible; others are. For example, if you get fit because of exercise prescribed by coaches and physical education teachers, you are dependent on them for the benefit you gain from the exercise. You may also eat well because of choices made by a parent who buys the food and prepares most or all of your meals. It's good that others help you to be active and adopt healthy lifestyles (step 1). It's also good when these lifestyles lead to fitness, health, and wellness (step 2). But it's not until you move to the third step in the stairway that you begin to make your own decisions.

## Step 3: Self-Assessment

Self-assessments help you set appropriate goals, make good decisions, and become more independent. A self-assessment is an evaluation that you make of yourself. You can evaluate (self-assess) your fitness, health, and wellness, as well as the lifestyle

choices that produce them. In this book, you'll try self-assessments of many kinds (one in each chapter). Once you learn to self-assess, you'll have reached the third step on the stairway. You can use the skill of self-assessment throughout your life to help you develop and implement your lifetime plan.

## Step 4: Self-Management Skills and Self-Planning

Self-management skills help you implement healthy lifestyle choices that lead to good fitness, health, and wellness. One self-management skill was discussed in the previous step—self-assessment—and many others are discussed throughout this book (one per chapter). A brief introduction to these self-management skills is provided in the next lesson of this chapter. After you've learned a variety of self-management skills, you'll be equipped to move on to the next step of the stairway.

## Step 5: Practicing a Self-Directed Healthy Lifestyle

With this step, you will move to the level of decision making and problem solving. You'll have learned *why* fitness, health, and wellness are important; *what* your personal needs are; and *how* to plan for a lifetime. Because no two people have identical needs, no two people will have exactly the same program. But you will now have the necessary tools (self-management skills) to succeed in independent planning. You'll be able to develop your own personal fitness, health, and wellness programs by implementing the healthy choices discussed in this book. In a way, then, this step is much like the first

**FITNESS TECHNOLOGY: Fitnessgram**

Fitnessgram is a fitness self-assessment program developed by a group of science advisors at the Cooper Institute in Dallas, Texas. The program provides instructions for assessing your fitness by using a variety of health-related test items. It also includes software that allows you to build a personal fitness report by entering your data into a computer. Fitnessgram has been adopted as the national assessment program for both the President's Council on Fitness, Sports, and Nutrition (PCFSN) and the Society of Health and Physical Educators (SHAPE America). You'll learn how to perform and practice the items in the Fitnessgram test battery in this chapter's Self-Assessment feature. Other chapters in this book provide more information about each test item and how to determine fitness ratings using Fitnessgram.

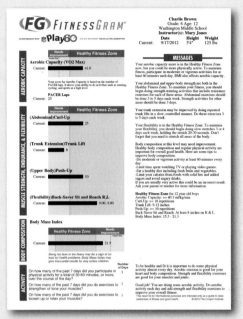

Reprinted by permission from Fitnessgram.

## Using Technology

From time to time, the Fitnessgram science advisors make changes based on new research related to the fitness test items or the method of rating fitness for each test. You can stay up to date with changes in Fitnessgram by accessing the student section of the Fitness for Life website.

step in the stairway, but now you're making your own decisions instead of having other people make decisions for you.

### Step 6: Achieving Lifelong Fitness, Health, and Wellness

When you reach the top step of the stairway, you will have taken responsibility for your own lifetime fitness, health, and wellness. You'll have moved from depending on others to making independent decisions, and you'll now implement the programs you developed in the previous step. You'll continue

to use self-assessment and other self-management skills (such as self-monitoring) to modify your plans as your needs and interests change. You'll also use other self-management skills to overcome barriers that might prevent you from sticking to your plan.

### Making Healthy Lifestyle Choices

This book and this class are designed to help you make healthy lifestyle choices that enable you to achieve lifetime fitness, health, and wellness. In the remaining chapters, you'll learn how to climb the stairway and reach the highest step.

## Lesson Review

1. What are the five types of determinants, and which are most in your personal control?
2. What are the major benefits of healthy lifestyle choices such as regular physical activity and good nutrition?
3. What is the Stairway to Lifetime Fitness, Health, and Wellness, and how can it be used?

In this book, you'll read about many physical fitness tests. The overall goal is to be able to select appropriate tests (self-assessments) to use both now and throughout your life. Several groups have developed physical fitness assessments specifically for young people. One of these, called Fitnessgram (see the Fitness Technology feature), is the most widely used test battery in the United States and is also used in many other countries. A test battery is a group of items designed to test several parts of fitness, and the Fitnessgram test battery assesses various parts of health-related physical fitness.

There are other test batteries in addition to Fitnessgram. The ALPHA-FIT test battery includes multiple test items that assess health-related physical fitness. It was developed in Europe and, like Fitnessgram, is used throughout the world. ALPHA-FIT contains some of the same items as Fitnessgram but also some different ones. For example, ALPHA-FIT includes the long jump and grip strength tests. These same two test items are included in the Institute of Medicine (IOM) Fitness Test

Battery developed for youth fitness surveys in the United States. Recent research has shown a relationship between grip strength and long jump tests and good health.

Before using a physical fitness test, learn about the test and what it measures, then practice each test item that you plan to use. Practice helps you get better at taking the test properly, so that you're truly measuring fitness rather than just learning test-taking skills. For best results, give your best effort when doing the self-assessment. For now, the goal is not to determine a score or rating on the test items but to practice the tests so that you know how to perform them properly. Since body composition assessments are not performance tests, they don't require practice and thus are not described here, but you'll learn more about them later.

Remember that self-assessment information is personal and is considered confidential. It should not be shared with others without the permission of the person being tested. Record your results as directed by your teacher.

# Test of Cardiorespiratory Endurance

## PACER
## (Progressive Aerobic Cardiovascular Endurance Run, or 20-meter shuttle run)

This test is included in Fitnessgram, ALPHA-FIT, and the IOM Fitness Test Battery.

1. The test objective is to run back and forth across a 20-meter (almost 22-yard) distance as many times as you can at a predetermined pace (pacing is based on signals from a special audio recording provided by your instructor).

2. Start at a line located 20 meters from a second line. When you hear the beep from the audio track, run across the 20-meter area to the second line, arriving just before the audio track beeps again, and touch the line with your foot. Turn around and get ready to run back.

3. At the sound of the next beep, run back to the line where you began. Touch the line with your foot. Make sure to wait for the beep before running back.

4. Continue to run back and forth from one line to the other, touching the line each time. The beeps will come faster and faster, causing you to run faster and

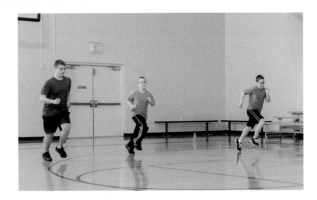

The PACER is a good test of cardiorespiratory endurance.

faster. The test is finished when you twice fail to reach the opposite side before the beep.

### Practice Tips
- Practice running at the correct pace so that you arrive just before the beep that signals you to change directions.
- Practice adjusting your pace as the beeps come faster and faster.

# Tests of Muscle Fitness

## Curl-Up (abdominal muscle strength and muscular endurance)

This test is included in Fitnessgram.

1. Lie on your back on a mat or carpet. Bend your knees approximately 140 degrees. Your feet should be slightly apart and as far as possible from your buttocks while still allowing your feet to be flat on the floor. (The closer your feet are to your buttocks, the more difficult the movement is.) Your arms should be straight and parallel to your trunk with your palms resting on the mat.

2. Place your head on a piece of paper. The paper will help your partner judge whether your head touches down on each repetition. Place a strip of cardboard (or rubber, plastic, or tape) 4.5 inches (about 11.5 centimeters) wide and 3 feet (about 1 meter) long under your knees so that the fingers of both hands just touch the near edge of the strip. You can tape the strip down or have a partner stand on it to keep it stationary.

3. Keeping your heels on the floor, curl your shoulders up slowly and slide your arms forward so that your fingers move across the cardboard strip. Curl up until your fingertips reach the far side of the strip.

4. Slowly lower your back until your head rests on the piece of paper.

5. Repeat this procedure so that you do one curl-up every three seconds. A partner can help you by saying "up, down" every three seconds.

### Practice Tips

- Practice keeping your buttocks and heels in the same location (that is, not moving them) as you do repetitions.
- Practice doing one repetition (up, down) every three seconds.
- Practice reaching to the end of the strip for each repetition.
- Practice lowering your head to the mat on each repetition.
- Next, practice as many repetitions as you can (up to 15). Have a partner check your form to make sure you are performing each curl-up correctly.

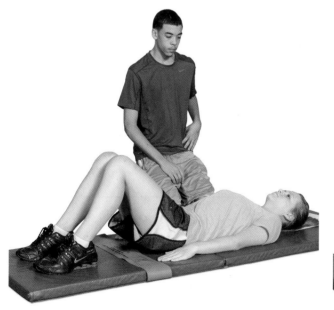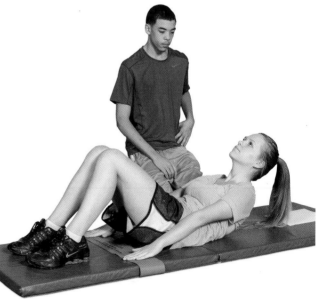

When properly performed, the curl-up is a good measure of muscle fitness of the abdominal muscles.

# Push-Up (upper body strength and muscular endurance)

This test is included in Fitnessgram.

1. Lie facedown on a mat or carpet with your hands (palm down) under your shoulders, your fingers spread, and your legs straight. Your legs should be slightly apart and your toes tucked under.

2. Push up until your arms are straight. Keep your legs and back straight. Your body should form a straight line from your head to your heels.

3. Lower your body by bending your elbows until your upper arms are parallel to the floor (elbows at a 90-degree angle), then push up until your arms are fully extended. Do one push-up every three seconds. You may want to have a partner say "up, down" every three seconds to help you.

**Practice Tips**

- Practice lowering until your elbows are bent at 90 degrees. You may want to have a partner hold a yardstick parallel to the floor (at the elbow) to help you determine when your elbows are properly bent.

- Practice pushing up all the way so that your arms are at full extension at the top of each push-up.

- Practice doing one repetition (up, down) every three seconds.

- Next, practice as many repetitions as you can (up to 15). Have a partner check your form to make sure you are performing each push-up correctly.

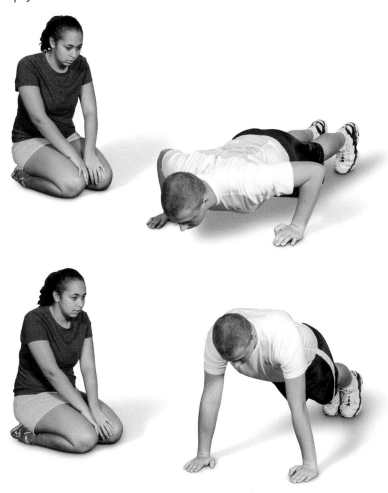

The 90-degree push-up is a measure of muscle fitness of the upper body.

## Handgrip Strength (isometric hand and arm strength)

This test is included in ALPHA-FIT and the IOM Fitness Test Battery.

1. Use a dynamometer to measure isometric strength. Adjust the dynamometer to fit your hand size.
2. Squeeze as hard as possible for two to five seconds. Your arm should be extended with your elbow nearly straight. Do not touch your body with your arm or hand.
3. Repeat with each hand. Alternate hands to allow a rest between each attempt.
4. Results are most often reported in kilograms (a kilogram equals about 2.2 pounds). To get your score in pounds, multiply your score in kilograms by 2.2.

**Practice Tips**

- Try the grip at different settings to see which enables you to perform the best.
- Try bending your knees a bit as you squeeze to help maintain good balance, which may help your score.

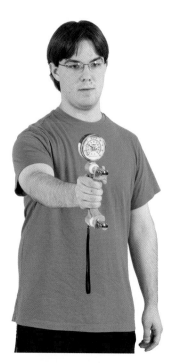

**The handgrip strength test measures muscle fitness, and scores are related to total body strength.**

## Standing Long Jump (leg power, or explosive strength)

This test is included in ALPHA-FIT and the IOM Fitness Test Battery.

1. Use masking tape or another material to make the necessary line on the floor.
2. Stand with your feet shoulder-width apart behind the line on the floor. Bend your knees and hold your arms straight in front of your body at shoulder height.
3. Swing your arms downward and backward, then vigorously forward as you jump forward as far as possible, extending your legs.
4. Land on both feet and try to maintain your balance on landing. Do not run or hop before jumping.

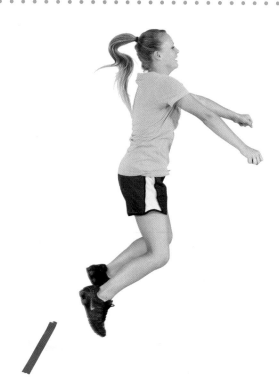

**The standing long jump is a test of power (explosive strength).**

### Practice Tips

- For best performance, lean forward just before you jump. Practice to get the best timing of the lean followed by the forward arm swing just before you jump.
- Try the test several times so that you can land without losing your balance. To help you avoid falling when you land, keep your arms extended in front of you. Also bend your knees when you land to help you absorb the shock of landing and to help you maintain your balance.
- Try bending your knees more or less before different jumps to see which amount of knee bend gives you the best jump.

# Test of Muscle Fitness and Flexibility

## Trunk Lift (back muscle fitness and back and trunk muscle flexibility)

This test is included in Fitnessgram.

1. Lie facedown with your arms at your sides and your hands under or just beside your thighs.
2. Lift the upper part of your body very slowly so that your chin, chest, and shoulders come off the floor. Lift your trunk as high as possible, to a maximum of 12 inches (30 centimeters). Hold this position for three seconds while a partner measures how far your chin is from the floor. Your partner should hold the ruler at least 1 inch (2.5 centimeters) in front of your chin. Look straight ahead so that your chin is not tipped abnormally upward.

Caution: The ruler should not be placed directly under your chin, in case you have to lower your trunk unexpectedly.

### Practice Tips

- Practice lifting your trunk 12 inches (30 centimeters) off the floor. Hold the trunk off the floor at 12 inches (do not lift higher) for three seconds.
- Practice three to five times to see if you are able to hold the lift for the required three seconds.
- Practice looking straight ahead so that your chin is not tipped up.

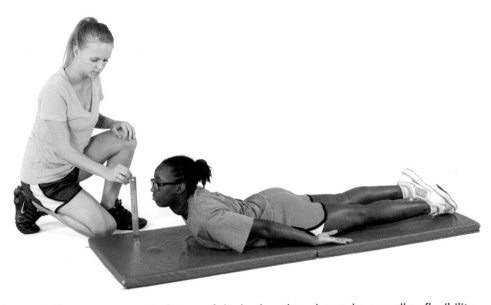

**The trunk lift measures muscle fitness of the back and trunk muscles as well as flexibility.**

# Test of Flexibility

## Back-Saver Sit-and-Reach (range of motion, or flexibility, of the hip)

This test is included in Fitnessgram.

1. Place a measuring stick, such as a yardstick or meter stick, on top of a box that is 12 inches (30 centimeters) high with the stick extending 9 inches (23 centimeters) over the box and the lower numbers toward you. You may use a flexibility testing box if one is available.

2. To measure the flexibility of your right leg, fully extend it and place your right foot flat against the box. Bend your left leg, with the knee turned out and your left foot 2 to 3 inches (5 to 8 centimeters) to the side of your straight right leg.

3. Extend your arms forward over the measuring stick. Place your hands on the stick, one on top of the other, with your palms facing down. Your middle fingers should be together with the tip of one finger exactly on top of the other.

4. Lean forward slowly; do not bounce. Reach forward with your arms and fingers, then slowly return to the starting position. Repeat four times. On the fourth reach, hold the position for three seconds and observe the measurement on the stick below your fingertips.

5. Repeat with your left leg.

### Practice Tips

- Do the PACER practice or another general warm-up before practicing this test.
- Practice keeping your extended leg straight (a very slight bend is okay).
- Practice keeping your other leg bent and the foot of that leg about 2 to 3 inches (5 to 8 centimeters) from your straight leg.
- Practice keeping one middle finger on top of the other.
- Practice holding your stretch for three seconds.
- Practice three to five times with each leg.

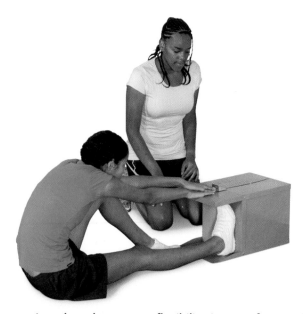

The back-saver sit-and-reach measures flexibility (range of motion) of the hip.

# Learning Self-Management Skills

**Lesson Objectives**

After reading this lesson, you should be able to

1. describe the stages of change in adopting a healthy lifestyle,
2. describe several self-management skills, and
3. explain how to use self-management skills for living a healthy life.

**Lesson Vocabulary**

exercise, motor skill, physical activity, sedentary, skill

In the first lesson of this chapter, you learned about what it means to live a healthy lifestyle. You also learned about many determinants of health, fitness, and wellness. In this lesson, you'll learn about making lifestyle changes to enhance your fitness, health, and wellness. First, you'll learn about the stages of change. People do not change overnight; change takes time, and people who are making a change typically progress through five stages. These stages were identified by psychologists working to help people stop smoking. They found that most smokers do not quit all at once but go through stages instead. Later, exercise psychologists and nutrition scientists found that these five stages of change apply to other lifestyle choices, such as physical activity and nutrition. Understanding these stages can help you make positive changes in your lifestyle.

## FIT FACT

Physical activity refers to movement that uses your large muscles. Thus it includes a wide range of pursuits, such as sport, dance, recreational activities, and activities of daily living. Exercise is a form of physical activity specifically designed to improve your fitness.

## Stages of Change for a Healthy Lifestyle

Healthy lifestyle behaviors—such as being active, eating well, and managing stress—are within your control. With effort, most anyone can make healthy lifestyle changes in these areas. There are five stages of change for modifying behaviors to improve fitness, health, and wellness: precontemplation (not thinking of change), contemplation, planning for change, taking action to change, and maintenance. Figure 2.3 shows the five stages of change for physical activity.

- **Precontemplation:** A person at stage 1 chooses not to be active. Another word for being inactive is **sedentary**, and more than one-third of all adults are sedentary and thus are included in this stage. You might think there are no sedentary teens, but there are. It's true that this category includes fewer teens than adults, but nearly one in four teens can also be included here. In an ideal world, all people would be active exercisers, but sometimes people move slowly from one stage to the next.

- **Contemplation:** A sedentary person might read about the importance of physical activity and even start to think about being active—but take no action. This person has moved from being sedentary to being an inactive thinker (stage 2). An inactive thinker does little physical activity but is thinking about becoming active.

- **Planning:** At stage 3, a person starts planning to be active. For example, he or she might visit an exercise facility or buy a new tennis racket. The person has now become a planner, even though he or she is not yet active.

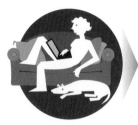
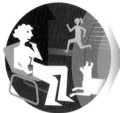
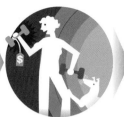
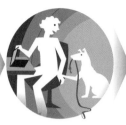
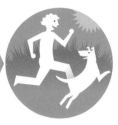

**Sedentary**
I'm inactive, and I plan to stay that way.

**Inactive thinker**
I'm inactive, but I'm thinking about becoming active.

**Planner**
I'm taking steps to start to be active.

**Activator**
I'm active, but not yet as active as I should be.

**Active exerciser**
I'm regularly active and have been for some time!

**FIGURE 2.3** The five stages of change for physical activity.

- **Taking action:** Stage 4 involves actually becoming active. The person, now an activator, goes to the exercise facility to work out, for example, or plays tennis with a friend.
- **Maintenance:** Stage 5 involves maintaining regular activity. The ultimate goal is to help all people progress to the stage of the active exerciser (stage 5). When this stage is reached, a person is active on a regular basis for a long time (at least several months).

The same five stages of change apply to other healthy lifestyle choices. For example, figure 2.4 shows the stages as they might relate to eating well. Only about 1 in every 4 teens eats the recommended number of fruits and vegetables each day, and about 1 in 10 have avoided eating meals for as long as 24 hours. Teens who do not eat well are at stage 1, whereas those who do eat well on a regular basis are at stage 5. For any healthy lifestyle choice, the goal is to move to stage 5.

Living a healthy lifestyle means making good choices in various areas of your life. You can be at one level of change in one area and at another level in a different area. For example, perhaps you're not active on a regular basis but are thinking about becoming more active; therefore, you're at stage 2 for physical activity. At the same time, you might regularly eat well and therefore be at stage 5 for healthy eating.

**FIT FACT**

Changes in behavior don't always occur from stage 1 to 5 without interruption. Sometimes people move forward a few stages, then fall back a stage, and then move forward again. With effort, progress is made gradually from one stage to another.

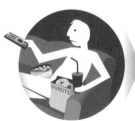
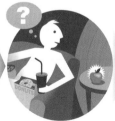
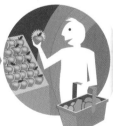
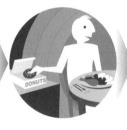
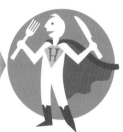

**Unhealthy eater**
I don't eat well, and I don't plan to.

**Thinker**
I don't eat well, but I'm thinking about eating better.

**Planner**
I'm taking steps to eat better.

**Improved eater**
I eat well some of the time, but I need to do better.

**Healthy eater**
I regularly eat healthy meals and avoid empty calories.

**FIGURE 2.4** The five stages of change for eating well.

# Self-Management Skills: Adopting a Healthy Lifestyle

How do you change your lifestyle? How do you move from stage 1 to stage 5 for being active or eating well?

The best way is to learn self-management skills for change. A **skill** is an ability that allows you to perform a specific task effectively. You improve your skills through practice. For example, writing and typing are skills that help you communicate; if you practice them, you get better at doing them. Similarly, **motor skills**—such as throwing, kicking, and catching—help you perform better in sports and games. They also improve with practice.

Self-management skills are abilities that help you change your lifestyles. There are <u>three kinds</u>: those that help you begin to change, those that help you make change, and those that help you maintain change (see figure 2.5).

> **"** Happiness lies, first of all, in health. **"**
>
> —George William Curtis,
> author and social reformer

## Skills That Help You Think About Change

Table 2.1 lists the names and descriptions of 21 self-management skills. Some of these are especially helpful to people who need to make changes but have not begun a plan of action (people in stages 1 and 2). *Self-assessment* skills, for example, help you see that you need to make changes and determine what changes to make. *Building knowledge and understanding* helps you see why it is important to change. Knowing the benefits of healthy lifestyle choices—such as being active and eating right—can also motivate you to make positive changes. More specifically, *identifying risk factors* for disease helps you see the need to adopt a healthy lifestyle not only for now but also for your future.

Two other self-management skills that help you begin to change are *positive attitude* and *self-confidence*. If you think you can make a change and you feel good about the change, then you're more likely to be motivated to actually do it! You'll learn more about the self-management skills that help you start making changes as you progress through this book.

## Skills That Help You Make Changes

Once you have reached stage 3 of the change process, you're ready to take action, but you must

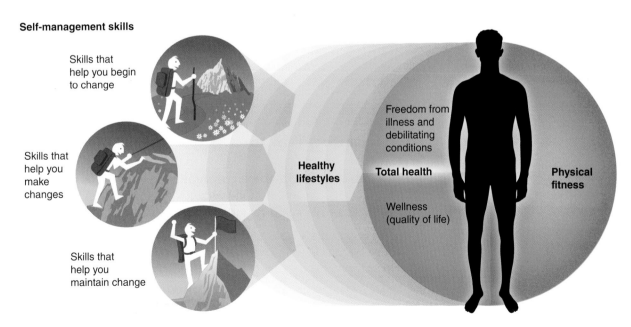

**Self-management skills**

Skills that help you begin to change

Skills that help you make changes

Skills that help you maintain change

Healthy lifestyles

Total health

Freedom from illness and debilitating conditions

Wellness (quality of life)

Physical fitness

**FIGURE 2.5** Self-management skills help you change your lifestyles to improve your fitness, health, and wellness.

**TABLE 2.1   Self-Management Skills for Fitness, Health, and Wellness**

| | Skill | Description |
|---|---|---|
| | **Skills that help you think about change** | |
| 1 | Self-assessment | This skill helps you see where you are and what to change in order to get where you want to be. |
| 2 | Building knowledge and understanding | You can use a modified form of the scientific method to solve problems—such as how to make healthy changes in your life. |
| 3 | Identifying risk factors | Identifying your health risks enables you to assess and then reduce them. |
| 4 | Positive attitude | This skill helps position you to succeed in adopting healthy lifestyles. |
| 5 | Self-confidence | This skill helps you build the feeling that you're capable of making healthy changes in your lifestyles. |
| | **Skills that help you make changes** | |
| 1 | Goal setting and self-planning | These skills create a foundation for developing your personal plan by setting goals that are SMART (specific, measurable, attainable, realistic, and timely) and preparing a written schedule. |
| 2 | Time management | This skill helps you be efficient so that you have time for the important things in your life. |
| 3 | Choosing good activities | This skill involves selecting the activities that are best for you personally so that you will enjoy and benefit from doing them. |
| 4 | Learning performance skills | This skill helps you to perform well and with confidence. For example, learning motor skills helps you become active, learning stress management skills helps you avoid or reduce stress, and learning nutrition skills helps you eat well. |
| 5 | Improving self-perception | This skill helps you think positively about yourself so that you're more likely to make healthy lifestyle choices and feel that they will make a difference in your life. |
| 6 | Stress management | This skill involves preventing or coping with the stresses of daily life. |
| | **Skills that help you maintain changes** | |
| 1 | Self-monitoring | This skill involves keeping records (logs) to see whether you are in fact doing what you think you're doing. |
| 2 | Overcoming barriers | This skill helps you find ways to stay active despite barriers, such as lack of time, temporary injury, lack of safe places to be active, inclement weather, and difficulty in selecting healthy foods. |
| 3 | Finding social support | This skill enables you to get help and support from others (such as your friends and family) as you adopt healthy behaviors and work to stick with them. |
| 4 | Saying no | This skill helps keep you from doing things you don't want to do, especially when you're under pressure from friends or other people. |
| 5 | Preventing relapse | This skill helps you stick with healthy behaviors even when you have problems getting motivated. |
| 6 | Thinking critically | This skill enables you to find and interpret information that helps you make good decisions and solve problems in living a healthy lifestyle. |
| 7 | Resolving conflicts | This skill helps you solve problems and avoid stress. |
| 8 | Positive self-talk | This skill helps you perform your best and make healthy lifestyle choices such as being active by thinking positive thoughts rather than negative ones that detract from success. |
| 9 | Developing good strategy and tactics | This skill helps you focus on a specific plan of action and successfully execute the plan. |
| 10 | Finding success | Finding success is not technically a skill, but it comes from using a variety of self-management skills to change behavior. If you use the self-management skills described here and believe that they will help you succeed, you are much more likely to achieve success. |

know how to take the *right* action. Six of the self-management skills help you begin to actually make the lifestyle changes that are right for you (see table 2.1). *Goal setting and self-planning* skills help you design a plan for change. *Time management* skills help you make time for carrying out your personal plan. Goal setting, self-planning, and time management skills apply to all types of lifestyle change.

Other self-management skills that help you become more active are *choosing good activities* and *learning performance skills*. As you do so, the skill of *improving self-perception* helps you think positively about yourself. Also, people who think positively and know how to *manage stress* are more likely to make changes because they believe that change is possible and aren't worried about confronting change.

## Skills That Help You Maintain Changes

The remaining self-management skills presented in table 2.1 help you stick with your healthy lifestyle changes. Once you've made a lifestyle change (that is, achieved stage 4 or 5 in that area of your life), these skills help you stay there. *Self-monitoring* helps you track your progress. You can also learn to *overcome barriers*, *find support from others*, and *say no* to those who might deter you. And you can learn specific skills that help keep you from quitting your healthy lifestyle (*preventing relapse*).

Several other skills can also help you stay on the right track. Learning to *think critically* helps you

make good decisions and avoid mistakes that can hurt your health. Learning to *resolve conflicts* helps you avoid stress. Using *positive self-talk* and *good strategy and tactics* helps you *find success* so that you are much more likely to stick with your lifestyle plan.

This book is intended to help you live an active, healthy life. To accomplish this goal, you must learn about and practice each of the self-management skills listed in table 2.1.

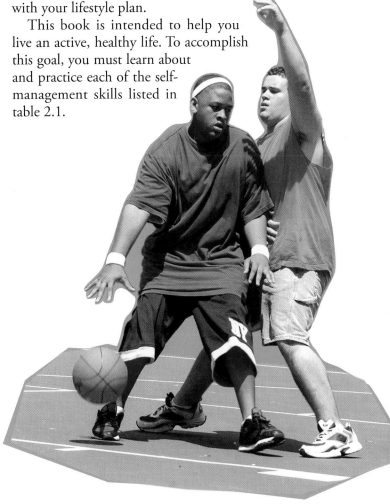

## Lesson Review

1. What are the five stages of change, and how are they useful to you?
2. What are some examples of self-management skills for each of the different stages of change?
3. How can you use self-management skills for living a healthy life?

47

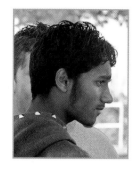

Anish's mother, Mrs. Bhalla, made a New Year's resolution to be more active. She did not know a lot about how to exercise, so she searched the web for information about fitness programs. She found a website with the following claim: "Get fit in five minutes a day without getting sweaty!" Anish was concerned because he had learned in class that it takes weeks of regular exercise to improve fitness.

Anish told his mom, "I think you need to get more knowledge and understanding about fitness and physical activity before you get started." But his mother decided to try the plan. Several months later, her fitness had not improved, and she felt discouraged.

At this point, she talked with Anish about the fitness and activity strategies he was learning at school. They both decided that it was important for her to gain good knowledge about fitness before trying a new program. Anish had also learned the value of understanding the

"why" of exercise if a person wants to get best results: Why should I exercise (what are the benefits)? Why is this plan best for me (what are my personal needs)?

Anish and his mother agreed that she would learn along with him as he studied fitness and physical activity at school so that she could do things right the next time she tried.

## For Discussion

Mrs. Bhalla made one good decision and one bad decision. How can someone who wants to make a healthy New Year's resolution avoid making a bad decision about fitness and physical activity? Why do you think people choose programs such as the one Mrs. Bhalla tried? Is it possible to get fit in five minutes a day? How might Anish help his mother in the future? Consider the guidelines presented in the following Self-Management feature as you answer these discussion questions.

Knowledge based on sound information can help you make good decisions. But knowledge alone does not always lead to good decisions. You must understand the information you take in. A person with knowledge knows facts, but a person with understanding comprehends the significance of the facts and can use that understanding to make good decisions.

In this book, you learn knowledge about fitness, health, and wellness. You also build higher-level understanding that helps you apply the information you've learned. The following guidelines will help you use this book to build both your knowledge and your understanding.

- **Learn the facts first.** Learning the facts is a necessary first step toward building higher-level understanding.

- **Use the scientific method.** Investigate (collect information) to gain as many facts as possible. The facts help you analyze and test hypotheses. For example, you might have a hypothesis that you can get fit in five minutes a day. After gaining the facts and analyzing them, you would learn that the hypothesis is false. The scientific method helps you understand the information you learn and make sound decisions.

- **Ask why.** When studying healthy lifestyle choices, ask yourself "why" questions: Why do I need this? Why should I believe this information? Why will this information be beneficial?

- **Consult reliable sources.** Whether you're consulting a website, magazine article, or book, check with trusted people to help you find good sources. Your knowledge and understanding are only as good as the sources you use. The chapter titled Making Good Consumer Choices provides more information about how to find reliable source material.

- **Try to apply.** When learning new information, ask, "How can I apply this?" Applying new information to real situations helps you understand it, which in turn helps you apply it more effectively. For example, regarding the dangers of fat in your diet, ask yourself questions like these: What else do I need to know? How much fat is too much? What changes can I make in my diet to reduce my fat intake?

- **Put it all together.** When you learn about something new, you often find many pieces of information. Taking time to fit the pieces together will help you make sense of what you've learned. Another word for "putting all the facts together" is *synthesizing*. For example, if you know you feel stressed out, and you know that there are several reasons for the stress, how do you use all of the information together—synthesize it—to make a good decision?

## ACADEMIC CONNECTION: Accurate Use of Words

English language arts is an area of academic study that focuses on preparing students who are college and career ready in reading, writing, speaking, listening, and language. Learning to use words accurately and knowing how similar words differ are important in the study of the English language and in achieving literacy (being educated).

In this chapter, and in other parts of this book, factors influencing fitness, health, and wellness are discussed. Health experts typically refer to the factors as determinants. The word *sex* is used throughout the book to describe whether you are biologically male or female. Your sex is one determinant that influences your fitness, health, and wellness. The word *gender* has a similar but slightly different meaning. It refers to social or cultural roles of people (masculine or feminine). For example, in the past some activities were identified as gender appropriate for males only (masculine) or females only (feminine). Over time, stereotypes have diminished, opening up more activity opportunities for both males and females. In this book, activities are not identified as masculine or feminine. Activities are considered appropriate for both sexes (male and female). *Gender* is also a word used in grammar to categorize pronouns (such as *he* or *she*) and other parts of speech.

The use of words sometimes changes over time. In recent years the word *gender* has been used more frequently to indicate a person's sex (male or female). In the sciences, the preferred term is *sex* rather than *gender* when indicating whether a person is male or female, and for this reason *sex* is the term used in this book (in this context).

Fresh air, nature, and fitness? Yes, please! Most communities have natural spaces where you can walk, jog, run, or bike. Some communities have also created fitness trails—pathways through parks or woodlands designed especially for walking, jogging, and running. Some fitness trails include human-made or natural structures intended for particular exercises. These structures allow walkers, joggers, and runners to mix their movement activity with muscle fitness and flexibility exercises. Fitness trails are sometimes considered "outdoor gyms," and there's probably one near you!

**Take action** by learning about, visiting, or even helping create a fitness trail near you. Many fitness trails are already well established by city or county park and recreation departments or federal agencies such as the U.S. National Park Service. Although they may differ from remote trails, urban areas can have fitness trails.

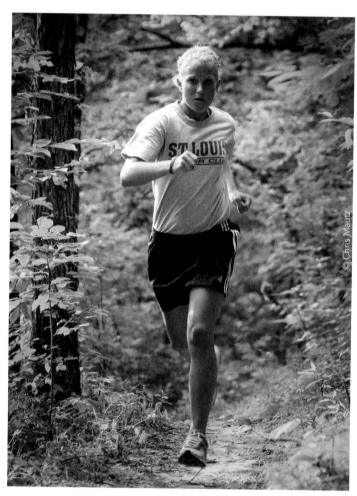

**Being outdoors dramatically increases the amount of activity that people perform.**

## Reviewing Concepts and Vocabulary

As directed by your teacher, answer items 1 through 5 by correctly completing each sentence with a word or phrase.

1. Factors that affect your fitness, health, and wellness are called _____.
2. Factors influencing fitness, health, and wellness over which you have little control are called _____.
3. Factors influencing fitness, health, and wellness over which you have the most control are called _____.
4. The steps that lead you from dependence to independence are referred to together as the _____.
5. The fitness test used to assess cardiorespiratory endurance by running when signaled by a beep is called the _____.

For items 6 through 10, as directed by your teacher, match each term in column 1 with the appropriate phrase in column 2.

6. sedentary person
7. inactive thinker
8. planner
9. activator
10. active exerciser

a. just bought exercise equipment
b. is active most days of the week
c. is sometimes active
d. is considering becoming active
e. is inactive

For items 11 through 15, as directed by your teacher, respond to each statement or question.

11. Explain what a self-management skill is and why it can be useful.
12. What are some of the fitness test items used in major fitness test batteries such as Fitnessgram, and what do they measure?
13. Describe the five stages of change.
14. What are fitness trails, and how can they be useful in staying active?
15. What are some guidelines for building knowledge and understanding?

## Thinking Critically

Write a paragraph to answer the following question.

Of all the self-management skills described in lesson 2, which one would most help *you* be more active or eat better? Give the reasons for your answer.

## Project

Assume that you are the head of a marketing company assigned to create an ad campaign promoting healthier eating and more active living. Prepare a script for a television commercial for the promotion. If resources are available, create a video of the commercial.

# 3

# Goal Setting and Program Planning

**In This Chapter**

 **Student Web Resources**
www.fitnessforlife.org/student

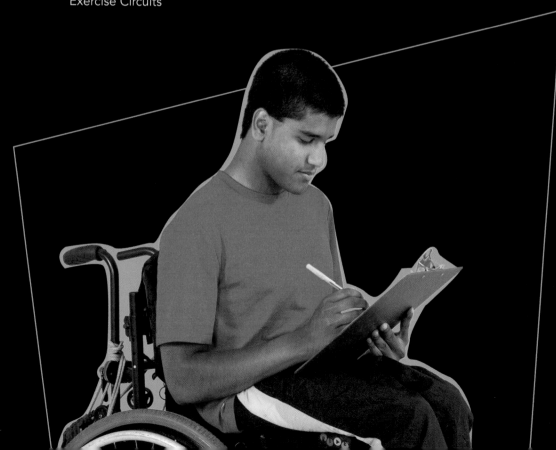

# Lesson 3.1
# Goal Setting

## Lesson Objectives

After reading this lesson, you should be able to
1. explain the SMART formula for setting goals,
2. explain how long-term and short-term goals differ, and
3. describe process and product goals and explain how they differ.

## Lesson Vocabulary

acronym, goal setting, long-term goal, mnemonic, process goal, product goal, short-term goal, SMART goal

**How** do you turn your dreams into realities? Successful people use **goal setting** as part of their overall planning to achieve success; they decide ahead of time what they plan to accomplish, then go about doing it. You can use goals to plan a personal fitness program, a program of good eating, or any other type of program. In this lesson, you'll learn to use long-term and short-term goals. You'll also learn about other goals that can help you make good lifestyle choices, such as being physically active and eating well.

## SMART Goals

You may have learned about **SMART goals** in middle school. Here's a quick review to help you remember the five rules for setting goals as you work your way through this book and set your own goals.

**S** = specific. Your goal should include details of what you want to accomplish.

**M** = measurable. You should be able to measure your progress and accurately determine whether you've accomplished your goal.

**A** = attainable. Your goals should challenge you. They should not be too easy or too hard.

**R** = realistic. You should be able to reach your goal if you put in the time and effort and have the necessary resources.

**T** = timely. Your goal should be useful to you at this time in your life and can be met in the time allotted.

## FIT FACT

A mnemonic (pronounced ni-mon'-ik) is a trick for remembering something. The mnemonic SMART helps us remember five guidelines for creating goals. Specifically, SMART is an acronym, which means that each letter in the word is the first letter of a key word related to goal setting.

## SMART Long-Term Goals

**Long-term goals** take you months or even years to accomplish, whereas you can reach **short-term goals** in a short time, such as a few days or weeks. One example of a long-term goal is saving money to help pay for college expenses. If you plan to save $2,400, you could make your long-term goal earning that amount.

In order to earn that much, you might have to work on weekends and during summers throughout high school. Saving money takes time. If your job allowed you to save $100 a month, it would take you two years to save the $2,400. Now let's see whether this would be a SMART goal.

**S**pecific. $2,400 is a very specific long-term goal. You know the amount of money you need.

**M**easurable. The $2,400 goal is measurable. You can count your money to see how close you are to reaching your goal.

Attainable. The goal might be too hard for a person without a job, but you have one. It won't be easy, but you make enough money each hour to make your goal possible.

Realistic. For someone else, the $2,400 goal might not be realistic. But if you put in the time and stick with your job, saving $100 a month for two years is possible. You must also consider other commitments, such as homework, activities, and family responsibilities.

Timely. The goal of saving $2,400 in two years has a specific and workable time line that fits your planned entrance into college.

## SMART Short-Term Goals

Short-term goals can usually be reached in a few days or weeks. Thus you might set a series of short-term goals to help you accomplish a long-term goal. For example, to meet your long-term goal of saving $2,400, you might set a short-term goal of working five hours a week at $8 an hour for two weeks. Doing so would be a manageable way to start working toward meeting your long-term goal. After completing this short-term goal, you could establish a new one.

Let's now consider whether this short-term goal would be a SMART one.

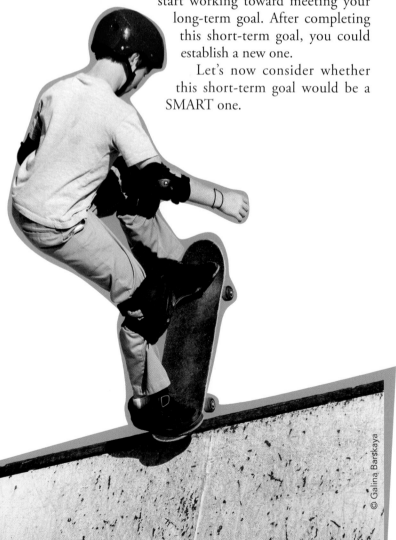
© Galina Barskaya

Specific. You've made the goal specific by listing the number of weeks and the number of hours worked per week.

Measurable. You can measure your progress toward the goal by tracking your work hours each week.

Attainable. Your short-term goal is attainable because it depends only on your making the effort to fulfill your work schedule. You could have set a goal of working more hours per week, but that might not be attainable.

Realistic. Setting a realistic number of work hours depends on other factors, such as homework, activities, and family responsibilities. However, you have the time to work five hours a week and still meet other responsibilities, so this is a realistic goal.

Timely. Working five hours a week for two weeks is a timely goal because you've specified the time frame for completing the goal and it fits your current schedule.

## Product and Process Goals

The long-term goal of earning $2,400 is a **product goal**. A product is something tangible that results from work or effort. It's not what you do, but what you get as a result of what you do. Examples of product goals for fitness, health, and wellness include being able to perform 25 push-ups, being able to run a mile in six minutes, and losing five pounds (figure 3.1a). In each case, the goal is a product or outcome of work and effort. Product goals make

### FIT FACT

Each year, millions of Americans make New Year's resolutions to eat better and exercise more. And each year, many of them fail to stick with their resolutions. Scientists have discovered that one of the main reasons for this failure is that people choose long-term goals that cannot be accomplished in the time allotted. In other words, they fail to set SMART goals. This pattern illustrates why scientists urge people to focus short-term goals on lifestyle change rather than on results such as fitness or weight loss.

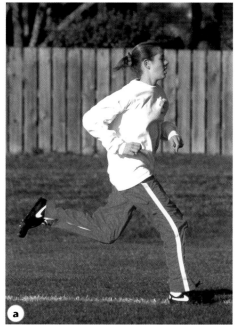
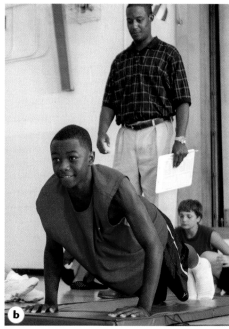

**FIGURE 3.1** Product and process goals: *(a)* Running a mile in eight minutes is a product goal, and *(b)* doing five push-ups a day for three weeks is a process goal.

appropriate long-term goals because it may take you a fair amount of work and time to reach them.

**Process goals** involve performing a behavior, such as working a certain number of hours to earn money. Process refers to what you do rather than to the product resulting from what you do. Examples for fitness, health, and wellness include exercising 60 minutes and eating five fruits and vegetables every

 **FITNESS TECHNOLOGY: Smartphones and Tablet Computers**

The first computers were so large that they filled entire rooms. Over time, computers got smaller and smaller. Today's smartphones are very small computers that can do many tasks that formerly required desktop or laptop computers. Smartphones use software, or applications (also known as apps), to perform a wide variety of functions. Some companies have developed smartphone apps that can help you plan and monitor your physical activity and nutrition. For example, you can record your self-assessment results and your program schedule and track your exercise and food intake. These apps can also be used on tablet computers, which are larger than smartphones but still very portable.

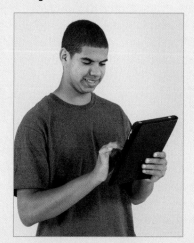

Smartphone and computer tablets have apps that help you meet healthy lifestyle goals.

**Using Technology**

Create an idea for a fitness or health app. Describe the app and how it would be used.

## SCIENCE IN ACTION: Optimal Challenge

Scientists in many fields have collaborated to find ways to help people stay active, eat well, and stick with other healthy lifestyle behaviors. They have discovered that in order to be successful, you must set goals that provide "optimal challenge." The key is giving effort (trying hard). If a challenge is too easy, there's no need to try hard—it's not really a challenge. On the other hand, if a goal is too hard, we fail, which may lead us to give up or quit because our effort seems hopeless (see figure 3.2).

An optimal challenge requires *reasonable* effort. Meeting an optimal challenge provides us with success and makes us want to try again. In fact, providing optimal challenge is one reason that video games are so popular. They challenge you by making the task more difficult as you improve, and this optimal challenge makes you want to play again and again. You can use optimal challenge when setting your own goals to help yourself succeed.

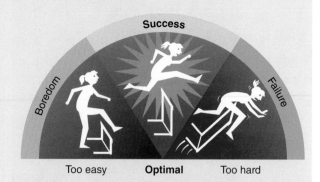

**Figure 3.2** Some challenges can lead to boredom or failure, but optimal challenges can lead to success.

### Student Activity

Imagine that you want to help a friend learn a skill—for example, hitting a tennis ball or a golf ball. How could you use optimal challenge to help your friend learn the skill?

day (figure 3.1*b*). Process goals make good short-term goals because you can easily monitor your progress and, with effort, succeed. In contrast, *product* goals do not make especially good short-term goals, because they can be discouraging, especially for a person who is just beginning to change. For example, if you chose a product goal of performing, say, 25 push-ups, it might (depending on your current fitness level) take you so long to meet the goal that you would give up. But a short-term process goal—such as performing 5 to 10 push-ups each day for two weeks—would be possible for you to achieve with effort. Thus, as you meet a series of short-term process goals, you work toward meeting long-term product goals.

The Taking Charge and Self-Management features in this chapter focus on setting goals for physical activity and building physical fitness. Elsewhere in the book, you'll get the chance to set long-term goals for fitness, health, and wellness (product goals) and for making healthy lifestyle changes (process goals) that lead to good fitness, health, and wellness. You'll also get the chance to set short-term goals that help you move toward achieving your long-term goals.

If you want to live a happy life, tie it to a goal, not to people or things. **"**

—Albert Einstein, Nobel Prize–winning physicist

### Lesson Review

1. How does the SMART formula help you set goals?
2. How can you use long-term and short-term goals to plan your program? In your answer, use fitness and physical activity examples.
3. What is the difference between a process goal and a product goal? In your answer, use fitness and physical activity examples.

This book's chapters on fitness, health, wellness, and self-management skills introduce you to national and international fitness test batteries and give you a chance to practice test items to make sure that you know how to do them properly. In this self-assessment, you'll perform four of the tests that measure your muscle fitness: curl-up, push-up, handgrip strength, and long jump. For each item, you'll learn how to rate your performance. Later, when you've taken all of the tests included in Fitnessgram, you can use your scores and ratings to prepare a Fitnessgram report. For the tests included in this chapter, you'll record your scores and ratings as directed by your teacher so that you can use the information when you plan your personal fitness program. If you're working with a partner, remember that self-assessment information is personal and considered confidential. It shouldn't be shared with others without the permission of the person being tested.

# Curl-Up
# (abdominal muscle strength and muscular endurance)

1. Lie on your back on a mat or carpet. Bend your knees approximately 140 degrees. Your feet should be slightly apart and as far as possible from your buttocks while still allowing your feet to be flat on the floor. Your arms should be straight and parallel to your trunk with your palms resting on the mat.

2. Place your head on a piece of paper. Place a strip of cardboard (or rubber, plastic, or tape) 4.5 inches (about 11.5 centimeters) wide and 3 feet (about 1 meter) long under your knees so that the fingers of both hands just touch the near edge of the strip.

3. Keeping your heels on the floor, curl your shoulders up slowly and slide your arms forward so that your fingers move across the cardboard strip. Curl up until your fingertips reach the far side of the strip.

4. Slowly lower your back until your head rests on the piece of paper.

5. Repeat the curl-up procedure so that you do one curl-up every three seconds. A partner could help you by saying "up, down" every three seconds. You are finished when you can't do another curl-up or when you fail to keep up with the three-second count.

6. Record the number of curl-ups you completed, then find your rating in table 3.1 and record it.

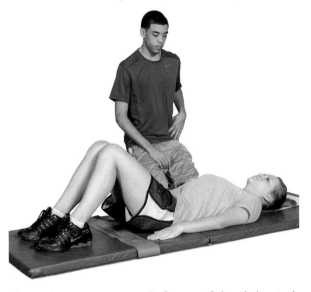
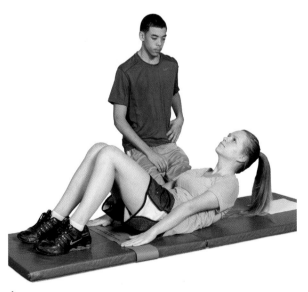

The curl-up assesses muscle fitness of the abdominal muscles.

**TABLE 3.1  Rating Chart: Curl-Up (Number of Repetitions)**

| | 13 years old | | 14 years old | | 15 years or older | |
|---|---|---|---|---|---|---|
| | Male | Female | Male | Female | Male | Female |
| High performance | ≥41 | ≥33 | ≥46 | ≥33 | ≥48 | ≥36 |
| Good fitness | 21–40 | 18–32 | 24–45 | 18–32 | 24–47 | 18–35 |
| Marginal fitness | 18–20 | 15–17 | 20–23 | 15–17 | 20–23 | 15–17 |
| Low fitness | ≤17 | ≤14 | ≤19 | ≤14 | ≤19 | ≤14 |

Data based on *Fitnessgram*.

# Push-Up (upper body strength and muscular endurance)

1. Lie facedown on a mat or carpet with your hands (palm down) under your shoulders, your fingers spread, and your legs straight. Your legs should be slightly apart and your toes tucked under.

2. Push up until your arms are straight. Keep your legs and back straight. Your body should form a straight line from your head to your heels.

3. Lower your body by bending your elbows until your upper arms are parallel to the floor (elbows at a 90-degree angle), then push up until your arms are fully extended.

4. Do one push-up every three seconds. You may want to have a partner say "up, down" every three seconds to help you. You are finished when you are unable to complete a push-up with proper form for the second time or are unable to keep the pace for a second time.

5. Record the number of push-ups you performed, then find your rating in table 3.2 and record it.

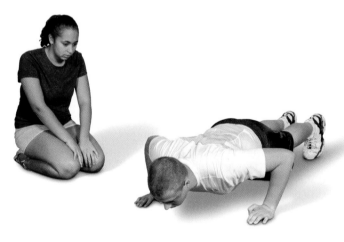
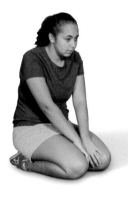
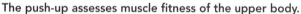
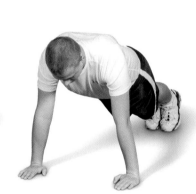

The push-up assesses muscle fitness of the upper body.

**TABLE 3.2    Rating Chart: Push-Up (Number of Repetitions)**

| | 13 years old | | 14 years old | | 15 years old | | 16 years or older | |
|---|---|---|---|---|---|---|---|---|
| | Male | Female | Male | Female | Male | Female | Male | Female |
| High performance | ≥26 | ≥16 | ≥31 | ≥16 | ≥36 | ≥16 | ≥36 | ≥16 |
| Good fitness | 12–25 | 7–15 | 14–30 | 7–15 | 16–35 | 7–15 | 18–35 | 7–15 |
| Marginal fitness | 10–11 | 6 | 12–13 | 6 | 14–15 | 6 | 16–17 | 6 |
| Low fitness | ≤9 | ≤5 | ≤11 | ≤5 | ≤13 | ≤5 | ≤15 | ≤5 |

Data based on *Fitnessgram*.

# Handgrip Strength (isometric hand and arm strength)

1. Use a dynamometer to measure isometric strength. Adjust the dynamometer to fit your hand size.
2. Squeeze as hard as possible for two to five seconds. Your arm should be extended with your elbow nearly straight. Do not touch your body with your arm or hand.
3. Results are most often reported in kilograms (a kilogram equals about 2.2 pounds). To get your score in pounds, multiply your score in kilograms by 2.2.
4. Do two tests with each hand. Record your best score for each hand. Add your best right-hand score to your best left-hand score, then divide the total by two to get your average score.
5. Record your average score, then find your rating in table 3.3 and record it.

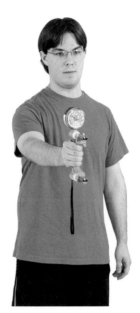

The handgrip strength test assesses isometric hand and arm strength.

**TABLE 3.3    Rating Chart: Handgrip Strength in Pounds**

| | 13 years old | | 14 years old | | 15 years old | | 16 years old | | 17 years or older | |
|---|---|---|---|---|---|---|---|---|---|---|
| | Male | Female | Male | Female | Male | Female | Male | Female | Male | Female |
| High performance | ≥65 | ≥57 | ≥80 | ≥60 | ≥91 | ≥61 | ≥107 | ≥62 | ≥112 | ≥71 |
| Good fitness | 58–64 | 54–56 | 71–79 | 58–59 | 82–90 | 59–60 | 100–106 | 60–61 | 104–111 | 65–70 |
| Marginal fitness | 52–57 | 50–53 | 63–70 | 55–57 | 74–81 | 56–58 | 93–99 | 57–59 | 97–103 | 59–64 |
| Low fitness | ≤51 | ≤49 | ≤62 | ≤54 | ≤73 | ≤55 | ≤92 | ≤56 | ≤96 | ≤58 |

Ratings are based on the average of the best right-hand and left-hand scores.

# Standing Long Jump (leg power, or explosive strength)

1. Use masking tape or another material to make the necessary line on the floor.

2. Stand with your feet shoulder-width apart behind the line on the floor. Bend your knees and hold your arms straight in front of your body at shoulder height.

3. Swing your arms downward and backward, then vigorously forward as you jump forward as far as possible, extending your legs.

4. Land on both feet and try to maintain your balance on landing. Do not run or hop before jumping.

5. Perform the test two times. Record the better of your two scores in inches (1 inch equals 2.54 centimeters), then find your rating in table 3.4 and record it.

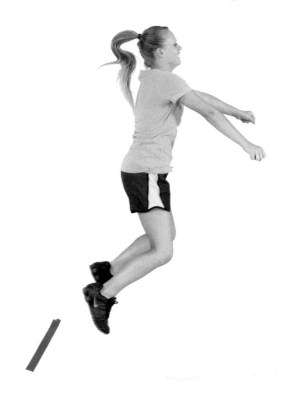

The standing long jump assesses leg power.

### TABLE 3.4   Rating Chart: Standing Long Jump in Inches

|  | 13 years old | | 14 years old | | 15 years old | | 16 years old | | 17 years or older | |
|---|---|---|---|---|---|---|---|---|---|---|
|  | Male | Female | Male | Female | Male | Female | Male | Female | Male | Female |
| High performance | ≥73 | ≥59 | ≥80 | ≥60 | ≥85 | ≥61 | ≥88 | ≥62 | ≥91 | ≥68 |
| Good fitness | 67–72 | 57–58 | 73–79 | 58–59 | 78–84 | 59–60 | 82–87 | 60–61 | 86–90 | 63–67 |
| Marginal fitness | 61–66 | 54–56 | 67–72 | 55–57 | 73–77 | 56–58 | 77–81 | 57–59 | 80–85 | 58–62 |
| Low fitness | ≤60 | ≤53 | ≤66 | ≤54 | ≤72 | ≤55 | ≤76 | ≤56 | ≤79 | ≤57 |

<h1>Lesson 3.2</h1>

<h1>Program Planning</h1>

## Lesson Objectives

After reading this lesson, you should be able to

1. describe the five steps in program planning,
2. describe and explain the purpose of a personal needs profile, and
3. describe what you would include in a written program plan.

 **Lesson Vocabulary**

personal lifestyle plan, personal needs profile, personal program

**Have** you ever prepared a written plan to change a healthy lifestyle? If not, would you know how to prepare a good plan? You can use self-management skills to help you adopt healthy lifestyles. You've already learned about the self-management skill of goal setting. In this lesson, you'll learn about another self-management skill—self-planning—in which you prepare personal plans for various aspects of a healthy lifestyle, such as being active, eating well, and managing stress. Eventually, you'll put all of these plans together to prepare a comprehensive **personal lifestyle plan**.

## The Five Steps of Program Planning

The steps used in program planning are similar to the steps used in the simplified scientific method. They are described in detail in the sections that follow.

### Step 1: Determine Your Personal Needs

The first step toward preparing a good **personal program** plan is to collect information about your personal needs. Throughout this book, you'll do many self-assessments of personal fitness, physical activity patterns, foods you eat, and other health-related areas. You'll use the information you gather to build a personal fitness, physical activity, or nutrition profile. This personal profile will help you focus on your own personal needs as you plan your program. If you don't know your needs, it will be difficult to perform the next steps in personal

program planning such as considering program options (step 2) or setting goals (step 3). For example, before planning a fitness and activity program, you assess your fitness level and physical activity patterns. Before planning a nutrition program, you assess your eating habits. In fact, before you plan to change *any* aspect of your lifestyle, you should perform a self-assessment in that particular area.

## FIT FACT

Nearly three in four Americans say they eat a balanced diet, but the typical teen eats less than a third of the recommended fruits and vegetables.

Once you complete your self-assessment in a specific lifestyle area, you summarize your scores and ratings in a chart called a **personal needs profile**. You'll build a personal needs profile for each healthy lifestyle plan you develop as you work your way through this book. The following example addresses muscle fitness and muscle fitness exercises. It will help you see what a profile looks like.

Jordan is a freshman in high school. She had always wanted to play on the lacrosse team and felt that improving her muscle fitness would help her be a better player. She also felt that building muscle fitness would help her look better. To evaluate her current muscle fitness, Jordan performed three self-assessments: the curl-up, the push-up, and the long jump. She also answered some questions about her current muscle fitness activities. She summarized her results in a personal needs profile (see figure 3.3).

| Activity self-assessment | Yes | No | Comment |
|---|---|---|---|
| Do you do muscle fitness exercises 2 or 3 days per week? | | ✔ | Stretch every day for 10 min. |
| **Fitness self-assessments** | **Score** | **Rating** | |
| Push-up | 6 | Marginal | |
| Curl-up | 19 | Good fitness | |
| Standing long jump | 57 in. (145 cm) | Marginal | |

**FIGURE 3.3** Jordan's personal needs profile.

## Step 2: Consider Your Program Options

After determining your personal needs, the next step is to consider your program options. For physical activity, you determine what types of activity are available to you. Since Jordan was interested in muscle fitness, she used a checklist of the muscle fitness activities available to her. As you can see from the chart (figure 3.4), there are many types of muscle fitness exercise. Jordan checked elastic band exercises, calisthenics, and isometric exercises because she could do them at home and had the necessary equipment. She decided to hold off on considering other types of exercise until she learned more about them.

| Elastic band exercises | | Calisthenics | Free weights | Resistance machine exercises | Isometric exercises | |
|---|---|---|---|---|---|---|
| ✔ | Arm curl | ✔ Prone arm lift | Bench press | Bench press | ✔ | Biceps curl |
| ✔ | Arm press | ✔ Push-up | Biceps curl | Biceps curl | ✔ | Bow exercise |
| ✔ | Upright row | ✔ Bridging | Dumbbell row | Lat pull-down | ✔ | Hand push |
| ✔ | Leg curl | ✔ Curl-up | Seated French curl | Seated row | ✔ | Back flattener |
| ✔ | Two-leg press | ✔ Trunk lift | Seated press | Triceps press | ✔ | Knee extender |
| ✔ | Toe push | ✔ High-knee jog | Half squat | Hamstring curl | ✔ | Leg curl |
| | | ✔ Side leg raise | Hamstring curl | Heel raise | ✔ | Toe push |
| | | ✔ Stride jump | Heel raise | Knee extension | ✔ | Wall push |
| | | | Knee extension | | | |

**FIGURE 3.4** Jordan's exercise options for muscle fitness.

## Step 3: Set Goals

The next step in self-planning is to set SMART goals. Jordan reviewed the example of writing SMART goals to save money for college, then used the SMART formula to write down her own long-term and short-term goals (see figure 3.5). She chose exercise (process) goals for her short-term goals. For her long-term goals, she listed fitness (product) goals.

> You are never too old to set another goal or to dream a new dream.
>
> —C.S. Lewis, author

| Short-term goals | Long-term goals |
|---|---|
| 1. Perform the push-up and elastic band biceps curl exercises 3 days a week. | 1. Perform 10 push-ups. |
| 2. Perform the long jump, the elastic band leg curl, and the elastic band toe push exercises 3 days a week. | 2. Long-jump 59 in. (about 1.5 m). |
| 3. Perform the curl-up exercise for the abdominal muscles 3 days a week. | 3. Perform 25 curl-ups. |

**FIGURE 3.5** Jordan's goals for fitness and physical activity included both short-term and long-term goals.

**S** = specific. Jordan set her goals for muscle fitness and physical activity by choosing specific exercises and a specific number of exercise days per week. She grounded these decisions in the information recorded in her personal needs profile.

**M** = measurable. Jordan made her goals measurable by deciding the number of weeks, the number of exercise days per week, and, for her long-term fitness goals, the number of repetitions or distance for each outcome.

**A** = attainable. To keep her goals attainable, Jordan's short-term goals addressed only activity (not fitness). She chose fitness goals for her long-term goals. She took this approach because muscle fitness takes time to build, which means that short-term fitness goals are often not attainable. In addition, for her long-term fitness goals, she chose scores that are higher than she can currently perform—but not too high. For her activity goals, Jordan chose two weeks of exercise as her short-term goal. In this way, she will first focus on her short-term goal as a step toward achieving her long-term goal. Jordan also sought out help from her physical education teacher in selecting her exercises and setting attainable goals.

**R** = realistic. Because Jordan has various commitments—such as homework, family activities, and school activities—she limited the number of her goals (both short- and long-term) so that she has a realistic chance to meet them all.

**T** = timely. Jordan also set a specific amount of time for reaching both her long-term and her short-term goals. Since she needs more muscle fitness to make the lacrosse team, she needs to improve her fitness in time for tryouts.

## Step 4: Structure Your Program and Write It Down

In the fourth step, you use information gained during steps 1, 2, and 3 to structure your program. Once you establish your goals, you prepare a detailed written plan. As you work through this book, you'll create written plans for several programs; they will all be similar to Jordan's planning.

Jordan used a chart to prepare her exercise plan for muscle fitness. Since muscle fitness exercises should not be done every day, Jordan's teacher helped her decide which days to do each exercise and how many to do. Her teacher also helped her select the right elastic band to use in her exercises. Jordan decided on the best time of day based on her free time and the times when she most enjoyed exercising. She also considered times when she was

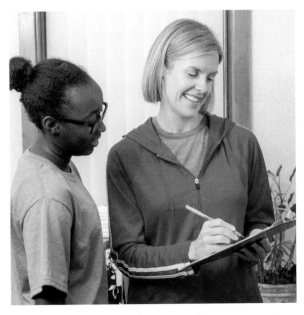

Experts can provide assistance in choosing exercises and determining how often to perform them.

| Day | Activity (exercise) | Time | Repetitions | Completed Week 1 | Completed Week 2 |
|---|---|---|---|---|---|
| Mon. | Warm-up (jog) | 4 p.m. | 5 min | ✔ | ✔ |
| | Biceps curl (exercise band) | | 3 sets of 10 | ✔ | ✔ |
| | Toe push (exercise band) | | 3 sets of 10 | ✔ | ✔ |
| | Curl-up | | 2 sets of 15 | ✔ | ✔ |
| | Long jump | | 3 sets of 10 | ✔ | ✔ |
| Tues. | Warm-up (walk) | 4 p.m. | 5 min | ✔ | ✔ |
| | Push-up | | 2 sets of 5 | ✔ | ✔ |
| | Leg curl | | 3 sets of 10 | ✔ | ✔ |
| Wed. | Warm-up (jog) | 4 p.m. | 5 min | ✔ | ✔ |
| | Biceps curl (exercise band) | | 3 sets of 10 | ✔ | ✔ |
| | Toe push (exercise band) | | 3 sets of 10 | ✔ | ✔ |
| | Curl-up | | 2 sets of 15 | ✔ | ✔ |
| | Long jump | | 3 sets of 10 | ✔ | ✔ |
| Thurs. | Warm-up (walk) | 4 p.m. | 5 min | ✔ | |
| | Push-up | | 2 sets of 5 | ✔ | |
| | Leg curl | | 3 sets of 10 | ✔ | |
| Fri. | Warm-up (jog) | 4 p.m. | 5 min | ✔ | ✔ |
| | Biceps curl (exercise band) | | 3 sets of 10 | ✔ | ✔ |
| | Toe push (exercise band) | | 3 sets of 10 | ✔ | ✔ |
| | Curl-up | | 2 sets of 15 | ✔ | ✔ |
| | Long jump | | 3 sets of 10 | ✔ | ✔ |
| Sat. | Warm-up (walk) | 4 p.m. | 5 min | ✔ | ✔ |
| | Push-up | | 2 sets of 5 | ✔ | ✔ |
| | Leg curl | | 3 sets of 10 | ✔ | ✔ |
| Sun. | No exercise | | | | |

**FIGURE 3.6** Jordan's two-week written program plan.

not likely to be interrupted. A sample of Jordan's written plan is shown in figure 3.6. The last column allowed Jordan to checkmark each day on which she did her exercises.

## Step 5: Keep a Log and Evaluate Your Program

After you've tried your program for some time (the exact amount of time depends on your goals), evaluate it. Did you meet your goals? Was your program plan a good one? After your evaluation, make a new plan using the program planning steps.

Jordan tried her plan for two weeks. She placed checkmarks beside the days on which she completed the exercises in her plan. As you can see in figure 3.6, she missed her planned exercises on only one day during the two-week period. Given this success, she decided to keep doing the same plan for another two weeks on her way to meeting her long-term goals. She hoped to reach her long-term goal in eight weeks.

**CONSUMER CORNER: Too Good to Be True**

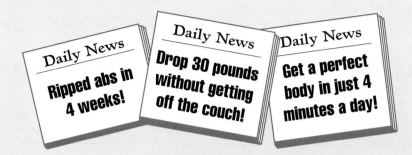

These are just a few examples of headlines you'll see in magazines, newspapers, and TV and web ads. The fitness and health industry is big business. Unfortunately, many companies try to make money by promising big results with little effort. They use marketing campaigns that prey on people who want quick results. As a student of Fitness for Life, you're becoming a critical consumer of fitness, health, and wellness information. Use the tips presented here to make good decisions and avoid falling victim to false claims.

| Consumer guideline | Consumer action |
| --- | --- |
| Evaluate the source of the information. | Avoid testimonials by famous people (such as athletes and movie stars) who are not experts.<br>Use information from experts in health, medicine, nutrition, and kinesiology who use the scientific method.<br>Use information from government sources (such as the U.S. Food and Drug Administration) and reliable professional organizations (such as the American Heart Association).<br>Use the scientific method to evaluate the information. |
| Be suspicious of claims that promise quick results and are inconsistent with information presented in this book. | Compare claims with facts you've learned from this book and other reliable sources.<br>Beware: If a claim seems too good to be true, it probably isn't true. |
| Be suspicious of "special offers" that say you must take advantage immediately or they will no longer be available. | Avoid quick action. "Special offers" that quickly expire are designed to get you to act fast without taking the time to make a good decision. |
| Check the credentials of the person or company doing the promotion. | Check to see if people who claim to be experts really are. Do they have a college degree or advanced degree? Are they certified by a well-known, legitimate organization? People with university degrees in kinesiology, physical education, and physical therapy are generally well equipped to give you sound advice about exercise. The same is true for a certified strength and conditioning specialist (CSCS), American College of Sports Medicine certified personal trainer (CPT), certified health fitness specialist (CHFS), certified group exercise instructor (CGEI), or registered clinical exercise physiologist (RCEP). For nutrition needs, a registered dietitian (RD) is well qualified to give you information. |

## Using Self-Planning Skills

You can use the five steps of program planning presented in this lesson to help you do your self-planning—that is, to plan your own program. Once you've developed a personal program plan, you're on your way to becoming independent rather than dependent on others.

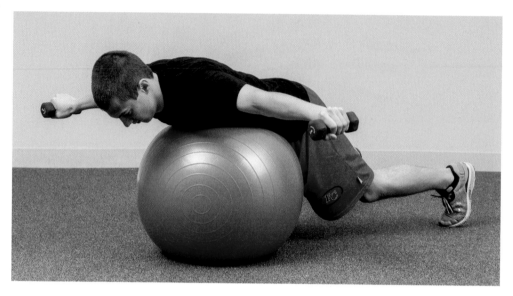

Keeping a log or journal of the activities you perform can help you determine if you have met your goals.

**Lesson Review**

1. What are the five steps in program planning? Describe each step.
2. What information do you need when preparing your personal needs profile?
3. What are some things you should write down when doing your personal program plan?

You probably know people who are sedentary or who eat a lot of unhealthy food. They may be in stage 1 of the process of change for physical activity or nutrition. They may have tried to make lifestyle changes but been ineffective because they failed to set good goals. This feature highlights SMART goals for physical activity.

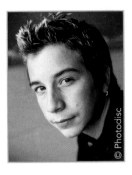

© Photodisc

Ms. Booker, a physical education teacher, noticed that Kevin seemed a bit listless in class. She stopped by his desk and asked, "Are you all right, Kevin? You seem a bit tired."

Kevin said, "I'm okay. I was in a hurry this morning so I missed breakfast."

Later, as she passed through the cafeteria, Ms. Booker couldn't help noticing that Kevin was eating food from a vending machine for lunch. He was sitting by himself at an isolated table.

Ms. Booker walked over, sat down, and asked, "Are you feeling better now?"

Kevin replied, "Yes, but I know I need to eat better."

Ms. Booker said, "Maybe you need to make a plan to eat better. Do you remember the SMART formula we learned in class? Maybe you could use the formula to set some goals." Kevin agreed that this was a good idea.

## For Discussion

How could Kevin use the SMART formula to set good nutrition goals? What might be some good long-term goals for him? What might be some good short-term goals? What kinds of advice do you think Ms. Booker gave Kevin about goal setting? What advice would you have for Kevin? Consider the guidelines presented in the following Self-Management feature as you answer these discussion questions.

##  SELF-MANAGEMENT: Skills for Setting Goals

Now that you know more about different types of goal setting, you can begin developing some goals of your own. Use the following guidelines to help you as you identify and develop your personal goals.

- **Know your reasons for setting your goals.** People who set goals for reasons other than their own personal improvement often fail. Ask yourself, *Why is this goal important for me?* Make sure you're setting goals for yourself based on your own needs and interests.

- **Choose a few goals at a time.** As you work your way through this book, you'll establish goals for fitness, physical activity, food choices, weight management, stress management, and other healthy lifestyle behaviors. But rather than focusing on all of these goals at once, you'll choose a few goals at a time. Trying to do too much often leads to failure.

Choosing a few goals at a time can help you be successful.

- **Use the SMART formula.** The SMART formula helps you set goals that are specific, measurable, attainable, realistic, and timely.

- **Set long-term and short-term goals.** The SMART formula helps you establish both long-term and short-term goals. When setting short-term goals, focus not on results but on making good lifestyle changes (that is, focus on process goals).

- **Put your goals in writing.** Writing down a goal represents a personal commitment and increases your chances of meeting that goal. You'll get the opportunity to write down your goals as you do the activities in this book.

- **Self-assess periodically and keep logs.** Doing self-assessments helps you set your goals and determine whether you've met them. Focus on improvement by working toward goals that are slightly higher than your current self-assessment results.

- **Reward yourself.** Achieving a personal goal is rewarding. Allow yourself to feel good. Congratulate yourself for your accomplishment.

- **Revise if necessary.** If you find that a goal is too difficult to accomplish, don't be afraid to revise it. It's better to revise your goal than to quit because you didn't reach an unrealistic goal.

- **Consider maintenance goals.** Improvement is not always necessary. Once you reach the highest level of change, setting a goal of maintenance can be a good idea. For example, an active, fit person cannot continue to improve in fitness forever. At some point, enough is enough, and following a regular workout schedule to maintain good fitness is a reasonable goal. Likewise, once you achieve the goal of eating well, maintaining your healthy eating pattern is a worthwhile goal.

## ACADEMIC CONNECTION: Mnemonics and Acronyms

Earlier in this chapter, you learned the meaning of the words *mnemonic* and *acronym*. SMART is a mnemonic device, or memory aid, that helps you remember the five guidelines for creating goals. SMART is also an acronym because each letter in SMART is the first letter of a guideline for setting goals. FIT is another useful mnemonic and acronym that can be used to remember the frequency, intensity, and time of physical activity when the type of activity is already established.

Health organizations are often referred to using an acronym. For example, most people recognize that the acronym AMA refers to the American Medical Association. The AMA does not promote the use of the acronym, but people frequently use it. Since AMA does not have a separate meaning, as is the case for SMART and FIT, it is not considered a mnemonic.

Not all mnemonics are acronyms. In addition to acronyms, poems or rhymes, songs, lists, and other devices can be used as mnemonics.

For example, a rhyme is commonly used as a mnemonic to remember how many days there are in each month ("Thirty days have September, April, June, and November"), and the alphabet song is a mnemonic that helps children learn the alphabet. As you continue your study of fitness, health, and wellness, you may want to make up your own mnemonics and acronyms to help you remember important information.

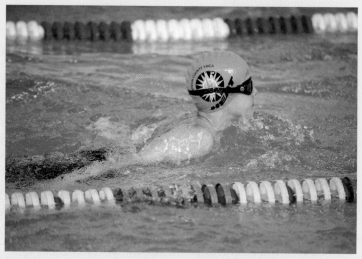

Swimmers on this team used the acronym TEAM (Together Everyone Achieves More) to help them achieve their goals.

An exercise circuit consists of several stations, each of which features a different exercise. Typically, you move from one station to the next without resting between them. Exercise circuits are popular because they include a variety of exercises, which helps make the workout interesting. Circuits can be designed to focus on either health-related or skill-related fitness components, and they can be performed in a variety of places—indoors or outdoors, at home or elsewhere. They also have the advantage of not requiring a lot of equipment, though you might enjoy bringing some favorite music to listen to while performing the circuit. **Take action** to create and use an exercise circuit. Try the following tips.

- Before starting the circuit, perform a dynamic warm-up.
- Plan stations that address all parts of your body: lower, middle, upper.
- Avoid having two stations in a row that challenge the same body part.
- Pace yourself so that you can be active for the whole time at each station and keep moving between stations.
- Use correct technique at each station; if your technique fails due to fatigue, take a break.
- After doing the circuit, perform a cool-down.

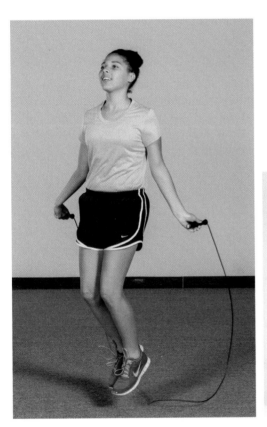
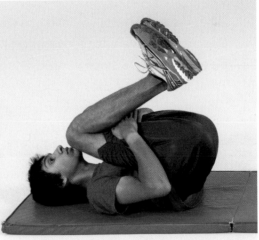

Exercise circuits use a variety of exercises at several stations.

## Reviewing Concepts and Vocabulary

As directed by your teacher, answer items 1 through 5 by correctly completing each sentence with a word or phrase.

1. The acronym used to remember the characteristics of effective goals is _____.

2. Performing several exercises three days a week for two weeks is an example of a _____-term goal.

3. Deciding to walk 30 minutes a day for the next two months is an example of a _____-term goal.

4. Being able to run a mile in six minutes (a kilometer in four) is an example of a _____ goal.

5. Deciding to do flexibility exercises three days a week is an example of a _____ goal.

For items 6 through 10, as directed by your teacher, match each term in column 1 with the appropriate phrase in column 2.

6. step 1
7. step 2
8. step 3
9. step 4
10. step 5

a. setting goals
b. considering program options
c. structuring your program
d. determining your personal needs
e. evaluating your program

For items 11 through 15, as directed by your teacher, respond to each statement or question.

11. What are some tests you can use to assess and rate your muscle fitness?
12. Describe the five rules for setting SMART goals.
13. Describe the five steps in program planning.
14. What are exercise circuits, and why are they useful in staying active?
15. What are some guidelines for using the self-management skill of goal setting?

## Thinking Critically

Write a paragraph to answer the following question.

Why is it important to understand the concept of optimal challenge when setting goals? Provide an example to help you make your point.

## Project

Imagine that you are hired as a health consultant in December to help clients make New Year's resolutions for eating better and being more active. Prepare a brief booklet that contains advice for making *effective* New Year's resolutions.

# UNIT II

# Becoming and Staying Physically Active

· · · · · · · · · · · · · · · · · · · · ·

**Healthy People 2020 Goals**

- Increase the percentage of teens who meet national physical activity guidelines.
- Increase aerobic activity among teens.
- Reduce the percentage of people who do no leisure-time physical activity.
- Increase daily physical education and out-of-school physical activity among teens.
- Reduce computer use to less than two hours a day for teens.
- Increase trips taken by walking and biking.
- Help people live high-quality, longer lives free from preventable disease, injury, and early death.
- Reduce heart disease, stroke, cancer, diabetes, high blood pressure, osteoporosis, and back problems.
- Increase the percentage of people who receive information about risk factors.

**Self-Assessment Features in This Unit**

- Body Composition and Flexibility
- PACER and Trunk Lift
- Assessing Skill-Related Physical Fitness

**Taking Charge Features in This Unit**

- Reducing Risk Factors
- Learning to Self-Monitor
- Improving Performance Skills

**Self-Management Features in This Unit**

- Skills for Reducing Risk Factors
- Skills for Learning to Self-Monitor
- Skills for Improving Performance

**Taking Action Features in This Unit**

- Walking for Health
- Physical Activity Pyramid Circuit
- Safe Exercise Circuit

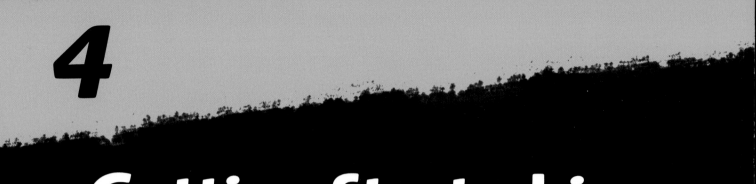

# 4

# Getting Started in Physical Activity

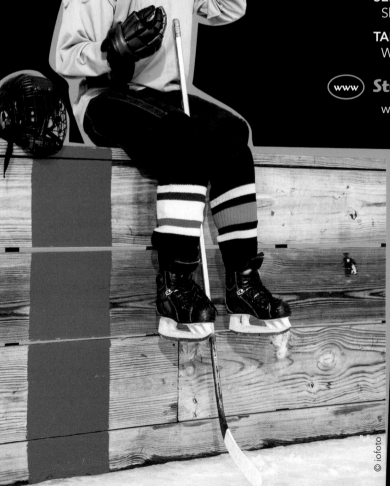

## In This Chapter

(www) **Student Web Resources**
www.fitnessforlife.org/student

© iofoto

# Lesson 4.1
## Safe and Smart Physical Activity

**Lesson Objectives**

After reading this lesson, you should be able to

1. describe medical readiness and explain how to assess it,
2. explain how the environment affects physical activity, and
3. describe some steps in dressing appropriately for physical activity in normal environments.

**Lesson Vocabulary**

air quality index, graded exercise test, heat index, humidity, hyperthermia, hypothermia, Physical Activity Readiness Questionnaire (PAR-Q), wind-chill factor

**Are** you prepared to be active? Whether you're a beginner or you've been physically active for some time, you need to know how to exercise safely in all conditions. If you're a beginner, the first step is to be physically and medically ready. As a young person, you probably won't have a problem with physical and medical readiness, but you should answer some simple questions about yourself just to be sure. You should also be ready for a variety of environmental conditions—such as heat, cold, pollution, and high altitude—that could necessitate a change in your exercise habits. In this lesson, you'll learn how to prepare yourself for physical activity.

> " An ounce of prevention is worth a pound of cure. "
>
> —Benjamin Franklin, statesman and scientist

## Medical Readiness

Have you ever been injured during physical activity? Do you know how to prepare yourself for exercise so as to avoid injury and participate safely? Before you begin a regular physical activity program for health and wellness, you should assess your medical and physical readiness. For this purpose, experts have developed a seven-item questionnaire called the **Physical Activity Readiness Questionnaire (PAR-Q)**. If you answer yes to any of the seven questions, you are advised to seek medical consultation before beginning or continuing an exercise program. You can get a copy of the questionnaire from your teacher. You may also want to show the PAR-Q to your parents or other adults who are important to you. Of course you should consider any current health problems as you prepare for exercise. For example, some people have short-term illnesses such as a cold or the flu that will alter their plans for exercise. Others, with chronic conditions such as asthma, will have to alter their exercise according to their doctor's instructions. Older people are more likely to be at risk when doing exercise. You may want to encourage older adults who are important to you to answer the PAR-Q questions before they begin an exercise program.

As for yourself, you may even be *required* to have a medical examination if you're going to participate in an interscholastic sport or other program of similar intensity, such as a community sport or other rigorous physical challenge. Medical exams help ensure that you are free from disease and can also help you prevent health problems in the future. You should also answer the questions included in the sport readiness questionnaire available from your teacher.

Later in life, you may need to do a **graded exercise test**, which is administered by a health professional and is sometimes called an exercise stress test. The test is done on a treadmill and can help identify people at high risk for health problems such as heart attacks (figure 4.1). It is an expensive test and is not necessary for everyone, and a health professional can use screening to determine whether it is appropriate for you. Even seemingly fit athletes can be at risk, although risk is low among

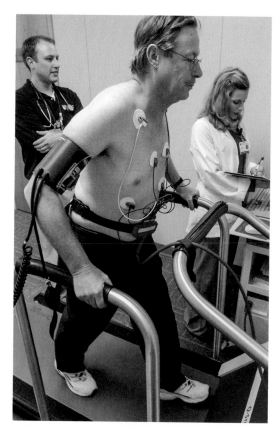

**FIGURE 4.1** The graded exercise test can be using to screen adults with risk factors.

will not perform this test unless it is recommended by a doctor after medical screening.

# Readiness for Extreme Environmental Conditions

Environmental conditions play an important role in determining when and how strenuously you should exercise. Whether you are just beginning a physical activity program or have been exercising for a while, you must understand how environmental conditions can affect your body during exercise. Your body can adapt to environmental factors such as heat, cold, altitude, and air quality. That adaptability is why people who have been exposed to an environment for a long time can function better in it than those who have just become exposed. This lesson presents guidelines to help you adapt to weather and other environmental factors in order to prevent injury and health problems. All people should follow these guidelines, but they are especially important for people who are new to exercise or new to a particular environment.

## Hot, Humid Weather

Be careful when performing physical activity in high heat and **humidity**, which can cause your body temperature to rise too high—a situation referred to as **hyperthermia** or overheating. When exercise causes your body temperature to rise, you start to perspire (sweat). As your sweat evaporates, your body is cooled. But when the humidity is high, evaporation is less effective in cooling your body, and hyperthermia is more likely to occur. Hyperthermia causes three main conditions, which are described in table 4.1.

young athletes. Nevertheless, outstanding runners and baseball and football players thought to be in good health have died from heart attacks, especially among older athletes. For example, Gaines Adams, a professional football player, died unexpectedly from an undetected heart condition in 2010. Jim Fixx, a famous runner and author, died of heart problems that could probably have been addressed if he had performed a graded exercise test. Most young people

### TABLE 4.1 Heat-Related Conditions

| Condition | Definition |
|---|---|
| Heat cramps | Muscle cramps caused by excessive heat exposure and low water consumption. |
| Heat exhaustion | Condition caused by excessive heat exposure and characterized by paleness, clammy skin, profuse sweating, weakness, tiredness, nausea, dizziness, muscle cramps, and possibly vomiting or fainting. Body temperature may be normal or slightly above normal. |
| Heatstroke | Condition caused by excessive heat exposure and characterized by high body temperature up to 106°F (41°C); hot, dry, flushed skin; rapid pulse; lack of sweating; dizziness; and possibly unconsciousness. This serious condition can result in death and requires prompt medical attention. |

# SCIENCE IN ACTION: Science Prepares Us for Safe Exercise

In the 1950s, people who had heart attacks were advised to stay in bed for months and avoid being active. Such myths about physical activity were common. For example, some athletes were told not to drink water during practice because it could make them "water-logged" and impair their performance. We have come a long way since then. Scientists who study medicine, nutrition, and kinesiology have made discoveries that make exercise safer and more effective. Here are two examples of science in action.

- **Exercise physiologists working with medical doctors developed cardiac rehabilitation programs.** They found that well-planned exercise after a heart attack is better than bed rest. In cardiac rehabilitation programs, people who have had a heart attack enroll in an exercise program under the care of a registered clinical exercise physiologist approved by the American College of Sports Medicine (ACSM). The physiologist works with a physician to plan an effective program of recovery for the patient. Exercise physiologists were also responsible for developing many of the tests now used in screening for heart disease, such as the graded exercise test described earlier in this chapter.

- **Nutrition scientists working with exercise physiologists have developed sport drinks that help people resist heat-related conditions.** The drinks contain electrolytes, which help the body retain fluid. They also contain a limited amount of sugar, which can be helpful for people performing long bouts of exercise. Scientists conducted many research studies to find the right combination of ingredients.

### Student Activity

Identify a product or program related to fitness or health that has been developed recently based on new scientific discoveries.

## FIT FACT

*Hyper* means too much or excessive, and *thermia* refers to heat, so *hyperthermia* means too much heat. *Hypo* means too little or less than normal, so *hypothermia* means too little heat.

Use the following guidelines to prevent and cope with heat-related conditions.

- **Begin gradually.** As your body becomes accustomed to physical activity in hot weather, it becomes more resistant to heat-related injury. Start with short periods of activity and gradually increase the duration.

- **Drink water.** In hot weather, your body perspires more than usual to cool itself. In order to replace the water your body loses through perspiration, you need to drink plenty of water before and after activity.

- **Wear proper clothing.** Wear porous clothing that allows air to pass through to cool your body. Also wear light-colored clothing—lighter colors reflect the sun's heat, whereas darker colors absorb it. Clothing made of fibers that wick away moisture and keep you cool (for example, Coolmax) are now available.

- **Rest frequently.** Physical activity creates body heat. Periodically stop to rest in a shady area to help your body lower its temperature.

- **Avoid extreme heat and humidity.** You can use the heat index chart shown in figure 4.2 to determine whether the environment is too hot and humid for activity. If the **heat index** is too high, you should postpone or cancel your activity. You should do physical activity in the caution zones only if you are well adapted to hot environments and follow all of the basic guidelines. The amount of time it takes to adapt to these conditions varies from person to person.

- **If heat-related injury occurs, get out of the heat and cool your body.** Find shade; apply cool, wet towels to your body; spray your body with water; drink water; and seek medical help if heatstroke occurs.

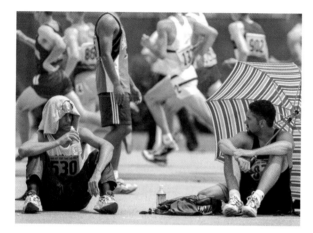

When you exercise in hot weather, wear light-colored clothing and drink plenty of water to help cool your body.

## Cold, Windy, and Wet Weather

It can also be dangerous to exercise in cold, windy, and wet weather. Extreme cold can result in **hypothermia**, or excessively low body temperature. Hypothermia is accompanied by shivering, numbness, drowsiness, muscular weakness, and confusion or disorientation. Extreme cold can also cause

a condition called frostbite, in which a body part becomes frozen. A person with frostbite often feels no pain, thus making the condition even more dangerous. Use the following guidelines when exercising in cold, windy, and wet weather.

- **Avoid extreme cold and wind.** Before dressing for physical activity, use the chart in figure 4.3 to determine the **wind-chill factor**. Exercising when the temperature is cold and the wind is blowing is especially dangerous because the air feels colder. The wind-chill chart shows how long it takes to get frostbite when your skin is exposed to various wind-chill levels. Experts agree that if the time to frostbite is 30 minutes or less, you should postpone activity. If you're active when the wind-chill factor is excessive, be sure to dress properly and be aware of the symptoms of frostbite:
  - Skin becomes white or grayish yellow and looks glossy.
  - Pain may be felt early and then subside, though often feeling is lost and no pain is felt.
  - Blisters may appear later.
  - The affected area feels intensely cold and numb.
- **Dress properly.** Wear several layers of lightweight clothing rather than a heavy jacket or coat. The clothing closest to your body (base layer) helps wick away body moisture to keep

### Heat index
As humidity increases, air can feel hotter than it actually is.
This chart shows how hot it feels as humidity rises.

| Relative humidity (%) | 70 | 75 | 80 | 85 | 90 | 95 | 100 | 105 | 110 | 115 | 120 |
|---|---|---|---|---|---|---|---|---|---|---|---|
| 100 | 72 | 80 | 91 | 108 | 132 | | | | | | |
| 90 | 71 | 79 | 88 | 102 | 122 | | | | | | |
| 80 | 71 | 78 | 86 | 97 | 113 | 136 | | | | | |
| 70 | 70 | 77 | 85 | 93 | 106 | 124 | 144 | | | | |
| 60 | 70 | 76 | 82 | 90 | 100 | 114 | 132 | 149 | | | |
| 50 | 69 | 75 | 81 | 88 | 96 | 107 | 120 | 135 | 150 | | |
| 40 | 68 | 74 | 79 | 86 | 93 | 101 | 110 | 123 | 137 | 151 | |
| 30 | 67 | 73 | 78 | 84 | 90 | 96 | 104 | 113 | 123 | 135 | 148 |
| 20 | 66 | 72 | 77 | 82 | 87 | 93 | 99 | 105 | 112 | 120 | 130 |
| 10 | 65 | 70 | 75 | 80 | 85 | 90 | 95 | 100 | 105 | 111 | 116 |
| 0 | 64 | 69 | 73 | 78 | 83 | 87 | 91 | 95 | 99 | 103 | 107 |

Air temperature (°F)

☐ Caution zone
■ Danger zone

**FIGURE 4.2** Heat index chart.

Temperature (°F)

| Wind (mph) | 30 | 25 | 20 | 15 | 10 | 5 | 0 | −5 | −10 | −15 | −20 | −25 |
|---|---|---|---|---|---|---|---|---|---|---|---|---|
| 5 | 25 | 19 | 13 | 7 | 1 | −5 | −11 | −16 | −22 | −28 | −34 | −40 |
| 10 | 21 | 15 | 9 | 3 | −4 | −10 | −16 | −22 | −28 | −35 | −41 | −47 |
| 15 | 19 | 13 | 6 | 0 | −7 | −13 | −19 | −26 | −32 | −39 | −45 | −51 |
| 20 | 17 | 11 | 4 | −2 | −9 | −15 | −22 | −29 | −35 | −42 | −48 | −55 |
| 25 | 16 | 9 | 3 | −4 | −11 | −17 | −24 | −31 | −37 | −44 | −51 | −58 |
| 30 | 15 | 8 | 1 | −5 | −12 | −19 | −26 | −33 | −39 | −46 | −53 | −60 |
| 35 | 14 | 7 | 0 | −7 | −14 | −21 | −27 | −34 | −41 | −48 | −55 | −62 |
| 40 | 13 | 6 | −1 | −8 | −15 | −22 | −29 | −36 | −43 | −50 | −57 | −64 |
| 45 | 12 | 5 | −2 | −9 | −16 | −23 | −30 | −37 | −44 | −51 | −58 | −65 |
| 50 | 12 | 4 | −3 | −10 | −17 | −24 | −31 | −38 | −45 | −52 | −60 | −67 |
| 55 | 11 | 4 | −3 | −11 | −18 | −25 | −32 | −39 | −46 | −54 | −61 | −68 |
| 60 | 10 | 3 | −4 | −11 | −19 | −26 | −33 | −40 | −48 | −55 | −62 | −69 |

Frostbite occurs in 30 minutes or less

**FIGURE 4.3** Wind-chill chart.

you warm and dry. Silk and special wicking materials made of synthetic fibers such as Polartec are good for this layer. Cotton is not recommended for the base layer because it tends to get wet and stay wet. The second layer is often called the insulating layer. This layer helps retain body heat but should also wick away moisture. Polyester fleece and wool are good for this layer. The outer layer is designed to protect you against wind and moisture (rain, snow) but should also allow heat and moisture to be released. For this reason jackets made of plastic, rubber, or other materials that do not "breathe" are not recommended. Jackets made of synthetic fibers (for example, Gore-Tex) that breathe are recommended. Wearing a jacket with a zipper allows you to regulate heat retained and released by the body. Wear a high collar on one of the inner layers. If needed, wear a knit cap, ski mask, or mittens (which keep hands warmer than gloves do).

## FIT FACT

Health scientists recently discovered an inaccuracy in the wind-chill factor system that had been used for years. Specifically, the importance of wind had been overemphasized. Now, Canadian experts aided by U.S. scientists have developed a new formula, which is used in the wind-chill chart shown in figure 4.3.

- **Avoid exercising in weather that is icy or cold and wet.** These conditions can cause special problems. Your shoes, socks, and pant legs can get wet, which increases your risk of foot injuries and falls.

## Pollution and Altitude

The effectiveness and safety of your exercise can also be affected by conditions other than weather, such as air pollution and altitude. Air pollution can affect your ability to breathe, and experts have identified levels of pollution (ozone and particulate matter) that are unhealthful. Pollution levels are rated by means of an **air quality index** that ranges from good to very unhealthful. When the air pollution level is high, you can find warnings on radio, television, and reliable

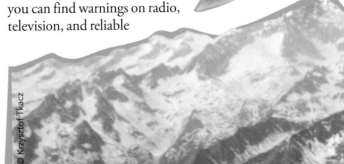
© Krzysztof Tkacz

websites. During such times, avoid exercising outdoors. A table showing air quality levels is available in the student section of the Fitness for Life website.

People who live at high altitude are able to exercise there with little trouble, but people who live at lower altitude may have trouble adjusting to being active at higher altitude. It takes time for the body to adjust, even for very fit people. For this reason, if you exercise at a higher altitude than you are used to (for example, if you go skiing), adjust the intensity of your physical activity until your body adapts.

# General Readiness: Dressing for Physical Activity

As you've seen, special environmental circumstances—such as intense heat and cold—require special dress for physical activity. But even under normal circumstances, the way you dress has a lot to do with your comfort and enjoyment. Consider the following guidelines when dressing for physical activity.

- **Wear comfortable and appropriate clothing for the environmental conditions.** Guidelines for dressing for cold and hot weather were presented earlier. In addition to following these guidelines, wearing comfortable clothing will make your workout more enjoyable.

- **Use sun screen or wear clothing that protects you from the sun.** These will help protect your skin from harmful ultraviolet rays.

- **Wash exercise clothing regularly.** Clean clothing is more comfortable than soiled clothing, and it reduces the chance of fungal growth and infection.

- **Dress in layers when exercising outdoors.** You can remove layers of clothing as you become warmer while exercising and put them back on when you cool down.

- **Wear proper socks.** Moisture-wicking fabrics are now used in making socks and other apparel (see the Fitness Technology feature). Socks made with these fabrics reduce foot moisture and can help prevent blisters. Thick socks made of cotton or another traditional fabric can help cushion your feet but are not as effective at keeping them dry.

- **Wear proper shoes.** Most people can use a good pair of multipurpose exercise or sport shoes. However, if you plan to do special activities, you might prefer shoes designed just for them. Try shoes on before buying them. When you try them on, wear the kind of socks you normally wear and walk around to see how the shoes feel. They should not feel too heavy, because extra weight makes exercise more tiring. Avoid vinyl or plastic shoes that do not let air pass through to help cool your feet. As an alternative to cloth and leather shoes (which do allow some air passage), new shoes made from fabrics that wick away excess moisture have proven effective in keeping feet dry. Before buying shoes, consider the features shown in figure 4.4.

- **Consider lace-up ankle braces.** Ankle braces can help prevent ankle injuries, especially for activities that involve quick changes in direction, such as basketball and racquetball. Studies show that lace-up ankle braces reduce the number of ankle injuries among those who have a history of them. Some people prefer high-top shoes for sports with high rates of ankle injury.

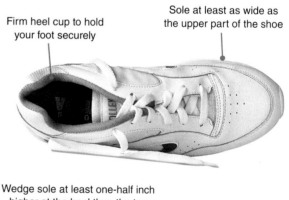

Firm heel cup to hold your foot securely

Sole at least as wide as the upper part of the shoe

Wedge sole at least one-half inch higher at the heel than the toe

Good arch support

**FIGURE 4.4** Characteristics of proper shoes.

# FITNESS TECHNOLOGY: High-Tech Exercise Clothing

Modern technology has produced clothing that is especially good for exercising in both hot and cold weather. As noted in the guidelines for exercising in hot or cold environments, clothing made of special synthetic fibers are available that wick moisture away from the body to help it stay cool (for example, Coolmax) or warm (for example, Polartec). Clothing made of wicking fibers can aid your performance in the heat and cold. Jackets made of a synthetic material such as Gore-Tex block the wind but allow your body heat to be released. This type of garment also works well as an outer layer in cold weather. These synthetic fibers are engineered to function in different ways.

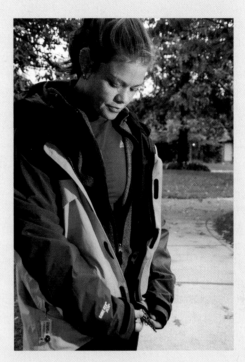

Wearing specially engineered clothing can help you when you exercise in the heat or cold.

---

**Using Technology**

Research one type of synthetic fiber used in making exercise clothing in hot or cold environments. What are the special characteristics of the fiber you selected?

---

## Other General Preparation Guidelines

In this chapter, you've learned about medical readiness, environmental factors that affect your activity, and dressing appropriately for activity. Here are some additional steps you can take to make your activity sessions safe and effective.

- **Get fit for your workout.** We all know that you do your workout to get fit. But you also need to be fit enough to do your workout without getting hurt. When you begin a new program, start gradually. As your fitness improves, you can do more. Safe exercise depends on good health-related fitness of all kinds.

- **Warm up before your workout.** Scientists have recently discovered that different types of warm-up are necessary for different kinds of activity. As you continue to study *Fitness for Life*, you'll try a variety of warm-up activities depending on the workout you plan to do.

- **Cool down after your workout.** The cooldown helps you recover after your workout.

---

**Lesson Review**

1. What are some steps you can take to make sure you're medically ready to participate in physical activity and sports?
2. What are some environmental factors that can make activity unhealthy or unsafe?
3. What are some guidelines for dressing properly for physical activity in normal environments?

In this self-assessment, you'll perform two tests: the body mass index (BMI) test and the back-saver sit-and-reach. The BMI is an indicator of your body composition. The back-saver sit-and-reach measures the flexibility of your lower back and your hamstrings (the muscles on the back of your thighs). If you have not done so already, practice this test before performing it for a score. You will have an opportunity later to do other self-assessments of body composition and flexibility. For these two tests, record your scores and fitness ratings as directed by your teacher. These tests give you information that you can use in preparing a Fitnessgram or other fitness report and your personal physical activity plan. If you're working with a partner, remember that self-assessment information is personal and considered confidential. It shouldn't be shared with others without the permission of the person being tested.

## Body Mass Index

1. Measure your height in inches (or meters) without shoes.

2. Measure your weight in pounds (or kilograms) without shoes. If you're wearing street clothes (as opposed to lightweight gym clothing), subtract 2 pounds (0.9 kilogram) from your weight.

3. Calculate your BMI using the chart or either of the following formulas.

$$\frac{\text{weight (lb)}}{\text{height (in.)} \times \text{height (in.)}} \times 703 = \text{BMI}$$

$$\frac{\text{weight (kg)}}{\text{height (m)} \times \text{height (m)}} = \text{BMI}$$

4. Use table 4.2 to find your BMI rating, and record your BMI score and rating.

Height

| Height | 90 | 95 | 100 | 105 | 110 | 115 | 120 | 125 | 130 | 135 | 140 | 145 | 150 | 155 | 160 | 165 | 170 | 175 | 180 | 185 | 190 | 195 | 200 | 205 | 210 | 215 | 220 | 225 | 230 | 235 | 240 | 245 | 250 |
|---|---|---|---|---|---|---|---|---|---|---|---|---|---|---|---|---|---|---|---|---|---|---|---|---|---|---|---|---|---|---|---|---|---|
| 4' 6" | 25 | 25 | 26 | 26 | 27 | 28 | 29 | 30 | 31 | 32 | 34 | 35 | 36 | 37 | 39 | 40 | 41 | 42 | 43 | 45 | 46 | 47 | 48 | 49 | 51 | 52 | 53 | 54 | 56 | 57 | 58 | 59 | 60 |
| 4' 7" | 24 | 24 | 25 | 25 | 26 | 27 | 28 | 29 | 30 | 31 | 32 | 34 | 35 | 36 | 37 | 38 | 39 | 40 | 41 | 43 | 45 | 46 | 47 | 48 | 49 | 50 | 51 | 52 | 54 | 55 | 56 | 57 | 58 |
| 4' 8" | 23 | 23 | 24 | 24 | 25 | 26 | 27 | 28 | 29 | 30 | 31 | 32 | 34 | 35 | 36 | 37 | 38 | 39 | 40 | 42 | 43 | 44 | 45 | 46 | 47 | 48 | 49 | 50 | 52 | 53 | 54 | 55 | 56 |
| 4' 9" | 22 | 22 | 23 | 23 | 24 | 25 | 26 | 27 | 28 | 29 | 30 | 31 | 32 | 34 | 35 | 36 | 37 | 38 | 39 | 40 | 42 | 42 | 43 | 44 | 45 | 47 | 48 | 49 | 50 | 51 | 52 | 53 | 54 |
| 4' 10" | 21 | 22 | 22 | 23 | 23 | 24 | 25 | 26 | 27 | 28 | 29 | 30 | 31 | 32 | 34 | 35 | 36 | 37 | 38 | 39 | 40 | 41 | 42 | 43 | 44 | 45 | 46 | 47 | 48 | 49 | 50 | 51 | 52 |
| 4' 11" | 20 | 21 | 21 | 22 | 22 | 23 | 24 | 25 | 26 | 27 | 28 | 29 | 30 | 31 | 32 | 33 | 34 | 35 | 36 | 37 | 38 | 39 | 40 | 41 | 42 | 43 | 45 | 46 | 46 | 47 | 48 | 49 | 50 |
| 5' 0" | 19 | 20 | 20 | 21 | 21 | 22 | 23 | 24 | 25 | 26 | 27 | 28 | 29 | 30 | 31 | 32 | 33 | 34 | 35 | 36 | 37 | 38 | 39 | 40 | 41 | 42 | 43 | 44 | 45 | 46 | 47 | 48 | 49 |
| 5' 1" | 18 | 19 | 19 | 20 | 21 | 22 | 23 | 24 | 25 | 26 | 26 | 27 | 28 | 29 | 30 | 31 | 32 | 33 | 34 | 35 | 36 | 37 | 38 | 39 | 40 | 41 | 42 | 43 | 43 | 44 | 45 | 46 | 47 |
| 5' 2" | 18 | 18 | 18 | 19 | 20 | 21 | 22 | 23 | 24 | 25 | 26 | 27 | 27 | 28 | 29 | 30 | 31 | 32 | 33 | 34 | 35 | 36 | 37 | 37 | 38 | 39 | 40 | 41 | 42 | 43 | 44 | 45 | 46 |
| 5' 3" | 17 | 18 | 18 | 19 | 19 | 20 | 21 | 22 | 23 | 24 | 25 | 26 | 27 | 27 | 28 | 29 | 30 | 31 | 32 | 33 | 34 | 35 | 35 | 36 | 37 | 38 | 39 | 40 | 41 | 42 | 43 | 43 | 44 |
| 5' 4" | 17 | 17 | 17 | 18 | 19 | 20 | 21 | 21 | 22 | 23 | 24 | 25 | 26 | 27 | 27 | 28 | 29 | 30 | 31 | 32 | 33 | 33 | 34 | 35 | 36 | 37 | 38 | 39 | 39 | 40 | 41 | 42 | 43 |
| 5' 5" | 16 | 17 | 17 | 17 | 18 | 19 | 20 | 21 | 22 | 22 | 23 | 24 | 25 | 26 | 27 | 27 | 28 | 29 | 30 | 31 | 32 | 32 | 33 | 34 | 35 | 36 | 37 | 37 | 38 | 39 | 40 | 41 | 42 |
| 5' 6" | 15 | 16 | 16 | 17 | 18 | 19 | 19 | 20 | 21 | 22 | 23 | 23 | 24 | 25 | 26 | 27 | 27 | 28 | 29 | 30 | 31 | 31 | 32 | 33 | 34 | 35 | 36 | 36 | 37 | 38 | 39 | 40 | 40 |
| 5' 7" | 15 | 15 | 16 | 16 | 17 | 18 | 19 | 20 | 20 | 21 | 22 | 23 | 23 | 24 | 25 | 26 | 27 | 27 | 28 | 29 | 30 | 31 | 31 | 32 | 33 | 34 | 34 | 35 | 36 | 37 | 38 | 38 | 39 |
| 5' 8" | 14 | 15 | 15 | 16 | 17 | 17 | 18 | 19 | 20 | 21 | 21 | 22 | 23 | 24 | 24 | 25 | 26 | 27 | 27 | 28 | 29 | 30 | 30 | 31 | 32 | 33 | 33 | 34 | 35 | 36 | 36 | 37 | 38 |
| 5' 9" | 14 | 15 | 15 | 15 | 16 | 17 | 18 | 18 | 19 | 20 | 21 | 21 | 22 | 23 | 24 | 24 | 25 | 26 | 27 | 27 | 28 | 29 | 30 | 30 | 31 | 32 | 32 | 33 | 34 | 35 | 35 | 36 | 37 |
| 5' 10" | 13 | 14 | 14 | 15 | 16 | 17 | 17 | 18 | 19 | 19 | 20 | 21 | 22 | 22 | 23 | 24 | 24 | 25 | 26 | 27 | 27 | 28 | 29 | 29 | 30 | 31 | 31 | 32 | 33 | 34 | 34 | 35 | 36 |
| 5' 11" | 13 | 14 | 14 | 15 | 15 | 16 | 17 | 17 | 18 | 19 | 20 | 20 | 21 | 22 | 22 | 23 | 24 | 24 | 25 | 26 | 26 | 27 | 28 | 29 | 29 | 30 | 31 | 31 | 32 | 33 | 33 | 34 | 35 |
| 6' 0" | 13 | 13 | 14 | 14 | 15 | 16 | 16 | 17 | 18 | 18 | 19 | 20 | 20 | 21 | 22 | 22 | 23 | 24 | 24 | 25 | 26 | 26 | 27 | 28 | 28 | 29 | 30 | 31 | 31 | 32 | 33 | 33 | 34 |
| 6' 1" | 12 | 13 | 13 | 14 | 15 | 15 | 16 | 16 | 17 | 18 | 18 | 19 | 20 | 20 | 21 | 22 | 22 | 23 | 24 | 24 | 25 | 26 | 26 | 27 | 28 | 28 | 29 | 30 | 30 | 31 | 32 | 32 | 33 |
| 6' 2" | 12 | 12 | 13 | 13 | 14 | 15 | 15 | 16 | 17 | 17 | 18 | 19 | 19 | 20 | 21 | 21 | 22 | 22 | 23 | 24 | 24 | 25 | 26 | 26 | 27 | 28 | 28 | 29 | 30 | 30 | 31 | 31 | 32 |
| 6' 3" | 11 | 12 | 12 | 13 | 14 | 14 | 15 | 15 | 16 | 17 | 17 | 18 | 19 | 19 | 20 | 20 | 21 | 22 | 22 | 23 | 24 | 24 | 25 | 26 | 26 | 27 | 27 | 28 | 29 | 29 | 30 | 31 | 31 |
| 6' 4" | 11 | 12 | 12 | 13 | 13 | 14 | 15 | 15 | 16 | 16 | 17 | 18 | 18 | 19 | 20 | 20 | 20 | 21 | 21 | 22 | 23 | 23 | 24 | 24 | 25 | 26 | 26 | 27 | 28 | 28 | 29 | 30 | 30 |

Weight

BMI calculation chart. Locate your height in the left column and your weight in pounds in the bottom row. The box where the selected row and column intersect is your BMI score.

## TABLE 4.2 Rating Chart: Body Mass Index

| | 13 years old | | 14 years old | | 15 years old | | 16 years old | | 17 years old | | 18 years old | |
|---|---|---|---|---|---|---|---|---|---|---|---|---|
| | Male | Female | Male | Female | Male | Female | Male | Female | Male | Female | Male | Female |
| Very lean | ≤15.4 | ≤15.3 | ≤16.0 | ≤15.8 | ≤16.5 | ≤16.3 | ≤17.1 | ≤16.8 | ≤17.7 | ≤17.2 | ≤18.2 | ≤17.5 |
| Good fitness | 15.5–21.3 | 15.4–22.0 | 16.1–22.1 | 15.9–22.8 | 16.6–22.9 | 16.4–23.5 | 17.2–23.7 | 16.9–24.1 | 17.8–24.4 | 17.3–24.6 | 18.3–25.1 | 17.6–25.1 |
| Marginal fitness | 21.4–23.5 | 22.1–23.7 | 22.2–24.4 | 22.9–24.5 | 23.0–25.2 | 23.6–25.3 | 23.8–25.9 | 24.2–26.0 | 24.5–26.6 | 24.7–27.6 | 25.2–27.4 | 25.2–27.1 |
| Low fitness | ≥23.6 | ≥23.8 | ≥24.5 | ≥24.6 | ≥25.3 | ≥25.4 | ≥26.0 | ≥26.1 | ≥26.7 | ≥27.7 | ≥27.5 | ≥27.2 |

Data based on *Fitnessgram*.

# Back-Saver Sit-and-Reach

1. Place a measuring stick, such as a yardstick or meter stick, on top of a box that is 12 inches (30 centimeters) high with the stick extending 9 inches (23 centimeters) over the box and the lower numbers toward you. You may use a flexibility testing box if one is available.

2. To measure the flexibility of your right leg, fully extend it and place your right foot flat against the box. Bend your left leg, with the knee turned out and your left foot 2 to 3 inches (5 to 8 centimeters) to the side of your straight right leg.

3. Extend your arms forward over the measuring stick. Place your hands on the stick, one on top of the other, with your palms facing down. Your middle fingers should be together with the tip of one finger exactly on top of the other.

4. Lean forward slowly; do not bounce. Reach forward with your arms and fingers, then slowly return to the starting position. Repeat four times. On the fourth reach, hold the position for three seconds and observe the measurement on the stick below your fingertips.

5. Repeat the test with your left leg straight.

6. Record your score to the nearest inch (1 inch equals 2.54 centimeters). Consult table 4.3 to determine your fitness rating for each side of your body.

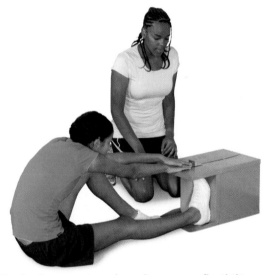

The back-saver sit-and-reach assesses flexibility.

## TABLE 4.3 Rating Chart: Back-Saver Sit-and-Reach (Inches)

| | 13 or 14 years old | | 15 years or older | |
|---|---|---|---|---|
| | Male | Female | Male | Female |
| High performance | ≥10 | ≥12 | ≥10 | ≥14 |
| Good fitness | 8–9 | 10–11 | 8–9 | 12–13 |
| Marginal fitness | 6–7 | 8–9 | 6–7 | 10–11 |
| Low fitness | ≤5 | ≤7 | ≤5 | ≤9 |

Data based on *Fitnessgram*.

# Lesson 4.2

# Health and Wellness Benefits

## Lesson Objectives

After reading this lesson, you should be able to

1. explain, using examples, how physical activity is related to hypokinetic conditions;
2. list some benefits of physical activity that contribute to health and wellness; and
3. explain, using examples, how physical activity is related to hyperkinetic conditions.

## Lesson Vocabulary

activity neurosis, atherosclerosis, blood pressure, cardiovascular disease (CVD), coronary artery disease (CAD), diabetes, diastolic blood pressure, eating disorder, heart attack, hyperkinetic condition, hypertension, metabolic syndrome, osteoporosis, peak bone mass, risk factor, stroke, systolic blood pressure

**Have** you ever wondered why many people now live twice as long as most people did a few hundred years ago? Do you know the leading causes of death today? Do you understand the roles played by physical activity and nutrition in living a long, high-quality life?

Prior to 1900, the leading cause of death in the United States and other developed countries was pneumonia, and infections from other bacteria and viruses accounted for many of the other common causes of death. Science has found cures or vaccinations for many of these conditions, and today they are no longer the leading health problems for people with access to modern health care. Instead, the leading health threats today are conditions that are hypokinetic—caused in part by sedentary living—such as heart disease, cancer, and stroke (in that order). In this lesson, you'll learn more about how physical activity reduces your risk of hypokinetic conditions and increases your personal wellness; similar benefits are provided by good nutrition.

## Hypokinetic Diseases and Conditions

Sedentary living costs the United States billions of dollars each year in health care expenses and loss of productivity. Even more alarming, thousands of people die prematurely every year because they are inactive. Reports issued by major health organizations, including the U.S. Office of the Surgeon General and the American Heart Association,

> In the United States, physical inactivity is the biggest health problem of the 21st century.
>
> —Dr. Steven Blair, past president of the American College of Sports Medicine

indicate that regular physical activity is one of the best ways to reduce illness and increase wellness in American society. The American College of Sports Medicine (ACSM) lists 27 different health benefits of regular exercise. Sometimes teenagers feel that these statistics are not relevant to them; they think illness happens only to old people. As you'll see next, however, many hypokinetic diseases are now prevalent among teens, and many teens are not active enough to resist these conditions.

## Cardiovascular Disease

Did you know that **cardiovascular disease (CVD)** has been the leading cause of death in the United States each year since 1920? In fact, CVD is a primary or contributing cause of more than half of all deaths in the United States. Currently, about one in every four Americans has at least one form of CVD.

CVD encompasses various conditions, such as **coronary artery disease (CAD)**. *Coronary* means related to the heart, and an *artery* is a kind of blood vessel. Your heart is a muscle that acts as a pump to push blood, and your arteries are the pipelines that carry your blood from your heart to various parts of your body. CAD exists when the arteries

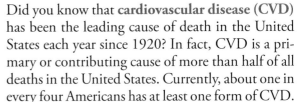

become clogged—a condition called **atherosclerosis**, which occurs when substances including fats, such as cholesterol, build up on the inside walls of the arteries. This build-up narrows the openings through the arteries. As a result, the heart must work harder to pump blood. See figure 4.5 for the difference between a clear artery and one that is partially blocked. Atherosclerosis typically develops with age but can begin early in life.

A **heart attack** occurs when the blood supply within the heart is severely reduced or cut off; as a result, an area of the heart muscle can die. The main reasons for heart attacks are arteries blocked by atherosclerosis, blood clots in narrowed arteries, spasms in the muscle of the artery, or a combination of these causes. During a heart attack, the heart may beat abnormally or even stop beating. Treatments often include medicines that stabilize the heartbeat and cardiopulmonary resuscitation (CPR) to restore circulation of oxygen.

Another form of cardiovascular disease is **stroke**, which is the third leading cause of early death in the United States and other developed countries. It occurs when the oxygen supply to the brain is severely reduced or cut off. A stroke can be caused when an artery that supplies blood to the brain bursts or is blocked by a blood clot or atherosclerosis. Because a stroke damages the brain, it can affect a person's ability to move, think, and speak. Some strokes are severe enough to cause death.

A primary risk factor for CVD is **hypertension**, or, as it is commonly called, high blood pressure.

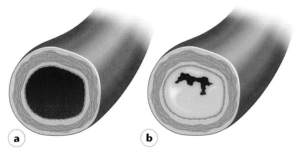

**FIGURE 4.5** *(a)* A healthy heart has open arteries. *(b)* An unhealthy heart has clogged arteries that can cause a heart attack.

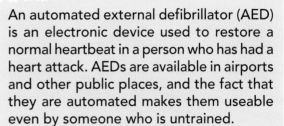

## FIT FACT

An automated external defibrillator (AED) is an electronic device used to restore a normal heartbeat in a person who has had a heart attack. AEDs are available in airports and other public places, and the fact that they are automated makes them useable even by someone who is untrained.

Each time your heart beats, it forces blood through your arteries, causing blood to push against your artery walls. The force of this pushing is called **blood pressure**. When the doctor checks your blood pressure, he or she looks for two readings. The pressure in your arteries immediately after your heart beats is called **systolic blood pressure**. It is the higher of the two readings. The lower of the two numbers, your **diastolic blood pressure**, is the pressure in your artery just before the next beat of your heart.

You can see what counts as normal blood pressure in table 4.4. The table also shows the range for prehypertension, a new category indicating blood pressure that is higher than normal but not high enough to be considered hypertension. People with prehypertension should take precautions to prevent developing even higher blood pressure. There are three stages of high blood pressure. Stage 1 is the least severe and stage 3 the most. When you have your blood pressure checked, you should be rested and relaxed. Blood pressure will be higher if you exercise immediately before taking a reading. Also, your blood pressure is often elevated when you're excited or anxious. The incidence of high blood pressure has decreased in recent years because of improved medicines and early screening. Because high blood pressure is a hypokinetic condition, regular physical activity can help decrease it. A healthy low-sodium diet is also helpful in reducing high blood pressure.

An active person's coronary arteries are more likely to be free from atherosclerosis and generally

## TABLE 4.4 Blood Pressure Readings

|  | Normal | Prehypertension | Stage 1 | Stage 2 | Stage 3 |
|---|---|---|---|---|---|
| Systolic | ≤119 | 120–139 | 140–159 | 160–179 | ≥180 |
| Diastolic | ≤79 | 80–89 | 90–99 | 100–109 | ≥110 |

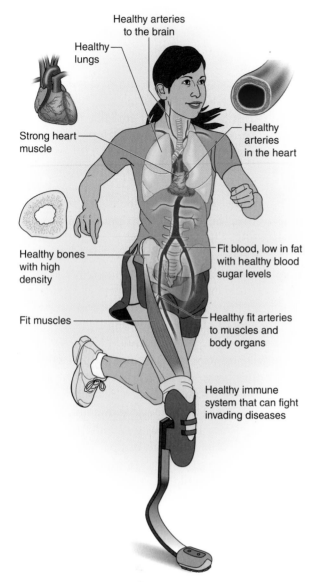

Healthy arteries
to the brain

Healthy
lungs

Strong heart
muscle

Healthy
arteries
in the heart

Healthy bones
with high
density

Fit blood, low in fat
with healthy blood
sugar levels

Fit muscles

Healthy fit arteries
to muscles and
body organs

Healthy immune
system that can fight
invading diseases

**FIGURE 4.6** Physical activity benefits associated with reduced risk of hypokinetic conditions and CVD.

healthy. An active person also has healthy arteries in his or her brain, muscles, and organs; has a strong heart muscle capable of pumping adequate blood to the body; has fit blood that is low in fat, such as cholesterol; and has blood pressure in the healthy range. Regular physical activity not only reduces your risk of heart attack and stroke but also is often prescribed by doctors to help people recovering from these conditions. Figure 4.6 illustrates some ways in which regular physical activity reduces the risk of hypokinetic conditions, including CVD.

People get CVD for many reasons, each of which is called a **risk factor**. The more risk factors you have, the more chance you have of getting a disease. Two kinds of risk factor exist: primary (more important) and secondary (less important). Because one primary risk factor is sedentary (inactive) living, cardiovascular disease is considered a hypokinetic condition. Other primary risk factors for heart disease include smoking, high blood pressure, high fat levels in the blood, too much body fat, and diabetes. Secondary risk factors include stressful living and excessive alcohol use. More information is available in the Taking Charge feature near the end of this chapter.

As you get older, your doctor will likely test your cholesterol, blood pressure, blood sugar, and other potential CVD risk factors. Your doctor will also provide you a rating or standard for each of these tests that indicates how those levels might affect your health. Research shows that your activity and nutrition influence conditions like high cholesterol, high blood pressure, and other risk factors.

## Cancer

According to the American Cancer Society, cancer includes more than one hundred types, all characterized by the uncontrollable growth of abnormal cells. Cancer's uncontrolled cells invade normal cells, steal their nutrition, and interfere with the cells' normal functioning.

Cancer is the second leading cause of death in the United States. When diagnosed early, many forms of cancer can be treated and even cured through surgery, chemical or radiation therapy, or medication. Many of the risk factors for cancer are the same as those for heart disease. We know that the death rate from all forms of cancer is lower in active people than in inactive people. Certain forms of cancer (breast, colon, prostate, and rectal) are considered hypokinetic conditions because people who are physically active are less likely to get them than people who are inactive. It is not clear why physical activity helps reduce the risk of cancer, but, as shown in figure 4.6, one of the health benefits of physical activity is an immune system that is more capable of fighting diseases that invade the body. Another good way to help prevent or minimize cancer is to get regular physical exams.

## Diabetes

When a person's body cannot regulate its sugar level, the person has a disease called **diabetes**. A person with diabetes has excessively high blood sugar unless he or she gets medical assistance. Diabetics may also have trouble using insulin effectively because the cells may become resistant to it. Insulin is a hormone made in the pancreas that helps control blood sugar level. Over time, diabetes can damage the blood vessels, heart, kidneys, and eyes. A very high level of sugar in the blood can cause coma and death. Fortunately, several effective medical treatments can help diabetic people regulate their blood sugar and lead a normal life.

There are two types of diabetes. Type 1, which accounts for about 10 percent of cases, is not a hypokinetic condition and is often hereditary. People with type 1 diabetes take insulin. In people without diabetes, the body automatically produce insulin to keep blood sugar in a normal range. At one time, it was thought that people with type 1 diabetes should avoid physical activity. Now we know that physical activity can help people manage diabetes. Most people with type 1 diabetes take a blood sample one or more times a day in order to test their blood sugar. If the level is high, they take insulin to lower their blood sugar. In the past, it was necessary to puncture the skin to take a blood sample, but new technology allows some people with diabetes to wear a computerized watch that automatically tests blood sugar without having to draw blood.

The most common kind of diabetes—type 2—is a hypokinetic condition because people who are physically active are less likely to have it. As shown in figure 4.6, active people are more likely to have a healthy level of blood sugar. Diabetes has many of the same risk factors as heart disease, including sedentary living. Exercise helps reduce your risk of type 2 diabetes by lowering your blood sugar level, helping your body tissues use insulin more efficiently, and helping control body fat. Having too much body fat is a major risk factor for type 2 diabetes. In fact, so many obese people have diabetes that one expert coined the term *diabesity*—a combination of the words *diabetes* and *obesity*.

## FIT FACT

Type 2 diabetes used to be called adult-onset diabetes because adults got it, not teens and children. This name is no longer used because in recent years the disease has become common among youth.

## Obesity

Obesity, in which a person has a high percentage of body fat, often results from inactivity, though many other factors can contribute. The American Medical Association now classifies obesity as a disease. Having too much body fat contributes to conditions such as heart disease and diabetes. Since 1980, the incidence of obesity among teens in the United States has almost quadrupled, rising from 5 percent to more than 18 percent, and a similar upward trend is found in other developed nations.

## Osteoporosis

**Osteoporosis** exists when bone structure deteriorates (see figure 4.7) and bones become weak. It is most common among older people but has its beginnings in youth. You develop your greatest bone mass—also called your **peak bone mass**—when you're young. People who exercise regularly develop stronger bones than those who are sedentary. Choose physical activities that cause you to bear weight and thus stress your bones in a healthy way. Examples of weight-bearing activities are walking, running, jumping, and resistance training. If you do the right kind of activity when you're young, you'll build a higher peak bone mass. As a result, even if you lose bone mass as you get older, you'll have stronger bones than if you hadn't exercised while young.

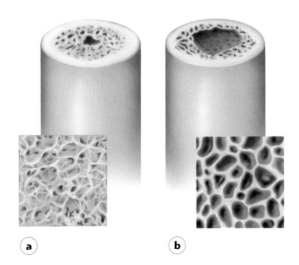

**FIGURE 4.7** Osteoporosis involves a decrease in bone density: *(a)* healthy bone in an active person; *(b)* unhealthy bone (osteoporosis) more common among sedentary people.

One contributor to osteoporosis is a lack of sufficient calcium in the diet, especially when a person is young. Women are more likely to have osteoporosis than men because the hormonal changes they experience later in life cause their body to absorb calcium less efficiently. Whether you are female or male, you can maximize your bone health throughout life by getting good nutrition, regular activity, and proper medical attention.

## Other Hypokinetic Conditions

Evidence suggests that regular physical activity can also reduce the risk or relieve the symptoms of the following diseases and conditions.

- **Mental health conditions.** One-third of all adults report that they often feel depressed, but people who do regular physical activity are less likely to be depressed. Being active can also help reduce feelings of anxiety and improve brain function in older people.

- **Back problems.** More than 80 percent of all adults experience back pain at some point, but exercise can help reduce the incidence of back problems.

- **Metabolic health conditions.** *Metabolism* is a word that refers to the many chemical reactions that allow the body, and the cells of the body, to live and function effectively. You are metabolically healthy when the chemical reactions work normally, allowing the cells to function well. When this does not happen metabolic problems occur. People with metabolic problems such as high blood fat (high cholesterol), high blood pressure, a large waistline, and high blood sugar have a condition called **metabolic syndrome.** This syndrome is associated with heart disease, diabetes, and other hypokinetic diseases. Regular exercise can improve metabolic health and reduce the symptoms of metabolic syndrome.

- **Immune system conditions.** Regular physical activity has been shown to enhance the function of the immune system, thus helping the body resist infections such as the common cold and the flu.

- **Arthritis.** Moderate activity has been shown to help reduce symptoms of some forms of arthritis.

- **Alzheimer's disease and dementia.** Research shows that doing regular exercise and challenging mental tasks can improve brain health and reduce the risk of memory loss disorders.

# Physical Activity and Wellness

As you can see, physical activity plays an important role in preventing hypokinetic diseases and conditions and thus is a key to good health. But remember—health is more than freedom from disease; it also includes positive health, or wellness. As a result, the U.S. government's Healthy People 2020 report incorporates wellness in two of its major goals: high quality of life and sense of well-being. Some of the benefits of physical activity that contribute to wellness are illustrated in figure 4.8.

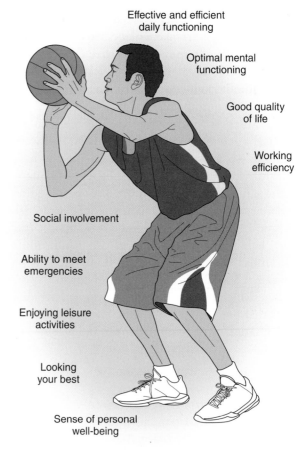

Effective and efficient daily functioning

Optimal mental functioning

Good quality of life

Working efficiency

Social involvement

Ability to meet emergencies

Enjoying leisure activities

Looking your best

Sense of personal well-being

**FIGURE 4.8** The wellness benefits of regular physical activity.

## FIT FACT

Studies conducted by experts in exercise physiology, exercise psychology, and physical activity show that teens who are fit and active enjoy multiple benefits. For example, they perform better in school and are less likely to be absent or cause discipline problems than unfit, inactive teens.

# Hyperkinetic Conditions

You've probably heard the saying "too much of a good thing can be bad." This saying can even be true of physical activity. The fact that some physical activity is good does not mean that more activity is always better. In some cases, people experience **hyperkinetic conditions**—health problems caused by doing too *much* physical activity.

## Overuse Injuries

Overuse injuries occur when you do so much physical activity that you suffer damage to a bone, muscle, or other tissue. Examples include stress fractures, shin splints, and blisters.

## Activity Neurosis ✓

Neurosis is a condition in which a person is overly concerned or fearful about something. People with an **activity neurosis** are overly concerned about getting enough exercise. They feel upset if they miss a regular workout and often continue physical activity when they are sick or injured. Activity neurosis is more common among aerobic dance instructors, bodybuilders, and runners than other active groups. Aerobic dance instructors often teach many classes and also take classes to improve their dance skills. Some experts believe this can lead to a compulsive need to exercise. Some bodybuilders seek perfection and continue to do more exercise in pursuit of this ideal. Reasons for activity neurosis among runners may be the desire to improve running times or distance.

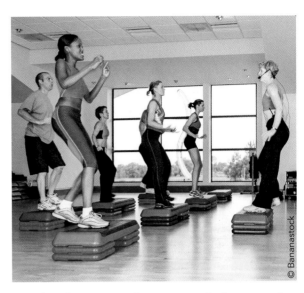

People who are overly concerned about getting enough exercise may have a condition called activity neurosis.

## Body Image and Eating Disorders

People with body image disorders try to achieve their idea of an ideal body by doing excessive exercise. This idealized body is unrealistic and distorted. People with this disorder often perform excessive resistance training and sometimes use dangerous supplements or substances such as steroids. Use of steroids and dangerous supplements or substances is most common among teenage boys and young adult men but can occur in both men and women of all ages. Teenage girls and young women, and to a lesser extent young men, often strive for extreme thinness, which is both unhealthy and unrealistic. An extreme desire to be abnormally thin is associated with several kinds of **eating disorders**. People with these conditions have dangerous eating habits and often resort to excessive activity to expend calories for fat loss. Eating disorders that include abuse of exercise are considered to be hyperkinetic conditions. People with body image disorders and eating disorders often need the help of an expert to overcome their problem.

## Lesson Review

1. Name and describe at least four hypokinetic conditions. How can physical activity reduce your risk of getting these conditions?
2. What are some health and wellness benefits of physical activity?
3. How is physical activity related to hyperkinetic conditions? Give examples.

A risk factor is any action or condition that increases your chances of developing a disease. Some risk factors, such as your age and your genetic makeup, are beyond your ability to control or change. But there are also risk factors that you can control—for example, your diet and physical activity. Therefore, your actions can affect the probability that you will get a disease.

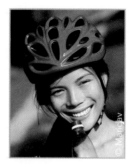

Here's an example. Last summer, Brenda's family took a trip to the mountains, where they planned to hike, raft the rivers, and ride bikes and horses. Unfortunately, Brenda's father did not get to enjoy all of the activities. Brenda was surprised: "I never thought my father had any health problems because he was always busy with work and taking care of the house. He never went to the doctor."

But Brenda's father was a smoker. And though he was busy, he didn't actually do much physical activity because he easily became short of breath. On the trip, Brenda's father found that he couldn't keep up with the rest of the family. While hiking, he became so short of breath that he almost fainted. While riding a bike, he fell far behind the others. And in the evening, while the rest of the family did other things, Brenda's father went to bed.

When they returned home, Brenda's father visited his doctor, who recommended that he change his lifestyle. Specifically, his doctor advised him to stop smoking and get more exercise. He also was warned that if he continued his present lifestyle, he was at risk for heart disease and other health problems.

### For Discussion

What controllable risk factors for heart disease did Brenda's father have? What can Brenda's father do to reduce his risk? Is there anything that Brenda can do to help her father reduce his risk? What can Brenda do now to minimize her own disease risk later in life? Consider the guidelines presented in the following Self-Management feature as you answer these discussion questions.

## ➔ SELF-MANAGEMENT: Skills for Reducing Risk Factors

Of the 10 leading causes of death, 6 can be considered hypokinetic conditions. Many of these conditions can be prevented if you adopt a healthy lifestyle early in life. You can take the following steps, even in your teen years, to reduce your risk of hypokinetic conditions.

- **Know how to identify important risk factors.** In order to lower your disease risks, you must first identify them. Risk factors for hypokinetic disease that are *not* in your control include heredity, sex, age, and diseases such as type 1 diabetes (which increases the risk of heart disease). You do have some control over risk factors such as your body fat, blood pressure, and blood fat, but they are also influenced by heredity. Risk factors over which you have more control are diet, physical activity, tobacco and alcohol use, and exposure to stress.

- **Periodically self-assess your risk factors.** You can't change risk factors if you don't know you have them. Doing a self-assessment helps you plan for reducing your risks and lets you know when you need to seek medical help. Because risk increases with age, it becomes even more important to check your risk factors as you grow older.

- **Learn about your family history.** Heredity is a factor over which you have no control. You can, however, check to see what diseases or conditions your parents or grandparents have had—and thus which ones you may inherit a tendency to develop (for example, heart disease, diabetes, and some forms of cancer). You can then pay special attention to controllable risk factors for those diseases.

- **Take steps to change risk factors that are partially in your control.** Some risk factors are influenced by heredity but can also be modified through healthy lifestyle choices. These risk factors include your blood pressure, your blood fat, your body's ability to regulate sugar, and your body fatness. You can influence these factors through choices such as getting regular physical activity, eating properly, and seeking proper medical care. If you have a family history of any of these risk factors, seek medical help and professional advice about how to make lifestyle changes to reduce your risk.

- **Take steps to change risk factors that are fully in your control.** Some risk factors are well within your control—for example, physical activity, what you eat, tobacco and alcohol use, and your stress level.

- **Use the self-management skills you learn in this book to make lifelong changes.** You'll learn many self-management skills throughout this book. Use them to change the risk factors that you identify.

 # ACADEMIC CONNECTION: Statistics

Statistics is a branch of mathematics dealing with the collection, analysis, and interpretation of data (numerical information). Mathematic literacy is important for meeting college and career readiness standards. Understanding and using some basic statistical concepts can help you not only as you prepare for a career or college and university studies but also in understanding health risks.

The average person is said to be typical. In math, *average* refers to measures of central tendency such as

- the mean, or the sum of all scores divided by the number of scores (11 scores in the following example);

- the median, or the middle score in a number of scores (in the following example, the sixth score from the lowest or sixth score from the highest); and

- the mode, or the most common score in a number of scores (in the following example, the only score that was common to two people).

Calculate the mean, median, and mode for a group of 11 people with the following systolic blood pressure readings in mmHg: 120, 125, 130, 130, 135, 140, 145, 150, 155, 160, 165. Remember that systolic blood pressure is the higher of the two blood pressure numbers and reflects the pressure in your arteries just after the heart beats.

A systolic blood pressure of 120 mmHg is considered to be healthy. Knowing this, would you want to have your blood pressure equal to the average for this group (using any of the three measures of central tendency)?

**Check Your Answers**

Mean = 141.36; median = 140; mode = 130

# TAKING ACTION: Walking for Health

Walking can be done by most people, in most places, and with little or no equipment. Research shows that 30 minutes or more of daily walking can

- help you maintain a healthy weight,
- reduce your risk of hypokinetic disease,
- improve your wellness and mental health,
- strengthen your bones and muscles, and
- increase your chances of living longer.

Because walking is a moderate-intensity activity, it can typically be done while talking with others. As a result, you can use it as a way of not only relaxing and helping your body but also building healthy relationships as you walk and talk with friends and family members. If you have not been active up until now, walking is also a great way to slowly build your fitness before you start an exercise program. In fact, some people have begun with a walking program and ended up running a marathon. If you want to start looking and feeling your best but don't know where to start, **take action** and try walking!

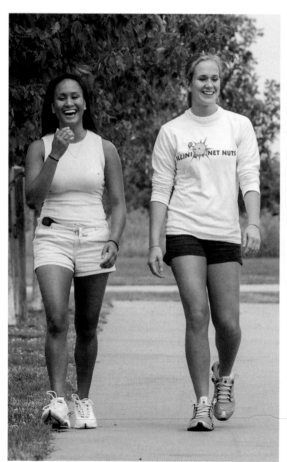 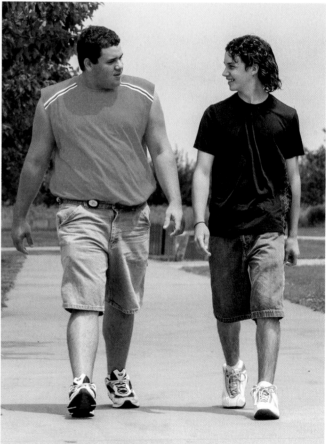

**Taking action by walking can improve health and promote social relationships.**

# CHAPTER REVIEW

## Reviewing Concepts and Vocabulary

As directed by your teacher, answer items 1 through 5 by correctly completing each sentence with a word or phrase.

1. The seven questions used to determine readiness for physical activity are called the _____.
2. The two factors used to determine the heat index are _____.
3. The measure used to determine whether it is too cold to exercise is called the _____.
4. Symptoms of frostbite include _____.
5. Hot, dry, flushed skin; rapid pulse; and lack of sweating are symptoms of _____.

For items 6 through 10, as directed by your teacher, match each term in column 1 with the appropriate phrase in column 2.

6. electrolytes
7. diabetes
8. air quality index
9. hypothermia
10. BMI

a. inability to regulate blood sugar
b. body composition measure
c. minerals that help prevent heat injuries
d. extremely low body temperature
e. indicator that helps determine whether it is safe to exercise

For items 11 through 15, as directed by your teacher, respond to each statement or question.

11. Describe the three types of heat-related conditions.
12. What are the benefits of physical activity in preventing heart disease?
13. Describe two hyperkinetic conditions.
14. Describe two wellness benefits of physical activity.
15. What are some benefits of walking 30 minutes or more each day?

## Thinking Critically

Write a paragraph to answer the following question.
Why is inactivity a primary risk factor for many diseases?

## Project

You have been asked to give a speech to a local civic club on the health benefits of physical activity. Prepare a presentation using 10 or more slides.

# 5

# How Much Is Enough?

## In This Chapter

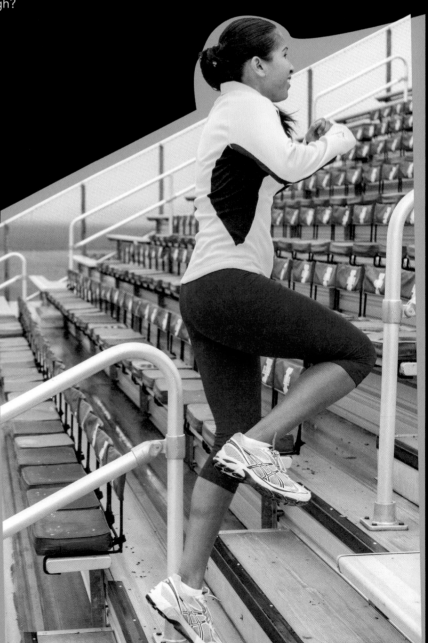

**www** **Student Web Resources**
www.fitnessforlife.org/student

# Lesson 5.1
## How Much Physical Activity Is Enough?

**Lesson Objectives**

After reading this lesson, you should be able to

1. name and describe the three principles of exercise;
2. describe the four parts of the FITT formula and discuss how they relate to threshold of training, target ceiling, and fitness target zone; and
3. describe the five types of physical activity included in the Physical Activity Pyramid.

**Lesson Vocabulary**

fitness target zone, FITT formula, frequency, intensity, Physical Activity Pyramid, principle of overload, principle of progression, principle of specificity, target ceiling, threshold of training, time, type

**How** much physical activity is enough? This question might seem very simple, but the answer can be complicated, especially if you're just beginning an activity program. In this lesson, you'll develop an understanding of three basic exercise principles as a good first step in answering the question of how much is enough.

## Principles of Physical Activity

Consider this example. Mia has been exercising for several months. Every day, she does the same physical activities for about 15 minutes. Her activity program has not changed since she started. Initially, Mia saw some positive results from her program: She was no longer tired at the end of her exercise, and a self-assessment showed that her cardiorespiratory endurance had improved. Lately, however, Mia has felt disappointed because her strength and flexibility haven't been improving as much as they did at first. Mia wants to know what she's doing wrong. For some clues to the answer, let's look at the three principles of exercise: overload, progression, and specificity.

### Principle of Overload

The most basic law of physical activity is the **principle of overload**, which states that the only way to produce fitness and health benefits through physical activity is to require your body to do more than it normally does. Increased demand on your body—overload—forces it to adapt. Your body was designed to be active, so if you do nothing (underload), your fitness will decrease, and you will increase your risk of hypokinetic disease.

Since Mia is no longer overloading when she exercises, she is maintaining but no longer gaining increased fitness and health benefits. If she wants to continue improving her strength and flexibility, she'll have to increase the amount of her physical activity.

### Principle of Progression

The **principle of progression** states that the amount and intensity of your exercise should be increased gradually. After a while, your body adapts to an increase in physical activity (load), and the activity gets easier for you to perform. When this happens, you can gradually increase your activity.

Figure 5.1 shows the minimum overload you need in order to build physical fitness. This amount is called your **threshold of training**. Performing activity above your threshold builds your fitness and promotes your health and wellness. Since Mia has exercised for several months at the same level, she may now be exercising below her threshold of training for at least some parts of fitness.

This correct range of physical activity is called your **fitness target zone**, typically shortened to just *target zone*. It begins with the threshold of training and has an upper limit called the **target ceiling**. Exercise below the threshold is not enough to produce benefits. Activities above the target ceiling (excessive exercise) can increase risk of injury and

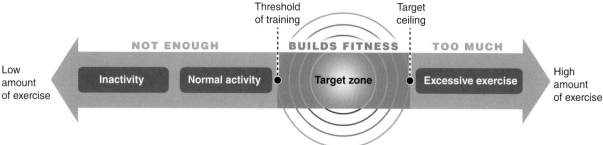

Threshold of training

Target ceiling

NOT ENOUGH          BUILDS FITNESS          TOO MUCH

Low amount of exercise

Inactivity     Normal activity     Target zone     Excessive exercise

High amount of exercise

**FIGURE 5.1**   The fitness target zone.

soreness and may produce less than optimal benefits. Some people think you have to experience pain in order to gain fitness, but the principle of progression provides the basis for rejecting the theory of "no pain, no gain." If you experience pain when you exercise, you're probably overloading too much or too quickly for your body to adjust.

## Principle of Specificity

The **principle of specificity** states that the particular type of exercise you perform determines the particular benefit you receive. Different kinds and amounts of activity produce very specific and different benefits. An activity that promotes health benefits in one part of health-related fitness may not be equally good in promoting high levels of fitness in another part of fitness. For example, Mia jogs on a track several days a week, but she does not do stretching exercises as often as she should. She may also need to use more resistance in her muscle fitness exercises.

In addition, exercises performed for specific body parts, such as the calf muscles, may provide benefits only for those parts. For example, if Mia does exercises only for her calf muscles, she will not build the muscles in her back, shoulders, arms, or other parts of her legs.

> "
> Knowing is not enough; we must apply. Willing is not enough; we must do.
> "
>
> —Johann Wolfgang von Goethe, writer and artist

## FITT Formula

You know that you must do more physical activity than normal to build fitness. You also know that

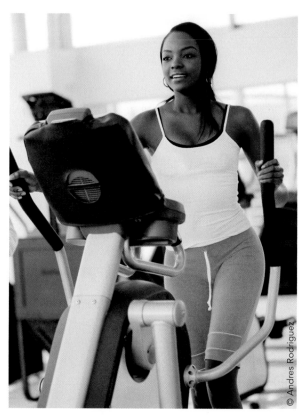

Applying the principle of specificity is important for getting optimal benefits.

you should gradually increase your physical activity in order to stay within your fitness target zone. But how much physical activity do you need?

To help you apply the principles of exercise, you can use the **FITT formula**. Some people refer to it as the FITT *principle*, but we use the term *formula* in this book because a formula refers to a prescription or recipe. In this case, the prescription is for determining the right amount of physical activity for applying the three exercise principles. In fact, each letter in the acronym FITT represents a key factor in determining how much physical activity is enough: frequency, intensity, time, and type.

- **Frequency refers to how often you do physical activity.** For physical activity to be beneficial, you must do it several days a week. Optimal **frequency** depends on the type of activity you're doing and the part of fitness you want to develop. To develop strength, for example, you might need to exercise two days a week. To lose fat, you should exercise daily.

- **Intensity refers to how hard you perform physical activity.** If the activity you do is too easy, you will not build fitness or gain other benefits. But remember—extremely vigorous activity can be harmful if you don't work up to it gradually. **Intensity** is determined differently depending on the type of activity you do and the type of fitness you want to build. For example, you can use your heart rate to determine your intensity of activity for building cardiorespiratory endurance, whereas you would use the amount of weight you lift to determine the intensity for building strength.

- **Time refers to how long you do physical activity.** As with frequency and intensity, the length of **time** for which you should do physical activity depends on the type of activity you're doing and the part of fitness you want to develop. For example, to build flexibility you should exercise for 15 seconds or more for each muscle group, whereas to build cardiorespiratory endurance you need to be vigorously active for a minimum of 20 minutes.

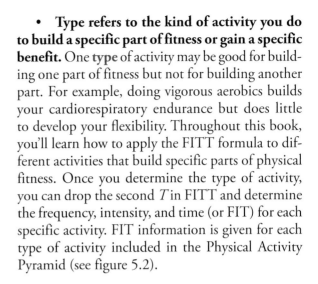

- **Type refers to the kind of activity you do to build a specific part of fitness or gain a specific benefit.** One **type** of activity may be good for building one part of fitness but not for building another part. For example, doing vigorous aerobics builds your cardiorespiratory endurance but does little to develop your flexibility. Throughout this book, you'll learn how to apply the FITT formula to different activities that build specific parts of physical fitness. Once you determine the type of activity, you can drop the second *T* in FITT and determine the frequency, intensity, and time (or FIT) for each specific activity. FIT information is given for each type of activity included in the Physical Activity Pyramid (see figure 5.2).

## FIT FACT

FITT is a mnemonic acronym or formula used to remember four key factors in applying the overload principle and related principles: frequency, intensity, time, and type.

## Volume and Progression

The American College of Sports Medicine (ACSM) uses the FITT formula for prescribing how much physical activity is enough. It's also important to consider the total amount of physical activity you perform (volume) and the need for progression (principle of progression) in your program, so ACSM sometimes includes the letters VP after FITT, thus making it FITT-VP. In this version, V stands for the volume (amount) of exercise, which is a function of intensity and time. Consider your total volume of activity when developing a personal activity plan. For example, you can do moderate activity for a longer time and do the same volume of activity as for vigorous activity done for a shorter time. As you learn more about the FITT formula you will learn how volume of exercise can be adjusted by altering the intensity and time of the workout. Over a longer time, such as a week, the frequency of exercise also contributes to volume. Doing the same workout four days a week will have twice the volume as doing the workout two days a week.

The P in FITT-VP is to remind people of the importance of progression—that is, applying the FITT formula gradually. As you work through this book, you'll see only the acronyms FIT and FITT, but you should also keep volume and progression (VP) in mind as you develop your personal activity plan.

## The Physical Activity Pyramid

National physical activity guidelines for youth developed by the U.S. Department of Health and Human Services (USDHHS) recommend at least 60 minutes of physical activity each day. The five steps of the **Physical Activity Pyramid** (figure 5.2) help you understand the five kinds of physical activity, which build different parts of fitness and produce different health and wellness benefits (recall the principle of specificity). To meet the recommended 60 minutes of daily activity, you can choose from the different types of activity. For optimal benefits, you should perform activities from all parts of the pyramid each week. As you can see, activities at or near the bottom of the pyramid may need to be done more frequently or for a longer time than those near the top of the pyramid to get the same volume of activity.

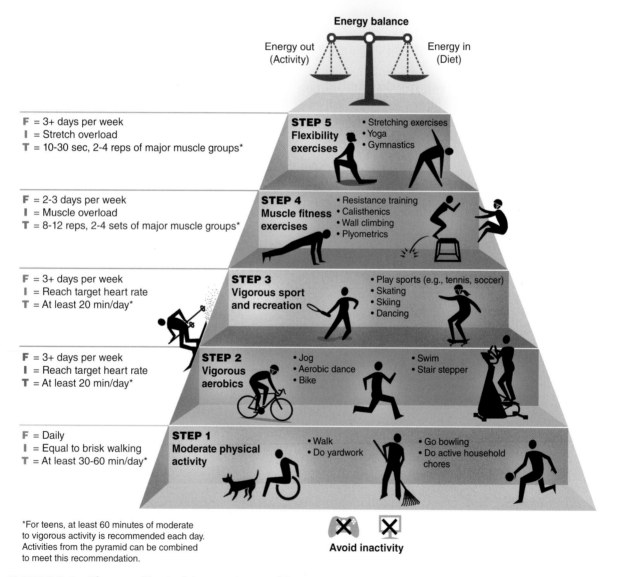

**Energy balance**

Energy out (Activity) — Energy in (Diet)

**F** = 3+ days per week
**I** = Stretch overload
**T** = 10-30 sec, 2-4 reps of major muscle groups*

**STEP 5**
**Flexibility exercises**
• Stretching exercises
• Yoga
• Gymnastics

**F** = 2-3 days per week
**I** = Muscle overload
**T** = 8-12 reps, 2-4 sets of major muscle groups*

**STEP 4**
**Muscle fitness exercises**
• Resistance training
• Calisthenics
• Wall climbing
• Plyometrics

**F** = 3+ days per week
**I** = Reach target heart rate
**T** = At least 20 min/day*

**STEP 3**
**Vigorous sport and recreation**
• Play sports (e.g., tennis, soccer)
• Skating
• Skiing
• Dancing

**F** = 3+ days per week
**I** = Reach target heart rate
**T** = At least 20 min/day*

**STEP 2**
**Vigorous aerobics**
• Jog
• Aerobic dance
• Bike
• Swim
• Stair stepper

**F** = Daily
**I** = Equal to brisk walking
**T** = At least 30-60 min/day*

**STEP 1**
**Moderate physical activity**
• Walk
• Do yardwork
• Go bowling
• Do active household chores

*For teens, at least 60 minutes of moderate to vigorous activity is recommended each day. Activities from the pyramid can be combined to meet this recommendation.

**Avoid inactivity**

**FIGURE 5.2** The new Physical Activity Pyramid for Teens.
Source: C.B. Corbin

## Moderate Physical Activity

Moderate physical activity is the first step in the Physical Activity Pyramid, and it should be performed daily or nearly every day. Moderate activity involves exercise equal in intensity to brisk walking. It includes some activities of normal daily living (also called lifestyle activities), such as yardwork (for example, raking leaves or mowing the lawn) and housework (for example, mopping the floor). It also includes sports that are not vigorous, such as bowling and golf. Some other sports can be either moderate or vigorous; for example, shooting basketballs is typically a moderate activity, whereas playing a full-court game is vigorous. National guidelines recommend 60 minutes of moderate to vigorous activity each day for teens. Moderate activity should account for some of this time each day (30 minutes a day is recommended for adults). It is also associated with many of the health benefits of activity described in this book, such as controlling your level of body fat, and is well suited for people of varying abilities.

## Vigorous Aerobics

Step 2 of the Physical Activity Pyramid represents vigorous aerobics, which includes any exercise that you can do for a long time without stopping and that is vigorous enough to increase your heart rate, make you breathe faster, and make you sweat. Thus these activities are more intense than moderate activities such as brisk walking. Vigorous aerobics, such as jogging and aerobic dance, are typically continuous in nature. Like moderate activity, they provide many health and wellness benefits, and they're especially helpful for building a high level of cardiorespiratory endurance. You should perform vigorous aerobics (or vigorous sport or recreation) at least three days a week for at least 20 minutes each day in order to meet national activity guidelines.

## FIT FACT

The word *aerobic*, meaning "with oxygen," is a scientific term that has been used for decades. It was popularized in the 1968 book *Aerobics*, written by Dr. Ken Cooper, whose work over the years has helped everyday people around the world understand how much activity is needed for fitness and health benefits. In fact, in Portuguese, the English word *jogging* is translated as "coopering"! Dr. Cooper also founded the Cooper Institute, a world-famous health and fitness research organization based in Dallas, Texas.

## Vigorous Sport and Recreation

Like vigorous aerobics, vigorous sport and recreation (represented in step 3 of the Physical Activity Pyramid) require your heart to beat faster than normal and cause you to breathe faster and sweat more. As your muscles use more oxygen, your heart beats faster, and you breathe faster and more deeply to meet the oxygen demand. Unlike vigorous aerobics, however, vigorous sport and recreation often involve short bursts of activity followed by short bursts of rest (as in basketball, football, soccer, and tennis). When done for at least 20 minutes a day in bouts of 10 minutes or more at a time, these activities provide similar fitness, health, and wellness benefits to those of vigorous aerobics. They also help you build motor skills and contribute to healthy weight management. As with vigorous aerobics, you can use vigorous sport and recreation to meet national activity recommendation when you do them for at least 20 minutes a day on three days a week.

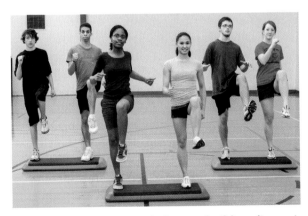

**Vigorous aerobic activity helps you build cardiorespiratory endurance.**

# FITNESS TECHNOLOGY: Activitygram

You can use computer technology to keep track of your daily physical activity. Activitygram is a computer program that helps you track your physical activity over a three-day period. You enter any activity you perform for every 30-minute block of time during your waking hours. You also record the type of activity you do and whether its intensity level is resting, light, moderate, or vigorous. The program generates a report showing your total number of activity minutes each day, the amount of activity you did at each step of the Physical Activity Pyramid, and the amounts of moderate activity and vigorous activity you performed.

### Using Technology

Locate the Activitygram portion of the student section of the Fitness for Life website. Open the document that explains Activitygram and use the information you find there to estimate the amount of activity you get from each of the different types shown in the pyramid. Ask your instructor for more information about Activitygram.

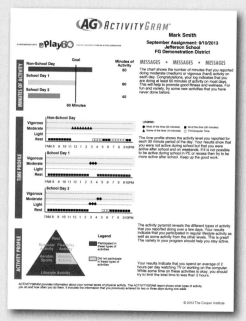

Reprinted by permission from Cooper Institute, 2003, *Activitygram* (Champaign, IL: Human Kinetics).

## Muscle Fitness Exercises

Step 4 in the Physical Activity Pyramid represents muscle fitness exercises, which build your strength, muscular endurance, and power. Muscle fitness exercises include both resistance training (with weights or machines) and moving your own body weight (as in rock climbing, calisthenics, and jumping). This type of exercise produces general health and wellness benefits, as well as better performance, improved body appearance, a healthier back, better posture, and stronger bones. These exercises can be used to meet national activity guidelines and should be performed on two or three days a week.

## Flexibility Exercises

Step 5 of the Physical Activity Pyramid represents flexibility exercises. According to ACSM, flexibility exercises improve postural stability and balance. There is also some evidence that flexibility exercises may reduce soreness, prevent injuries, and reduce risk of back pain. Flexibility exercises also improve your performance in activities such as gymnastics and dance. They also are used in therapy to help people who have been injured. Two examples of flexibility exercise are stretching and yoga (figure 5.3). To build and maintain flexibility, you should perform flexibility exercise at least three days a week.

## Avoiding Inactivity

Just below the Physical Activity Pyramid (see figure 5.2) you'll notice pictures of a television set and a video game controller with an X over them. This illustration emphasizes the fact that being sedentary, or inactive, poses a health risk.

Just as you should do 60 minutes of physical activity each day, drawing from the five types of activity presented in the pyramid, you should also avoid the inactivity that is common among people who log too much "screen time" on a daily basis. Screen time refers to time spent in front of a TV, computer game, phone screen, or any other device that substitutes inactivity for activities from the pyramid. A recent survey of children and teens in the United States found that they watch TV for an average of nearly four hours a day! Sixty-eight

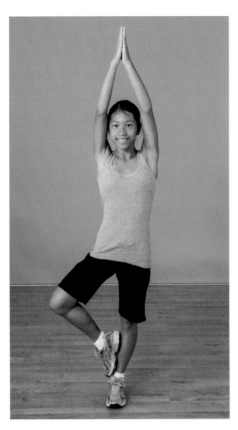

**FIGURE 5.3** Yoga is one type of physical activity for improving flexibility.

percent of teens have a TV in their room, and of course many also spend screen time on computers, video games, movies, and cell phones, more than doubling the amount of time they spend watching a screen. Research shows that screen time results in inactivity and increases health risk.

We all need to take time to recover from daily stresses and prepare for new challenges, so periods of rest and sleep are important for good health. Some activities of daily living—such as studying, reading, and even a moderate amount of screen time—are appropriate. But general inactivity or sedentary living is harmful to your health. Your choices from active areas of the pyramid should exceed your choices from the inactivity area.

## Balancing Energy

The top of the pyramid presents a balance scale illustrating the need to balance the energy you take in (food) with the energy you put out (activity). Energy balance means that the calories in the food you eat each day are equal to the calories you expend in exercise each day. Balancing your energy in this way is essential to maintaining a healthy body composition.

# Patterns of Moderate and Vigorous Activity

A pattern is a schedule you use to accumulate minutes of activity from the pyramid each day and each week. One pattern is continuous activity, in which you do all of your physical activity for the day in one continuous session (for example, 30 minutes of continuous moderate activity).

The second pattern is accumulated activity, in which you do sessions of 10 minutes or more in order to accumulate your targeted daily total (for example, 10 + 10 + 10 = 30). Bouts of less than 10 minutes may provide some health benefits but are not recommended for use in accumulating your recommended daily activity time, because bouts of less than 10 minutes are considered below the threshold of training for getting benefits.

The ACSM refers to a third pattern as that of the "weekend warrior." This pattern is marked by inactivity during most of the week punctuated by relatively long sessions of activity—sometimes for several hours at a time and often all in one day. Adults often do this extended activity on weekends because of their work commitments during the week—thus the name "weekend warrior." This pattern is not recommended and can even be dangerous for people with risk factors because it violates the principle of progression and can lead to soreness and injury. Thus you should do your activity on most days of the week using a continuous or accumulated pattern.

## Lesson Review

1. What are the three principles of exercise, and why are they important?
2. What are the four parts of the FITT formula as represented by the letters in the acronym FITT? How are they related to the following concepts: threshold of training, target ceiling, and fitness target zone?
3. What are some characteristics and examples of the five types of activity included in the Physical Activity Pyramid?

In this assessment, you'll perform two tests: one to assess your cardiorespiratory endurance and another to measure the flexibility and fitness of your back and trunk muscles. If you have not done so already, practice each test before performing them for a score. Record your scores and fitness ratings for the two tests as directed by your teacher. Performing these tests will provide information that you can use in preparing a Fitnessgram report and in preparing your personal physical activity plan. If you're working with a partner, remember that self-assessment information is personal and considered confidential. It shouldn't be shared with others without the permission of the person being tested.

## PACER (Progressive Aerobic Cardiovascular Endurance Run, or 20-meter shuttle run)

This test of cardiorespiratory endurance was originally called the 20-meter shuttle run, and that name is still used in many countries. The name PACER, as it is called in Fitnessgram, was the winning entry, submitted by Dr. Jack Rutherford, in a contest designed to create a new name for the test that would be easy to remember.

The test is scored differently by different test batteries. In this book, you'll use the number of laps you perform as the score on which your fitness rating is based; laps are also used for scoring by the ALPHA-FIT test. Using laps makes it easy for you to see if you improve after performing your personal activity plan. If you want to do a Fitnessgram report, you'll need to convert your laps score to an aerobic capacity score as described in the student section of the Fitness for Life website.

### Directions

1. The test objective is to run back and forth across a 20-meter (almost 22-yard) distance as many times as you can at a predetermined pace (pacing is based on signals from a special audio recording provided by your instructor).

2. Start at a line located 20 meters from a second line. When you hear the beep from the audio track, run across the 20-meter area to the second line, arriving just before the tape beeps again, and touch the line with your foot. Turn around and get ready to run back.

3. At the sound of the next beep, run back to the line where you began. Touch the line with your foot. Make sure to wait for the beep before running back.

4. Continue to run back and forth from one line to the other, touching the line each time. The beeps will come faster and faster, causing you to run faster and faster. The test is finished when you twice fail to reach the opposite side before the beep.

5. Your score is the number of laps you ran (the number of times you ran the 20-meter distance from one line to the other) before your test was finished. Using laps as your score allows you to easily test yourself to see how you improve over time. This method of scoring provides you with a good indicator of your cardiorespiratory endurance, which is a measure of functional fitness—your ability to function effectively in daily living.

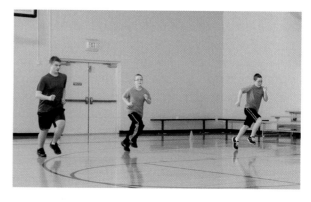

The PACER test assesses cardiorespiratory endurance and can be used to estimate aerobic capacity.

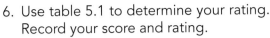

6. Use table 5.1 to determine your rating. Record your score and rating.

7. If you or your teacher would like to prepare a Fitnessgram report card, aerobic capacity score will be used. Aerobic capacity refers to your body's ability to supply oxygen during sustained aerobic activity and is best determined using a treadmill test. Your lap score can be used to estimate your aerobic capacity score. You can use Fitnessgram software with the help of your teacher; alternatively, you can use the charts presented in the student section of the Fitness for Life website to determine your aerobic capacity score and fitness rating. Aerobic capacity is discussed further in the Cardiorespiratory Endurance chapter.

### TABLE 5.1 Rating Chart for PACER

|  | 13 years old | | 14 years old | | 15 years old | | 16 years old | | 17 years or older | |
|---|---|---|---|---|---|---|---|---|---|---|
|  | Male | Female | Male | Female | Male | Female | Male | Female | Male | Female |
| High performance | ≥36 | ≥31 | ≥45 | ≥34 | ≥54 | ≥38 | ≥60 | ≥40 | ≥67 | ≥50 |
| Good fitness | 29–35 | 25–30 | 36–44 | 27–33 | 42–53 | 30–37 | 47–59 | 32–39 | 54–66 | 38–49 |
| Marginal fitness | 23–28 | 19–24 | 28–35 | 21–26 | 32–41 | 23–29 | 36–46 | 25–31 | 42–53 | 30–37 |
| Low fitness | ≤22 | ≤18 | ≤27 | ≤20 | ≤31 | ≤22 | ≤35 | ≤24 | ≤41 | ≤29 |

Scores in this table refer to the number of completed laps.

Based on data provided by G. Welk.

## Trunk Lift (upper back)

1. Lie facedown with your arms to your sides and your hands under your thighs.

2. Lift the upper part of your body very slowly so that your chin, chest, and shoulders come off the floor. Lift your trunk as high as possible, to a maximum of 12 inches (30 centimeters). Hold this position for three seconds while a partner measures how far your chin is from the floor. Your partner should hold the ruler at least 1 inch (2.5 centimeters) in front of your chin. Look straight ahead so that your chin is not tipped abnormally upward.

3. Do the trunk lift two times (lifting slowly) and record how far from the floor you can lift and hold your chin (for three seconds). Do not record scores above 12 inches (30 centimeters).

   Caution: The ruler should not be placed directly under your chin, in case you have to lower your trunk unexpectedly.

4. Use table 5.2 to determine your fitness rating. Record your score and rating.

### TABLE 5.2 Rating Chart for Trunk Lift

| Rating | Inches |
|---|---|
| High performance | 11–12 |
| Good fitness | 9–10 |
| Marginal fitness | 7–8 |
| Low fitness | ≤6 |

To convert inches to centimeters, multiply by 2.54.

Data based on Fitnessgram.

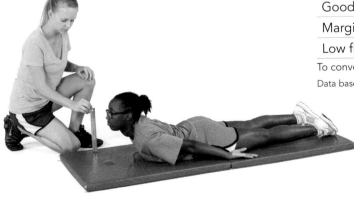

This test measures the flexibility of your back and trunk muscles, as well as the muscle fitness of your back muscles.

# Lesson 5.2

# How Much Fitness Is Enough?

## Lesson Objectives

After reading this lesson, you should be able to

1. describe the four fitness rating categories and how they apply to your physical activity program,
2. identify factors that contribute to fitness, and
3. explain how a person can attain good health and fitness even if some factors make it difficult to succeed.

## Lesson Vocabulary

criterion-referenced health standard, maturation

**You** now know that physical activity is necessary to build each part of physical fitness. But exactly how much fitness do you need? In this lesson, you'll learn some ways to decide how much fitness is enough for you.

## Fitness Standards and Rating Categories

Sometimes people judge their fitness by comparing themselves with others. If they score higher on a fitness test than most other people, they consider themselves fit. This type of comparison creates several problems. First, it suggests that only a few people can be fit. Second, it suggests that only high test scores are adequate for fitness. In this lesson, you'll learn why neither of these suggestions is true.

Most experts agree that you should judge fitness using **criterion-referenced health standards**. The word *standard* refers to an established amount or quantity. The word *criterion* is a marker used to establish the standard (as it relates to health). So a criterion-referenced standard for health-related fitness refers to the amount of fitness you need in order to achieve good health. This type of standard does not require you to compare yourself with others. It does require you to have enough fitness to

- reduce your risk of health problems,
- achieve wellness benefits,
- function effectively in your daily life,
- meet emergencies, and
- enjoy your free time.

As noted in this chapter's Science in Action feature, you'll learn to do many self-assessments for each of the health-related parts of physical fitness. In this book, we use a rating system based on criterion-referenced health standards. It is similar to the rating systems used in test batteries such as Fitnessgram, and we use it here so that you can rate your fitness in all of the tests included in this book by means of the same system.

To rate yourself in each of the six parts of health-related physical fitness, you'll use one of the following four categories. If you attain a rating of "good fitness" for all six fitness areas, you'll achieve the basic health and wellness standards of physical fitness.

- **Low fitness.** If you have a low fitness rating, you have an above average risk of developing health problems. You also might not look your best, feel your best, or work and play as efficiently as you could. If you have a low fitness rating, you should work to achieve a marginal fitness rating.

- **Marginal fitness.** Moving from the low to the marginal rating shows important progress in fitness. However, if you have a marginal rating, you should try to get a good fitness rating.

- **Good fitness.** This rating indicates that you have the fitness needed to live a full, healthy life. In fact, achieving a good fitness rating is the goal of most people. To maintain this level of fitness, you'll need to continue being physically active.

## ⚛ SCIENCE IN ACTION: Personal Fitness Assessment

Experts in physical education and exercise physiology have worked together to develop various physical fitness test batteries. A battery is a group of tests designed to assess all parts of physical fitness. As you've learned, Fitnessgram is one fitness test battery used in many schools in the United States and throughout the world. Fitnessgram has been adopted as the national assessment program for both the President's Council on Fitness, Sports, and Nutrition (PCFSN) and the Society of Health and Physical Educators (SHAPE America). ALPHA-FIT is a fitness test battery widely used in Europe. The two batteries contain some similar tests and some that differ from each other.

In this book, you'll try many fitness tests. The goal is to help you select test items for your own personal fitness test battery that you can use throughout your life to self-assess your fitness. You will perform all of the test items in the

Fitnessgram and ALPHA-FIT batteries, as well as several other tests. For all tests in this book, you'll use the Fitness for Life rating system, but you can also learn how to use standards and ratings from other test batteries. What's most important is that you learn to test your own fitness and use your personal self-assessment results to plan your own fitness and physical activity.

### Student Activity

On the Fitness for Life website, find the information about the Fitnessgram and ALPHA-FIT test batteries. Specifically, read the information about the two batteries' standards. Compare the standards to see how they differ. Prepare a report in writing or present your report to the class.

---

- **High performance.** Most experts agree that many health benefits can be achieved without reaching a high performance rating. However, performing the amount of physical activity necessary to reach this rating has additional health benefits because you get more benefits with a greater volume of activity (when not overdone). It should be noted that the fitter you get, the harder it is to improve. Achieving a high performance rating is necessary if you want to be an athlete or perform a physically demanding job, such as firefighter, soldier, or police officer.

## Factors Influencing Physical Fitness

Physical activity is the most important thing you can do to improve or maintain your health-related physical fitness. Fortunately, it is also something that you can control. You can choose the kinds of activity you want to do and schedule a regular time to do them. But as figure 5.4 shows, physical activity is not the only factor that contributes to your physical fitness. Other important factors are **maturation**, age, heredity, environment, and lifestyle choices such as nutrition and stress management.

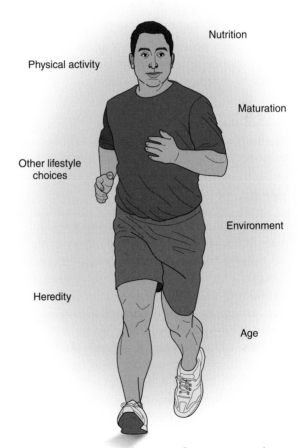

**FIGURE 5.4** Various factors influence your physical fitness.

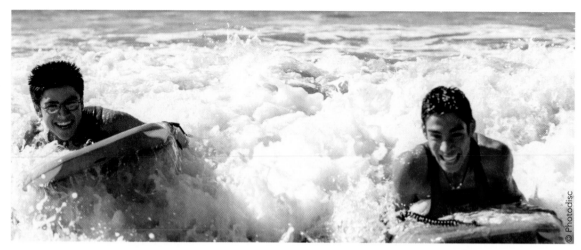

**Compare your fitness with criterion-referenced health standards rather than with your friends' fitness levels.**

## Maturation

Physical maturation means becoming physically full grown and developed. It begins in earnest in your early teen years because of hormones that promote the growth and development of tissues such as muscle and bone. Some people mature earlier than others, and early developers often do better on physical fitness tests than those who mature later. But ultimately time is the great equalizer. We all develop fully over time, and it is not unusual for late developers to achieve fitness levels that equal or exceed those who develop early.

## Age

Studies show that older teens perform better on fitness tests than younger teens. Even in the same class,

## FIT FACT

The amount of medicine prescribed for an illness is often referred to as a dose. Similarly, the amount of activity you need in order to get health benefits is sometimes referred to as an exercise prescription, or an Ex Rx (Ex for exercise and Rx for prescription), and it can be measured in doses. Up to a certain point, people who do more doses get more benefits, but, as with medicine, too many doses of activity can be harmful. To help yourself get just the right number of activity doses for good health and fitness, follow the FIT formula for each type (the last *T* in FITT) of physical activity.

those who are older typically do better than those who are younger. This difference results mostly from the fact that the older you are, the more you've grown and the more physically mature you're likely to be. As you learned earlier, age and maturation do not always parallel each other. However, sometimes one person matures earlier than another, and in such cases a younger but more physically mature person could have an advantage in performing physical fitness tests.

 Do not let what you cannot do interfere with what you can do.

—John Wooden, basketball coach

## Heredity

Heredity involves the characteristics we inherit from our parents, including the physical characteristics that influence how we perform on physical fitness tests. For example, some people have more fat cells than others because of heredity. Similarly, some people have more of the muscle fibers that help them run fast, whereas others have more of the muscle fibers that help them run a long time without fatigue. Each person's heredity enables better performance in some areas and makes it harder to perform well in others. Fortunately, fitness is composed of many different parts. Your heredity helps determine the parts of fitness in which you do well and the parts in which you may not do as well.

## Environment

Your fitness is also affected by environmental factors, such as where you live (city, suburbs, country), your school environment, and the (un)availability of places to play and do other types of physical activity. Even your social environment can affect your fitness, including the friends you choose. For example, people who live near parks and those who have active friends are typically more active than those who don't.

## FIT FACT

Teens who walk or ride a bicycle to school are more active overall than those who do not. Specifically, they get an average of 16 minutes more activity each day, and that difference in itself is more than 25 percent of the recommended amount of daily activity.

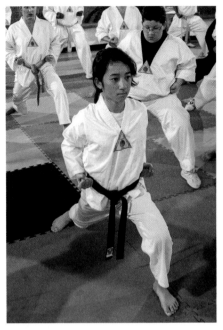

Find an activity that you enjoy and will be able to do later in life.

## Anyone Can Succeed

Because many factors contribute to physical fitness, it is possible for some people who do relatively little physical activity to achieve relatively good fitness scores while they are in their teens. These people probably matured early and inherited physical characteristics that help them do well on physical fitness tests. However, they may also be in danger of concluding that they don't need to do physical activity. This may be true enough if they care only about doing well on fitness tests while they're young, but it will not be true for a lifetime. As people get older, they can no longer gain a fitness advantage from early physical maturation or the energy of youth. Sooner or later, physical inactivity will catch up with even those who enjoy a hereditary advantage. Therefore, if you want lifetime fitness, health, and wellness, you need to perform regular physical activity and make healthy lifestyle choices.

Just as some people enjoy fitness advantages because of age, maturation, and heredity, others face disadvantages. For some people, even if they do physical activity, they still find it hard to get high fitness scores, and they may become discouraged. If you're one of these people, avoid comparing yourself with others. Try to achieve a good fitness rating rather than worrying about getting a high performance rating. Good fitness may be harder to achieve for some people than others, but all people can do it. In fact, studies show that people who are good at sports in school but do not remain active later in life are less healthy and die earlier than those who do regular activity throughout their lives—even if they were not especially good performers when they were young.

Anyone can do physical activity. And no matter who you are, physical activity is crucial to your fitness, health, and wellness. With regular physical activity, you can achieve a good fitness rating in all parts of fitness.

## Lesson Review

1. What are the four fitness ratings? How do they apply to your physical activity program?
2. What factors contribute to fitness?
3. How can a person attain good health and fitness even if he or she has factors that make it difficult to build a high level of fitness?

An activity log is a written account of your physical activities during a specified time. It's a way to keep track of what you do so that you can tell whether you're meeting your activity goals. Self-monitoring refers to any of a variety of techniques for keeping track of your behavior (for example, a log, diary, or step counter).

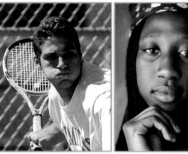

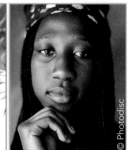

Mark enjoyed playing tennis on the weekends. He would start out full of energy, but he lacked the endurance to play well for a complete match. His instructor suggested that he do some daily activities to improve his endurance. For several weeks, Mark reported that he faithfully engaged in the activities. But Mark's instructor was a little skeptical based on his level of improvement. Finally, she suggested that Mark keep a log of all the times that he did the activities, and the results were eye opening: "Boy, was I surprised," said Mark. "I usually didn't spend as much time as I thought on each activity. I really thought I was doing well until I saw the results written down."

Erica's situation was different. She had knee surgery and was ordered to limit both the kinds and the amount of her activity and to follow a schedule of rehabilitation exercises. She was also supposed to elevate her leg whenever possible. Erica's leg was often swollen and sore at the end of the day, so her physical therapist suggested that she keep a daily log. Erica discovered that she was spending much more time on her feet than she had intended. As a result, she realized that she had to continue doing her rehabilitation exercises but curtail her other activities so that her knee could heal.

## For Discussion

How did keeping a log help Mark and Erica? What are some other ways in which a log might help someone? What other ways might Mark and Erica self-monitor their physical activity levels? Consider the guidelines presented in the following Self-Management feature as you answer these discussion questions.

One of the truths of human nature is that adults tend to underestimate how much they eat and overestimate how much physical activity they get. People also make other errors in estimating what they do. For example, we often underestimate how much television we watch and how much money we spend on nonessential items. One name for keeping track of what we do is "self-monitoring." We all self-monitor our behavior in informal ways, but sometimes it's necessary to make formal assessments if we want accuracy. You can self-monitor your behaviors to help you set goals and make plans—and to evaluate whether you're meeting your goals and fulfilling your plans. Self-monitoring of physical activity is sometimes referred to as "record keeping" or "keeping an activity log." Use the following guidelines to effectively monitor your physical activity.

- **Keep a written log.** Make a formal record of your physical activities by using an activity log or a computer program such as Activitygram.

- **Consider using an activity monitor.** Two examples are pedometers and heart rate watches. A pedometer counts the number of steps you take; it is typically worn on your belt or arm. A heart rate monitor uses a strap around your chest and a watchlike device on your wrist. Either of these devices gives you objective information that you can record in your activity log.

- **Record information as frequently as possible.** The longer you wait before you write down what you do, the more likely you are to make an error. Write

- things down as soon as possible after you do them.
- **Start by self-monitoring your current activity pattern.** To get an accurate picture of your activity level, monitor yourself for at least three days. At least one of the days should be a weekend day, since most people's activity pattern is different on weekends than on weekdays.
- **Use your current activity pattern to help you determine your goals and plans.** People who are already active can set higher goals than those who are less active (or just beginning).

- **Determine how much activity you do in each area of the Physical Activity Pyramid.** For each type of activity included in the pyramid, determine your frequency, intensity, and time (FIT).
- **Write down your goals and plans and keep records to see whether you fulfill them.** Putting your goals and plans in writing can help you self-monitor. Keep records to see whether you did what you planned to do. Keep a diary or an activity chart.

You can also use these guidelines to self-monitor other behaviors, such as your eating patterns.

 # ACADEMIC CONNECTION: Percentages

The term *percentage* is used to express a portion or part of a whole. The whole is 100 percent. In a group of 100 people, one person represents 1 percent of the whole group. As an example, we often describe the activity levels of teens and adults in terms of percentages. Among adults in the United States, 20 percent meet national activity guidelines (150 minutes a week) and 80 percent do not. The percentage of teens meeting national activity guidelines (60 minutes a day) is 29 percent; 71 percent of teens do not meet the goal. You can calculate the percentage of a group that meets a health standard by dividing the number of people in the group who meet the standard by the total number of people in the group.

Scores for the trunk lift test for one group of teens are presented in the following table. A score of nine or higher (shown in boldfaced type) is required to meet the good fitness standard for this test. To determine the percentage of teens meeting the good fitness standard for the trunk lift, count the number who met the standard and divide it by the total number of teens in the group. What percentage of teens in the group meet the good fitness standard?

### Distribution of Trunk Lift Test Scores for One Group

|   |   |   |   |   | 8 |   |    |    |    |
|---|---|---|---|---|---|---|----|----|----|
|   |   |   |   | 7 | 8 |   |    |    |    |
|   |   |   |   | 7 | 8 | 9 | 10 |    |    |
|   |   |   | 6 | 7 | 8 | 9 | 10 | 11 |    |
|   |   | 5 | 6 | 7 | 8 | 9 | 10 | 11 |    |
| 3 | 4 | 5 | 6 | 7 | 8 | 9 | 10 | 11 | 12 |
| 3 | 4 | 5 | 6 | 7 | 8 | 9 | 10 | 11 | 12 |

### Check Your Answers

40 percent (16 students met the standard, and there are 40 total students; 16 ÷ 40 = 0.40)

The Physical Activity Pyramid illustrates how much physical activity you need of different types in order to build fitness, health, and wellness. For example, you need to perform moderate physical activity (the first step of the pyramid) almost every day to get health benefits, whereas you need to perform muscle fitness activities only two or three times per week. The area *below* the pyramid represents inactivity or sedentary living. Aside from sleeping, you should minimize your daily sedentary time. A Physical Activity Pyramid circuit is an exercise circuit with stations that provide opportunities for you to **take action** by performing activities from each step of the Physical Activity Pyramid.

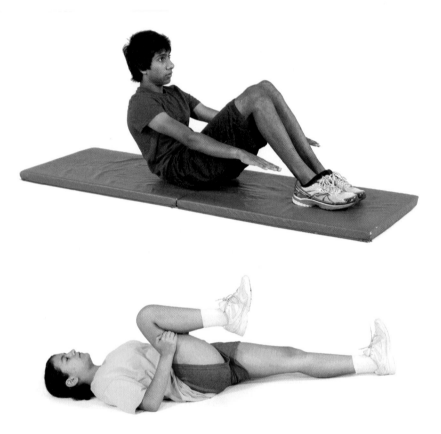

The Physical Activity Pyramid circuit includes activities from each step of the pyramid, including step 4 (muscle fitness) and step 5 (flexibility).

# CHAPTER REVIEW

## Reviewing Concepts and Vocabulary

As directed by your teacher, answer items 1 through 5 by correctly completing each sentence with a word or phrase.

1. The diagram with five steps that helps you understand the types of physical activity is called the _____.
2. The minimum amount of overload needed to achieve physical fitness is called the _____.
3. Age, maturation, _____, and the environment are factors that affect your physical fitness.
4. If you achieve a _____ fitness rating, you're probably at the level of fitness you need in order to live a full, healthy life.
5. The preferred standard used to rate fitness based on health is called a _____.

For items 6 through 10, as directed by your teacher, match each term in column 1 with the appropriate phrase in column 2.

6. target ceiling
7. intensity
8. progression
9. specificity
10. overload

a. how hard you perform physical activity
b. gradual increase of exercise
c. upper limit of your physical activity
d. performing more exercise than you normally do
e. exercising for one fitness part

For items 11 through 15, as directed by your teacher, respond to each statement or question.

11. What is the FITT formula, and what does each of the four letters mean?
12. Why should you develop a lifetime physical activity plan even if you're in the good fitness zone now?
13. Explain why your physical activity program should include activities from all steps of the Physical Activity Pyramid.
14. What are some guidelines for self-monitoring physical activity?
15. Explain why you shouldn't compare yourself with others when assessing fitness.

## Thinking Critically

A friend tells you that it's important for everyone to attain a high performance fitness rating. Your friend says that if a good rating is the goal, then a high performance rating must be even better. How would you respond? Write a paragraph to explain your answer.

## Project

Investigate places in your school and community that offer facilities and equipment for performing activities in the Physical Activity Pyramid. Compile a directory of places, their addresses and phone numbers, their websites, and their facilities and equipment. Distribute the directory to class members or post it on a website that other students can access.

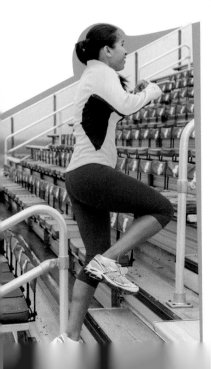

# 6

# Skill Learning and Injury Prevention

## In This Chapter

 **Student Web Resources**
www.fitnessforlife.org/student

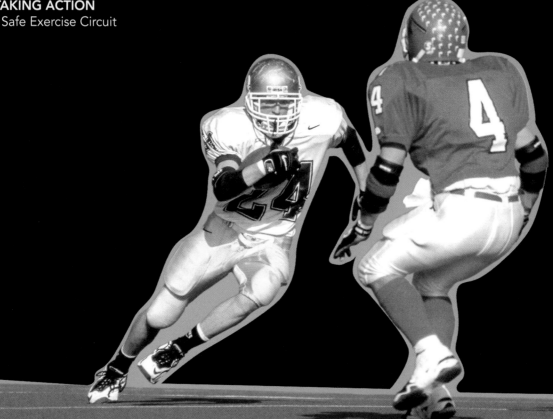

# Lesson 6.1

# Skills and Skill-Related Physical Fitness

## Lesson Objectives

After reading this lesson, you should be able to

1. describe the five parts of skill-related fitness and give examples of each,
2. describe the factors that influence skill-related fitness and explain how to build a skill-related fitness profile,
3. define *motor skill* and describe the factors that influence it, and
4. define *teamwork* and *leadership* and describe some guidelines for building these skills.

## Lesson Vocabulary

agility, balance, coordination, feedback, leadership, motor unit, reaction time, skill, skill-related physical fitness, speed, teamwork

**Do** you have good skill-related physical fitness? Do you have good skills? Do you know the difference between skill-related fitness and skills? In this lesson, you will learn more about skill-related fitness and skills.

## Skill-Related Fitness

You already know that physical fitness is divided into two categories: health-related physical fitness and **skill-related physical fitness**. Health-related fitness is considered the most important because it helps you maintain good health and wellness and perform well in physical activities. Skill-related fitness refers to a group of basic abilities that helps you perform well in sports and activities requiring certain physical skills. These are the five parts of skill-related fitness:

- **Agility:** The ability to change the position of the body quickly and control your body's movements
- **Balance:** The ability to keep an upright posture while standing still or moving
- **Coordination:** The ability to use your senses together with your body parts or to use two or more body parts together
- **Reaction time:** The amount of time it takes you to move once you recognize the need to act

- **Speed:** The ability to perform a movement or cover a distance in a short time

A **skill** is a capability for doing a task that is acquired through knowledge and practice. Skills are specific tasks that people perform. Skills such as those in sports and games are sometimes referred to as physical or motor skills (motor refers to muscles and nerves working together). Physical (or motor) skills include sport and recreational skills such as catching, throwing, swimming, and batting, as well as certain other skills (such as dancing). As you can see, skill-related fitness abilities and physical skills are not the same thing. The various parts of skill-related fitness help you learn particular skills, but they are not skills. If you have good skill-related fitness abilities—such as speed and agility—you'll be able to learn running skills used in football more

## FIT FACT

Power was formerly considered to be a part of skill-related fitness because it is important in sport and other physical activities. However, the U.S.-based Institute of Medicine now classifies power as a health-related part of fitness. Ultimately, all parts of fitness are important for both health and skill performance, but the link to health for teens is more established for the health-related parts of fitness than it is for the skill-related parts.

easily. Similarly, if you have good balance, you'll be able to learn gymnastics skills more easily. You'll learn more about skills later in this lesson.

Learning about your own skill-related fitness will help you determine which sports and lifetime activities will be easiest for you to learn and enjoy. Because people differ in their levels of each part of skill-related fitness, different people find success in different activities. In this lesson, you'll learn how to assess your skill-related fitness so that you can choose activities that match your abilities, work to improve your abilities, and find activities that you can enjoy for a lifetime. You'll also learn about skills and how to acquire them.

Factors affecting skill-related fitness include heredity, age, maturation, sex, and training. Figure 6.1 shows how these factors are related.

## Heredity

Skill-related fitness abilities are influenced by heredity. For example, some people are able to run fast or react quickly because they inherited these traits from their parents. A person who did not inherit these tendencies may have more difficulty performing well on skill-related fitness tests. However, it is still possible for such a person to improve his or her skill-related fitness by using special training techniques (discussed a bit later). In addition, lack of inherited ability can sometimes be made up for by desire and motivation.

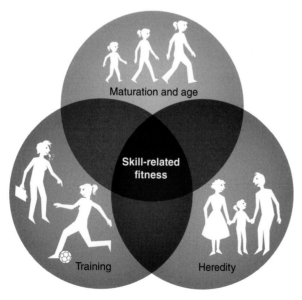

**FIGURE 6.1** Various factors influence skill-related fitness.

## Maturation and Age

In general, teens who mature early perform better on skill-related fitness tests than those who mature later. Because older teens in the same grade or on the same team are typically more mature, they also often have an advantage in skill-related fitness. Late-maturing teens typically catch up as they grow older.

## Training

It has long been thought that changing one's skill-related fitness is hard to do. Because of heredity, this is somewhat true. But recent research has shown that with the right kind of training, you can improve your skill-related fitness, though it takes considerable effort and strong motivation to do so.

# The Principle of Specificity

Skill-related fitness is also subject to the principle of specificity. Excelling in one part of skill-related fitness does not mean that you will excel in another. This is often true even when abilities seem closely related, such as reaction time and speed. For example, you might have great speed, meaning you can run fast, but lack good reaction time and thus be unable to get a good start. Apply the principle of specificity to choose a sport or activity that requires the specific skill-related fitness abilities you perform best.

The principle of specificity also tells you that you get what you train for. So if you want to build a specific part of skill-related fitness, train specifically for it.

# Assessing Skill-Related Fitness

If you want to learn a lifetime sport or physical activity, a good first step is to assess your skill-related fitness abilities. Doing so helps you to determine your strengths and weaknesses. Self-assessments have two other benefits. They help you choose activities that can improve your skill-related fitness and they help you match your abilities to activities in which you have the greatest chance of success. As you perform the skill-related fitness assessments presented in this chapter, remember that skill-related fitness has many subparts. For example, coordination is a skill-related

## ♥ FITNESS TECHNOLOGY: Motion Analysis Systems

Many technological advances have helped people become more skilled at a variety of sport activities. One of the most noteworthy is the use of motion analysis systems, which can be as simple as a basic video camera and playback system or as complicated as a high-speed video camera and software that helps analyze whether a performer's movements (biomechanics) are efficient and effective. Whether simple or complex, a motion analysis system video-records a person performing a sport or activity. Next, a skill-learning expert, such as a sport pedagogist or coach, views the video and analyzes the performer's movements. For example, football players and coaches routinely review game footage together to look at defensive and offensive formations, as well as opponents' tactics. High-powered systems allow users to analyze the action in very slow motion and generate computer analysis to provide information that helps the performer make corrections. Motion analysis systems can be used for many kinds of activity (such as softball pitching and tennis) but are especially popular among golfers, who use the biomechanical feedback to improve their swings.

### Using Technology

Make a video of your performance of a motor skill. Analyze the performance using information you've learned from an instructor or from information gained in the Science in Action student activity.

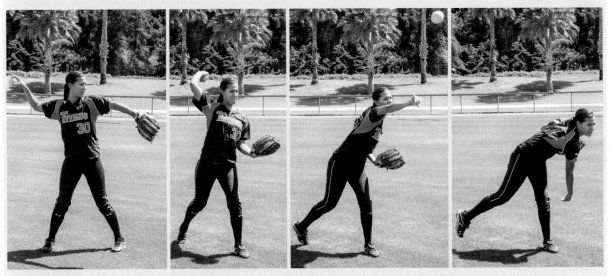

**Movement sequences can be studied to provide feedback for improved performance.**

ability that includes both eye–hand coordination (the ability to use your hands and eyes together, as in hitting a ball) and eye–foot coordination (the ability to use your eyes and feet together, as in kicking a ball). You may be good in one area but not as good in another. In addition to working on the areas that need improvement, you should consider selecting activities for your program that match your strengths.

Once you've assessed your skill-related fitness abilities, you can develop a profile of your results to help you select lifetime sports and other activities.

In this lesson, you'll learn both how to do that and how to make plans for becoming proficient in your chosen activities.

## Building a Skill-Related Fitness Profile

One student, Sue, did all of the skill-related physical fitness assessments presented in this chapter, then developed a profile for her skill-related fitness (see table 6.1). Sue's profile helped her identify her strengths and weaknesses, and she used her profile to develop her fitness program.

You can see that Sue has better ability in some parts of fitness than in others. One way she used her profile was to identify areas where she needed to improve her skill-related fitness. She used table 6.2 to choose activities that provided the most benefit for the parts of skill-related fitness that she wanted to improve. For example, Sue didn't do well in agility and balance, so she decided to take tai chi lessons to help her improve. She also didn't do well in reaction time and speed, but she realized that because of her heredity she probably would never be a really fast person with good reaction time. Still, she thought that tai chi might help her improve these abilities to some degree. She also decided not to worry if she wasn't as able as some other people in these parts of fitness.

The second way in which Sue can use her profile is to point her toward physical activities that are well suited to her abilities. Activities that provide the most benefit in a specific part of skill-related fitness also *require* the most fitness in that specific part. For example, Sue scored well in coordination, and bowling is excellent for building coordination, which means that it's also an activity in which a person with good coordination is likely to succeed.

Sue also decided to include bicycling in her activity program because it doesn't require high levels of skill-related fitness and therefore didn't require her to learn new skills. At the same time, bicycling does offer good health benefits.

You can develop your own skill-related fitness profile similar to the one Sue developed (refer back to table 6.1). Use your profile to determine which activities can help you improve where you need to and which activities you can most easily learn and enjoy.

# Physical or Motor Skills

To review, a skill is a capability for doing a task that is acquired through knowledge and practice. Physical skills are also referred to as motor skills because learning a skill requires you to use "motor units" in your body. A **motor unit** is made up of nerves that cause muscles to contract and the muscle fibers that do the contracting and thus cause movement. If motor units are used over and over again (as when you practice a skill), you learn to use the nerves and muscles to move efficiently and thus improve your skills.

## Skill Learning

The five parts of skill-related fitness are abilities that help you to learn physical skills. For this reason, factors that affect your skill-related fitness such as heredity, maturation, and age also affect your skill learning (see figure 6.1). However, the two factors that affect skill learning the most are knowledge and practice.

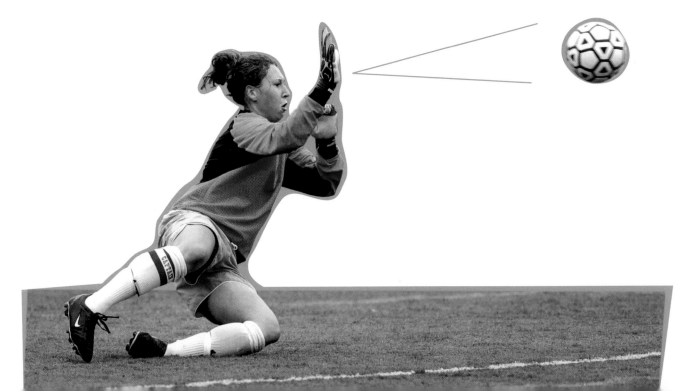

### TABLE 6.1   Sue's Skill-Related Fitness Profile

| Part of fitness | Low | Marginal | Good | High |
|---|---|---|---|---|
| | | | Skill-related performance rating | |
| Agility | ✔ | | | |
| Balance | | ✔ | | |
| Coordination | | | | ✔ |
| Speed | | ✔ | | |
| Reaction time | | ✔ | | |

### TABLE 6.2   Skill-Related Benefits of Sports and Other Activities

| Activity | Balance | Coordination | Reaction time | Agility | Speed |
|---|---|---|---|---|---|
| Badminton | Fair | Excellent | Good | Good | Good |
| Baseball | Good | Excellent | Excellent | Good | Good |
| Basketball | Good | Excellent | Excellent | Excellent | Good |
| Bicycling | Excellent | Fair | Fair | Fair | Fair |
| Bowling | Good | Excellent | Poor | Fair | Fair |
| Circuit training | Fair | Fair | Poor | Fair | Fair |
| Dance (aerobic or social) | Fair | Good | Fair | Good | Poor |
| Dance (ballet or modern) | Excellent | Excellent | Fair | Excellent | Poor |
| Fitness calisthenics | Fair | Fair | Poor | Good | Poor |
| Extreme sports | Good | Good | Excellent | Excellent | Good |
| Football | Good | Good | Excellent | Excellent | Excellent |
| Golf (walking) | Fair | Excellent | Poor | Fair | Poor |
| Gymnastics | Excellent | Excellent | Good | Excellent | Fair |
| Interval training | Fair | Fair | Poor | Poor | Fair |
| Jogging or walking | Poor | Poor | Poor | Poor | Poor |
| Martial arts | Good | Excellent | Excellent | Excellent | Excellent |
| Racquetball or handball | Fair | Excellent | Good | Excellent | Good |
| Rope jumping | Fair | Good | Fair | Good | Poor |
| Skating (ice or roller) | Excellent | Good | Fair | Good | Good |
| Skiing (cross-country) | Fair | Excellent | Poor | Good | Fair |
| Skiing (downhill) | Excellent | Excellent | Good | Excellent | Poor |
| Soccer | Fair | Excellent | Good | Excellent | Good |
| Softball (fastpitch) | Fair | Excellent | Excellent | Good | Good |
| Swimming (laps) | Poor | Good | Poor | Good | Poor |
| Tai chi | Excellent | Good | Fair | Excellent | Good |
| Tennis | Fair | Excellent | Good | Good | Good |
| Volleyball | Fair | Excellent | Good | Good | Fair |
| Weight training | Fair | Fair | Poor | Poor | Poor |

## Knowledge

Practice helps you to learn skills. But first you have to have basic information (knowledge) about how to perform skills and how best to practice. Throughout this book you will gain information about biomechanical principles that are important for skill learning. You will also learn how to practice properly. For example, the Science in Action feature in this lesson provides information about feedback, or information used to help you perform and practice properly.

## Practice

All people, regardless of their skill-related fitness, can learn skills with practice. However, it takes some people longer than others to learn skills, and some people will be better at performing skills than others. Not everyone can become an Olympic athlete, but with practice everyone can learn the basic skills necessary to enjoy some sports and

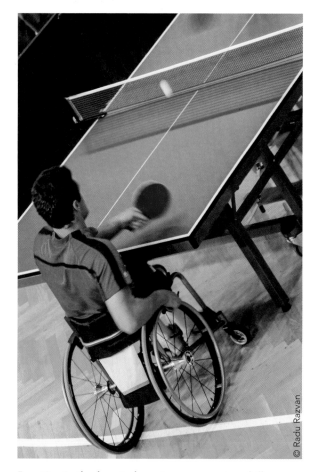

Practice is the key to learning new motor skills.

to perform physical tasks efficiently. Considerable evidence shows that people who are dedicated and willing to work hard can even overcome hereditary disadvantages and outperform people who have a hereditary advantage. The key is practice.

Practice involves repeating a skill over and over again. If you repeat a skill, such as a tennis serve, and do it correctly, you will become better at that skill. You'll learn more about skill development in this chapter's Taking Charge and Self-Management features.

## Three Stages of Skill Learning

When learning to perform a motor skill, you typically move through three stages. The first stage is called the *cognitive stage* because you have to think about what you're doing and apply knowledge to help you perform the skill. During this stage, movements are inefficient and typically slower than at later stages. Verbal feedback helps you to perform the skill properly. The second stage is called the *associative stage* because you begin to associate the knowledge of the skill with the actual movements. You still have to think about what you're doing, but skills start to become more automatic and your performance becomes more efficient and consistent. The final stage of skill learning is called the *autonomous stage* because you perform independent of cognitive control. (*Autonomous* is a word that refers to performing independently without outside control.) You do the movements automatically, and they are much more accurate and efficient.

Practice is the most important factor in skill learning, but practicing a skill *incorrectly* can be

## FIT FACT

Having too much feedback can cause "paralysis by analysis," a state of mind in which you can't focus on the few things that are really important. For example, if a softball batter is given too much information—keep your eyes level, keep your elbows up, stride straight forward, lead with your hips, keep your eye on the ball—she may swing and miss the ball entirely. Too much feedback all at once can be more harmful than helpful.

**SCIENCE IN ACTION: Feedback**

Motor learning is an area of study in the field of kinesiology. Experts in motor learning study the best ways to learn skills. One key to motor or skill learning is **feedback**. Feedback refers to information you receive about your performance that includes suggestions for making changes in order to perform better. Feedback helps you use practice effectively. One of the best forms of feedback is from experts such as teachers and coaches. After watching your performance, they can give you specific comments about how to improve. Another way to receive feedback is to watch a video recording of your performance. Motor learning experts suggest that when you practice, you use one piece of feedback at a time.

### Student Activity

Choose a skill used in one of the activities included in the Physical Activity Pyramid. Ask an expert to watch you perform the skill and give you feedback. Write down key points to remember when practicing the skill.

harmful to your skill learning because it may cause you to perform the skill incorrectly. Practice doesn't make perfect—*perfect practice* makes perfect. So it is crucial that you know both what to practice and how to practice it correctly. When first learning a skill (stage 1), you gain knowledge about the skill so that you know what to practice. You rely on cognitive information, including feedback from instructors (see the Science in Action feature). As you improve, you continue to refine your skills but focus more on repeating the skill rather than thinking about it. Even highly skilled athletes, who typically perform at the autonomous stage, practice regularly to keep their skills sharp and to make their performances more consistent and reliable.

> " The more I practice, the luckier I get. "
>
> —Gary Player, Hall of Fame golfer (and others)

## Teamwork and Leadership Skills

Performance in sport and other activities depends, of course, on motor skills. But teamwork and leadership skills are also important for success, especially in team sports. Team sports require team members to work together, follow the team leader, and play their designated roles so that the team can enjoy success. No team can succeed without good leaders, but even the best leader is ineffective without teammates who play other important roles.

**Leadership** involves motivating people in a group to work toward a common goal. **Teamwork** involves all team members striving to achieve that common goal through cooperative effort. Team members can play different roles in different situations, perhaps leading in one instance and following in another. This pattern is good because it allows all people to play a variety of roles and helps them enjoy their involvement. Here are some ways to learn and develop your leadership and teamwork skills.

- **Learning and accepting your role.** Listening to coaches and more experienced players can help you define the role that is best for you. Carrying out that role is the best way for you to help your team.

- **Sacrifice.** Success often depends on a team member's willingness to sacrifice personal gain for the benefit of the team.

- **Communication.** Part of being a good leader is being able to convey your ideas clearly—for example, communicating specific feedback to your teammates in a respectful manner. Being a good communicator also involves positive nonverbal communication, such as appearing upbeat instead of dejected after something bad happens. Another important part of communication is good listening, which can help you understand team goals and personal roles and thus exercise effective leadership.

- **Sensitivity.** Teams work best when all members are sensitive to each other's feelings and concerns. Ways to build sensitivity include listening (for example, hearing what others have to say rather than only telling others what to do) and communicating in nonthreatening language (for example, giving positive comments rather than harsh criticism).

- **Trust and respect.** Good leaders are respected because they can be trusted. They keep their promises and are sensitive to fellow team members' feelings. Good leaders communicate and interact effectively with all team members. Trust is built when everyone feels a part of the team.

- **Decision making.** Teams perform best when team members, especially leaders, use critical thinking skills to make good decisions. This can be demonstrated by explaining why decisions are made and how they will help the team.

- **Observation.** Good leaders learn by observing effective leaders and teams that use good teamwork. By observing, you can learn to identify the specific behaviors of good leaders.

- **Practice.** Leadership and teamwork skills are learned in the same way that motor skills are learned—with practice. The reason that team leaders are often older and more experienced is that their experiences have allowed them to practice and develop their leadership skills.

## Lesson Review

1. What are the five parts of skill-related fitness, and what are some examples of each part?
2. What factors influence skill-related fitness? How do you build a skill-related fitness profile?
3. What is a motor skill, and what factors influence motor skill?
4. What is involved in teamwork and leadership? What are some guidelines for building these skills?

You can assess your skill-related fitness abilities by using the following tests. Use tables 6.3 and 6.4 to get your ratings. Record your scores and ratings as directed by your teacher. Keep the following points in mind, especially if you score low.

- You can improve all parts of your skill-related fitness, but it is often harder to improve skill-related fitness abilities than health-related fitness abilities.

- Due to the principle of specificity, you may excel in some and do less well in others.

- Some activities, such as jogging, do not require a high level of skill-related fitness.

- You do not need to excel in skill-related fitness in order to enjoy physical activity.

If you're working with a partner, remember that self-assessment information is personal and considered confidential. It shouldn't be shared with others without the permission of the person being tested.

## Part 1: Side Shuttle (agility)

Use masking tape or another material to make five parallel lines 2 to 3 feet (61 to 91 centimeters) long on the floor; space the lines 3 feet apart. Have a partner count while you do the side shuttle. Then count while your partner does it.

1. Stand with the first line to your right. When your partner says "go," step to the right with the right foot, and then slide the left foot over to the right foot. Continue to step-slide until your right foot steps over the last line. Then reverse direction, stepping with the left foot and sliding with the right until your left foot steps over the first line.
   Caution: Do not cross your feet.

2. Repeat the exercise, moving from side to side as many times as possible in 10 seconds. Only one foot must cross the last line.

3. When your partner says "stop," freeze in place until he or she counts your score. Score 1 point for each line you crossed in 10 seconds. Subtract 1 point for each time you crossed your feet.

4. Do the side shuttle twice and record the better of your two scores. Use table 6.3 to determine your rating. Record your rating.

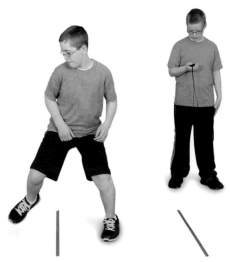

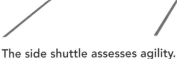

The side shuttle assesses agility.

# Part 2: Stick Balance (balance)

You may take one practice try before doing each test for a score.

## Test 1

1. Use a square stick (1.5 inches, or about 4 centimeters) that is 1 foot long (30 centimeters). Place the balls of both feet across a stick so that your heels are on the floor.

2. Lift your heels off the floor and maintain your balance on the stick for 15 seconds. Hold your arms out in front of you for balance. Once you begin, do not allow your heels to touch the floor (off of the stick) or your feet to move on the stick.

   Hint: Focus your eyes on a stationary object in front of you.

3. Try the test twice. Give yourself 2 points if you succeed on the first try but fail on the second, 1 point if you fail on the first try but succeed on the second, and 3 points if you succeed on both tries.

4. Record your scores.

## Test 2

1. Stand on the stick with either foot. Your foot should run the length of the stick.

2. Lift your other foot off the floor. First, balance for 10 seconds with your base foot flat. Then rise onto the ball of your base foot (with your heel off the stick) and continue balancing for 10 seconds.

   Hint: Balance on your dominant leg—the one you use to kick a ball.

3. Try the test twice. Give yourself 1 point if you balance flat-footed for 10 seconds, 1 point if you balance on the ball of your foot for 10 seconds, and another point if you successfully performed both trials. Your maximum score is 3 points.

4. Add the scores from both stick tests. Use table 6.3 to determine your rating.

5. Record your scores and rating.

The two stick balance tests assess balance.

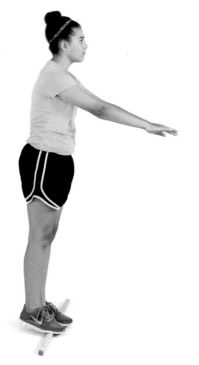
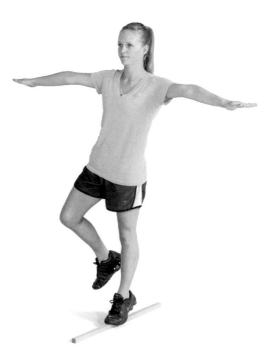

# Part 3: Wand Juggling (coordination)

1. Take three practice tries before doing this test for a score. Hold a stick in each hand. Have a partner place a third stick across the sticks held in your hands.

2. Using the two sticks you're holding, toss the third stick into the air so that it makes a half turn. Catch it with the sticks you're holding. The tossed stick should not hit your hands.

3. Do this test five times by tossing the stick to the right, then five times by tossing the stick to the left. Score 1 point for each successful catch.

   Hint: Absorb the shock of the catch by giving with the held sticks, as you might do when catching an egg or something breakable.

4. Record your results and use table 6.3 to determine your rating. Record your rating.

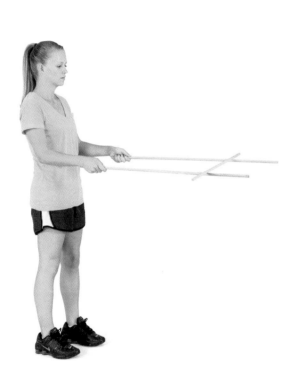

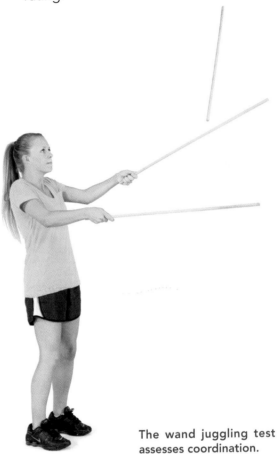

The wand juggling test assesses coordination.

## TABLE 6.3 Rating Chart: Agility, Balance, and Coordination

| | Side shuttle | | Stick balance | Wand juggling |
|---|---|---|---|---|
| | Male | Female | Male or female | Male or female |
| Excellent | ≥31 | ≥28 | 6 | 9 or 10 |
| Good | 26–30 | 24–27 | 5 | 7 or 8 |
| Fair | 19–25 | 15–23 | 3 or 4 | 4–6 |
| Poor | ≤18 | ≤14 | ≤2 | ≤3 |

# Part 4: Stick Drop (reaction time)

1. Have a partner hold the top of a yardstick (or meter stick) with his or her thumb and index finger between the 1-inch (2.5-centimeter) mark and the end of the stick.

2. Position the 24-inch (61-centimeter) mark on the stick between your thumb and fingers. Do not touch or grip the stick. Your arm should rest on the edge of a table with only your fingers over the edge.

3. When your partner drops the stick without warning, catch it as quickly as possible between your thumb and fingers.
   Hint: Focus on the stick, not your partner, and be very alert.

4. Try this test three times. Your score for each try is the number on the stick at the place where you catch it. Record your scores. Your partner should be careful

not to drop the stick after the same waiting period each time. In other words, you should not be able to guess when the stick will drop.

5. Use table 6.4 to determine your rating based on your middle score (the one between your lowest and highest scores). Record your rating.

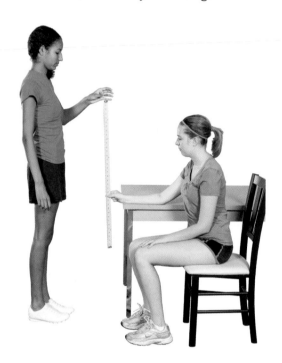

The stick drop test assesses reaction time.

# Part 5: Short Sprint (speed)

Use masking tape or other materials to make 10 lines on the floor that are 2 to 3 feet long (61 to 91 centimeters). The first line is a starting line; the second is 10 yards (9.1 meters) from the starting line. The remaining lines are 2 yards (1.8 meters) apart beginning after the 10-yard (9.1-meter) line for a total distance of 26 yards (23.8 meters). Work with a partner who will time you and blow a whistle to signal you to stop.

Try the test once for practice without being timed, then do it for a score.

1. Stand two or three steps behind the starting line.

2. When your partner says "go," run as far and as fast as you can. Your partner will start a stopwatch when you cross the starting line. Three seconds later, your partner will blow the whistle. When the whistle sounds, do not try to stop immediately, but do begin to slow down.

3. Your partner should mark where you were when the three-second whistle blew. Measure the distance to the nearest line. If you were more than halfway to a line, count that line when scoring. Your score is the distance you covered in the three seconds after crossing the starting

line. For example, if you cross five lines after the starting line plus 1 foot, your score is 18 yards because 1 foot is less than half the distance to the next line.

4. Record your score and use table 6.4 to determine your rating. Record your rating.

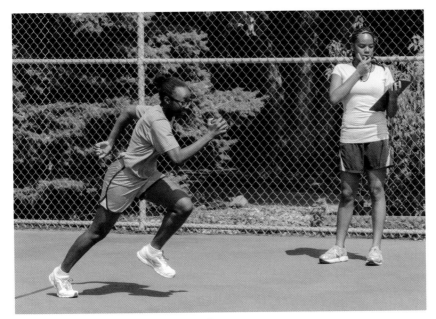

The short sprint test assesses speed.

### TABLE 6.4   Rating Chart: Reaction Time and Speed

| | Stick drop (inches) | Short sprint (yards run) | |
| --- | --- | --- | --- |
| | Male or female | Male | Female |
| Excellent | ≥22 | ≥24 | ≥22 |
| Good | 19–21 | 21–23 | 19–21 |
| Fair | 14–18 | 16–20 | 15–18 |
| Poor | ≤13 | ≤15 | ≤14 |

To convert inches to centimeters, multiply by 2.54. To convert yards to meters, multiply by 0.91.

The rating categories for skill-related physical fitness describe levels of performance ability, not health or wellness.

# Lesson 6.2
# Physical Activity and Injury

**Lesson Objectives**

After reading this lesson, you should be able to

1. list and describe some activity-related physical injuries,
2. list some guidelines for preventing injury during physical activity,
3. explain how to apply the RICE formula for treating physical injuries, and
4. identify types of risky exercise.

 **Lesson Vocabulary**

biomechanical principles, extension, flexion, ligament, microtrauma, overuse injury, RICE, side stitch, sprain, strain, tendon

**Would** you know what to do if you sprained your ankle? If you were performing a yoga pose that is risky, would you know it? At this point, you certainly know that physical activity provides many benefits for your health and wellness. But if you don't do it properly, you can injure yourself; fortunately, most injuries are minor and can be prevented by being careful.

Before you start a physical activity program, be sure you're prepared for exercise and know how to exercise safely. In this lesson, you'll learn about some common minor injuries, as well as some basic precautions you can take to avoid them. You'll also learn about some exercises that are considered too risky and about safer alternatives that you can use.

 ## Common Injuries

If you've ever suffered a sport- or exercise-related injury, you may already know that an injury can be quite painful even if it's not serious. Some of the more common minor injuries related to sport and exercise are sprains, strains, blisters, bruises, cuts, and scrapes. More serious but less common injuries include joint dislocation and bone fracture. The body parts injured most commonly in physical activity are the skin, feet, ankles, knees, and leg muscles (see figure 6.2). Parts less likely to be injured are the head, arms, trunk, and internal organs, such as the liver and kidneys.

One type of injury, called an **overuse injury**, occurs when you repeat a movement so much that your body suffers wear and tear. You're most likely

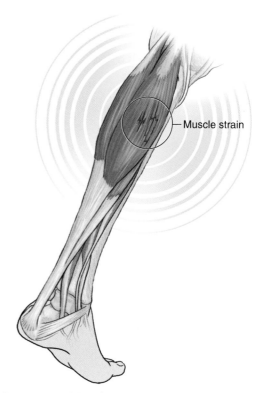

**FIGURE 6.2** Muscle strains are a common injury in sport and physical activity.

familiar with one very common overuse injury—a blister. Another example is shin splints, which involves soreness in the front of the lower leg. Small muscle tears or muscle spasms resulting from overuse are probably the cause. A third example, runner's heel, also involves soreness, in this case usually caused by running or jumping activities that require the heel to repeatedly hit the ground. These injuries are especially common among long-distance runners and other people whose activities involve repeated foot impact.

A **side stitch** is a pain in the side of the lower abdomen that people often experience when participating in a sport (especially running activities). No one is exactly sure what causes the side stitch, but one theory is a spasm in the diaphragm, the muscle tissue involved in breathing. Side stitches are most common among people who are not accustomed to vigorous activity. A side stitch is not really an injury, because the pain goes away if you stop the activity or continue at a more moderate pace. To help relieve a side stitch, press firmly at the point of the pain with your hand while bending forward or backward.

Another type of injury is called **microtrauma**. *Micro* means small—so small it may not show up on an X ray or exam—and *trauma* is another word for injury. So a microtrauma is an invisible injury. This injury often causes no immediate pain, but, with repeated use, symptoms of the damage eventually appear. Many adults today experience back problems, neck aches, and stiff or painful joints caused by microtrauma suffered when they were younger. Some risky exercises that can cause microtrauma are discussed later in this chapter.

## FIT FACT

Anabolic steroids are illegal supplements taken by some athletes, including some teens. People who take steroids are trying to enhance their performance but often end up experiencing the opposite effect. Steroids have been identified as a significant cause of injury to tendons and ligaments. Leading sports medicine doctors indicate that steroid use causes athletes to miss many games and can result in career-ending injury or serious health problems.

## Preventing Injury

Your body is made up of more than two hundred bones that connect at joints. Different kinds of joints allow different types of movement. For example, synovial joints allow free movement; they include hinge joints (such as your knees and elbows) that allow only **flexion** and **extension**, as well as ball

and socket joints (such as your hips and shoulders) that allow additional movements such as rotation. Cartilaginous joints (such as the vertebrae in your back) allow only limited movement. Fibrous joints are referred to as immoveable or fixed; examples are the joints where the bones of your skull connect.

When your muscles contract, they pull your tendons and make your bones move. Your bones act as levers to allow body movement. For example, contracting the muscles at the top of your upper arms (your biceps muscles) provides force that pulls on the tendons connecting to the bones (levers) of your lower arms, thus causing your elbows (hinge joints) to bend as shown in figure 6.3. When used properly, the levers of your body help you move efficiently, but when used incorrectly they can produce forces that cause injury to a joint or other body part.

Different types of injury can affect different types of tissue. A **sprain** is an injury to a ligament that typically results in swelling and pain around the joint. As illustrated in figure 6.4, **ligaments** are

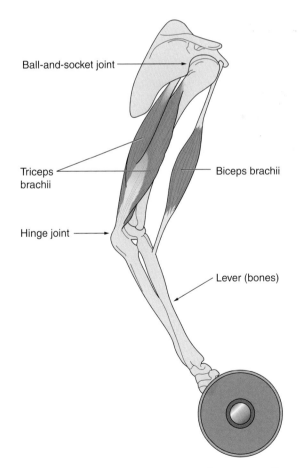

Ball-and-socket joint

Triceps brachii

Biceps brachii

Hinge joint

Lever (bones)

**FIGURE 6.3** Your bones act as levers to allow body movement.

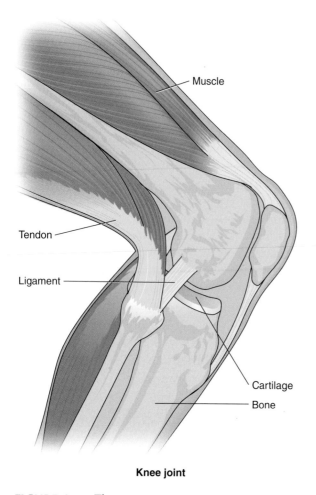

**Knee joint**

**FIGURE 6.4** These tissues are commonly injured.

- **Listen to your body.** Injury can occur when you ignore signs and symptoms that your body is giving you. If you experience pain, pay attention to it. Until you know what is causing the pain, slow your exercise or stop altogether. Most blisters and shin splints can be avoided if you listen to your body.

- **Be fit!** One of the best ways to avoid injury is to be physically fit. A person with a fit heart and lungs and long, strong muscles is less likely to be injured than one who is unfit. Proper physical activity builds total physical fitness, which helps you prevent injury.

- **Use moderation.** Overuse causes many minor injuries in physical activity. For example, about 40 percent of regular runners and 50 percent of aerobic dancers experience injury at some point, usually due to using a body part too intensely or for too long a time.

- **Dress properly.** Some injuries are caused by improper dress; for example, wearing poor shoes and socks can cause blisters or runner's heel. Make sure you dress properly, wear proper shoes, and replace them when they begin to wear down.

- **Avoid risky exercises.** Injury can be caused by certain exercises that violate the rules of biomechanics (see risky exercise descriptions later in this lesson).

tough tissues that hold your bones together. The other types of tissue you see in the figure are tendons, muscles, and bones; **tendons** connect muscles to bones. A **strain**, sometimes called a pulled muscle, is an injury to tendon or muscle resulting from tears in the tissues. Like sprains, strains often result in pain and swelling.

Experts in sports medicine have studied injuries that occur in a wide variety of activities, including all of those included in the Physical Activity Pyramid. They have developed the following guidelines to help you prevent injury.

- **Start slowly.** Injuries are more common among beginners. If you haven't been exercising regularly, follow the principle of progression: start slowly, then gradually build up to more vigorous activity.

## FIT FACT

People who are just beginning a physical activity program sometimes get a type of soreness called delayed onset muscle soreness (DOMS). This soreness occurs 24 to 48 hours after a vigorous workout, such as a sport practice. DOMS is caused by microscopic muscle tears. Unlike microtrauma, these tears do not cause permanent damage. To avoid DOMS, progress gradually when you begin an exercise program. It is okay to continue to exercise when you're sore, but if pain persists or is sharp rather than general in nature, stop exercising and seek medical advice.

## Simple Treatment of Minor Injuries

When injury occurs, it is often necessary to seek medical help. However, you can take immediate steps to reduce pain and prevent complications—if you know basic first aid and thus can take the right steps. For muscle strains, sprains, and bruises, which are common in sport and other activities, you can follow the **RICE** formula. Each letter in the formula represents a step taken to treat a minor injury:

- **R is for rest.** After first aid has been given, the injured body part should be immobilized for two or three days to prevent further injury. The length of rest depends on the severity of the injury and the response to treatment.

- **I is for ice.** A body part that has been sprained or strained should be immersed in cold water or covered with ice that is wrapped in a towel or placed in a plastic bag. Icing for 20 minutes immediately after injury helps reduce swelling and pain. Apply ice or cold several times a day for one to three days. To relieve the pain of shin splints, apply the ice bag and towel to the front of your leg until the pain subsides (no longer than 20 minutes at a time).

- **C is for compression.** Use an elastic bandage to wrap the injured area in order to help limit swelling. For a sprained ankle, keep the shoe laced and the sock on the foot until compression can be applied with a bandage (the shoe and sock compress the injury). To avoid restricting blood flow, remove the bandage for a few minutes or loosen it if you feel throbbing or it feels too tight.

- **E is for elevation.** Raise the injured body part above the level of your heart to help reduce swelling.

> " The more injuries you get, the smarter you get. "
>
> —Mikhail Baryshnikov, professional dancer

## Risky Exercises

Biomechanics experts who study the body's levers and tissues have developed several rules to help you avoid improper movement and therefore prevent injury.

1. Avoid movements that stretch your ligaments.

2. Avoid movements that twist your joints or force them to move in other ways for which they were not designed.

3. Avoid movements that use your body's levers improperly.

4. Balance your muscle development on both sides of your joints so that all of your muscles develop properly. For example, look back at figure 6.3, which shows the muscles of the upper arm. If you overdevelop your biceps muscle with no attention to your triceps, you may eventually become unable to fully extend your arm (your triceps may not be strong enough). You also increase your risk of straining your triceps muscle because this weak muscle will be overstressed by the pull of the stronger biceps.

Some exercises are considered risky because they cause your body to move in ways that violate these rules and basic **biomechanical principles**. Doing these exercises may not cause immediate injury and pain, but if you do them repeatedly they put you at risk for microtrauma. They can result in pain, joint problems, wear-and-tear injuries such as inflammation of tendons and bursas (cushioning tissues in your joints), and wearing away of joint cartilage. Over time, microtrauma caused by risky exercise can result in crippling arthritis or back and neck pain—a leading medical complaint in the United States.

Generally speaking, you should avoid the following exercises (you'll perform some safe substitutes in the Taking Action section). Of course, some athletes may find it impossible to avoid all potentially harmful exercises. For example, gymnasts must perform stunts that require back arching, and softball and baseball catchers must do full squats. These athletes do extra flexibility and strength exercises to prepare their bodies for these activities; in addition, if pain occurs when exercising, they should get medical help immediately.

## Hyperflexion Exercises to Avoid

*Hyper* means too much, and *flexion* means bending at the joint. Hyperflexion exercises cause you to use joints in ways that they are not intended to be used; specifically, they violate rules 1 and 2 because they bend your joints too far and overstretch your ligaments. For example, deep knee bends involve hyperflexion of the knee (figure 6.5). Other hyperflexing exercises to avoid include duckwalks, bicycles (also called shoulder stands), yoga ploughs, sit-ups with the hands behind the neck, and knee pull-downs. Some safer alternatives include the curl-up with the hands across the chest, the half squat, and the hip and thigh stretch.

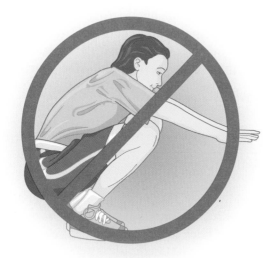

**FIGURE 6.5** Avoid hyperflexion exercises, such as deep knee bends.

## Hyperextension Exercises to Avoid

Hyperextension is the opposite of hyperflexion. As mentioned earlier, *hyper* means too much. *Extension* means increasing the angle of the bones at a joint. So *hyperextension* means increasing the angle of the joint too much. For example, having some curve in the back is normal, but arching the lower back more than normal involves hyperextension. Exercises that create hyperextension violate rules 2 and 3 because they cause joints such as the vertebrae to move in ways for which they are not intended and because they cause the levers of the body to apply force inappropriately.

Some back arching exercises tend to stretch your abdominal muscles and can injure your spinal discs and joints. These exercises also violate rule 4 because they may shorten your back muscles, which are already too short in most people. Particular caution should be used by people with swayback, weak abdominal muscles, a protruding abdomen, or back problems. (You can learn more about swayback and other back problems in the chapter titled Muscle Fitness Applications.) Risky hyperextension exercises include straight-leg sit-ups, back bends (figure 6.6), rocking horses, cobras, prone swan positions, excessive upper back lifts, and incorrect weightlifting positions in which the back is arched. Safe alternatives include the curl-up, knee-to-nose touch, and the hip and thigh stretch. Some other exercises that hyperextend the spine are neck hyperextensions, neck circling to the rear (figure 6.7),

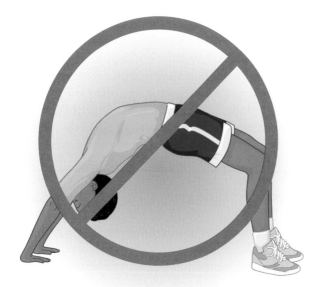

**FIGURE 6.6** Avoid hyperextension exercises, such as back bends.

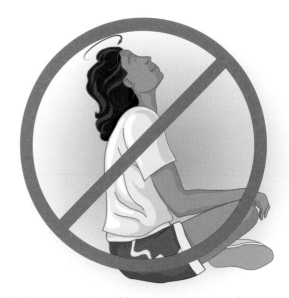

**FIGURE 6.7** Avoid hyperextension and exercises that cause friction, such as neck circling to the rear.

rear double-leg lifts, donkey kicks, landing from a jump with the back arched, wrestler's bridges, and backward trunk circling.

## Joint-Twisting, Compression, and Friction Exercises to Avoid

Some exercises cause the joints to twist excessively (such as standing windmill toe touches and heroes). Others cause compression at the joints or cause certain structures to rub against each other, creating friction that results in wear and tear. Examples of exercises in this category are hurdle sits, heroes (figure 6.8), double-leg lifts, sit-ups with the hands behind the head, standing straight-leg toe touches, and arm circling with the palms down. Safe alternatives include the back-saver hamstring stretch, the reverse curl, the curl-up, knee-to-nose touch, and the hip and thigh stretch.

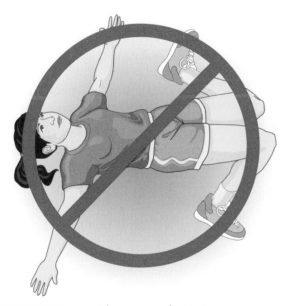

**FIGURE 6.8** Avoid exercises that twist or compress your joints, such as heroes.

## Improper Strengthening or Stretching Exercises

Some exercises can result in muscle imbalance (thus violating rule 4) because they build muscles that are not especially in need of development rather than muscles that are needed for good health and wellness. These exercises are not risky but are still poor choices. For example, forward arm circling develops already-strong pectorals, but backward arm circling with your palms up is a better choice because it

works on the weaker back muscles. Other improper exercises strengthen the already-too-strong muscles that go across the front of your hip joints. These exercises can cause disc injury, abdominal tears, tendon tears, and loose ligaments. Examples of this type of risky exercise include straight-leg sit-ups and double-leg lifts (figure 6.9). Safe alternatives include the curl-up and the reverse curl.

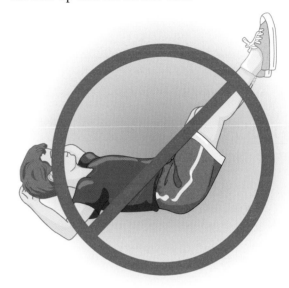

**FIGURE 6.9** Avoid exercises that strengthen muscles that may already be too strong, such as the double-leg lift.

# Concussions and Other Sport Injuries

Sports medicine is a branch of medical science. Sports medicine experts study injuries in sport to help people take steps to prevent them. One serious sport injury is concussion, a brain injury that occurs when a blow to the head causes the brain to crash into the bones of the skull. Concussions range in severity from mild to severe. A mild concussion may result in dizziness and confusion. A more severe concussion can cause you to pass out; it can also result in temporary or long-term loss of functions such as speaking and moving your muscles and cause other severe symptoms. Fortunately, most sport-related concussions are not severe, and symptoms usually disappear within hours or days. However, having one concussion increases the risk of having another. Repeated blows or jolts to the head can cause cumulative damage even when a concussion is not present.

## 👥 CONSUMER CORNER: Putting Technology Into Action

Advances in technology have limited the amount of physical activity that many people get each day. Often, they get screen time instead. At the same time, however, technological advances have produced wonderful tools for use in almost every part of our lives, and some of these tools can help you implement the Fitness for Life program.

You can use software (sometimes called applications or "apps") for smartphones, tablets, and computers to help you achieve the objectives of the Fitness for Life program. You can also access exercise video clips to see how to perform exercises properly. And you can use devices such as pedometers, accelerometers, and heart rate monitors to help with your self-assessment and self-monitoring.

If you decide to use one or more of these devices, consider the following consumer guidelines.

- **Apps.** Check the app to determine if it adheres to the exercise principles described in this book.

- **Exercise videos.** View the video. Check to see if it includes any risky exercises. Check to see if the video follows exercise principles described in this book.

- **Pedometers.** Check the accuracy of a pedometer with a simple walk test. Set the pedometer to zero, then walk and count exactly 100 steps. Check the pedometer to see if it counted 100 steps; an error of up to 3 steps in 100 is considered acceptable. You may also find that a pedometer counts more accurately in one location on your body than in another. Test the accuracy in different positions on your belt. If the unit does not count accurately in any position, try a different pedometer.

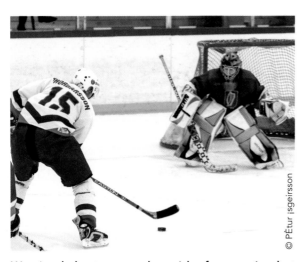

Wearing helmets can reduce risk of concussion but doesn't eliminate it.

Concussions are more prevalent in collision sports such as hockey and football, but they also occur in other sports, such as soccer and basketball. Examples include head-to-head or head-to-ball contact in soccer and falls and blows to the head in basketball. Repeated concussions increase a person's risk of suffering permanent damage. This is why boxers have a higher incidence of permanent damage than athletes in other sports. Sports medicine experts have developed guidelines for preventing concussions and for allowing athletes to return to action after a concussion.

### Lesson Review

1. What are some activity-related physical injuries, and what are the characteristics of the injuries?
2. What steps can you take to prevent injury during physical activity?
3. How can the RICE formula be used to treat physical injuries?
4. What are some types of risky exercise, and why are they considered risky?

To enjoy a physical activity, you must possess the specific skills needed for that particular sport or game. Performance skills such as kicking, throwing, hitting, and swimming can be learned by most people with practice. It does, however, take some people longer than others to learn skills. Here's an example.

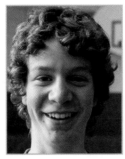

Zack felt that he was never really good at sports. He tried several activities and found that he was not as good at them as other people he knew. He even tried out for sport teams at school—first soccer, then swimming—but didn't make either one. His biggest problem was that he had not learned to play sports when he was young, and now he was behind others who had learned.

Zack wanted to learn a sport but was afraid that he'd be unsuccessful again and that his friends would laugh at him. He performed a self-assessment of his skill-related abilities and was surprised to find that he did pretty well on most of the assessments. He did especially well in coordination and agility, though his speed was not very high.

Before trying out for another team, Zack thought it would be best to try to learn the skills needed for a sport that matched his abilities. His size seemed to be an advantage—he was over 6 feet (1.8 meters) tall and weighed 180 pounds (82 kilograms)—but he wanted to get stronger, and he was not sure which sport would be best for him. He wanted to be on a team but also wanted to learn something that would be fun and interesting.

## For Discussion

What advice would you give Zack for choosing a sport? Once he makes his choices, what steps could he take to improve his performance skills? Who could he talk to for help? Zack knew that he needed to practice but wasn't sure exactly *what* to practice. What practice advice would you give him? Consider the guidelines presented in the Self-Management feature as you answer the discussion questions.

# SELF-MANAGEMENT: Skills for Improving Performance

Experts in sport pedagogy and motor learning have studied the best ways to learn sport skills. They have developed guidelines that can help you as you work to improve your skills.

- **Get good instruction.** If you learn a skill incorrectly, it will be hard to improve, even with practice. Good instructors provide feedback that you can use to correct errors and improve your performance.

- **Practice.** Good practice is the key to improving your skills. It involves repeated performance focused on correct technique. Good instruction helps you perform good practice. Many people do not like to practice skills—they just want to play the game. But just playing the game doesn't provide practice in a particular skill, and if you

play a game without the proper skills you often develop bad habits that hinder your success.

- **Practice all skills, not just those that you already do well.** Sport requires more than a few skills to become proficient. For example, basketball requires shooting, dribbling, passing, catching, and defensive skills. In order to succeed, you must practice all necessary skills.

- **At first, don't worry about details.** When you first learn a skill, concentrate on the skill as a whole. You can deal with the details after you learn the main skill. As you improve, concentrate on one detail at a time. If you try to concentrate on too many details at once, you may develop what is called "paralysis by analysis," a condition in which you analyze an activity and try to correct several problems all at once. For example, if you're learning the tennis serve, don't try to work on your ball toss, grip, backswing, and follow-through at the same time. Instead, practice the parts of the skill one at a time.

- **Avoid competing while learning a skill.** Although competition can be fun, competing while you're learning a skill is stressful and does not promote optimal learning. When you compete you only try skills that you are already good at, so you often don't make improvements in areas of need.

- **Think positively.** Experts have shown that if you think negatively, you're likely to perform poorly. But if you think positively while you practice, you'll learn

faster and become more confident in your abilities.

- **Choose an activity that matches your skill-related fitness.** As you may recall, heredity can play a role in your sport success. Use the information in your self-assessment of skill-related fitness to help you select a sport in which you're most likely to succeed.

- **Consider mental practice.** Doing mental practice involves imagining that you're performing a skill. Research shows that practicing a skill mentally can improve your performance. You can do mental practice even when you can't do regular practice due to factors such as bad weather or lack of a suitable location or facility.

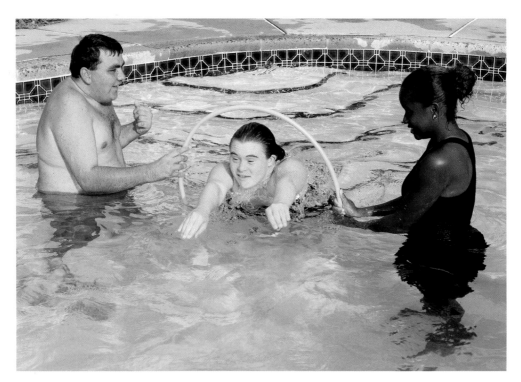

Good instruction and good practice can help you learn new skills.

You now know about risky exercises. Some safe substitutes were listed but not described in detail. You can **take action** by trying some of the safe exercises using a safe exercise circuit.

The exercises in the circuit are safe to perform and give you the benefits of risky exercises without the risk. Additional safe exercises are described throughout this book.

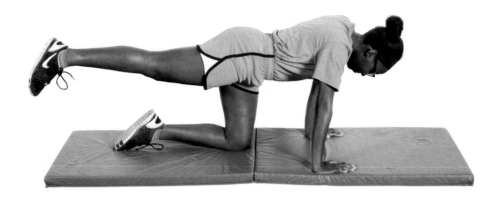

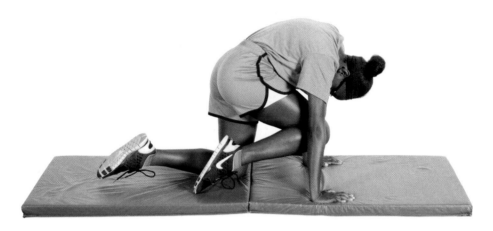

Take action by doing a safe exercise circuit that includes only safe alternatives to risky exercises.

# CHAPTER REVIEW

## Reviewing Concepts and Vocabulary

As directed by your teacher, answer items 1 through 5 by correctly completing each sentence with a word or phrase.

1. Fitness that improves your ability to learn skills is called _____.
2. Software programs used on smartphones to help with fitness are called _____.
3. Information you receive about your performance that helps you improve is called _____.
4. Invisible body damage caused by heavy repetition of a movement is called a _____.
5. Soreness that occurs 24 to 48 hours after a workout is called _____.

For items 6 through 10, as directed by your teacher, match each term in column 1 with the appropriate phrase in column 2.

6. joint
7. ligament
8. tendon
9. skills
10. practice

   a. connects muscle to bone
   b. repetition of a skill to aid improvement
   c. holds bones together at a joint
   d. catching, throwing
   e. place where bones connect

For items 11 through 15, as directed by your teacher, respond to each statement or question.

11. What are some ways to self-assess your skill-related physical fitness?
12. What is the difference between skill and skill-related physical fitness?
13. Explain how to follow the RICE formula when treating a minor injury.
14. Describe two risky exercises and explain why they are risky.
15. Describe several guidelines for effective skill learning.

## Thinking Critically

Write a paragraph to answer the following question.

You're about to begin an exercise program with a group of friends. The leader of your group has selected the exercises. How can you determine whether the exercises are safe?

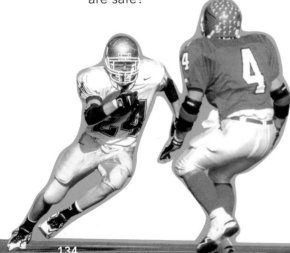

## Project

Look through some magazines for articles that feature exercises. Evaluate two exercises to determine whether you think they are safe. Report your findings to your class and discuss the criteria you used to make each evaluation.

# UNIT III

# Moderate and Vigorous Physical Activity

● ● ● ● ● ● ● ● ● ● ● ● ● ● ● ● ● ● ● ● ● ●

**Healthy People 2020 Goals**

- Increase the percentage of teens who meet aerobic activity guidelines.
- Increase overall cardiovascular health.
- Reduce the risk of heart disease and other chronic diseases.
- Increase education to promote health-enhancing behaviors and reduce health risks.
- Reduce the percentage of teens with high blood pressure and other health risks.
- Improve teens' understanding of health promotion and disease prevention.
- Reduce overweight and obesity among teens.
- Reduce sport and recreation injuries.
- Improve community facilities (such as parks) and environment (such as sidewalks).
- Increase physical education in schools.
- Increase the percentage of teens who do in-school and out-of-school activity.
- Improve health literacy and increase the number of high-quality health-related websites.

**Self-Assessment Features in This Unit**

- Walking Test
- Step Test and One-Mile Run Test
- Assessing Jogging Techniques

**Taking Charge Features in This Unit**

- Learning to Manage Time
- Self-Confidence
- Activity Participation

**Self-Management Features in This Unit**

- Skills for Managing Time
- Skills for Building Self-Confidence
- Skills for Choosing Good Activities

**Taking Action Features in This Unit**

- Your Moderate Physical Activity Plan
- Target Heart Rate Workouts
- Your Vigorous Physical Activity Plan

# 7

# Moderate Physical Activity

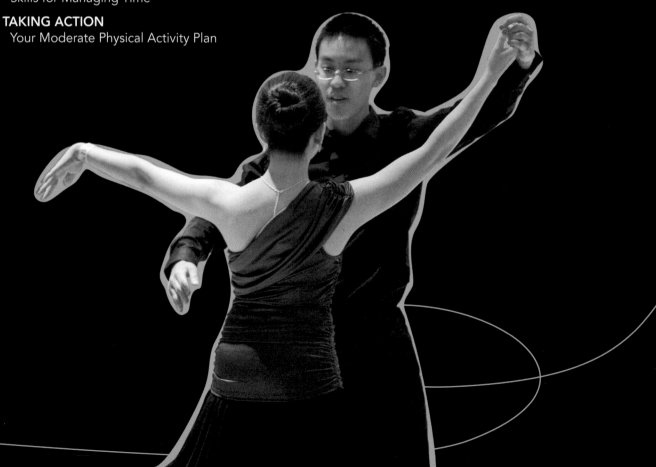

# Lesson 7.1
## Moderate Physical Activity Facts

**Lesson Objectives**

After reading this lesson, you should be able to

1. describe the meaning of the term *MET* and why it is important,
2. describe various types of moderate physical activity,
3. describe the FIT formula for moderate physical activity, and
4. describe several methods of self-monitoring moderate activity.

**Lesson Vocabulary**

accelerometer, lifestyle physical activity, metabolic equivalent (MET), moderate physical activity, pedometer

**Have** you ever wondered if you can be healthy without feeling pain and getting sweaty during exercise? Do you know the minimum amount of weekly physical activity you need for good health? While it's good to choose activities from each of the five steps of the Physical Activity Pyramid, public health scientists place a high priority on the first step—moderate physical activity. The reason is that moderate physical activities provide many of the health benefits described in this book. These activities are easy to do and can be performed by people of all ages and ability levels. They are sometimes referred to as the foundation of health-enhancing physical activity and thus are appropriately placed at the base of the Physical Activity Pyramid.

> " Walking is [our] best medicine. "
>
> —Hippocrates, Greek physician and originator of modern medicine

## What Are Moderate Physical Activities?

The term **metabolic equivalent (MET)** comes from the word *metabolism*, which refers to the amount of energy (oxygen) necessary to sustain life. You can use the abbreviated term *MET* to help you determine the intensity of any type of exercise. One MET represents the energy expended while sitting at rest. Physical activities are rated according to their MET value from very light to maximal. The harder the body works, the higher the MET level. For teens, activities requiring less than 2 METs are considered to be very light—for example, eating, reading, and using a computer. Activities that require 2 to 3.9 METs are considered to be light activities; examples include making a bed, washing dishes while standing, preparing food, and walking slowly. These activities are not intense enough to be considered as health-enhancing as those presented in the Physical Activity Pyramid (figure 7.1). However, as you've learned, research has shown that some activity is better than none, and performing light or very light activity does expend energy and thus helps you maintain a healthy weight.

### FIT FACT

The amount of energy (the number of METs) used in an activity depends in part on your fitness level. Fit people use fewer METs than unfit people use for the same activity.

**Moderate physical activity** requires you to use four to seven times as much energy as being sedentary (thus 4 to 7 METs). For most teens, a good example of moderate physical activity is brisk walking. Moderate physical activities are often divided into the following categories: **lifestyle physical activities** done as part of daily life (such as walking to school and doing yardwork or housework), moderate sports (such as bowling and golf), moderate

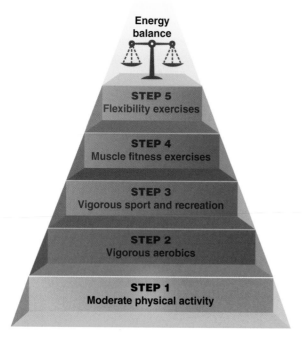

**FIGURE 7.1** Step 1 of the Physical Activity Pyramid, moderate physical activity, provides a foundation for all other activities.

as carpentry or landscaping). Table 7.1 presents examples in each of these categories along with the METs for each activity. Some of the activities can require more than 7 METs, and when they are performed at that level they are considered vigorous activities.

# Where Do You Get Energy for Moderate Physical Activities?

The human body uses three systems to provide energy for physical activity. For short bursts of very vigorous activity, such as sprinting (for 10 seconds or less), the body uses a high-energy fuel (ATP-PC) stored in the muscles to provide energy. This system is called the ATP-PC system. When the high-energy fuel is used up, a second system takes over. For vigorous activities that last between 11 seconds and about 90 seconds, such as running up and down a soccer field several times or lifting a heavy weight many times, the body uses the glycolytic system to provide energy. A carbohydrate called glucose is stored in the muscles and liver as glycogen, which provides energy to perform vigorous activity in this second system.

recreational activities (such as social dancing and biking slowly), and occupational activities (such

### TABLE 7.1   Moderate Physical Activities for Teens

| Activity type | Description | METs |
|---|---|---|
| Lifestyle activities | Walking (brisk) | 4.0–5.5 |
| | **Yardwork** | |
| | Wood chopping | 6.0–7.0 |
| | Push mower (hand) | 6.0–7.0 |
| | Push mower (power) | 4.0–5.0 |
| | Leaf raking | 3.0–4.0 |
| | Shoveling | 5.0–7.0 |
| | **Housework** | |
| | Floor mopping | 3.0–4.0 |
| | Cleaning (heavy) | 3.0–4.0 |
| Moderate sports | Bowling | 3.0–4.0 |
| | Golf (walking) | 3.5–4.5 |
| | Basketball (shooting only) | 4.0–5.0 |
| Moderate recreation | Bicycling (slow) | 3.0–5.0 |
| | Bicycling (brisk) | 5.0–7.0 |
| | Fishing (standing in water) | 3.5–4.5 |
| | Social dance | 3.0–6.0 |
| Occupational activities | Bricklaying | 3.5–4.5 |
| | Carpentry | 3.5–5.5 |
| | Heavy assembly work | 5.0–6.0 |

METs for people with low fitness will be higher than those shown in the table; likewise, they will be lower for people with high fitness.

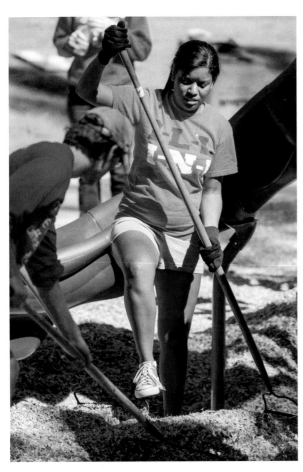

Many moderate activities are lifestyle activities, such as yardwork and housework.

For sustained activity of moderate intensity, such as brisk walking, the body uses the oxidative system (also called the aerobic system) to provide energy. This system allows you to perform activity for many minutes or even hours. Like the glycolytic system, this system uses glucose to provide energy. But since adequate oxygen is available to convert carbohydrate and fat in the body into glucose during moderate activity, the body does not have to rely primarily on glycogen (glucose) stored in the muscles and liver. More information about energy systems is available on the student section of the Fitness for Life website.

## Why Should I Do Moderate Physical Activities?

Experts used to think that in order to gain health benefits you had to do vigorous physical activity (using more than 7 METs). We now know that many health benefits can be achieved by doing moderate physical activity. Here's a summary of the benefits of moderate physical activity.

- Reduced risk of hypokinetic disease, such as heart disease, cancer, diabetes, and other chronic diseases
- Improved bone health
- Fitness benefits for people in the low and moderate fitness zones (whereas vigorous activity is required for fitness improvement in people in the good fitness and high performance zones)
- Healthy weight maintenance as a result of adequate energy expenditure
- Improved wellness and functional fitness, including feeling good, enjoying free time, and doing the things you want to do without undue fatigue
- Improved academic performance (such as improved mental performance resulting from physical activity done before taking a test)

## How Much Moderate Physical Activity Is Enough?

National physical activity guidelines in the United States recommend 60 minutes of daily activity for teens. Some of the recommended activity should be vigorous activity performed on at least three days a week, and some should be activity that promotes muscle fitness and bone building performed on at least two days a week. Moderate activity is recommended every day, and for most teens it will be the easiest way to meet the 60-minute recommendation. For adults, the recommendation is 150 minutes of moderate activity per week, which translates to 30 minutes per day on five days a week. For this reason, many experts recommend that teens get at least 30 minutes of moderate activity each day so that they develop the habit of meeting the adult activity guideline.

You need to be familiar with the FIT formulas for moderate physical activity for both teens and adults (see table 7.2). The teen guidelines apply, of course, while you're in school, and the adult guidelines will apply for the rest of your life after school.

# SCIENCE IN ACTION: Sedentary Living

Exercise physiologists have recently learned that extended periods of inactivity can be harmful to your health—the more time people spend sitting, the higher their rate of chronic disease. For this reason, scientists now refer to excessive sedentary living as the "sitting disease." One major reason for sitting among teens today is screen time (whether it be with a television, computer, smartphone, or other device). In fact, teens spend more time sitting now than in the past, and from age 12 to age 16 the amount of sitting and inactivity increases by more than 100 percent.

The danger posed by the sitting disease is the reason that the words "Avoid inactivity" are included under the first step of the Physical Activity Pyramid. Physical activity guidelines published by the Society of Health and Physical Educators (SHAPE America) indicate that youth should not go more than two hours without an activity break. Among adults, many companies now offer activity breaks to reduce sitting time, and some companies provide treadmills beside computers to encourage employees to move while working.

> **Student Activity**
>
> Keep track of the daily time you spend in front of a screen. Do you need to reduce your screen time? If so, how could this be done?

For teens, the goal is to accumulate at least 60 minutes each day, but more is better. Moderate activities can be combined with other activities from the pyramid to meet the goal. Experts now agree that it is best to get your 60 minutes in bouts or activity sessions lasting at least 10 minutes each. In other words, you could do six 10-minute bouts, three 20-minute bouts, two 30-minute bouts, or other combinations that total 60 minutes a day. Accumulating 60 minutes in bouts shorter than 10 minutes each is better than doing nothing, but it does not give you optimal benefits.

### TABLE 7.2    FIT Formulas for Health and Wellness Benefits From Moderate Physical Activity

| FIT formula | Threshold of training | Target zone |
|---|---|---|
| **Teens** | | |
| Frequency | Most days of the week | Daily |
| Intensity | 4 METs<br>Moderate activity equal in intensity to brisk walking | 4–7 METs<br>At least as intense as brisk walking but less intense than normal jogging |
| Time | 60 min of total activity, some of which should be moderate activity in bouts of ≥10 min* | 60 min to several hr of total activity, some of which should be in bouts of ≥10 min* |
| **Adults** | | |
| Frequency | Most days of the week | Daily or most days of the week |
| Intensity | 4 METs**<br>Moderate activity equal in intensity to brisk walking | 4–7 METs<br>At least as intense as brisk walking but less intense than normal jogging |
| Time | 30 min in bouts of ≥10 min*** | 30–60 min in bouts of ≥10 min*** |

*Using 30 of the 60 minutes on moderate activity would meet the teen and adult guidelines.

**Less fit adults may use activities of 3 to 4 METs.

***At least 150 minutes per week, spread over multiple days.

For adults, the recommendation is for 150 minutes per week because this amount provides many health benefits with a minimum of effort. As with teens, moderate exercise is best done on several days a week (see table 7.2) and in bouts of at least 10 minutes each. Doing more than 30 minutes at a time gives additional benefits and is recommended for maintaining a healthy weight and for achieving good fitness, health, and wellness. Adults can substitute 75 minutes per week of vigorous exercise for the 150 minutes of moderate activity; they can also meet the guidelines by combining moderate and vigorous activity.

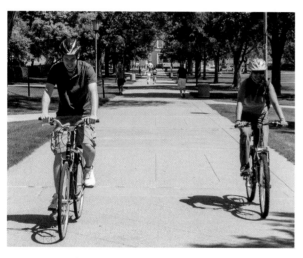

Recreational biking is an example of a moderate physical activity. It's one of many activities you can choose to accumulate your 60 minutes of daily physical activity.

## Counting Steps and Movement

Another way to determine how much moderate physical activity you perform is to count the steps you take each day. You can do so by using a pedometer (see the Fitness Technology feature), which automatically tracks your step count; the disadvantage is that a pedometer counts *all* steps that you take, regardless of whether they come in very light, light, or even vigorous activity. Still, wearing a pedometer can help you see how active you really are; you may have the opportunity to wear one in school. The American College of Sports Medicine states that moderate physical activity requires a step rate of 100 steps per minute.

For adults, some experts believe that taking 10,000 steps each day is necessary to be in the target zone for moderate physical activity. Other experts are concerned about this advice because you can reach 10,000 steps without doing any sustained activity (bouts of 10 minutes or more). On the other hand, some people can do 60 minutes of moderate activity each day and still not reach a 10,000-step count. Rather than setting an absolute daily step count, most experts recommend monitoring your activity for a full week and then determining your average daily step count. People who want to increase their activity level can then establish a realistic step goal that is 500 to 1,000 steps per day higher than their average step count. Once they reach this goal, they can, if desired, gradually increase their step count to higher levels.

Studies show that children average 12,500 steps a day (13,000 for boys and 12,000 for girls), whereas teens average 10,000 steps a day (11,000 for boys and 9,000 for girls). To meet the national physical activity guidelines of 60 minutes a day, most teens would require 12,000 steps. However, if you're just beginning, remember the principle of progression. Instead of starting with a high goal such as 12,000 steps per day, work gradually toward a realistic step goal.

## FIT FACT

On average, Americans of all ages take about 5,000 steps per day. This is considerably less than the averages in some other countries—for example, 9,000 or more in Australia and Switzerland and 7,000 or more in Japan—where obesity rates are much lower.

The President's Council on Fitness, Sports, and Nutrition offers the Presidential Active Lifestyle Award for people who do regular physical activity. Many types of physical activity can be used to earn the award, including moderate physical activity in which steps are counted with a pedometer.

You can also monitor moderate physical activity by means of other devices, such as an accelerometer (see the Fitness Technology feature) and a heart rate monitor. An accelerometer both counts your steps and gives you a better idea of your exercise intensity than a pedometer can. You can determine the distance you've walked by determining the length of your step (your stride length), then multiplying it by the number of steps you take.

## ♥ FITNESS TECHNOLOGY: Pedometers and Accelerometers

A **pedometer** is a small, battery-powered device that can be worn on your belt. It counts each step you take and displays the running count on a meter. You simply open the face of the pedometer or push a button to see how many steps you've taken. Some pedometers also contain a small computer that allows you to enter the length of your step (your stride length) and your body weight so that the computer can estimate the distance you walk and the number of calories you expend. More expensive pedometers can also track the total time you spend in activity during the day and the number of bouts of activity that you perform lasting 10 minutes or longer. Less expensive pedometers must be reset at the end of the day, but some more expensive ones can store steps for several days.

**Accelerometers** are similar to pedometers but measure physical activity in more detail. Specifically, accelerometers can record the *intensity* of your movements (for more about intensity, see the discussion of METs and recall the I in the FITT formula), as well as the amount of *time* (the first T in the FITT formula) you spend at

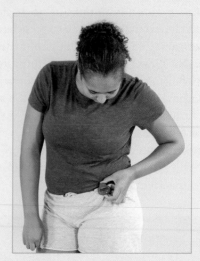

A pedometer counts steps and is a good way to self-monitor moderate activity.

different intensities. Like a pedometer, an accelerometer is worn on your belt and contains a small computer and a device (the accelerometer itself) that measures the intensity of your movements. Most accelerometers can count your steps taken per day and estimate the calories you expend in activity.

### Using Technology

Estimate the number of steps you take on a typical weekday and a typical weekend day. Then wear a pedometer to see how many steps you actually take (weekday and weekend day). See if you're as active as you think you are!

## Counting Physical Activity Calories

We know that moderate activity should be done according to the FIT formula summarized in table 7.2. Another way to determine whether you perform enough moderate activity is to count the calories you expend in activity. For example, a teen who weighs 150 pounds (68 kilograms) would expend 300 to 400 calories during 60 minutes of moderate activity, such as brisk walking. Therefore, this number of calories expended per day would be a good goal for moderate activity. You can learn more about counting calories in the chapter titled Choosing Nutritious Food.

### Lesson Review

1. What does the term *MET* mean, and how is it useful?
2. What are some types of moderate physical activity, and what benefits do they provide?
3. What is the FIT formula (in terms of the threshold of training and target zone) for gaining health and wellness benefits from moderate physical activity?
4. What are some methods of self-monitoring moderate activity?

Many of the self-assessments you perform in this course require very intense physical activity. If you're a very active person and are quite fit, the mile run or PACER may be the best way to estimate your cardiorespiratory endurance, but the walking test is also a good one. The test is especially good for people who are beginners, who haven't done a lot of recent activity, or who are regular walkers but do not regularly get more vigorous activity. The walk test is also good for older people and for those who cannot do running tests due to joint or muscle problems. As directed by your teacher, record your scores and fitness ratings for the walking test. You can then use the information in preparing your personal physical activity plan. If you're working with a partner, remember that self-assessment information is personal and considered confidential. It shouldn't be shared with others without the permission of the person being tested.

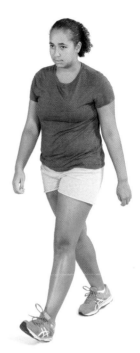

**The walking test is a good assessment for beginners or people who don't do a lot of vigorous activity.**

1. Walk a mile at a fast pace (as fast as you can go while keeping approximately the same pace for the entire walk).

2. Immediately after the walk, count your heartbeats for 15 seconds. Multiply the result by four to calculate your one-minute heart rate.

3. Use the appropriate chart to determine your walking rating. Locate your heart rate in the left column of the chart and your walking time along the bottom row. Find the point where the row and column intersect to determine your rating.

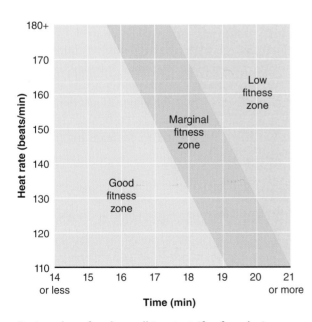

**Rating chart for the walking test (for females).**

Adapted from the *One Mile Walk Test* with permission of author James M. Rippe, M.D.

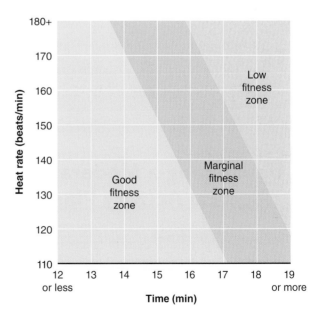

**Rating chart for the walking test (for males).**

Adapted from the *One Mile Walk Test* with permission of author James M. Rippe, M.D.

# Lesson 7.2

# Preparing a Moderate Physical Activity Plan

## Lesson Objectives

After reading this lesson, you should be able to

1. prepare a moderate physical activity plan using the five planning steps, and
2. carry out your moderate activity plan for several days.

 **Lesson Vocabulary**

calisthenics, habituate

---

**Have** you ever created your own fitness plan? Have you ever tracked your daily activities? In this lesson, you'll use the five steps of program planning to develop a moderate physical activity plan for yourself. You'll then carry out that plan. Implementing a good plan will help you meet national physical activity guidelines—both now and later in your life. The most popular physical activities among adults are moderate ones, including walking, biking, yardwork, and home **calisthenics**. If you establish the habit of doing moderate physical activity early in your life, you're more likely to be active as you grow older. And people who **habituate** to activity get multiple health benefits over the course of a lifetime.

> Walking is the best possible exercise. Habituate yourself to walk very fast.
>
> —Thomas Jefferson, U.S. president

## Developing a Moderate Physical Activity Plan

Javier used the five steps of program planning to prepare a moderate physical activity program. Because he created the plan as an assignment for his physical education class, it covered only two weeks. Later, he would get the opportunity to prepare a longer plan. Notice that in doing his planning, Javier used steps similar to those of the scientific method. You can prepare a similar plan.

## Step 1: Determine Your Personal Needs

To get started, Javier collected some basic information. First, he answered questions about his moderate physical activity levels in the past week. He also wrote down his fitness test results that related to moderate physical activity. He recorded his results in figure 7.2.

Javier had a good fitness rating for both the PACER and the walking test (see figure 7.2). He also met the national activity guideline of 60 minutes a day on three days of the previous week. His moderate activity included mostly walking to and from school (20 minutes each weekday) and riding his bike for 10 minutes two days a week (Tuesday and Thursday). He also performed 10 minutes of vigorous calisthenics (Tuesday, Thursday, and Saturday). On Saturday he played tennis in addition to his calisthenics. Still, his physical activity profile told him that if he wanted to meet national activity guidelines, he needed to increase his physical activity.

### FIT FACT

Walking, a moderate physical activity, is the most popular type of activity in the United States. More than 145 million adults report walking at least 10 minutes a day, most commonly for transportation, for fun, for exercise, or for walking the dog. People with a dog walk more frequently than people who don't have a dog.

| Physical fitness profile | | | |
|---|---|---|---|
| Fitness self-assessments | Score | Rating | |
| Walking test | Time: 15:00 Heart rate: 140 | Good fitness | |
| PACER | 41 laps | Good fitness | |
| Physical activity profile | | | |
| Day | Moderate activity (min) | All activity (min) | Met guideline |
| Mon. | 30 | 30 | |
| Tues. | 30 | 60 | ✔ |
| Wed. | 30 | 30 | |
| Thurs. | 30 | 60 | ✔ |
| Fri. | 30 | 60 | ✔ |
| Sat. | 30 | 30 | |
| Sun. | 0 | 0 | |

**FIGURE 7.2** Javier's physical activity and fitness profiles.

## Step 2: Consider Your Program Options

Javier looked at the list of moderate physical activities presented in table 7.1 and created a list of other moderate activities that were easily available to him.

**Lifestyle Activities**

- More walking in addition to walking to and from school
- Yardwork at home

**Moderate Sports**

- Bowling
- Shooting baskets

**Moderate Recreation**

- Fishing
- More bike riding

**Occupational or School Activity**

- Physical education class activities

## Step 3: Set Goals

Since two weeks was too short a time for setting long-term goals, Javier developed only short-term goals for his moderate physical activity plan; as a result, all of his goals were physical activity goals. He did this because he knew that activity goals (process goals) work best as short-term

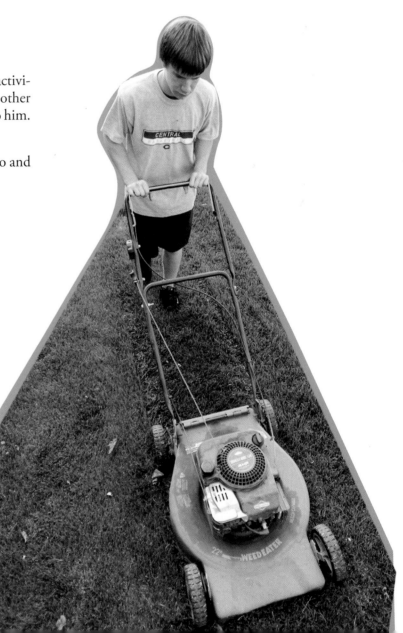

goals. He also knew that if he met his activity goals he would be making progress toward his fitness (product goals). Later, when he prepares a longer plan, he will develop long-term goals, including physical fitness goals. For these first two weeks, Javier decided to focus on moderate activity through the following goals.

1. Continue to perform the same activities that he has regularly been doing.

2. Walk to school and back three days a week (30 minutes each day).

3. Perform 30 minutes of moderate activity on three days each week in physical education class.

4. Rake the yard for 30 minutes on one day every two weeks.

5. Shoot baskets for 30 minutes two days a week.

6. Bike with friends for 30 minutes on two days a week.

7. Mow the neighbor's yard once every two weeks (60 minutes).

8. Go fishing one day a week (includes walking for 60 minutes).

9. Walk with family for 15 minutes on two days a week.

Javier remembered to use SMART goals. His goals listed *specific* activities and amounts of time because he wanted to be able to *measure* his progress. He also tried to make his goals challenging but *attainable* and *realistic*. Finally, he wanted his goals to be *timely*—just right for his life at this time and able to be achieved in the time allotted.

## Step 4: Structure Your Program and Write It Down

Javier's plan included at least the recommended 60 minutes of moderate physical activity on each day during the two-week period. On several days, he planned to do more than 60 minutes. As shown in figure 7.3, he wrote down the activities and the times when he planned to perform them.

| Week 1 | | | | Week 2 | | | |
|---|---|---|---|---|---|---|---|
| Day | Activity | Time | ✔ | Day | Activity | Time | ✔ |
| Mon. | Walk to school*<br>Walk home*<br>Shoot baskets | 7:45–7:55 a.m.<br>3:30–3:40 p.m.<br>3:45–4:15 p.m. | | Mon | Walk to school*<br>Walk home*<br>Shoot baskets | 7:45–7:55 a.m.<br>3:30–3:40 p.m.<br>3:45–4:15 p.m. | |
| Tues. | Walk to school*<br>PE class activity*<br>Walk home* | 7:45–7:55 a.m.<br>10:00–10:30 a.m.<br>3:30–3:40 p.m. | | Tues. | Walk to school*<br>PE class activity*<br>Walk home* | 7:45–7:55 a.m.<br>10:00–10:30 a.m.<br>3:30–3:40 p.m. | |
| Wed. | Walk to school*<br>Walk home*<br>Ride bike | 7:45–7:55 a.m.<br>3:30–3:45 p.m.<br>3:45–4:00 p.m. | | Wed. | Walk to school*<br>Walk home*<br>Ride bike | 7:45–7:55 a.m.<br>3:30–3:45 p.m.<br>3:45–4:00 p.m. | |
| Thurs. | Walk to school*<br>PE class activity*<br>Walk home* | 7:45–7:55 a.m.<br>10:00–10:30 a.m.<br>3:30–3:40 p.m. | | Thurs. | Walk to school<br>PE class activity*<br>Walk home* | 7:45–7:55 a.m.<br>10:00–10:30 a.m.<br>3:30–3:40 p.m. | |
| Fri. | Walk to school*<br>PE class activity*<br>Walk home* | 7:45–7:55 a.m.<br>10:00–10:30 a.m.<br>3:30–3:45 p.m. | | Fri. | Walk to school<br>PE class activity*<br>Walk home* | 7:45–7:55 a.m.<br>10:00–10:30 a.m.<br>3:30–3:40 p.m. | |
| Sat. | Mow the grass*<br>Ride bike | 9:00–9:30 a.m.<br>1:00–1:30 p.m. | | Sat. | Rake the yard*<br>Ride bike | 9:30–10:30 a.m.<br>1:00–1:30 p.m. | |
| Sun. | Bowling<br>Family walk | 2:30–3:30 p.m.<br>6:30–6:45 p.m. | | Sun. | Bowling<br>Family walk | 2:30–3:30 p.m.<br>6:30–6:45 p.m. | |

*Activities that Javier was already doing.

**FIGURE 7.3** Javier's two-week written program plan.

## FIT FACT

Canadian laws provide tax incentives for increasing regular physical activity. Families that enroll children and teens in youth activity programs get an income tax break, and people who buy bicycles get a reduction in sales tax.

## Step 5: Keep a Log and Evaluate Your Program

Over the next two weeks, Javier will self-monitor his activities and place a checkmark beside each activity he performs. At the end of two-week period, he'll evaluate his performance to see whether he met his goals. He can then use that evaluation to help him make another activity plan.

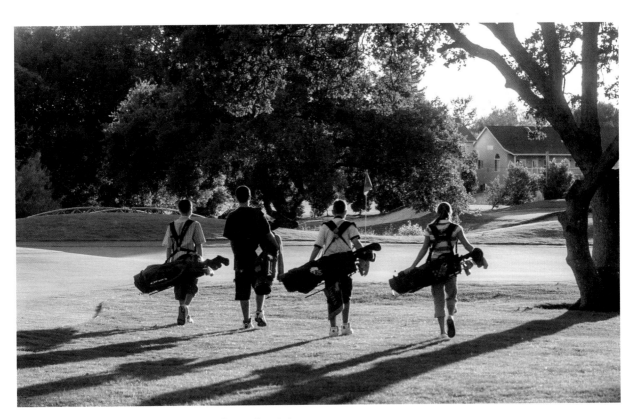

Golfing is a good form of moderate physical activity.

## Lesson Review

1. How do you use the five steps in planning to prepare a personal moderate physical activity plan?
2. How can you best implement your personal plan over a span of several days?

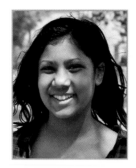

Why can some people always find time for an added activity while others barely have time to do their regularly scheduled activities? For a lot of people, the answer is time management. Good time managers know how to make the best use of their time. They efficiently control their daily schedule in order to complete their activities without wasting time. These people are more likely to find time for regular physical activity.

Here's an example of poor time management. Jennifer lives near some good cross-country ski trails. In the winter, her friends spend a few hours skiing every Monday and Wednesday after school; they also go skiing on weekends. Although they always ask her to join their fun, Jennifer usually refuses. Her common excuse is, "I just don't have the time. I really love skiing, but with three honors classes, homework, and my job at the mall, I barely have time to eat, let alone ski. I wish I could go with you, but I can't. It's impossible! I'll ski next year when my schedule is easier. Then I'll have more spare time."

Jennifer's friends are used to her excuses. In fact, she used many of the same ones last year. Her friends have the same classes and work hours that Jennifer has, but they complete their homework assignments and handle their jobs with time to spare. They do not understand why Jennifer can't manage to find the time to go skiing with them.

### For Discussion

What can Jennifer do to manage her time better so that she can do things with her friends? What can her friends do to help? What suggestions can you make to help anyone who would like to manage time better? Consider the time management strategies presented in this chapter's Self-Management feature when answering the discussion questions.

## SELF-MANAGEMENT: Skills for Managing Time

How many times do you hear yourself and others say, "I don't have the time"? It seems to be a common complaint. If you're one of those who seems to have too little time, how can you remedy the problem? Many experts believe that learning to manage time is a good solution. In this lesson, you'll learn how to manage your time so that you can be more active.

In 1900, the average person worked more than 60 hours a week. Now the average work-week is less than 40 hours. Similarly, in 1900, many young people were not enrolled in school and were already working long hours in factories and on farms. Now most teens are in school, and those who work limit their work hours.

Fewer working hours has made free time much more abundant now than it was years ago. But work and school aren't the only things that take time. Most of us make other time commitments when we aren't working or going to school. For example, you might have to care for a brother or sister, or you might have committed to a school or community activity such as a club, band, chorus, or sport team. And of course you also spend time on necessary activities such as eating, sleeping, dressing, and getting to and from school or work. The time you spend in all of these activities is called committed time.

Free time, on the other hand, is the time left over after accounting for your school and work time and your other committed time. Some people make so many commitments that they have very little free time. Often, people who say they don't have time for physical activity have not planned their time carefully. Active people manage their time effectively so that they can commit regularly to being active. If you're in the group of people who often say, "I don't have time," the following guidelines can help you.

- **Keep track of your time.** The best way to start managing your time more efficiently is to see what you're doing with it now. You can do this by keeping records (self-monitoring your use of time). Write down what you do during the course of each day. Record when you sleep, when you eat, when you're in school, when you're at work, and when you do all of the other things you do. You might use three categories: school and work, other committed time, and free time. Most people who keep records of their time use are surprised by the results. For example, some people who say they don't have time to exercise spend several hours a day watching television. Others find that they spend a lot of time doing nothing.

- **Analyze your use of time.** Once you've tracked your time for several days, review your records to see how many hours you spend in each of the three categories. You can also identify exactly how you spend your committed time and your free time. Doing so will help you decide whether you're using your time in the way you really want to use it.

- **Decide purposefully what to do with your time.** After you determine how much time you spend doing various activities, decide whether you're managing your time efficiently. Efficient time management enables you to do the things you think are most important. To decide what's most important to you, answer the following questions.
  - What activities did you spend more time on than you wanted to?
  - How much less time could you spend on each?
  - Are the activities you would like to change under your control?
  - What activities do you want to spend more time on?
  - How much more time would you like to spend on these activities?

- **Schedule your time.** After you decide how you would like to spend your time, create a schedule to ensure that you make time for the things you identified as most important. If you feel that regular physical activity is important, you will commit time to doing it. Plan a schedule for one day, making sure you have time to do the most important things.

Sometimes good scheduling allows you to do two things at once. For example, since you have to get to school somehow, what if you did so by walking or riding a bicycle? Thus you would be effectively committing that time to two different purposes. Similarly, if you join a sport team or activity club, the time you commit to that group is also committed to doing physical activity.

**TAKING ACTION: Your Moderate Physical Activity Plan**

Prepare a two-week moderate physical activity plan using the five steps described in this chapter. Like Javier, consider moderate activities from each activity category: lifestyle activity, moderate sports, moderate recreation, and occupational or school activity. The goal is to accumulate at least 60 minutes of activity each day, including a considerable portion that involves moderate activity. Prepare a written plan and carry out it over a two-week period. Your teacher may give you time in class to do some of the activities in your plan. Consider the following suggestions for **taking action** and building moderate activity into your plan.

- **Lifestyle activity.** Walk or bike to school. If driving, park away from your destination and walk the rest of the way. When you have a choice, take the stairs. Walk while talking on the phone. Work in the yard.
- **Moderate sports.** Consider bowling or shooting baskets with friends.
- **Moderate recreation.** Walk with friends at lunch or go for a walk in the park.
- **Occupational or school activity.** Do yardwork for pay, take an optional physical education class, participate in intramural activities, or start a walking club.

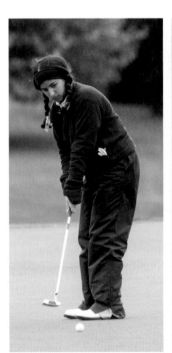 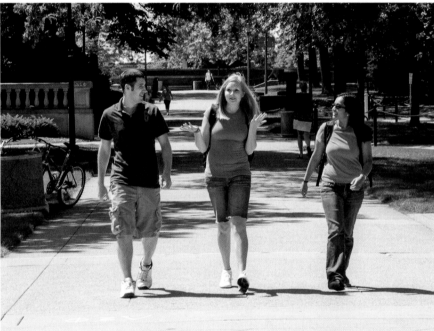

Lifestyle activities can be part of your plan for taking action.

## Reviewing Concepts and Vocabulary

As directed by your teacher, answer items 1 through 5 by correctly completing each sentence with a word or phrase.

1. Activity that is equivalent to brisk walking in intensity is considered to be _____ physical activity.
2. An activity done as part of daily life is called a/an _____ activity.
3. A device worn on your belt that counts steps is called a/an _____.
4. Intensity of activity can be expressed in units called _____.
5. Considering your program options is step _____ of the planning process.

For items 6 through 10, as directed by your teacher, match each term in column 1 with the appropriate word or phrase in column 2.

6. excessive inactivity      a. mopping
7. yardwork      b. carpentry
8. recreational activity      c. sitting disease
9. occupational work      d. bowling
10. housework      e. mowing

For items 11 through 15, as directed by your teacher, respond to each statement or question.

11. What does *sedentary* mean, and what can be done to reduce sedentary living among teens?
12. Describe several devices that can be used to self-monitor physical activity.
13. How much moderate physical activity is enough?
14. List and describe the five steps for planning a moderate physical activity program.
15. Describe several guidelines for managing time effectively.

## Thinking Critically

Write a paragraph to answer the following question.

Teens are often more vigorously active than adults. For this reason, some people say that teens should begin to do more moderate activity to increase their chance of staying active later in life. Do you think you will become more or less active as you grow older? What types of activity do you think you'll do as you grow older?

## Project

National polling groups regularly conduct surveys to learn people's opinions about various issues, including health and fitness. Assume that you work for a polling company. Develop a list of questions about moderate activity and ask at least six people to answer them. Try to interview people from different age groups. Analyze your results and prepare a brief news article reporting the results.

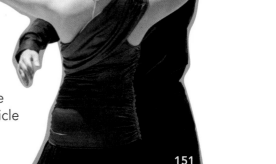

# 8

# Cardiorespiratory Endurance

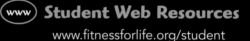 **Student Web Resources**
www.fitnessforlife.org/student

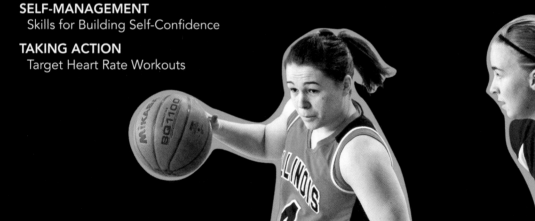

# Cardiorespiratory Endurance Facts

## Lesson Objectives

After reading this lesson, you should be able to

1. describe the health and wellness benefits of cardiorespiratory endurance;
2. explain how physical activity benefits the cardiovascular, respiratory, and muscle systems;
3. describe some methods for assessing your cardiorespiratory endurance; and
4. determine how much cardiorespiratory endurance is enough.

## Lesson Vocabulary

aerobic capacity, artery, cardiorespiratory endurance, cardiovascular system, cholesterol, fibrin, graded exercise test, high-density lipoprotein (HDL), lipoprotein, low-density lipoprotein (LDL), maximal oxygen uptake, respiratory system, vein

**Do** you have good cardiorespiratory endurance? Do you do enough regular vigorous physical activity to build good cardiorespiratory endurance? Of the 11 parts of fitness, cardiorespiratory endurance is the most important because it gives you many health and wellness benefits, including a chance for a longer life. In addition, the activity that you do to improve your cardiorespiratory endurance helps you look your best. As shown in figure 8.1, cardiorespiratory endurance requires fitness of your heart, lungs, blood, blood vessels, and muscles. In this lesson, you'll learn how proper physical activity improves your cardiorespiratory endurance. You'll also learn how to assess your cardiorespiratory endurance.

**Cardiorespiratory endurance** is the ability to exercise your entire body for a long time without stopping. It requires a strong heart, healthy lungs, and clear blood vessels to supply your large muscles with oxygen. Examples of activities that require good cardiorespiratory endurance are distance running, swimming, and cross-country skiing. Cardiorespiratory endurance is sometimes referred to by other names, including cardiovascular fitness, cardiovascular endurance, and cardiorespiratory fitness. The term *aerobic capacity* is also used to describe good cardiorespiratory function, but it is not exactly the same as cardiorespiratory endurance (see this chapter's Science in Action feature).

This book uses the term *cardiorespiratory endurance*. The first word in the term is *cardiorespiratory* because two vital systems are involved. Your

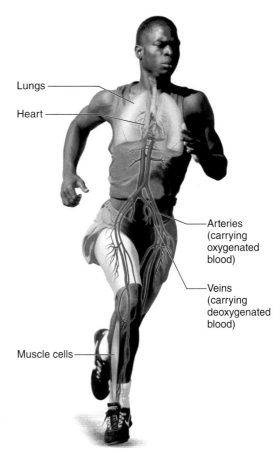

Lungs

Heart

Arteries (carrying oxygenated blood)

Veins (carrying deoxygenated blood)

Muscle cells

**FIGURE 8.1** Cardiorespiratory endurance requires fitness of many parts of the body, including heart, lungs, muscles, and blood vessels.

**cardiovascular system** is made up of your heart, blood vessels, and blood. Your **respiratory system** is made up of your lungs and the air passages that bring air, including oxygen, to your lungs from outside of your body. In your lungs, oxygen enters your blood, and carbon dioxide is eliminated. Your cardiovascular and respiratory systems work together to bring your muscle cells and other body cells the materials they need and to rid the cells of waste. Together, the two systems help you function both effectively (with the most benefits possible) and efficiently (with the least effort).

The second word in the term *cardiorespiratory endurance* refers to the ability to sustain effort. Together, then, these two words—*cardiorespiratory* and *endurance*—refer to the ability to sustain effort, which hinges on fitness of the cardiovascular (cardio) and respiratory systems.

# Benefits of Physical Activity and Cardiorespiratory Endurance

Doing regular physical activity can help you look better by controlling your weight, building your muscles, and helping you develop good posture. Regular physical activity also produces changes in your body's organs, such as making your heart muscle stronger and your blood vessels healthier. These changes improve your cardiorespiratory endurance and wellness and reduce your risk of hypokinetic diseases, especially heart disease and diabetes.

 Physical activity provides benefits for both your cardiovascular and respiratory systems. In this lesson, you'll learn how each part of these systems benefits and how all the parts work together to promote optimal functioning and good health.

## FIT FACT

In the early 1900s, medical doctors referred to an enlarged heart as the "athlete's heart" because athletes' hearts tend to be large, and enlarged hearts were associated with disease. By midcentury, research showed that the large heart muscle of a trained athlete was a sign of health, not disease.

## Heart

Because your heart is a muscle, it benefits from exercise and activities, such as jogging, swimming, and long-distance hiking. Your heart acts as a pump to deliver blood to cells throughout your body. When you do vigorous physical activity, your muscle cells need more oxygen and produce more waste products. Therefore, your heart must pump more blood to supply the additional oxygen and remove the additional waste. If your heart is unable to pump enough blood, your muscles will be less able to contract and will fatigue more quickly.

Your heart's capacity to pump blood is crucial when you're doing physical activity, especially for an extended length of time. Your heart has two ways to get more blood to your muscles—by beating faster and by sending more blood with each beat (this is called stroke volume).

Your resting heart rate is determined by counting the number of heartbeats per minute when you're relatively inactive. A person who does regular physical activity might have a resting heart rate of 55 to 60 beats per minute, whereas a person who does not exercise regularly might have a resting heart rate of 70 or more beats per minute. As a result, a very fit person's heart beats approximately 9.5 million fewer times each year than that of the average person. As you can see in figure 8.2, a fit person's heart works more efficiently by pumping more blood with fewer beats.

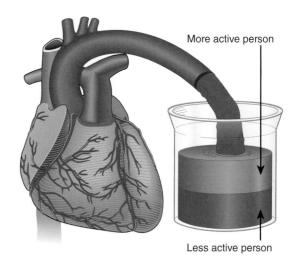

More active person

Less active person

**FIGURE 8.2** The heart muscle of a fit, active person pumps more blood per heartbeat than that of a less active person.

## Lungs

When you inhale, air enters the lungs, causing them to expand. In the lungs, oxygen is transferred from the air to the blood for transport to the tissues of the body. When you exhale, air leaves the lungs. The diaphragm (a band of muscular tissue located at the base of your lungs) and abdominal muscles (which help move the diaphragm) work to allow you to breathe in and out (figure 8.3a). Fit people can take in more air with each breath than unfit people because they have more efficient respiratory muscles. As shown in figure 8.3b, a fit person gets more air in the lungs with each breath and therefore can transport the same amount of air to the lungs in fewer breaths. Healthy lungs also have the capacity to easily transfer oxygen to the blood. Together healthy lungs and fit respiratory muscles contribute to good cardiorespiratory endurance.

## Blood

Although your body needs a certain amount of fat, excessive amounts trigger formation of fatty deposits along your artery walls. **Cholesterol**—a waxy, fat-like substance found in meat, dairy products, and egg yolk—can be dangerous because high levels can build up in your body without your noticing it.

Cholesterol is carried through your bloodstream by particles called **lipoproteins**. One kind, **low-density lipoprotein (LDL)**, is often referred to as "bad cholesterol" because it carries cholesterol that is more likely to stay in your body and contribute to atherosclerosis. An LDL count below 100 is considered optimal for good health. Another kind, **high-density lipoprotein (HDL)**, is often referred to as "good cholesterol" because it carries excess cholesterol out of your bloodstream and into your liver for elimination from your body. Therefore, HDLs appear to help prevent atherosclerosis. An HDL count above 60 is considered optimal for good health.

In addition to being free of fatty deposits, healthy arteries are free from inflammation, which contributes to arterial clogging. Blood tests can pick up markers of inflammation.

Regular physical activity helps you improve your health and resist disease by reducing your LDL (bad cholesterol) and increasing your HDL (good cholesterol). It also helps reduce inflammation in your arteries and can help prevent the formation of blood clots by reducing the amount of **fibrin** in your blood. Fibrin is a substance involved in making your blood clot, and high amounts of fibrin can contribute to the development of atherosclerosis.

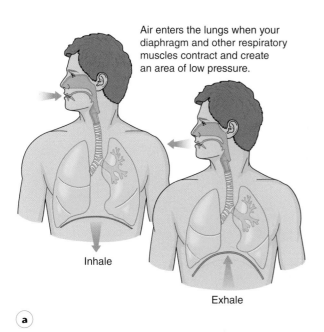

Air enters the lungs when your diaphragm and other respiratory muscles contract and create an area of low pressure.

Inhale

Exhale

**a**

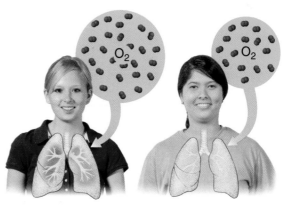

The average lung holds 3 to 5 liters of air.

Trained individuals take bigger breaths, thus requiring fewer breaths to get the same amount of oxygen.

Untrained individuals take shallow breaths and thus need more breaths to get sufficient oxygen.

**b**

**FIGURE 8.3** (a) The lungs and diaphragm during inhalation and exhalation; (b) fit people can breathe more efficiently than unfit people.

## Arteries

Each **artery** carries blood from your heart to another part of your body. The beating of your heart forces blood through your arteries. Therefore, a strong heart and healthy lungs are not very helpful if your arteries are not clear and open. As you now know, fatty deposits on the inner walls of an artery lead to atherosclerosis. An extreme case of atherosclerosis can totally block the blood flow in an artery. The hardened deposits can also allow the formation of blood clots, severely blocking your blood flow. In either case, your heart muscle does not get enough oxygen, and a heart attack occurs.

Regular physical activity also provides other cardiovascular benefits. Scientists have found that people who exercise regularly develop more branching of the arteries in the heart. Figure 8.4 shows that the heart muscle has its own arteries (coronary arteries), which supply it with blood and oxygen. People who exercise regularly develop extra coronary arteries. The importance of this richer network of blood vessels can be shown in two examples.

- After astronaut Ed White died in a fire while training for a mission, an autopsy was performed. Doctors found that one of the major arteries in his heart was completely blocked due to atherosclerosis. However, because of all the physical training that astronauts perform, scientists think White's body had developed an extra branching of arteries in his heart muscle. Therefore, he didn't die of a heart attack when a main artery was blocked. Instead, he had been able to continue a high level of physical fitness training without signs of heart trouble.

- Like White, professional hockey player Richard Zednik had very good cardiorespiratory endurance. This fact became crucial to his survival during a hockey game when his carotid artery was cut by an opponent's skate. For most people, this would be a deadly injury. However, the doctor who performed the rescue surgery reported that because of Zednik's fitness level, he had very healthy and elastic arteries that were large and easy to repair. Zednik made a full recovery.

## Veins

Each **vein** carries blood filled with waste products from the muscle cells and other body tissues back to the heart. One-way valves in your veins keep the blood from flowing backward. Your muscles squeeze the veins to pump the blood back to your heart. Regular exercise helps your muscles squeeze your veins efficiently. Lack of physical activity can cause the valves, especially those in your legs, to stop working efficiently, thereby reducing circulation in your legs.

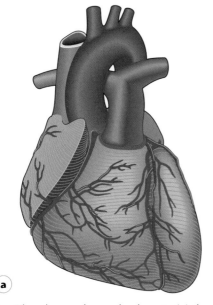
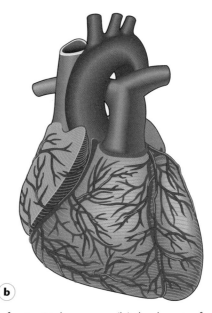

(a)    (b)

**FIGURE 8.4** Blood vessels on the heart: (a) the heart of a typical person; (b) the heart of a person who exercises regularly.

> " If you don't do what's best for your body, you're the one who comes up on the short end. "

—Julius Erving (Doctor J),
Hall of Fame basketball player

## Nerves of Your Heart

Your heart muscle is not like your arm and leg muscles. When your arm and leg muscles contract, nerves in them are responding to a message sent by the conscious part of your brain. In contrast, your heart is not controlled voluntarily; it beats regularly without your consciously telling it to do so. Instead, your heart rate is controlled by a part of it called a pacemaker, which sends out an electrical current telling it to beat regularly. People who do regular vigorous aerobic exercise often develop a slower heart rate because the heart pumps more blood with each

beat—meaning it has greater stroke volume—and therefore can beat less often. Thus, if you exercise properly, your heart works more efficiently because each heartbeat supplies more blood and oxygen to your body than if you did not exercise. You can also function more effectively during an emergency or during vigorous physical activity.

## Muscle Cells

In order to do physical activity for a long time without getting tired, your muscle cells must also function efficiently and effectively. Regular physical activity helps your cells be effective in their use of oxygen and in getting rid of waste materials. Physical activity also helps your muscle cells use blood sugar, with the aid of the hormone called insulin, to produce energy. This function is important for good health.

 **FITNESS TECHNOLOGY: Heart Rate Monitors**

One way to count your heart rate is to use your wrist or neck pulse. But it's difficult to do so while you're exercising, so pulse is typically counted after exercise.

To count your pulse during activity, you can use a high-tech device called a heart rate monitor. One type requires you to wear a band around your chest. The band contains sensors that detect electrical stimulation from your heart's nervous system (similar to how an electrocardiogram works). A transmitter in the chest band sends a signal to a receiver located in a special watch worn on your wrist. The receiver picks up the signal and displays your heart rate on the watch. Another type of monitor counts your pulse and displays your heart rate on a watch located on your arm. It does not require the band around your chest.

You can set a heart rate watch to tell you whether you're exercising in your heart rate target zone. You can also set it to keep track of how many minutes you stay in your target zone. Heart rate monitors vary in cost, and some are better than others, so consult with your teacher

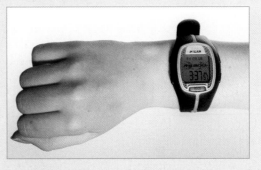

**A heart rate watch is helpful for counting your pulse during activity.**

or another reliable source before buying one. If your school has heart rate watches, you might want to use one to monitor your heart rate during vigorous activity.

### Using Technology

Use a variety of sources to evaluate several heart rate monitors. Consider cost, reliability, and ease of use, then decide which monitor would be the best buy.

## Summary of Benefits

As noted in the previous sections, regular physical activity benefits many different body systems. A summary of these benefits is presented in figure 8.5.

# Cardiorespiratory Assessment

You might be curious about your own cardiorespiratory endurance. How good is it? Several tests can help you find the answer.

You can assess the fitness of your cardiorespiratory systems in two settings: in the laboratory and in the field (such as in a gym and or on an athletic field). Two types of laboratory test are the **maximal oxygen uptake** test (also referred to as the $\dot{V}O_2$max test) and the **graded exercise test**.

The maximal oxygen uptake test is considered the best for assessing fitness of the cardiovascular and respiratory systems. It measures how much oxygen you can use when you're exercising very vigorously. To take the test, you run on a treadmill while connected to a special gas meter (figure 8.6). The difficulty increases as the treadmill goes faster

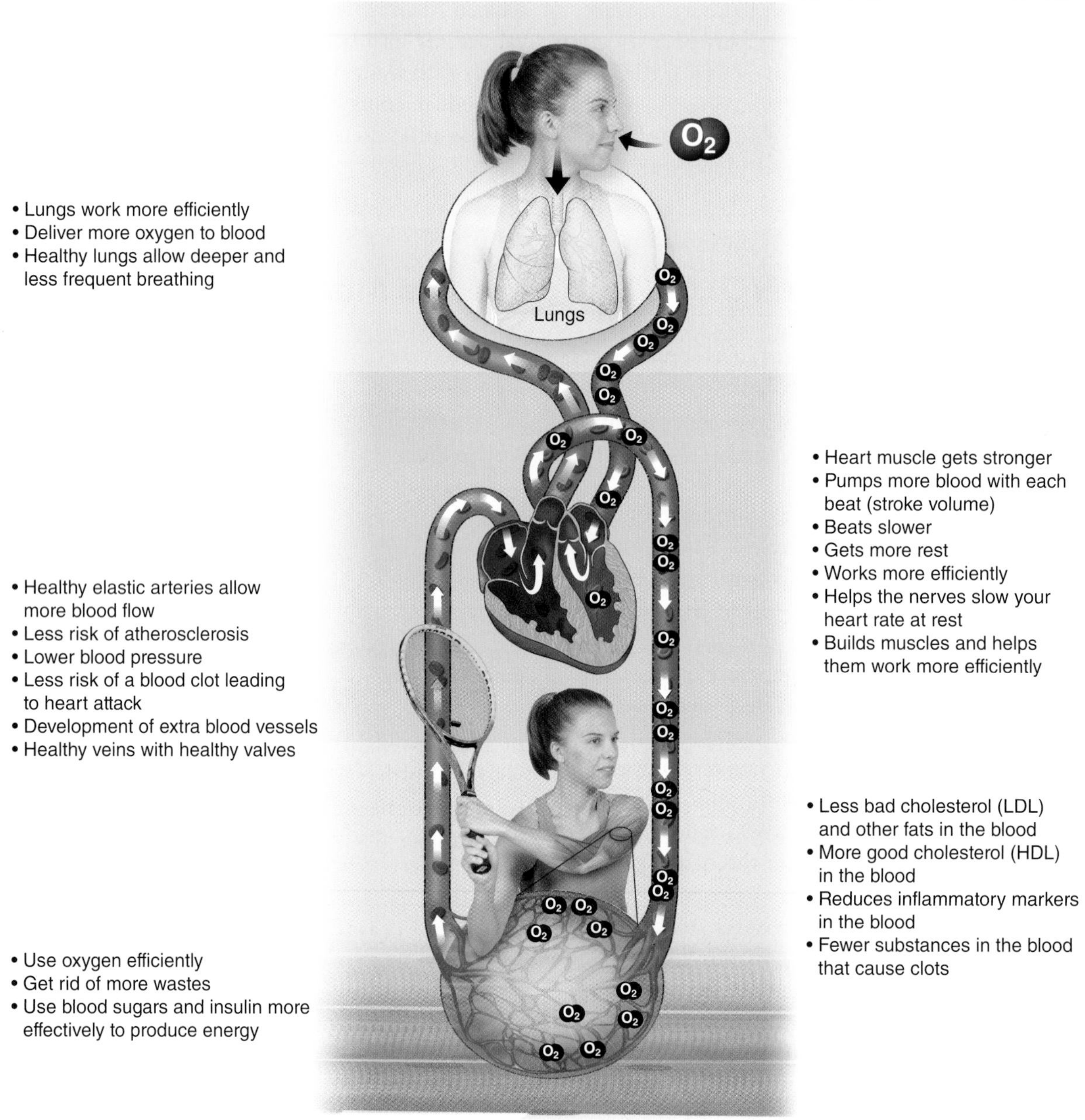

- Lungs work more efficiently
- Deliver more oxygen to blood
- Healthy lungs allow deeper and less frequent breathing

- Healthy elastic arteries allow more blood flow
- Less risk of atherosclerosis
- Lower blood pressure
- Less risk of a blood clot leading to heart attack
- Development of extra blood vessels
- Healthy veins with healthy valves

- Use oxygen efficiently
- Get rid of more wastes
- Use blood sugars and insulin more effectively to produce energy

- Heart muscle gets stronger
- Pumps more blood with each beat (stroke volume)
- Beats slower
- Gets more rest
- Works more efficiently
- Helps the nerves slow your heart rate at rest
- Builds muscles and helps them work more efficiently

- Less bad cholesterol (LDL) and other fats in the blood
- More good cholesterol (HDL) in the blood
- Reduces inflammatory markers in the blood
- Fewer substances in the blood that cause clots

**FIGURE 8.5** Benefits of physical activity for the cardiovascular and respiratory systems.

rather than on the amount of oxygen you can use. Examples include the PACER, the walking test, the step test, and the one-mile run test.

## FIT FACT

Studies show that endurance athletes— such as cross-country skiers, cyclists, and distance runners—typically have very high aerobic capacity and score well on field tests of cardiorespiratory endurance.

## Interpreting Self-Assessment Results

Self-assessments are not as accurate as laboratory tests of fitness; therefore, you should perform more than one self-assessment for cardiorespiratory endurance. However, self-assessments do give a good estimate of your fitness level, and each assessment has its own strengths and weaknesses. For example, the results of the PACER and the one-mile run (included in this chapter) are influenced by your motivation; if you don't try very hard, you won't get an accurate score. Because these tests require a high level of exertion, they may not be the best tests for people who have not been exercising regularly or who have low fitness.

The walking test, on the other hand, is a good indicator of fitness for most people but is not best for assessing very fit people. It would be a good test for a beginner. The step test (included in this chapter) uses heart rate; therefore, motivation does not influence its results as much as it does some other assessments. But step test results can be distorted if you've done other exercise that might elevate your heart rate before doing the assessment. Your heart rate can also be influenced by emotional factors (stress) and nutritional factors (caffeine) that cause it to be higher than normal. Finally, your results may vary depending on the time of day the assessment is done. For example, fatigue associated with daily activities may result in poorer scores late in the day.

Regardless of which tests you do, practice them before using them to assess your fitness. Practice allows you to pace yourself properly during the test and enables you to perform the tests properly so that you get accurate assessments. Because you may get different ratings on different tests of cardiorespiratory endurance, consider the strengths and weaknesses of each test when making decisions

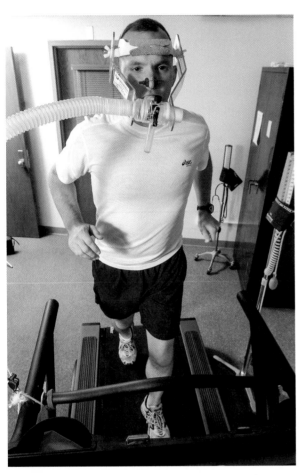

**FIGURE 8.6** The maximal oxygen uptake test measures the amount of oxygen you use while running on a treadmill.

and you begin to run uphill. As you exercise, the gas meter measures the amount of oxygen you use each minute. The amount (volume) of oxygen you can use during the hardest minute of exercise is considered your $\dot{V}O_2$max score (see Science in Action).

Medical doctors and exercise physiologists sometimes use another laboratory test called a graded exercise test (or an exercise stress test). This test is used to detect potential heart problems. During the test, your heart is monitored by means of an electrocardiogram while you run on a treadmill.

Both the graded exercise test and the maximal oxygen uptake test are done in a laboratory and require special equipment and people who are trained to administer them. Most people, however, assess their cardiorespiratory endurance using practical nonlaboratory tests called field tests. These tests require little equipment and can be done at home or at school. Scores are determined based on your ability to function (your functional fitness)

# SCIENCE IN ACTION: Aerobic Capacity

After extensive research, the Institute of Medicine recommended the use of the term *cardiorespiratory endurance* for performance on field tests such as the PACER. Because of this recommendation, we use the term *cardiorespiratory endurance* in this book rather than some of the other commonly used terms (such as *cardiovascular fitness* or *aerobic fitness*). Cardiorespiratory endurance reflects a person's functional fitness—the ability to perform tasks of daily life such as enjoying leisure-time activities and the ability to meet emergencies without undue fatigue.

As noted earlier, the term **aerobic capacity** is similar to, but not exactly the same as, cardiorespiratory endurance. The only true measure of aerobic capacity is your score on a laboratory based maximal oxygen uptake test. Your score on the maximal oxygen uptake test ($\dot{V}O_2$ max test) is recorded in liters of oxygen per minute. You may want to adjust your aerobic capacity score (in liters) to account for body size because big people use more liters of oxygen simply because of their size. So aerobic capacity scores are commonly reported as milliliters of oxygen per kilogram of body weight per minute (mL/kg/min).

You can also get an idea of your aerobic capacity in other ways. For example, when used with the Fitnessgram report card, your cardiorespiratory endurance score is converted to an estimated aerobic capacity score. You can find more information and tables for estimating aerobic capacity from PACER scores at the student section of the Fitness for Life website.

### Student Activity

Estimate your aerobic capacity score in milliliters of oxygen per kilogram of body weight per minute (mL/kg/min) using your PACER score. Tables for converting PACER scores to aerobic capacity scores are available in the student section of the Fitness for Life website.

about which score best represents your fitness. After you've done regular exercise over time, test yourself again to see how much you've improved.

# How Much Cardiorespiratory Endurance Is Enough?

To get the health and wellness benefits associated with cardiorespiratory endurance, you should achieve the good fitness zone in the rating charts that accompany each self-assessment in this book. Health benefits are associated with moving out of the low and marginal zones and into the good fitness zone. The risk of hypokinetic diseases is greatest for people in the low fitness zone.

Some people aim for especially high cardiorespiratory endurance because they want to perform at a high level in a sport or a physically demanding job, such as being a Marine or a police officer. To be properly fit for such challenges, you must train harder than most people. Achieving the high performance zone will be difficult for some people, and doing so is not necessary in order to get many of the health benefits of fitness. Nevertheless, the higher your cardiorespiratory endurance score, the lower your risk of hypokinetic disease.

## Lesson Review

1. What are some health and wellness benefits of cardiorespiratory endurance?
2. How does physical activity affect the various parts of your cardiovascular and respiratory systems?
3. What are some methods for assessing cardiorespiratory endurance and aerobic capacity, and how are they done?
4. How much cardiorespiratory endurance is enough?

As you've learned, the maximal oxygen uptake test is the best test of fitness of the cardiovascular and respiratory systems. But if you want a quicker, easier, and less expensive test, try the step test or the one-mile run test. Then, after you've done regular exercise over time, test yourself again to see how much you've improved. As directed by your teacher, record your scores and fitness ratings for either test (or both). You can then use the information in preparing your personal physical activity plan. If you're working with a partner, remember that self-assessment information is personal and considered confidential. It shouldn't be shared with others without the permission of the person being tested.

## Step Test

1. Use a bench that is 12 inches (30 centimeters) high. Step up with your right foot. Step up with your left foot.

2. Step down with your right foot. Step down with your left foot.

3. Repeat this four-count pattern (up, up, down, down). Step 24 times each minute for three minutes.

4. Immediately after stepping for three minutes, sit and count your pulse. Begin counting within five seconds. Count for one minute.

5. Use table 8.1 to determine your cardiorespiratory endurance rating. Record your heart rate, minutes of stepping, and rating.

Note: The height of the bench and the rate of stepping are both crucial to getting an accurate test result. Sit calmly for several minutes before the test to assure that your resting heart rate is normal.

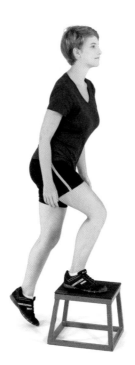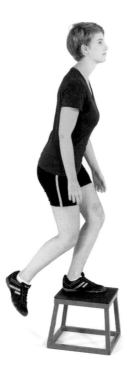

The step test assesses cardiorespiratory endurance.

## TABLE 8.1   Rating Chart: Step Test (Heartbeats per Minute)

| | 13 years old | | 14–16 years old | | 17 years or older | |
|---|---|---|---|---|---|---|
| | Male | Female | Male | Female | Male | Female |
| High performance | ≤90 | ≤100 | ≤85 | ≤95 | ≤80 | ≤90 |
| Good fitness | 91–98 | 101–110 | 86–95 | 96–105 | 81–90 | 91–100 |
| Marginal fitness | 99–120 | 111–130 | 96–115 | 106–125 | 91–110 | 101–120 |
| Low fitness | ≥121 | ≥131 | ≥116 | ≥126 | ≥111 | ≥121 |

Those who cannot step for 3 minutes receive a low fitness rating.

# One-Mile Run

An alternative test of cardiorespiratory endurance is the one-mile (1.6-kilometer) run. Remember that this test is for your own information; it's not a race. Your goal is a good fitness rating, which indicates reduced risk of hypokinetic disease and enough fitness to function effectively. Some people may strive to achieve the high performance zone, which provides additional health benefits and allows you to perform sports and jobs requiring strong cardiorespiratory endurance.

1. Run or jog for one mile (1.6 kilometers) in the shortest possible time. A steady pace is best. Try to set a pace that you can keep up for the full run. If you start too fast and then have to slow down at the end, you will probably not be able to run for the entire distance. You can use target heart rate or ratings of perceived exertion (RPE) to help you set a good pace. Another indicator is the talk test. If you are unable to talk comfortably while running (for example, talking with a friend), then you are probably running too fast.

2. Your score is the amount of time it takes you to run the full distance. Record your time in minutes and seconds.

3. Find your rating in table 8.2 and record it.

## TABLE 8.2   Rating Chart: One-Mile (1.6-Kilometer) Run (Minutes:Seconds)

| | 13 years old | | 14 years old | | 15 years old | | 16 years old | | 17 years or older | |
|---|---|---|---|---|---|---|---|---|---|---|
| | Male | Female | Male | Female | Male | Female | Male | Female | Male | Female |
| High performance | ≤7:45 | ≤8:40 | ≤7:30 | ≤8:25 | ≤7:15 | ≤8:10 | ≤7:00 | ≤7:45 | ≤6:50 | ≤7:35 |
| Good fitness | 7:46–10:09 | 8:41–10:27 | 7:31–9:27 | 8:26–10:15 | 7:16–9:00 | 8:11–9:58 | 7:01–8:39 | 7:46–9:46 | 6:51–8:26 | 7:36–9:31 |
| Marginal fitness | 10:10–12:29 | 10:28–13:03 | 9:28–11:51 | 10:16–12:48 | 9:01–11:14 | 9:59–12:27 | 8:40–10:46 | 9:47–12:11 | 8:27–10:37 | 9:32–11:54 |
| Low fitness | ≥12:30 | ≥13:04 | ≥11:52 | ≥12:49 | ≥11:15 | ≥12:28 | ≥10:47 | ≥12:12 | ≥10:38 | ≥11:55 |

Based on data provided by G. Welk.

# Lesson 8.2

# Building Cardiorespiratory Endurance

## Lesson Objectives

After reading this lesson, you should be able to

1. define *vigorous aerobic activity* and give several examples,
2. describe the FIT formula for developing cardiorespiratory endurance,
3. describe how to count your resting heart rate and determine your maximal heart rate, and
4. explain how to use two methods for determining your threshold of training and your target zone for building cardiorespiratory endurance.

## Lesson Vocabulary

aerobic activity, heart rate reserve (HRR), maximal heart rate, vigorous aerobics

**You** now know that physical activity is important to your cardiorespiratory endurance. But how much physical activity do you have to do to improve your cardiorespiratory endurance? In this lesson, you'll learn about the best types of activity for building cardiorespiratory endurance. You'll also learn to determine how much physical activity you need in order to build your own cardiorespiratory endurance.

> To keep the body in good health is a duty; otherwise, we shall not be able to keep our mind strong and clear.
>
> —The Buddha

## Physical Activity and Cardiorespiratory Endurance

The term *aerobic* means "with oxygen," and **aerobic activity** is activity that is steady enough to allow your heart to supply all the oxygen your muscles need. Moderate physical activities are considered to be aerobic because you can do them for a long time without stopping. Moderate activities provide many health benefits and can build cardiorespiratory endurance in low-fit people, but they are not intense enough to build cardiorespiratory endurance for most people.

**Vigorous aerobics**, represented on the second step of the Physical Activity Pyramid for Teens, is the most effective way to build cardiorespiratory endurance. Vigorous aerobic activities are intense enough to elevate your heart rate above your threshold of training and into your target zone for cardiorespiratory endurance. National physical activity guidelines for teens recommend doing vigorous activity on at least three days a week because they promote benefits beyond those provided by moderate activity.

Vigorous sport and recreation activities, represented on the third step of the Physical Activity Pyramid for Teens (figure 8.7), also build cardiorespiratory endurance. Vigorous sports often involve quick bursts of vigorous activity followed by rest, and for this reason they are not totally aerobic. However, they offer the same benefits as vigorous aerobic activity. To be considered vigorous, sports and recreation activities must be intense enough to elevate your heart rate above your threshold of training and into your target zone for cardiorespiratory endurance.

## How Much Vigorous Activity Is Enough?

As you're already aware, teens should accumulate 60 minutes of physical activity each day of the week. Some of that recommended activity should be of

Energy balance

**STEP 5**
Flexibility exercises

**STEP 4**
Muscle fitness exercises

**STEP 3**
Vigorous sport and recreation

**STEP 2**
Vigorous aerobics

**STEP 1**
Moderate physical activity

**FIGURE 8.7** Vigorous activities from steps 2 and 3 are best for building cardiorespiratory endurance.

The FIT formula for building cardiorespiratory endurance is shown in table 8.3. As you can see, both the threshold of training and the target zone are different for people who are sedentary than for people who are regularly active. Sedentary people exercise at a lower intensity and use a different target heart rate zone than more active people.

When using table 8.3, first find your current physical activity level among the options listed in the table's second row. Rows below indicate frequency and length of exercise in days and minutes. The intensity of your exercise is determined by one of two methods of counting heart rate; these two methods are described in the next section of this chapter. Once you learn how to count your heart rate using one of the two methods, you can use table 8.3 to determine your exercise intensity.

a vigorous nature. Specifically, you should perform vigorous activity at least three days a week in exercise sessions totaling at least 20 minutes per day. Vigorous activity should be of a high enough intensity that it increases your heart rate above your threshold level and into your target zone.

## FIT FACT

Another way (besides heart rate) to determine intensity is to use rating of perceived exertion (RPE). In this method, you estimate the intensity of your exertion during exercise using numbers from 6 (no exertion) to 20 (maximal exertion). An RPE of 12 to 14 is typically equal to the target zone for cardiorespiratory endurance (see table 8.3). RPE can be used to help you determine your pace during vigorous aerobic activity.

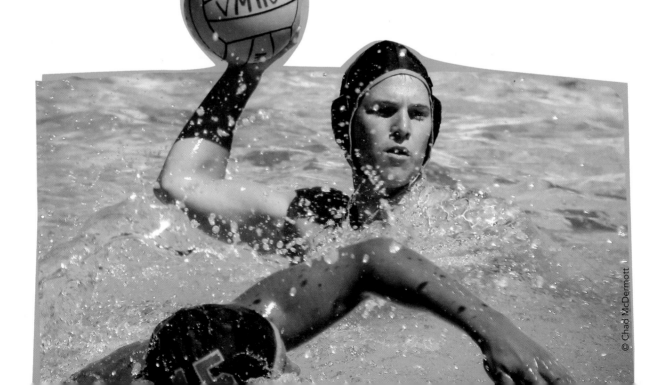

**TABLE 8.3  Threshold of Training and Target Heart Rate Zones (FIT Formula) for People With Different Activity Levels**

| | Threshold of training | | | Target heart rate zone | | |
|---|---|---|---|---|---|---|
| Current activity level | No regular vigorous activity | Some vigorous activity | Regular vigorous activity | No regular vigorous activity | Some vigorous activity | Regular vigorous activity |
| Frequency | 3 days a week for all fitness levels | | | 3–6 days a week for all fitness levels | | |
| Intensity | Percentage | | | Percentage | | |
| HRR* | 50 | 60 | 70 | 50–70 | 60–80 | 70–89 |
| % max HR** | 70 | 80 | 84 | 70–85 | 80–91 | 84–95 |
| Time | 20 min for all activity levels*** | | | 20–90 min for all activity levels*** | | |

*HRR indicates heart rate reserve.

**% max HR indicates percent of maximal heart rate.

***Sessions of at least 10 minutes can be combined to meet time recommendations.

Based on ACSM exercise prescription guidelines.

# Heart Rate and Intensity of Physical Activity

Monitoring heart rate is a common technique for determining exercise intensity. This is because taking a pulse count to determine your heart rate is relatively easy to do. But what exactly are we looking for when we take a pulse count? In order to build cardiorespiratory endurance, you need to overload the cardiovascular and respiratory systems. Calculating a target heart rate zone, including your threshold of training and target ceiling, is the scientific approach to providing optimal overload. Once you know your target heart rate zone, you know how high you need to elevate your heart rate to pace your exercise for building cardiorespiratory endurance. The American College of Sports Medicine (ACSM) recommends two methods for determining your target heart rate zone. The first is the percent of heart rate reserve (% HRR) method and the second is the percent of maximal heart rate (% max HR) method.

In this lesson, you'll learn how to use both of these methods to calculate your threshold target heart rate zone. After learning both methods, you'll choose one to use. You can then count your heart rate during or right after exercise to determine whether you're exercising at the right intensity for your target zone.

## Counting Resting Heart Rate

To determine your target heart rate zone, you first need to determine your resting heart rate, which is the number of times your heart beats when you're relatively inactive. Use the following instructions.

1. Sit and take your heart rate by using the first and second fingers of your hand to find a pulse at your opposite wrist (your radial pulse) (figure 8.8a). Do not use your thumb. Practice so that you can locate your pulse quickly.

2. Count the number of pulses for one minute. Record your one-minute heart rate.

3. Take your resting (seated) heart rate again, this time counting the pulse at your neck (figure 8.8b). This is your carotid pulse. Use two fingers (index and middle) of either hand. Place the fingers on the side of your neck. Move until you locate the pulse. Press only as hard as necessary to feel the pulse; be careful not to press too hard.

4. Now take both your wrist and your neck pulse while you are standing. Repeat the pulse count (both wrist and neck) while sitting. Compare your results. Usually, your standing pulse is faster than your sitting pulse.

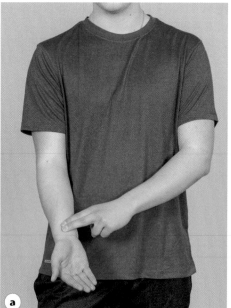 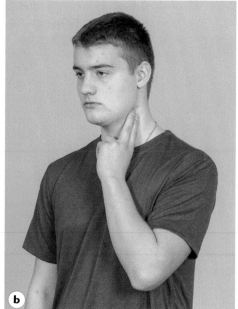

**FIGURE 8.8**  Use your first and second finger to find a pulse *(a)* at your wrist and *(b)* at your neck.

5. Take a partner's pulse while your partner takes your pulse (both standing). Compare your self-counted heart rate with your heart rate as determined by your partner. You may use different methods of counting, but use the same one as your partner when making comparisons.

6. As directed by your teacher, record your resting heart rate using the methods just described.

## Determining Maximal Heart Rate (Max HR)

**Maximal heart rate** (max HR) is the highest heart rate that a person can reach during the most vigorous exercise. To estimate your max HR, you can count your heart rate after a very vigorous exercise session; or, to determine a more accurate max HR, you can wear a heart rate monitor to see how high your heart rate gets during very vigorous exercise. Be aware, however, that people who are unfit or are not regularly active should *not* do an exercise session vigorous enough to determine max HR.

Because determining a true max HR requires very vigorous activity that isn't appropriate for some people, exercise physiologists have developed several formulas for estimating max HR without doing exercise. Five different formulas are listed by the ACSM for estimating max HR. Each has advantages and disadvantages. Here we use the formula that is most commonly used by exercise experts. It's simple to use, and the estimated max HRs from the formula are very similar to those calculated using a more complex formula for young people including teens. You can use the formula below or estimate your max HR by using table 8.4.

220 – age in years = maximal heart rate

Example for 16-year-old: 220 – 16 = 204

As directed by your teacher, record your estimated max HR. You'll use it when determining your heart rate target zone.

## Counting Exercise Heart Rate

It can be difficult to count your pulse during activities such as jogging, but you can get a good estimate of your heart rate during a physical activity by determining your heart rate immediately after exercising. To estimate your heart rate during exercise based on your after-exercise pulse count, use the following instructions.

1. Immediately after exercise, locate your pulse (within 5 seconds).

2. Use either your wrist or neck pulse to count your heart rate for 15 seconds. Multiply your

15-second count by 4 to get your 1-minute heart rate. This method is useful because you can do it quickly and because your heart rate slows down quickly when you stop exercising, which means the longer counts may underestimate what your heart rate was during the exercise. On the other hand, counting for a shorter time can result in error because a single counting mistake is multiplied. You can use table 8.5 to help you determine your 1-minute heart rate from your 15-second count.

3. While you count your heart rate, you may want to continue to walk slowly because slow walking can help you recover faster. If you have trouble counting your heart rate while walking, stand still when you count, then begin moving.

## Percent of Heart Rate Reserve Method for Determining Target Heart Rate

To build cardiorespiratory endurance, you must elevate your heart rate above your threshold of training and into your target zone (see table 8.3). The percent of heart rate reserve (% HRR) is one of two methods for determining target heart rate. This method is considered the most accurate, but it is a bit more difficult to calculate than the other method. To use this method, you must know your resting and maximal heart rates and your **heart rate reserve (HRR)**. Table 8.6 provides an example of the calculations for a 16-year-old who has a resting heart rate of 67 and is in the good fitness zone for cardiorespiratory endurance.

1. Begin by determining your resting and max HR as described earlier in this chapter. In the example, the resting HR is 67 and the max HR is 204.

2. Next, determine your heart rate reserve by subtracting your resting heart rate from your maximal heart rate (max HR). In the example, the resting heart rate is 67, so the heart rate reserve is 137.

3. To calculate the threshold heart rate, multiply the heart rate reserve (HRR) by a percentage of the max HR—60 percent (0.6) in the example. As shown in table 8.3, different percentages are used for people of different activity levels; use the percentage that fits your current activity level. This number is

### TABLE 8.4 Estimated Maximal Heart Rates

| Your age (years) | 12 | 13 | 14 | 15 | 16 | 17 | 18 | 19 |
|---|---|---|---|---|---|---|---|---|
| Max HR | 208 | 207 | 206 | 205 | 204 | 203 | 202 | 201 |

Find your age in the top row, then find your estimated max HR immediately below your age.

### TABLE 8.5 Heart Rate in 15-Second and 1-Minute Intervals

| 15-sec rate | 1-min rate | 15-sec rate | 1-min rate | 15-sec rate | 1-min rate |
|---|---|---|---|---|---|
| 15 | 60 | 27 | 108 | 39 | 156 |
| 16 | 64 | 28 | 112 | 40 | 160 |
| 17 | 68 | 29 | 116 | 41 | 164 |
| 18 | 72 | 30 | 120 | 42 | 168 |
| 19 | 76 | 31 | 124 | 43 | 172 |
| 20 | 80 | 32 | 128 | 44 | 176 |
| 21 | 84 | 33 | 132 | 45 | 180 |
| 22 | 88 | 34 | 136 | 46 | 184 |
| 23 | 92 | 35 | 140 | 47 | 188 |
| 24 | 96 | 36 | 144 | 48 | 192 |
| 25 | 100 | 37 | 148 | 49 | 196 |
| 26 | 104 | 38 | 152 | 50 | 200 |

Find your 15-second heart rate in a shaded column; your 1-minute heart rate is in the white column to the immediate right of it.

then added to the resting heart rate. In the example, the threshold is 149.

4. The target ceiling heart rate is calculated by repeating steps 1 through 3, but in step 3 multiply by a higher percentage—80 percent (0.8) in the example. Refer to table 8.3 to find the percentage you should use for your target zone based on your currently activity level. Then add your resting heart rate. In the example, the target ceiling heart rate is 177.

5. Thus the target heart zone is 149 to 177 (60 to 80 percent of HRR) in the example of the 16-year-old who is in the good fitness zone.

## Percent of Maximal Heart Rate Method for Determining Target Heart Rate

The second method, percent of maximal heart rate (% max HR), is not quite as accurate as the HRR method but is easier to calculate. In this method, you do not use your resting heart rate. Table 8.7 provides an example using the % max HR method for a 16-year-old in the good fitness zone for cardiorespiratory endurance.

1. Estimate your maximal heart rate. In the example, the maximal heart rate is 204.

2. In this example, the max HR (204) was multiplied by 80 percent (0.8) to find the threshold heart rate. As noted in table 8.3, different percentages are used for people of different activity levels; use the percentage that fits your current activity level. In the example, the threshold is 163.

3. To calculate the target ceiling rate, repeat steps 1 and 2, but in step 2 multiply by 91 percent (0.91). This number will vary based on your activity level (see table 8.3). In the example, the ceiling rate is 186.

**TABLE 8.6　Calculating Heart Rate Target Zone (% HRR Method)**

| Threshold HR | Step 1: | 204 (max HR)* |
| | Step 2: | − 67 (resting HR) |
| | | 137 (HRR) |
| | Step 3: | × 0.6 (threshold %) |
| | | 82 |
| | | + 67 (resting HR) |
| | | 149 (threshold HR) |
| Target ceiling | Step 1: | 204 (max HR)* |
| | Step 2: | − 67 (resting HR) |
| | | 137 (HRR) |
| | Step 3: | × 0.8 (ceiling %) |
| | | 110 |
| | | + 67 (resting HR) |
| | | 177 (target ceiling HR) |
| Target HR zone | 149–177 beats per min | |

*The example is for a 16-year-old with a resting HR of 67 with cardiorespiratory endurance in the good fitness zone.

**TABLE 8.7　Calculating Heart Rate Target Zone (% max HR Method)**

| Threshold HR | Step 1: | 204 (max HR)* |
| | Step 2: | × 0.8 (threshold %) |
| | | 163 (threshold HR) |
| Target ceiling rate | Step 1: | 204 (max HR)* |
| | Step 2: | × 0.91 (ceiling %) |
| | | 186 (target ceiling rate) |
| Target HR zone | 163–186 beats per min | |

*The example is for a 16-year-old with a resting HR of 67 and cardiorespiratory endurance in the good fitness zone.

4. Thus the target heart rate zone is 163 to 186 (80 to 91 percent of max HR) in the example of the 16-year-old in the good fitness zone for cardiorespiratory endurance. Note that these numbers are slightly higher than those generated with the % HRR method.

## Exercise for Ellen

Ellen is a high school sophomore. She took the PACER and the walking test and got a marginal fitness rating in both. She was not surprised, because she rarely did vigorous exercise, but she did want to improve her cardiorespiratory endurance. To do so, she knew that she had to start doing more vigorous activity each week.

Specifically, based on information presented in table 8.3, Ellen learned that she needed to do vigorous exercise at least three (and up to six) days a week. She decided to begin with three, and she chose to jog for 20 minutes on each of the three days because table 8.3 recommended sessions of 20 minutes.

In class, Ellen learned how to use the % HRR and % max HR methods for determining her target heart rate zone. She decided to use the % HRR method. She first determined her maximal heart rate (204 beats per minute) and resting heart rate (67 beats per minute). She then determined that her heart rate reserve (HRR) was 137 by subtracting her resting heart rate from her maximum heart rate (204 − 67 = 137).

Next, she calculated her target heart rate zone, and she did so with the 50 percent to 70 percent range shown in table 8.3 for someone who does no regular vigorous activity. Specifically, she did the following calculations: 50 percent of 137 (her heart rate reserve) is 69, and 70 percent of 137 is 96. Ellen then added 67 (her resting heart rate) to each of these figures to get her threshold heart rate (69 + 67 = 136) and her upper heart rate (96 + 67 = 163). Thus she determined that her target heart rate zone was 139 to 163 beats per minute.

Immediately after each jogging session, Ellen counted her heart rate to see if it was in her target heart rate zone. On a few days, it was below the zone, so she ran a bit faster the next time. Over time, Ellen expects to improve her cardiorespiratory endurance so that she will be in the good fitness zone.

## Lesson Review

1. What is vigorous aerobic activity? Give several examples.
2. What is the FIT formula for developing cardiorespiratory endurance?
3. How can you determine your resting heart rate and estimate your max HR?
4. How can you determine your threshold of training and your target heart rate zone for building cardiorespiratory endurance? Describe two methods.

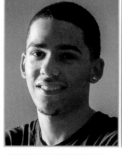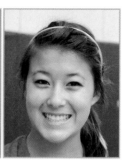

Self-confidence involves believing that you can be successful in an activity. If you think you'll succeed, you have more confidence than if you're unsure about how well you'll do. You're more likely to participate in an activity if your self-confidence is high.

Tony rarely takes part in any physical activity. He went through an awkward stage in his preteen years and thinks that people laugh at the way he runs: "My arms and legs don't seem to work together when I run. I think I look foolish."

Mei, on the other hand, loves any kind of physical activity. Every day, she shoots baskets or rides her bike, and she is a member of multiple teams. Even though she excels in sport, however, she would like to socialize more, but she feels shy around strangers: "I can't think of anything witty or even halfway intelligent to say. When I try to talk, I get tongue tied. It's easier for me to just avoid talking."

Tony and Mei both lack self-confidence but in two different situations. Tony wants to participate in physical activity, and Mei wants to socialize, but they both avoid situations where they might get involved because they feel uncomfortable. Both need to find a way to build their self-confidence so they can succeed in these situations.

## For Discussion

For different reasons, people like Tony may avoid trying new activities or may quit an activity prematurely. People like Mei who lack confidence in social situations may avoid them. What are some reasons that people lack self-confidence? How can they increase their self-confidence? What advice can you give Tony to get him to try new activities and stick with them? What advice can you give Mei to help her be more comfortable in social situations? Also consider the guidelines presented in the Self-Management feature when answering the discussion questions.

##  SELF-MANAGEMENT: Skills for Building Self-Confidence

A recent study of teenagers found that one of the best indicators of who will be physically active is self-confidence. A person is self-confident if he or she thinks *I can do that* rather than *I don't think I can*. Some people are not very confident when it comes to physical activity because they think they are not very good at it or that others are better than they are. Does it surprise you to learn that self-confident people are not always the best performers and that some good performers lack self-confidence? In fact, research done with teenagers in schools shows that all students can find some type of activity in which they can be successful, regardless of physical ability. In addition, people who think they can succeed in activity are nearly twice as likely to be active as people who don't think they can succeed.

Building self-confidence is a self-management skill that you can learn. You may want to assess your self-confidence using the worksheet supplied by your teacher. Then, if necessary, you can use the following guidelines to improve your self-confidence.

- **Learn a new way of thinking.** One major reason some people lack self-confidence is that they think their own success depends on how they compare with others. Practicing a new way of thinking means setting your own standards of success rather than comparing yourself with others. These guidelines are designed to help you build self-confidence by developing a new way of thinking.

- **Set your own personal standards for success.** Assess yourself and set standards for success related to your own improvement. Comparing yourself with others is not necessary for your success, and it can contribute to low self-confidence.

- **Avoid competition if it causes you a problem.** Some people like to compete, but others don't. If competition makes you feel less confident in a physical activity, try to find noncompetitive activities (such as walking, jogging, and swimming) that allow you to feel good about yourself.

- **Set small goals that you're sure to reach.** Setting goals that are a bit higher than your current level is a good idea, but don't set them too high. As you reach one small goal, you can set another. Reaching several small goals builds your self-confidence, whereas not reaching one unrealistic goal can make you less confident.

- **Think and act on positive—not negative—ideas.** When you're involved in a physical activity, think of how you can improve. Talk to yourself about what you did well and what you can practice to improve in the future. Avoid negative self-talk, such as berating yourself for what you didn't do well or referring to yourself in negative terms.

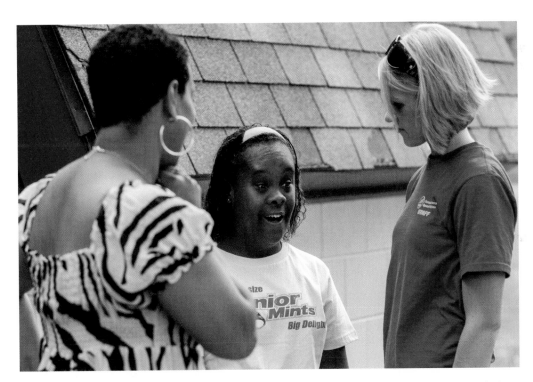

Setting a personal standard of success and getting reinforcement from others can help a person build self-confidence.

# TAKING ACTION: Target Heart Rate Workouts

Cardiorespiratory endurance is important for living a long and healthy life. It's also essential for competing, participating in your favorite physical activities, and maintaining a healthy body weight. As you've learned in this chapter, you must do vigorous physical activity above your threshold of training and in your target zone to build cardiorespiratory endurance. **Take action** by doing vigorous activity that fulfills the FIT formula: at least three days each week (addressing F for frequency in the FIT formula), in your target heart rate zone (addressing I for intensity), and for at least 20 minutes each session (addressing T for time). Consider the following tips as you take action by performing a target heart rate workout.

- Determine your target heart rate by using either the percent of heart rate reserve method or the percent of maximal heart rate method.
- Before choosing vigorous activities, consider your level of fitness.
- Before doing vigorous activity, perform a 5-minute cardiorespiratory general warm-up.
- Check your pulse rate or rating of perceived exertion periodically to make sure you're maintaining the intensity of your workout in your target heart rate zone.
- After your vigorous workout, perform a cool-down.

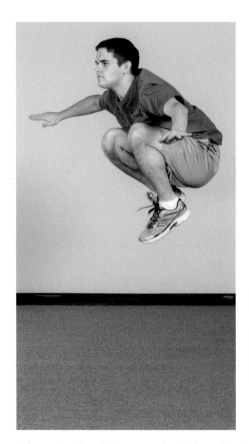
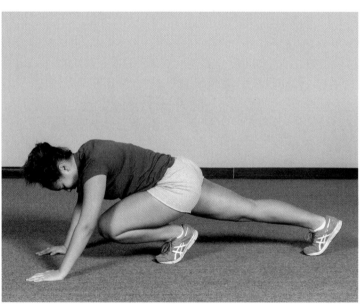

Take action by doing a workout that elevates your heart rate into the target zone.

## Reviewing Concepts and Vocabulary

As directed by your teacher, answer items 1 through 5 by correctly completing each sentence with a word or phrase.

1. Vessels that carry blood from the muscles back to the heart are called _____.

2. The body system that includes your heart, blood vessels, and blood is the _____ system.

3. The substance in your blood that helps it clot is called _____.

4. The method for determining exercise intensity by estimating it without measuring it is called rating of _____.

5. The highest your heart rate ever gets is called your _____.

For items 6 through 10, as directed by your teacher, match each term in column 1 with the appropriate phrase in column 2.

6. carotid                          a. waxy, fatlike substance in blood

7. cholesterol                     b. neck pulse

8. high-density lipoprotein        c. bad cholesterol

9. low-density lipoprotein         d. aerobic capacity

10. maximal oxygen uptake          e. carries bad cholesterol out of the bloodstream

For items 11 through 15, as directed by your teacher, respond to each statement or question.

11. Explain how cardiorespiratory endurance helps your cardiovascular and respiratory systems work more efficiently and thus helps to prevent cardiovascular disease.

12. Define *aerobic capacity*. How does it relate to cardiorespiratory endurance?

13. Describe the two field tests of cardiorespiratory endurance discussed in this chapter.

14. Describe two methods for determining your target heart rate zone.

15. Describe several guidelines for building self-confidence.

## Thinking Critically

Write a paragraph to answer the following question.

Sue has a resting heart rate of 76 beats per minute. Bill has a resting heart rate of 54. Assuming that neither has a disease or illness, what are some possible reasons that their resting heart rates differ so much?

## Project

Create a poster, slide presentation, or video describing the benefits of physical activity for the cardiovascular and respiratory systems.

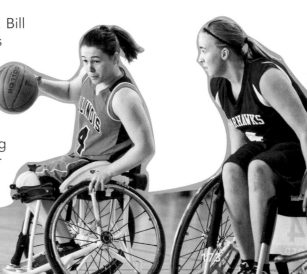

173

# 9

# Vigorous Physical Activity

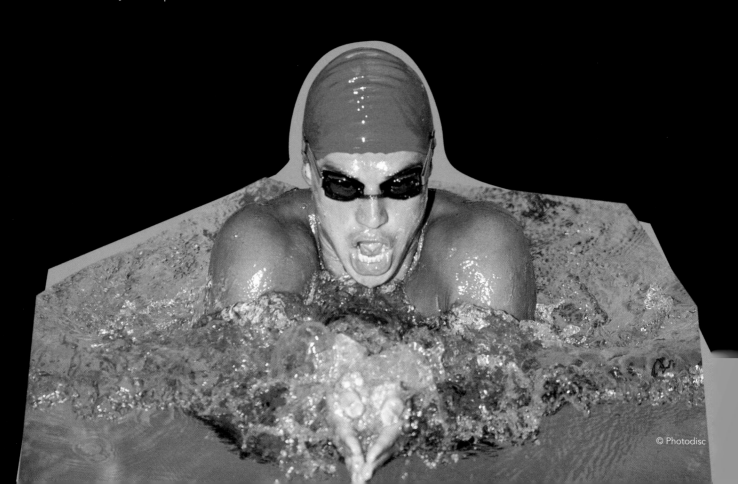

© Photodisc

# Lesson 9.1

# Vigorous Aerobics, Sport, and Recreation

## Lesson Objectives

After reading this lesson, you should be able to

1. describe the three types of vigorous activity (one from step 2 and two from step 3 of the Physical Activity Pyramid),
2. describe several types of vigorous aerobic activity (pyramid step 2),
3. define *sport* and describe the four categories of vigorous sport (pyramid step 3), and
4. define *recreation* and *leisure* and describe several types of vigorous recreation (pyramid step 3).

## Lesson Vocabulary

aerobic, anaerobic activity, anaerobic capacity, circuit training, leisure time, lifetime sport, recreation, sport, vigorous aerobics, vigorous recreation, vigorous sport

**How** often do you engage in activities that make you breathe hard and sweat? Did you know that building fitness increases your chances of living longer? The Physical Activity Pyramid shows two types of vigorous physical activity: vigorous aerobics (step 2) and vigorous sport and recreation (step 3) (figure 9.1). Activities included in these steps are more vigorous (requiring 7 METs or more) than the moderate activities included in step 1 (which require 4 to 7 METs) and are especially good for building cardiorespiratory endurance. (As discussed in the Moderate Physical Activity chapter, 1 MET represents the energy you expend when at rest.) The MET count increases as activity becomes more vigorous. Research shows that vigorous physical activity (7+ METs) provides the health benefits of moderate activity—and more. In this lesson, you'll learn more about the many types of vigorous activity.

## Vigorous Aerobic Activity

Most activities included in the Physical Activity Pyramid (including moderate activities) can be considered **aerobic**. But only activities that are intense enough to elevate your heart rate above your threshold of training and into your target zone are considered **vigorous aerobics**. Aerobic activities—such as jogging, aerobic dancing, cycling, and swimming—are among the most popular and

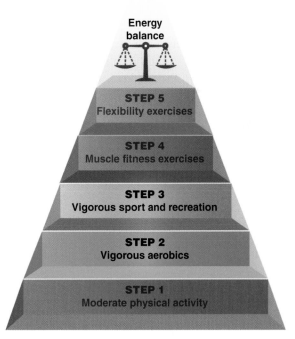

**FIGURE 9.1** Vigorous aerobics, sport, and recreation (steps 2 and 3) build cardiorespiratory fitness and have many other health benefits.

most beneficial of all the activities included in the Physical Activity Pyramid. Their popularity results from the following reasons.

- They often do not require high levels of skill.
- They frequently are not competitive.
- They often can be done at or near home.
- They often do not require a partner or group.

There are many types of vigorous aerobic activity. Some of the most popular are described in the following sections. Some activities could be classified in more than one section of the Physical Activity Pyramid. For example, swimming is a sport, a type of vigorous aerobic activity, and a type of vigorous recreation; in this book, it is classified as a vigorous aerobic activity. Each activity is described only once in this chapter, even if it could fit in multiple places.

## Aerobic Dance

Aerobic dance involves continuously performing various dance steps to music. Unlike social dancers, aerobic dancers typically dance by themselves, often following a leader or a video. This activity first became popular in the 1970s and remains one of the most popular forms of aerobic exercise. Forms of aerobic dance include low-impact, high-impact, and step aerobics. Low-impact aerobics is typically done with one foot staying on the ground at all times. This form is best for beginners because it leads to fewer injuries than other forms. High-impact aerobics is typically more vigorous and involves jumping. Step aerobics involves dance steps done on a step or box. Some types of aerobic dance use light weights, rubber bands, and other types of exercise equipment, as well as movements from other activities such as martial arts.

## Aerobic Exercise Machines

Types of aerobic exercise machines include treadmills, stair steppers, exercise bicycles, rowing machines, and ski machines. You can purchase these machines for use in your own home or use them in health clubs and schools. They can be effective if used properly, but some people do not find exercise on machines to be as enjoyable as activities that allow them to move more freely. For example, skiing may be more enjoyable than using a ski machine. On the other hand, exercise machines are often convenient and efficient.

## Bicycling

Bicycling could be classified as a sport because some people compete in it and as a recreational activity because some do it for fun. If done slowly, it can also be considered a form of moderate physical activity. It is included here because it is often done continuously at a consistent speed that elevates the heart rate. Some forms of cycling, such as BMX and downhill mountain biking, are considered extreme sports.

## Cooper's Aerobics

Dr. Ken Cooper, founder of the Cooper Institute in Dallas, Texas, created the term *aerobics*. He has been so successful in promoting physical activity that in Brazil and some other South American countries, some forms of aerobic activity (aerobics), such as jogging, are referred to as "coopering" or "doing the cooper." He also developed a system in which points can be earned for doing vigorous aerobic activities each week.

## Circuit Training

**Circuit training** involves performing several different exercises one after another. The performer does one exercise for a period of time, then moves to the next with only a brief time between exercises. The goal is to keep the heart rate in the target zone. Circuit training can use exercise machines, small equipment such as jump ropes or rubber bands, free weights, or no equipment at all (for example, calisthenics). Doing different activities helps build muscle fitness as well as cardiorespiratory endurance and can increase your enjoyment because of the variety. Sometimes people use music to determine how much time is spent on

© Getty Images

each exercise. A break in the music signals that it's time to move to the next exercise.

## Dance

Dance is one of the oldest art forms and has been a means of expression in many cultures. Some dance forms are not only enjoyable but also excellent forms of vigorous aerobic exercise. More traditional dance activities include modern, ballet, folk, and square dance. Another category of dance is social dance, which includes both more traditional types (such as the waltz, country dancing, and Latin dancing) and newer forms (such as hip-hop and line dancing). Some dance activities have been altered so that traditional steps are used in ways that are similar to aerobic dance. For example, Zumba uses Latin music and Latin dance steps in ways that resemble aerobic dance. All can be good forms of vigorous aerobics if you do them vigorously enough to elevate your heart rate.

## Jogging and Running

Jogging and running consistently rank among the most popular forms of vigorous aerobic activity.

Jogging is generally considered to be noncompetitive, whereas running is considered to be jogging that is done more seriously. Runners often participate in competitive events such as 5K and 10K races. Jogging and running are combined into one category here because they are very similar. You'll learn more about them in the self-assessment that follows this lesson.

## Martial Arts Exercise

Judo and karate are just two of the several hundred martial arts practiced around the world. Different countries throughout the world have different forms. Martial arts can build various parts of fitness, but they are not always good at building cardiorespiratory endurance because they may not involve enough continuous activity to keep the heart rate elevated. Some forms of martial arts, however, have been combined with aerobic dance to create martial arts exercises; examples include Tae Bo and cardio karate. These forms of exercise can build cardiorespiratory endurance but may not be as effective for learning self-defense as more traditional techniques.

## FITNESS TECHNOLOGY: Global Positioning System

The global positioning system (GPS) is a satellite-based system that communicates precise location information to places around the world. Satellites send signals to a receiver, which sends the signal to a computer that analyzes the information. The GPS was developed by the U.S. government to aid in national defense, but the technology is now available for consumer use. GPS technology is quite accurate and has been used in automobiles to help drivers find their way. It is now being used to help bikers, joggers, hikers, and others who perform outdoor physical activities. The GPS can also provide information about how fast you're moving, the distance you've traveled, the altitude you've gained or lost, and the average pace for your total workout. The first GPS systems for use in physical activity were complicated and required arm or leg straps with a receiver as well as a watchlike device worn on the arm. Others required a computer chip built into shoes to

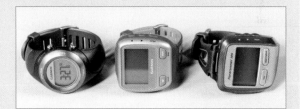

GPS technology can help track your physical activity—for example, these watches can track how far a jogger has run.

pick up the satellite signal. Technology changes rapidly, however, and now GPS devices for use in physical activity are more advanced.

### Using Technology

Research GPS technology for use in physical activity. Identify the device that you think would be the best buy and give reasons for your choice.

### Rope Jumping

Rope jumping has long been used by boxers and other athletes as a method of training. Because it requires moving the arms and legs, as well as the entire body, it can be quite vigorous. For this reason, people sometimes alternate rope jumping with other forms of exercise, such as calisthenics. Practitioners have developed many rope-jumping moves. Rope jumping is inexpensive and can easily be done at home or in your neighborhood. You can also easily transport the needed equipment when traveling.

### Swimming

Swimming is both a sport and a form of recreation. It is included here because it is one of the most popular fitness activities among adults and can serve as a good way to improve cardiorespiratory endurance for almost all people. Like water aerobics, it is a good choice for people who are overweight, elderly, or suffering from joint problems. For swimming to be an effective aerobic exercise, however, your heart rate must be elevated, which means that you must swim continuously for many minutes. Many people who swim do not meet either of these standards.

### Water Aerobics

Water aerobics, sometimes called aqua dynamics, involves doing calisthenics or dance steps in a

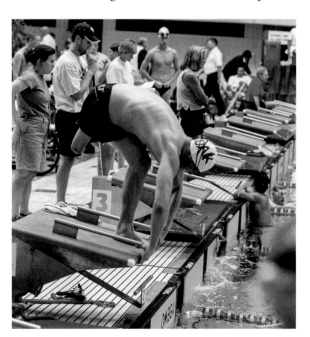

**Swimming can be a good form of vigorous aerobics.**

swimming pool. This form of aerobic exercise is especially good for people who are overweight, elderly, or suffering from arthritis or other joint problems because the water reduces stress on the joints. For stronger exercisers, water can also be used to provide resistance and thus increase the intensity of exercise.

# Vigorous Sport

**Sport** involves physical activity that is competitive (has a winner and loser) and follows well-established rules. Some sports, such as golf and bowling, are classified as moderate physical activity (step 1 of the Physical Activity Pyramid). **Vigorous sports** (step 3 of the pyramid) elevate the heart rate above the threshold level and into the target zone for cardiorespiratory endurance.

There are so many vigorous sports that it is impossible to mention them all here. We can, however, mention general categories: team sports; dual sports; individual sports; and outdoor, challenge, or extreme sports. Certain other sports are not considered here either because they are not among the most popular or because they have little relevance to a personal physical activity program (for example, auto racing and horse racing).

### Team Sports

Team sports such as football, hockey, soccer, volleyball, and basketball are among the most popular for high school students and for adult spectators. These activities can be very good for helping participants build fitness (though of course they do little for the fitness of spectators!). Team sports can be harder to do after your school years are completed because they require other participants (teammates), as well as special equipment and facilities. Even though baseball and softball involve some vigorous activity and training for these sports is often vigorous, they are usually considered to be moderate activities.

No team sport is among the 10 most popular types of physical activity performed by adults in the United States, but basketball is one of the few listed among the top 20. The 10 most popular activities are mostly either moderate physical activities or vigorous aerobics. Because relatively few people who play team sports when they are young continue to pursue them for a lifetime, it will be important for you to actively seek opportunities to continue

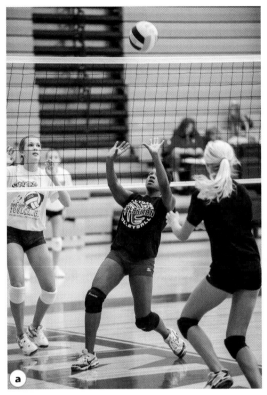
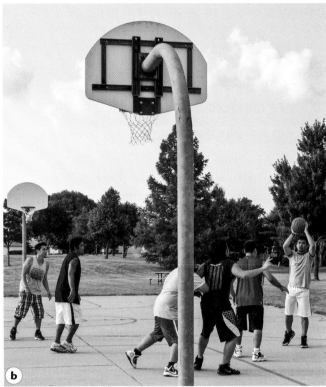

Team sports: *(a)* Volleyball is among the most popular team sports for high school students in the United States; *(b)* basketball is one of the few team sports listed among the top 20 physical activities performed by adults in the United States.

if you want to play team sports as you grow older. Another way to stay active is to begin learning an individual sport, a dual sport, or an aerobic activity that you can enjoy later in life.

## Dual or Partner Sports

Dual sports are those you can do with just one other person (the person you are playing against) or with a partner against another set of partners (for example, tennis doubles). Examples include tennis, badminton, fencing, and judo. Because they require fewer people than team sports, dual sports are often referred to as **lifetime sports** because they are easier to continue throughout your life. Tennis is often included in the top 10 participation activities in the United States, partly because it can be done with just one other person and because tennis courts are now available to most people.

Some dual sports are not activities that many people do as adults. For example, wrestling is considered a dual sport but is not often done as a lifetime sport, even though it does develop many important parts of health-related fitness. Dual sports

that are not done by many adults are not considered lifetime sports.

## Individual Sports

Individual sports are those that you can do by yourself. Golf, gymnastics, and bowling are truly individual sports because you do not have to have a partner or a team to perform them. Many of these sports are also lifetime sports because they are more likely to be done throughout life, although some, such as gymnastics, are not done by many people later in life (and gymnastics often requires a spotter). Skiing and skating are two forms of vigorous recreation that are also sometimes classified as individual sports.

## Outdoor, Challenge, or Extreme Sports

Many of the types of vigorous recreation can also be classified as sports. Some vigorous recreation activities are sometimes referred to as outdoor or challenge sports, such as mountain biking, rock climbing, sailing, and water skiing. Some other activities are sometimes referred to as extreme sports, such as snowboarding, skateboarding, surfing, and BMX cycling.

# Vigorous Recreation Activities

**Vigorous recreation** includes activities that are fun and, typically, noncompetitive. **Recreation** is something you do during your free time; therefore, recreational activities are sometimes called leisure activities. Recreation includes both physical activity and other pursuits, such as art and music. Here, of course, we focus on recreational activity that requires you to use your large muscles and involves considerable movement.

Many types of vigorous recreation are done outdoors because participants feel that the beauty of the setting and the fresh air help rejuvenate them. Examples of vigorous recreation include the following.

## Backpacking and Hiking

Hiking is particularly enjoyable because it takes place outdoors and can be done either independently or in a group. Most county, state, and national parks offer scenic trails for hikers of all levels of experience. Hiking usually involves a one-day trip, whereas backpacking often involves a multi-day venture that requires you to carry food, shelter, and other supplies on your back.

> " [Leave] all the afternoon for exercise and recreation, which are as necessary as reading; I will rather say more necessary, because health is worth more than learning. "
>
> —Thomas Jefferson, U.S. president

## Boating, Canoeing, Kayaking, and Rowing

Boating can be done in various forms that offer the enjoyment of water and the outdoors, free from the hassles of normal daily life. When done vigorously, these activities also help you build fitness and promote good health. Kayaking and rowing can be especially vigorous, and they require considerable skill to perform well and safely. Even when not done vigorously, boating activities can be relaxing and refreshing.

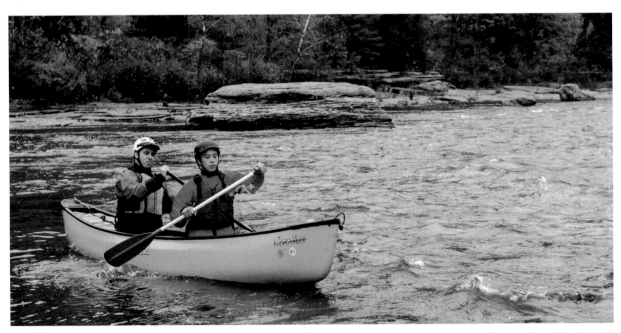

Boating can be a vigorous recreational activity that builds cardiorespiratory endurance and provides other health benefits.

## SCIENCE IN ACTION: Anaerobic Physical Activity

Unlike aerobic activity that can be sustained for long periods of time, **anaerobic activity** is activity that is so intense your body cannot supply adequate oxygen to sustain performance for more than a few seconds. Very vigorous anaerobic activity, such as an all-out sprint, can be sustained for only about 10 seconds and relies on high-energy fuel stored in the muscles (ATP-PC). Some vigorous activities (also anaerobic) are not "all-out" but are still very intense (they can be sustained for 11 to 90 seconds), and for those activities, the glycolytic system is used. Glucose (glycogen) stored in the muscles and liver provides the energy. Anaerobic activities are typically done in short bursts followed by rest periods. During the anaerobic activities your body builds up an oxygen debt because it can't take in enough oxygen to replenish the fuel needed to continue performance. After the activity is completed, oxygen is available to replenish the fuel stores—it repays the oxygen debt.

Your ability to perform anaerobic activity is referred to as **anaerobic capacity**. One of the most common tests of anaerobic capacity is the Wingate Test, which is done on a bicycle ergometer (stationary bicycle) and requires an all-out effort to pedal as fast as possible. This test is typically reserved for people interested in high-level anaerobic performance.

Sports such as basketball, football, and soccer involve sprints up the court or down the field. These sprints are anaerobic because they often require short but maximal effort. Sports allow time for recovery after these anaerobic bursts. This pattern means that players' heart rates may exceed the target zone during anaerobic sprints, then drop below the threshold of training during rest intervals (for example, when a free throw is taken in basketball). In fact, vigorous sports are not true aerobic activities, but when they are done for similar amounts of time they can be considered similar to vigorous aerobics. This is because they provide health benefits and improve cardiorespiratory endurance.

These sports offer the added advantage of building anaerobic capacity (also called *anaerobic power* and *anaerobic fitness*). Anaerobic capacity allows you to recover more quickly from anaerobic bursts and therefore improve your performance in certain sport activities. Some vigorous recreation activities, such as kayaking, are similar to vigorous sport activities in that they require good cardiorespiratory endurance as well as anaerobic fitness.

People who train for vigorous sport and recreation activities often use special anaerobic training techniques, such as interval training. Interval training involves repeated high-intensity exercise alternated with rest periods or bouts of lower-intensity exercise. There are many different kinds of interval training, including high-intensity interval training (HIIT) that alternates bouts of exercise at various intensities and lengths. The FIT formula for the most commonly used type of interval training is as follows.

- **F**requency = three to six days a week
- **I**ntensity = upper level of the target heart rate zone (because your exercise bouts are short)
- **T**ime = multiple exercise bouts of 10 to 60 seconds alternated with 1- to 2-minute rest periods or bouts of moderate exercise (totaling at least 10 minutes of exercise)

Depending on your goal, your length of exercise may vary from the durations given in the preceding formula. This type of training is appropriate for people who have already achieved the good fitness zone for cardiorespiratory endurance and who have regularly been doing vigorous activity. Before beginning this type of training, consult your teacher or coach or other qualified expert in kinesiology.

### Student Activity

While participating in an intermittent activity—such as basketball, soccer, or tennis—count your heart rate right after several vigorous bursts of activity. Determine whether the intensity of the activity is near the upper level of your target heart rate zone for aerobic activity.

## Orienteering

Orienteering combines walking, jogging, and skilled map reading. It is usually done in a rural area and might include hiking through rugged terrain. Participants depart from a starting point in staggered fashion every few minutes so that no participant can simply follow another. Each participant uses a compass and a map that describes a course up to 10 miles (16 kilometers) long. The compass is used to help locate several checkpoints marked by flags or other identifiers. At each checkpoint, the participant marks a card to indicate that he or she has located it. The activity can be competitive if the goal is to cover the course as fast as possible. Urban orienteering uses the same ideas and skills but in inner-city areas rather than rural settings.

## Rock Climbing and Bouldering

Many schools now teach rock climbing on climbing walls. Learning on a climbing wall allows you to get proper instruction with good spotting (protection against falling). More advanced climbers are skilled in using special safety ropes and equipment. Beginners and intermediate climbers should always climb with the help of an expert. When rock climbing is done properly with proper equipment, it is a relatively safe activity. It's also a good type of activity for building muscle fitness.

Bouldering is a type of rock climbing in which the climber tries to reach the top of a boulder using only gloves and special shoes (no special ropes or other equipment). Bouldering is most often done outside, but some clubs have artificial boulders for indoor climbing. The height of climbs is typically limited to 30 feet (about 9 meters). As with rock climbing, bouldering requires specials skills, so instruction is recommended for beginners.

## Skateboarding

As you probably know, skateboarding is a popular recreational activity among teens. Competitive skateboarding is now considered an extreme sport. Therefore, it can be considered both a recreational activity and a sport (for high-level competitors). Like in-line skating, skateboarding is a risky activity, so you should use proper safety equipment and seek proper instruction. You also need to find a proper place to perform skateboarding. Many skate hangouts are unsafe, and they are sometimes located in places where skating is prohibited. But many cities offer planned skate parks to provide safe places to skate.

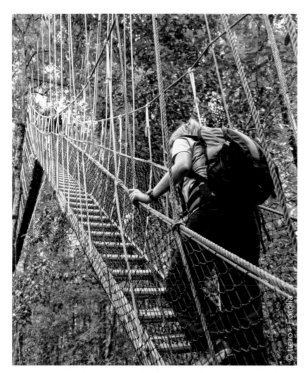

**Outdoor vigorous recreational activities have health benefits and help you meet national activity guidelines.**

### FIT FACT

Leisure time is more than free time. It is an attitude of declaring freedom from doing things you have to do. Similarly, the word *recreation* suggests refreshing or re-creating yourself. For this reason, a recreational activity is one that you do during your leisure or free time to refresh or re-create yourself. Recreational activities are done for fun and enjoyment. They need not be vigorous or purposeful. They can include watching TV, reading a book, playing chess, and doing many other relatively inactive pursuits. Some leisure activities—such as fishing, camping, and some forms of boating—can be considered moderate activities.

## Skating

Types of skating include in-line, roller, and ice. In-line skating is one of the fastest-growing activities in the United States. It was originally developed as a method of training for cross-country skiers in the summer, but its popularity has grown, and in-line sports (for example, hockey) have been developed. One study by a sports medicine group found that in-line skating was the most risky of the many participation activities studied, possibly because people fail to use proper safety equipment or because they try advanced skills too soon. The risk involved in skating activities makes it especially important for you to follow the safety guidelines described later in this chapter.

## Skiing

Kinds of skiing include cross-country skiing (a type of Nordic skiing), downhill skiing, snowboarding, and ski jumping. Cross-country skiing is typically done at a steady pace over a relatively long distance. For this reason, it could be considered a vigorous aerobic activity. Downhill skiing typically involves faster skiing, sometimes over moguls (bumps) and jumps. Snowboarding is like skateboarding on snow and has become extremely popular. It has joined the other forms of skiing as an Olympic sport, and some forms of snowboarding (halfpipe, superpipe, and slopestyle) can also be considered extreme sports. Ski jumping is also an Olympic sport, and it involves skiing down a ramp and jumping, trying to land as far down the hill as possible. All types of skiing

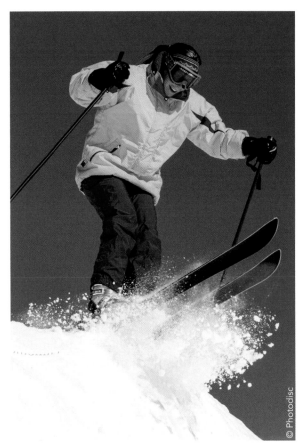

© Photodisc

**Skiing can be considered both a vigorous sport and a form of vigorous recreation.**

could be considered sports, but they are included here because so many people do them just for fun and recreation, although ski jumping isn't typically a recreational activity for most people.

---

### Lesson Review

1. What is vigorous aerobic activity, and what are the two major categories of vigorous activity included in the Physical Activity Pyramid?
2. What are some types of vigorous aerobic activity?
3. How is *sport* defined, and what are some categories of sport? Give an example of each.
4. How is *vigorous recreation* defined, and what are some examples?

If you're looking for an excellent vigorous activity that requires little skill and no equipment—except for a good pair of running shoes and proper clothing—then jogging might be for you. Millions of people jog (that is, run recreationally and noncompetitively), and millions more run competitively (and are called runners rather than joggers). Learning to jog properly can help you make the activity safe and fun. Guidelines for jogging have been developed on the basis of the principles of biomechanics and exercise physiology. Look over the two sets of principles, then study table 9.1 to learn about jogging guidelines.

### Biomechanical Principles

- Changing velocity (acceleration) is less efficient than maintaining a constant velocity.
- Applying force in the direction of movement is more efficient than moving to the side.
- Friction is necessary in order to apply force and to prevent slipping.
- Action (foot striking) results in a reaction (impact to the sole of the foot or heel).
- Stability requires a wide base of support.
- Proper leverage increases efficiency.
- Proper posture increases efficiency.

### Exercise Physiology Principles

- Muscle contractions not used to produce movement are inefficient.
- You must do more than normal to improve (this is the overload principle).

### Work With a Partner

- Jog about 100 yards (90 meters) while your partner stands behind you and checks your technique.
- Have your partner answer the questions in table 9.1 after watching you jog. Your instructor may provide a worksheet that contains the questions.
- Now have your partner jog while you evaluate his or her technique.
- Discuss the assessment with your partner.
- Both you and your partner can perform the jog a second time.
- Try to correct your technique and have your partner check you again. Do the same for your partner.

The self-assessment not only will help you jog more efficiently but also can reduce your risk of injury. Improper jogging technique can cause injuries such as sore shins, sore calves, and even a sore back. Having your feet and legs out of alignment can cause unnecessary strain on your joints and muscles.

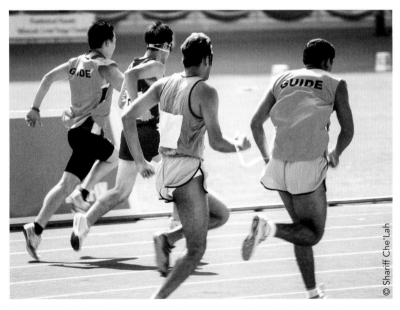

**Proper technique is important for everyone, from beginning joggers to elite runners.**

**TABLE 9.1   Jogging Self-Assessment Guidelines and Checklist**

| Guideline | Principle | Checklist | ✔ |
|---|---|---|---|
| Use proper foot action. Land on your heel or your entire foot. Then rock forward and push off with the ball of your foot and your toes. | Leverage | Do you land on your heel or whole foot? Do you push off with the ball of your foot and toes? | |
| Swing your legs and feet forward. Do not let your feet turn out to the sides. | Force application | Do your legs and feet swing and land straight ahead? | |
| Swing your arms forward and backward. Do not swing them across your body or to the sides. | Force application | Do your arms swing straight forward and backward? | |
| Keep your trunk fairly erect. When jogging, do not lean forward as you would when starting to run fast. Keep your head and chest up. | Proper posture | Is your body erect or leaning forward only slightly? Are your head and chest up? | |
| Use a longer step than your normal walking step. | Leverage | Is your jogging stride longer than your walking stride? | |
| Keep your arms bent at the elbow and your hands relaxed. Try to keep your shoulders relaxed. Avoid jogging with a clenched jaw to allow your upper body to relax more. | Efficient muscle use | Are your elbows bent properly (90 degrees) with your hands relaxed? Is your jaw relaxed? | |
| Jog at a steady pace. Avoid speeding up and slowing down. Correct jogging pace can vary from person to person. Find your own pace that elevates your heart rate into your target zone. If you are panting or gasping for breath, you are jogging too fast. | Velocity Overload | Is your pace steady? Is your heart rate in your target zone after several minutes of jogging? Is your pace slow enough to prevent gasping for breath? | |
| Wear shoes with a wide sole and heel, good heel cushions, and outer soles designed for running. | Stability Friction | Do your shoes have a wide heel and sole and good tread? | |

# Beginner's Jogging Workout

This workout helps you learn about how fast to jog in order to get a fitness benefit (by reaching your target heart rate). Try this workout after you've practiced your jogging technique.

1. Determine your target heart rate.

2. Jog for five minutes, trying to get your heart to the target level. Keep track of how long you run—how long you run is more important than how far. By using time instead of distance, you can jog anywhere. Set your own course. Try to jog half the time moving away from your starting point and the other half returning to your starting point. If you are not near your starting point at the end of five minutes, walk the rest of the way back.

3. Focus on using the jogging techniques that you learned earlier in this self-assessment.

4. At the end of five minutes, determine your one-minute exercise heart rate. Determine whether your rate was in your target heart rate zone.

5. Jog for five minutes again. If your exercise heart rate was lower than your target heart rate on the first jog, jog faster this time. If your exercise heart rate was higher than your target rate on the first jog, jog slower this time. If your exercise heart rate was in the target zone on the first jog, jog at the same speed this time. After your second run, count your exercise heart rate again.

6. As directed by your teacher, record your results.

# Preparing and Performing a Safe and Vigorous Physical Activity Program

**Lesson Objectives**

After reading this lesson, you should be able to

1. describe several guidelines for participating safely in vigorous physical activity,
2. collect information about your personal needs and build a fitness and activity profile,
3. set goals for vigorous physical activity, and
4. select vigorous activities and write a plan for vigorous activity.

**Lesson Vocabulary**

compendium, over-exercising

---

**Are** you prepared to do regular vigorous physical activity? In this lesson, you'll learn why it's important to be well prepared before you begin. You'll also use the five steps of program planning to prepare your personal plan for vigorous physical activity. Creating your plan will help you meet national physical activity guidelines both now and later in life. Vigorous activities can be some of the most enjoyable, and they also offer many health benefits.

## Fitness for Vigorous Aerobics, Sport, and Recreation

Just as vigorous physical activity contributes to good fitness, you also must stay fit in order to participate in vigorous activity. Some people mistakenly assume that fitness is not necessary for certain sports, especially if the sport itself does little to build fitness. For example, softball is not particularly good for developing fitness, but it does require good fitness. Similarly, some people snow-ski only once or twice a year and otherwise do not exercise regularly. Nevertheless, they believe they are fit enough to ski. In reality, these people should exercise regularly for at least several weeks before skiing in order to get ready for the activity and to reduce their chance of injury.

Participating in vigorous activity involves greater risk of injury than doing no activity or doing light or moderate activity. Even vigorous aerobics, which is relatively safe compared to other vigorous sport

and recreational activities, can result in injury if overdone. Jogging (or running) is one of the top five activities in terms of injury to participants, and regular participants in high-impact and step aerobics are also often injured. Unlike common sport injuries such as ligament sprains and muscle strains, the injuries typically experienced by joggers and aerobic dancers involve overuse—for example, heel bruises, sore shins, stress fractures in the legs and feet, and sometimes knee or back injury. Long distance runners and aerobic dance instructors also have a higher-than-normal rate of injury. More generally, the people most prone to injury are those who train every day or who participate in several vigorous aerobic activity sessions in a day.

**Safety Tips for Vigorous Physical Activity**

• **Warm up before your workout.** Use a low- to moderate-intensity general warm-up for 5 to 10 minutes, a series of dynamic exercises, or a stretching warm-up, depending on the activity to be performed. For a stretching warm-up, remember to hold stretches no more than 30 seconds prior to strength, power, and speed activities.

• **Cool down after the workout.** A cool-down helps you recover more quickly.

• **Wear proper safety equipment.** For example, bikers and skaters should wear helmets, and skaters should also wear hand and knee pads. Dress appropriately for the weather.

• **Use safe equipment.** Bikes should have lights and reflectors. Backpacking equipment should fit your body size, and loads should not be too heavy. Skis and other equipment should be in good repair, properly sized, and equipped with proper releases or other safety features. Boaters should wear life preservers. Rock climbers should use appropriate safety equipment. When doing any vigorous activity, especially in the heat, drink water regularly.

• **Get proper instruction.** Whether you're skiing, in-line skating, boating, rock-climbing, or doing some other activity, you should get proper instruction before participating. Performing an activity improperly has caused many people to get injured or have an accident.

• **Perform within the limits of your current skills.** Many injuries occur because people try to perform beyond their skill limits; for example, beginning skiers should not attempt to ski advanced slopes. For all activities, start with simple skills and then gradually attempt to perform more difficult skills as your abilities improve.

• **Don't overdo it.** Taking at least one day a week to rest can help you avoid injury, especially if you're participating in a vigorous aerobic activity such as aerobic dance or running. Most injuries can be prevented simply by not **over-exercising** (doing so much exercise that you increase your risk of injury or soreness).

• **Plan ahead.** If you're going on a hike, make sure that you have a map and know where you're going. Carry an emergency phone. If you're going skiing, make sure that the trail is open, and don't ski in restricted areas. When backpacking, carry enough food and water to supply you if you get lost. When traveling in an unfamiliar area, stay with your group.

For most vigorous sport and recreation activities, you must have good fitness in order to perform well. For example, a baseball player must sprint between bases, slide into bases, and jump to catch the ball. Each of these actions could result in an injury if the player is not physically fit. Good or high-performance fitness is especially necessary for activities with the following characteristics.

## FIT FACT

Each year, participation in common recreational activities leads to two million medically treated injuries among youth in the United States. Medical groups state that you can dramatically decrease your risk of injury by following simple safety tips when participating in physical activity.

• Physical contact (football, rugby, wrestling, ice hockey)

• Sprinting (baseball, softball, soccer, ultimate)

• Sudden fast starts and stops (volleyball, racquetball, track, basketball)

• Vigorous jumping (basketball, high jumping, soccer)

• Danger of falling (skiing, skating, judo)

• Danger of overstretching muscles (tennis, football, squash)

## Finding the Best Vigorous Activities for You

In this class, you'll get the opportunity to try many types of vigorous activity, such as aerobic dance, step

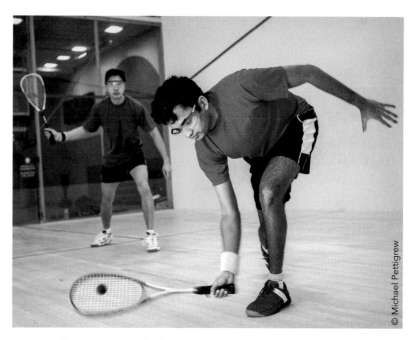

© Michael Pettigrew

**Exercise helps you get fit, but you must also be fit to perform physical activities safely.**

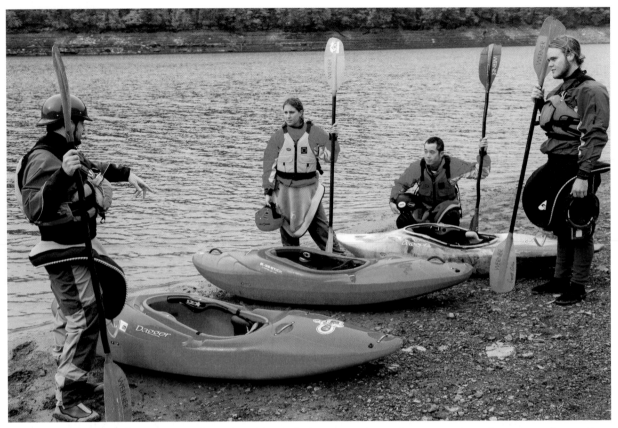

Important safety tips for vigorous physical activity include using safe equipment and getting proper instruction.

aerobics, line dancing, jogging, exercise circuits, and rope jumping. Try a variety of activities to discover which ones you like best. For any given activity, try it more than once before you decide whether to do it in the future. It takes time to decide what you like and don't like. If you're going to stick with an activity over the long term, it must be enjoyable. To help you enjoy an activity, consider finding good instruction, wearing appropriate clothing, getting good equipment (if necessary), and finding others with whom you can participate.

## Preparing a Vigorous Physical Activity Plan

Lin Su used the five steps of program planning to prepare a vigorous physical activity program. She had been doing some regular moderate activity but wanted to do more vigorous activity. Her program is described in the following sections of this chapter.

### FIT FACT

Teen boys are more likely than teen girls to be vigorously active at least three times a week, and high school girls are especially likely to become less active as they grow older. Health experts are interested in finding ways to help teen girls be more physically active.

### Step 1: Determine Your Personal Needs

To get started, Lin Su wrote down her fitness test results that related to vigorous physical activity. She also made a list of the vigorous physical activities that she had performed over the past week. Her results are shown in figure 9.2.

Lin Su's cardiorespiratory endurance ratings showed that she was in the marginal category for each of the self-assessments that she performed. She

| Physical fitness profile | | | |
|---|---|---|---|
| **Fitness self-assessment** | **Score** | **Rating** | |
| Walking test | Time: 18:30 Heart rate: 150 | Marginal | |
| PACER | 37 mL/kg/min | Marginal | |
| Step test | Heart rate: 104 | Marginal | |
| One-mile (1.6 km) run | No score | No rating | |
| Physical activity profile | | | |
| **Day** | **Vigorous activity (min)** | **All activity (min)** | **Met 60 min guideline?** |
| Mon. | 0 | 40 | |
| Tues. | 20 | 60 | ✔ |
| Wed. | 0 | 40 | |
| Thurs. | 20 | 60 | ✔ |
| Fri. | 20 | 40 | |
| Sat. | 0 | 20 | |
| Sun. | 0 | 20 | |

**FIGURE 9.2**   Lin Su's vigorous physical activity and fitness profiles.

met the national activity guideline of 60 minutes per day on two days of the previous week. She did vigorous activity for 20 minutes on Tuesday and Thursday in her physical education class. On Friday she jogged for 20 minutes with her friend Eric, but she didn't do that regularly. She had also walked to and from school (20 minutes each way), and this moderate activity combined with her physical education activities and jogging totaled 60 minutes. On the other days, she did only moderate activity (walking to and from school) totaling less than 60 minutes, except on Friday when she had physical education class. Lin Su knew that she needed to be more active and especially wanted to do more vigorous activity.

## Step 2: Consider Your Program Options

Lin Su wanted to include activities that would help her build her cardiorespiratory endurance and that offered other health-fitness benefits. She also wanted to focus on activities that she thought she would enjoy. To select vigorous activities, she used table 9.2, which illustrates the health-related fitness benefits of a wide variety of vigorous activities. Even this list, however, includes only a sample of the most popular vigorous aerobics, sport, and recreation activities; it was adapted from a larger **compendium** of activities. A link to the compendium can be found in the student section of the Fitness for Life website.

After reviewing the list of activities, Lin Su wrote down her preferred activity options.

**Continue Current Activities**
- Walking to and from school
- Jogging
- Physical education class activities

**Vigorous Aerobics**
- More jogging
- Aerobic dance

**Vigorous Recreation**
- Hiking
- In-line skating

**Vigorous Sport**
- Tennis
- Badminton

**School**
- Before-school recreation
- After-school sports

## TABLE 9.2 Health-Related Benefits of Selected Vigorous Physical Activities

| Activity | Develops cardiorespiratory endurance | Develops strength | Develops muscular endurance | Develops flexibility | Helps control body fat |
|---|---|---|---|---|---|
| Aerobic dance*+ | Excellent | Fair | Good | Fair | Excellent |
| Aerobics machine+ | Excellent | Fair | Good | Poor | Excellent |
| Backpacking+ | Fair | Fair | Excellent | Poor | Good/Excellent |
| Badminton+ | Fair | Poor | Fair | Fair | Fair/Good |
| Baseball/Softball* | Poor | Poor | Poor | Poor | Poor/Fair |
| Basketball, half-court*+ | Fair | Poor | Fair | Poor | Poor/Fair |
| Basketball, full-court*+ | Excellent | Fair | Good | Poor | Excellent |
| Biking+ | Good | Fair | Good | Poor | Good/Excellent |
| BMX cycling | Good | Good | Excellent | Fair | Good |
| Canoeing+ | Fair | Fair | Fair | Poor | Fair/Good |
| Circuit training+ | Good | Good | Good | Fair | Good/Excellent |
| Football* | Fair | Good | Fair | Poor | Fair |
| Gymnastics | Fair | Excellent | Excellent | Excellent | Fair |
| Handball/Racquetball*+ | Good/Excellent | Fair | Good | Poor | Good/Excellent |
| Hiking | Fair | Fair | Fair/Good | Poor | Good |
| Hip-hop dance | Good/Excellent | Fair | Good | Fair | Good/Excellent |
| Horseback riding+ | Poor | Poor | Poor | Poor | Poor |
| Kayaking*+ | Good | Good | Good | Fair | Good |
| Martial arts*+ | Good | Fair | Fair | Fair | Fair |
| Mountain or rock climbing*+ | Good | Good | Good | Poor | Good |
| Racquetball*+ | Good/Excellent | Fair | Good | Poor | Good/Excellent |
| Rowing (crew)* | Excellent | Fair | Excellent | Poor | Excellent |
| Sailing+ | Poor | Poor | Poor | Poor | Poor |
| Skating (roller or ice)*+ | Good | Fair | Good | Fair | Good |
| Skiing (cross-country)*+ | Excellent | Fair | Good | Poor | Excellent |
| Skiing (downhill)*+ | Fair/Good | Fair | Good | Poor | Fair/Good |
| Snowboarding*+ | Fair/Good | Fair | Good | Fair | Fair/Good |
| Soccer* | Excellent | Fair | Good | Fair | Excellent |
| Social dance+ | Fair | Poor | Fair | Fair | Fair |
| Surfing*+ | Fair | Poor | Good | Fair | Fair/Good |
| Swimming+ | Good | Fair | Good | Fair | Good/Excellent |
| Table tennis*+ | Poor | Poor | Poor/Fair | Poor | Poor/Fair |
| Tennis*+ | Good/Excellent | Fair | Good | Poor | Good/Excellent |
| Volleyball*+ | Fair | Fair | Good | Poor | Fair/Good |
| Waterskiing*+ | Fair | Fair | Good | Poor | Fair/Good |

*Fitness needed to prevent injury.

+Lifetime activity.

## Step 3: Set Goals

For this vigorous activity plan, Lin Su chose a time period of two weeks. Since this was too short to accommodate long-term goals, she developed only short-term physical activity goals for the plan. Later, she will develop long-term goals, including some physical fitness goals, when she prepares a longer plan. For now, in developing her short-term goals for vigorous physical activity, she referred to her activity preferences decided in step 2. She also reviewed her work to be sure that she was setting SMART goals. She set the following goals.

1. Continue to jog one day a week for 20 minutes.
2. Continue to do vigorous activity in physical education class two days a week (20 minutes).
3. Play tennis for 60 minutes of moderate activity one day every other week.
4. Do aerobic dance for 30 minutes one day a week.
5. Go hiking for 60 minutes one day every other week.

## Step 4: Structure Your Program and Write It Down

Lin Su's written two-week plan for vigorous physical activity is shown in figure 9.3. Lin Su included most of the activities from her list. She didn't include badminton or in-line skating, and she didn't participate in before-school recreation or after-school sports. Her plan met the national activity guideline of at least 20 minutes of vigorous activity three days a week. In fact, her plan called for more than 20 minutes of vigorous activity on six days of the week. Lin Su decided to take a break from vigorous activity on Sunday. She also kept walking to and from school daily. Although this was moderate activity, she planned to keep doing it to help her meet the national activity goal of 60 minutes of moderate to vigorous physical activity each day.

## Step 5: Keep a Log and Evaluate Your Program

Over the next two weeks, Lin Su will self-monitor her activities and place a checkmark in her written plan beside each of the activities that she performs.

| Week 1 | | | | Week 2 | | | |
|---|---|---|---|---|---|---|---|
| Day | Activity | Time | ✔ | Day | Activity | Time | ✔ |
| Mon. | | | | Mon. | | | |
| Tues. | Physical education class | 10:30–11:15 a.m.* | | Tues. | Physical education class* | 10:30–11:15 a.m.* | |
| Wed. | Aerobic dance | 4:00–4:30 p.m. | | Wed. | Aerobic dance | 4:00–4:30 p.m. | |
| Thurs. | Physical education class | 10:30–11:15 a.m.* | | Thurs. | Physical education class | 10:30–11:15 a.m.* | |
| Fri. | Jog | 4:00–4:20 p.m. | | Fri. | Jog | 4:00–4:20 p.m. | |
| Sat. | Tennis | 9:00–10:00 a.m. | | Sat. | Hiking | 9:00–10:00 a.m. | |
| Sun. | No planned activity | | | Sun. | No planned activity | | |

*Only 20 minutes of the 45-minute class included vigorous activity.

**FIGURE 9.3**  Lin Su's written plan.

**CONSUMER CORNER:** **Using the Web for Fitness, Health, and Wellness Information**

One national health goal in the United States for the year 2020 is to increase the number of high-quality websites related to health. Health is the most common subject of web searches, and 75 percent of all teens and young adults seek health information on the web. But many websites, including popular web encyclopedias, contain incorrect information about health, which can result in injury, illness, failure to get adequate care, and loss of money spent on products and treatments that don't work. With all this in mind, one of the most important goals of *Fitness for Life* is to help you become a critical consumer of fitness, health, and wellness information. Consider the following guidelines when you search the web.

- Consider using websites provided by government agencies. They contain information supplied by experts based on scientific research. Most government website addresses end with the extension .gov. One example of a good governmental source for information is the U.S. Centers for Disease Control and Prevention.

- Consider using websites provided by universities and professional organizations (such as the American Medical Association). Professional organizations' website addresses typically end with the extension .org, and universities' addresses typically end with the extension .edu.

- Beware of websites with names intended to fool you. When the web was first developed, only a few extensions (such as .gov, .org, .edu, and .com) were available for use at the end of a web address. Now, many more extensions are in use, and some people take advantage of this variety to create copycat websites intended to fool you into thinking you're choosing a reliable site when in fact you're not. They do this by using the same name as a reliable website (or a similar name) but a different extension—for example, reliablewebsite.xyz instead of reliablewebsite.gov.

At the end of two weeks, she will evaluate her activity to see whether she met her goals, then use the evaluation to help her create another activity plan.

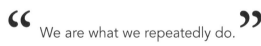
" We are what we repeatedly do. "

—Aristotle, Greek philosopher

In the Taking Action activity later in this lesson, you will get to use the same planning steps that Lin Su used to create a two-week personal plan for vigorous physical activity. Use tables similar to those used by Lin Su to help you in your planning. Then try out your program and see if you can meet your goals. The same steps can be used in the future to plan health goals or prepare for a special event, such as running a 10K race or participating on the cross-country team.

## Lesson Review

1. What steps can you take to make vigorous activity safe and fun?
2. How can you assess personal needs and build a fitness and activity profile?
3. What are some factors to consider in setting goals for vigorous physical activity?
4. How can you best select vigorous activities and write a plan for vigorous activity?

You can help yourself be active by choosing activities you're likely to do both now and throughout your life. One way to evaluate an activity is to find out the number of people who participate and how long they tend to stay involved. Here's an example.

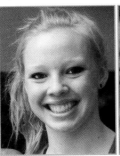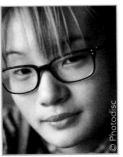

© Photodisc

At a recent high school reunion, the alumni enjoyed seeing their former classmates again. Everyone remembered Norma as an athlete. She had played soccer, basketball, and softball. What a surprise when her classmates discovered that 10 years later Norma was doing very little physical activity! The closest she got to participating in any sport was to watch her son's tee ball games. According to Norma, "It was just too hard to find people who wanted to play the team sports I used to enjoy."

Kim Lea was just the opposite. In high school, she had always gone to the games and cheered for the teams, but she had never dreamed of taking part in a sport. In fact, she would have been the first to admit that she was sedentary. Now, Kim Lea was biking with her two children and organizing her neighborhood aerobics class. She described it this way: "Every Tuesday and Thursday morning, we all get together and talk while we work out. No one cares how we dress or how good we are at doing the exercises. We all just seem to be energized as we go on to our next activities."

## For Discussion

Why did Norma feel that it was no longer feasible to continue participating in the sports she played in high school? What might help her get involved in a physical activity again? Why do you think Kim Lea started to participate in activities? What advice would you have for other people who want to get active later in life? Consider the guidelines presented in the Self-Management feature as you answer the discussion questions.

# SELF-MANAGEMENT: Skills for Choosing Good Activities

Research shows that the most active people in society are those who have identified specific activities that they enjoy. For example, many people love tennis, golf, or running and participate in their chosen activity on a regular basis. Others prefer variety, so they choose several activities. In both cases, these people might not have become so active if they were not doing activities that they especially enjoy. Use the following guidelines to help you find a physical activity (or activities) especially good for you.

- **Consider your physical fitness.** How well you do in an activity depends on all parts of fitness—both health related and skill related. Choose activities that match your abilities in both kinds of fitness. Also consider activities that help you build health-related fitness (see table 9.2).

- **Consider your interests.** Don't avoid an activity that you really enjoy or have always wanted to do just because it doesn't match your fitness profile. Do be aware, however, that even with practice it may take you longer than others to learn the activity. But finding an activity that is fun for you is very important, so consider a variety of activities.

- **Consider an activity that you can do with others.** Try to find others of your own ability so that you won't be discouraged if you don't learn the activity as quickly as you'd like.

- **Consider the activity's benefits.** As you progress through this book, you'll learn about the benefits of various activities. If you want to get optimal fitness, health, and wellness benefits, select activities from each area of the Physical Activity Pyramid.

- **Practice, practice, practice.** Becoming skilled in a sport or activity increases your enjoyment. If you choose an activity that is new to you, there is no substitute for practice. To make your practice more productive, consider taking lessons.

- **Consider activities that do not require high levels of skill.** Some activities do not require high levels of any part of skill-related fitness. Of the activities included in the Physical Activity Pyramid, sport provides the most benefit for skill-related fitness, but it also *requires* relatively high levels of both sport skill and skill-related fitness in order to play. Sport skills such as throwing, catching, hitting, and kicking are different from skill-related fitness abilities such as agility, balance, and coordination—though these do help you learn sport skills more easily. Learning sport skills requires a lot of practice in order to perform them well. Generally speaking, fewer skills are required for moderate and vigorous aerobic activities than for sport. As a result, even people with relatively low scores on most or all parts of skill-related fitness can find a moderate or aerobic activity to enjoy—for example, jogging, walking, or cycling. Because these activities don't require high skill levels, they also tend not to require extensive practice. Therefore, you might want to consider one of these activities if you're not willing to put in the necessary time to learn a more complicated one.

 ## ACADEMIC CONNECTION: Figurative Language

Part of meeting standards for English language arts is being able to describe the meaning of words and phrases, including figurative and literal meanings. Figurative language describes a person or thing by comparing it to another thing. Literal language describes people and things as they actually are (in real terms).

When studying fitness, health, and wellness, you might have come across figurative language. It has several categories. Following are some examples of the use of figurative language from various categories.

- She is strong as an ox (a simile—compares two things using the words *like* or *as*).

- He is a couch potato (metaphor—a phrase that doesn't make sense literally but uses similarities between two things to make a connection that is meaningful).

- He ran at the crack of the bat (onomatopoeia—uses words that mimic sounds or sound like their meaning).

- I was so tired you could have knocked me down with a feather (hyperbole—exaggerating to emphasize a point).

- The team's bright uniforms screamed for attention (personification—things or ideas are described as if they had human characteristics).

Try to think of other examples of figurative language associated with fitness, health, or wellness.

# TAKING ACTION: Your Vigorous Physical Activity Plan

Prepare a vigorous physical activity plan using the five steps described in the second lesson in this chapter. Like Lin Su, consider activities from all three categories: vigorous aerobics, vigorous sport, and vigorous recreation. Your goal should be to accumulate at least 20 minutes of vigorous physical activity on at least three days each week.

Prepare a written plan and carry out it over a two-week period. Your teacher may give you time in class to do some of the activities included in your plan. Consider the following suggestions for **taking action**.

- Before you do vigorous physical activity, perform a dynamic warm-up.
- Consider the tips presented in this chapter for safe vigorous activity.
- Consider the guidelines presented in this chapter for making good activity selections.
- Progress gradually. Don't try to do too much too soon.
- After your workout, perform a cooldown.

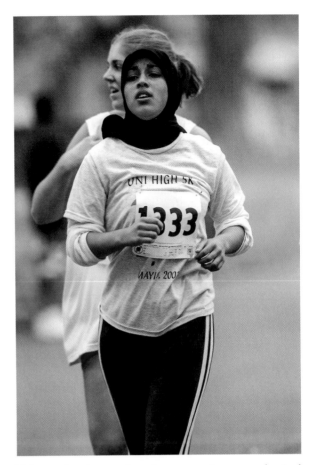

Take action by performing your vigorous physical activity plan.

# CHAPTER REVIEW

## Reviewing Concepts and Vocabulary

As directed by your teacher, answer items 1 through 5 by correctly completing each sentence with a word or phrase.

1. Vigorous activity is exercise that raises your heart rate above the _____.
2. Activities that are competitive and have rules are called _____.
3. Activities so intense that you can perform them for only a few seconds are called _____ activities.
4. Free time, or time free from work, is called _____.
5. A _____ is a list that tells you the intensity of various activities.

For items 6 through 10, as directed by your teacher, match each term in column 1 with the appropriate phrase in column 2.

6. water aerobics
7. orienteering
8. in-line skating
9. recreational activity
10. circuit training

a. aqua dynamics
b. several exercise stations
c. done for fun during free time
d. uses map-reading skills
e. has relatively high injury risk

For items 11 through 15, as directed by your teacher, respond to each statement or question.

11. What is the difference between individual and dual sports?
12. What are some examples of outdoor, challenge, and extreme sports? Why are these sports popular?
13. What is interval training and what are the best frequency, intensity, and time for performing it?
14. What are several safety tips for vigorous physical activity?
15. What are some guidelines for making good physical activity selections?

## Thinking Critically

Write a paragraph to answer the following question.

You have a friend who wants to avoid vigorous physical activity because of suffering frequent injuries in the past. What advice would you give your friend to help him or her avoid such problems in the future?

## Project

Create a vigorous aerobics exercise routine. Choose music paced at about 100 to 120 beats per minute and plan for the routine to last two to three minutes. You can do an aerobic dance routine, a hip-hop routine, or some other form of continuous exercise. Work with a group to perform a routine (yours or another group member's) in class.

© Photodis

# UNIT IV

# Muscle Fitness and Flexibility

**Healthy People 2020 Goals**
- Increase the percentage of teens who do regular muscle fitness exercises.
- Increase the percentage of adults who meet national guidelines for muscle fitness exercise.
- Reduce the percentage of teens who do no leisure physical activity.
- Increase out-of-school physical activity by teens.
- Decrease steroid use among teens.
- Reduce incidence of back problems.
- Reduce incidence of osteoporosis.
- Reduce sport and recreation injuries.
- Reduce overweight and obesity.

**Self-Assessment Features in This Unit**
- Muscle Fitness Testing
- Healthy Back Test
- Arm, Leg, and Trunk Flexibility

**Taking Charge Features in This Unit**
- Preventing Relapse
- Finding Social Support
- Overcoming Barriers

**Self-Management Features in This Unit**
- Skills for Preventing Relapse
- Skills for Finding Social Support
- Skills for Overcoming Barriers

**Taking Action Features in This Unit**
- Resistance Machine Exercises
- Your Muscle Fitness Exercise Plan
- Your Flexibility Exercise Plan

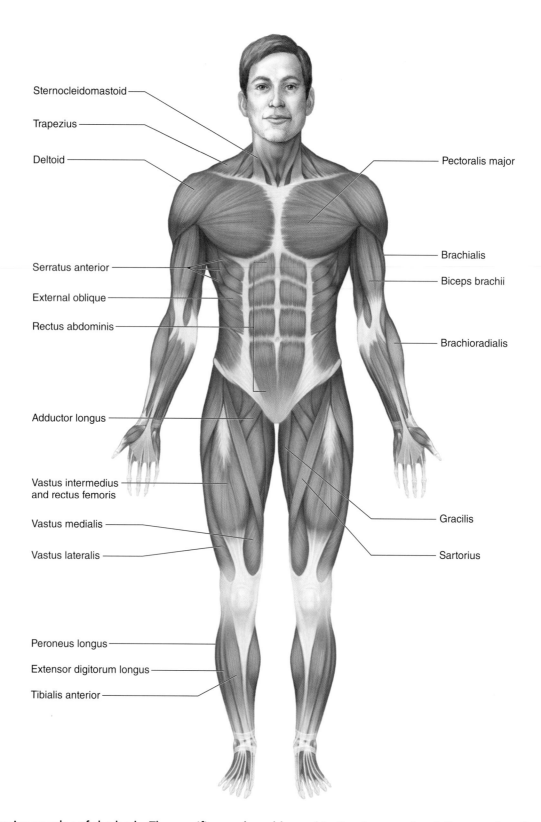

Sternocleidomastoid

Trapezius

Deltoid

Pectoralis major

Brachialis

Biceps brachii

Serratus anterior

External oblique

Rectus abdominis

Brachioradialis

Adductor longus

Vastus intermedius and rectus femoris

Gracilis

Vastus medialis

Vastus lateralis

Sartorius

Peroneus longus

Extensor digitorum longus

Tibialis anterior

**The major muscles of the body. The specific muscles addressed in the chapters that follow are described with each exercise. Refer to these two illustrations for exact muscle locations.**

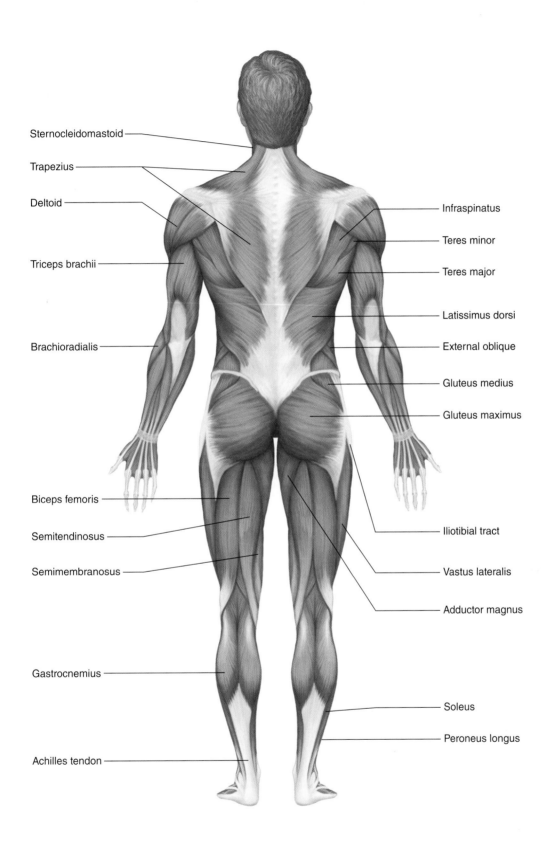

Sternocleidomastoid

Trapezius

Deltoid

Triceps brachii

Brachioradialis

Biceps femoris

Semitendinosus

Semimembranosus

Gastrocnemius

Achilles tendon

Infraspinatus

Teres minor

Teres major

Latissimus dorsi

External oblique

Gluteus medius

Gluteus maximus

Iliotibial tract

Vastus lateralis

Adductor magnus

Soleus

Peroneus longus

# 10

# Muscle Fitness Basics

## In This Chapter

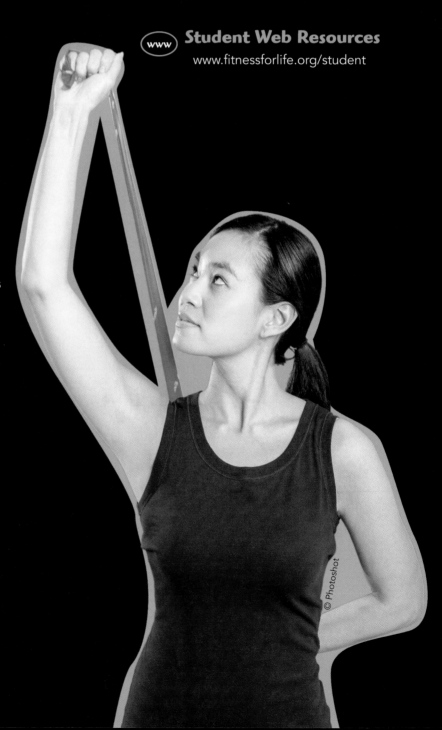

**www** **Student Web Resources**
www.fitnessforlife.org/student

© Photoshot

# Lesson 10.1
# Muscle Fitness Facts

## Lesson Objectives

After reading this lesson, you should be able to

1. explain the differences between strength, muscular endurance, and power;
2. describe how exercise principles apply to muscle fitness;
3. describe the types of muscle fitness exercise; and
4. describe several methods for assessing muscle fitness.

## Lesson Vocabulary

absolute strength, calisthenics, concentric, dynamometer, eccentric, fast-twitch muscle fiber, hypertrophy, intermediate muscle fiber, isokinetic exercise, isometric contraction, isometric exercise, isotonic contraction, isotonic exercise, 1-repetition maximum (1RM), plyometrics, principle of rest and recovery, progressive resistance exercise (PRE), relative strength, reps, set, slow-twitch muscle fiber

**Does** your favorite activity require muscle fitness? Do you have enough muscle fitness? Muscle fitness is made up of three health-related parts of physical fitness: strength, muscular endurance, and power.

## FIT FACT

Together strength, muscular endurance, power, and flexibility are referred to as *musculoskeletal fitness* because all four of these parts of fitness are associated with the muscular and skeletal systems. In this book, *muscle fitness* is used as a general term to describe the three parts of musculoskeletal fitness that require the muscles to produce force (strength, muscular endurance, and power).

Strength is the amount of force that a muscle can exert. The amount of weight that a group of muscles can lift one time is called a **1-repetition maximum (1RM)**, which is a good indicator of force exerted. This is considered the best measure of strength. Having good strength enables you to apply effective force in sports (such as football) and in tasks that require heavy lifting (figure 10.1*a*).

Muscular endurance is the ability to contract muscles many times without tiring or to hold a muscle contraction for a long time without fatigue. Muscular endurance allows you to resist muscle fatigue in recreational activities such as backpacking and to persist in work activities such as carrying a mailbag for hours at a time (figure 10.1*b*).

The third part of muscle fitness is power. Power is the ability to use strength (produce force) quickly; thus it involves both strength and speed. It is often referred to as explosive strength. Examples of power include jumping high or far and throwing objects a great distance. Research has shown that power is especially important to bone health and that bone health built in the teen years provides lifelong benefits (figure 10.1*c*).

All three components of muscle fitness—strength, muscular endurance, and power—are important to both health and good performance. This chapter includes exercises from step 4 of the Physical Activity Pyramid (figure 10.2) to develop muscle fitness.

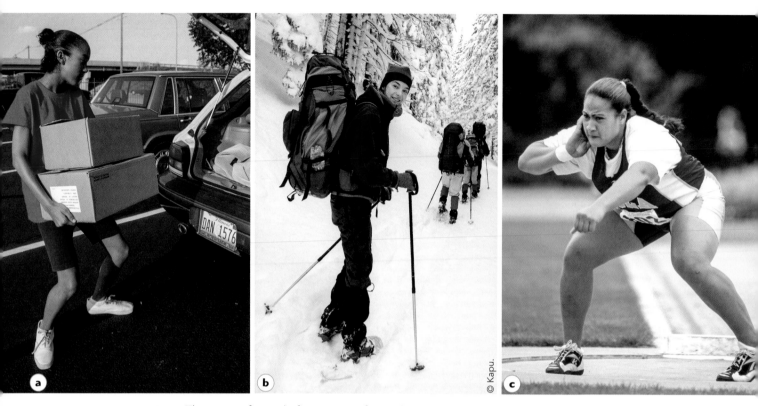

**FIGURE 10.1** The parts of muscle fitness: *(a)* Lifting a heavy object requires strength; *(b)* using your muscles for a long time requires muscular endurance; and *(c)* doing activities that involve fast application of force requires power.

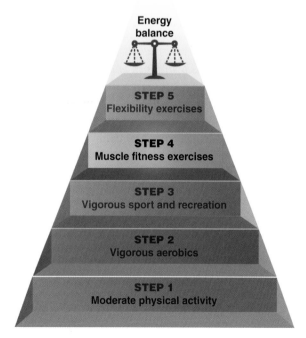

**FIGURE 10.2** Activities from step 4 of the Physical Activity Pyramid build muscle fitness.

## Muscle Fitness Terminology

You may have heard the terms *reps* and *sets* in relation to muscular fitness, and figure 10.3 can help you understand them. The term **reps** (short for *repetitions*) refers to the number of consecutive times you do an exercise. A **set** is one group of repetitions. For example, suppose you do an exercise 8 times, then rest; repeat it 8 times, then rest again; and repeat it another 8 times. You have just done 3 sets of 8 repetitions each.

## The Muscular Endurance–Strength Continuum

The exercises used to develop muscular endurance and strength differ only in the number of repetitions and the amount of resistance. The relationship between endurance and strength can be represented on a continuum such as the one shown in figure 10.4, which presents pounds of resistance on one edge and number of repetitions on the other.

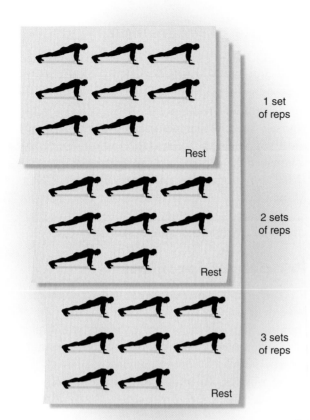

**FIGURE 10.3** Muscle fitness exercises are typically done in reps and sets.

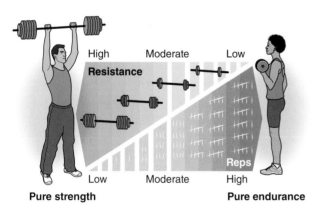

**FIGURE 10.4** Muscular endurance–strength continuum.

The continuum shows the resistance and repetitions that a person might use to build muscle fitness. To develop strength, you would use <u>high resistance</u> with fewer repetitions; to develop endurance, you would use low resistance with more repetitions; and to develop both strength and endurance, you

would use the resistance and repetitions shown in the middle of the continuum. This continuum also shows that usually when you train for strength you will also develop some endurance, and when you train for endurance you will also develop some strength.

# Cardiorespiratory Endurance and Muscular Endurance

Muscular endurance is one part of muscle fitness, and it is different from the other parts (strength and power). It is also different from cardiorespiratory endurance, which depends on your cardiovascular and respiratory systems to supply oxygen. Cardiorespiratory endurance is general (not specific to one area of the body), and good cardiorespiratory endurance allows your entire body to function.

Muscular endurance, on the other hand, is the ability to contract your muscles many times without tiring or to hold one contraction for a long time. Muscular endurance depends on the ability of your muscle fibers to keep working without getting tired. You can have good muscular endurance in one part of your body (such as your legs) without having it in another part of your body (such as your arms).

# Strength and Power

For years, power was considered to be a skill-related part of fitness. Sometimes it was referred to as a combined part of fitness because it involves both strength (the ability to exert force) and speed (the ability to cover a distance in a short time). Because it involves a strength component, power is often referred to as explosive strength. There is no doubt that both power and strength are important for performance, but today we understand that both are also important for your health. The Institute of Medicine reports that adults who lack power have a higher-than-normal risk of chronic disease, reduced lifespan, and poor functional health as they grow older. Exercise physiologists have also demonstrated that power—and activities that produce power—are very important in building healthy bones in youth. Because of these links to health, power is now classified as a health-related part of fitness.

# Fitness Principles and Muscle Fitness

The three basic fitness principles can be applied to muscle fitness exercise. These principles—overload, progression, and specificity—have been covered elsewhere in this book. They are discussed again in this chapter to show how they relate specifically to muscle fitness.

## Principle of Overload

To improve muscle fitness, a muscle must contract harder than normal. In other words, the muscle must work against a greater load than it normally bears in regular daily activity. High overload (high resistance) builds strength, whereas more moderate overload repeated many times builds muscular endurance. Exercises for power require overload for speed and strength. The reverse of the overload principle also applies—if you don't use your muscles, you'll lose muscle fitness. "Use it or lose it!"

## Principle of Progression

The principle of progression holds that you should gradually increase load or resistance over time in order to best improve your muscle fitness. If you try to use too much resistance too soon, you can injure yourself. Exercise that increases resistance (overload) until you reach the desired level of muscle fitness is referred to as **progressive resistance exercise (PRE)** or progressive resistance training (PRT). Many kinds of progressive resistance exercise—for example, weight training, resistance machine exercises, and plyometrics—are described later.

## Principle of Specificity

Strength, muscular endurance, and power each have their own FIT formula. The specific type of training that you perform determines which part of muscle fitness you build. In addition, you build specific muscles by doing exercises specifically for those muscles. To build your arm muscles, you must overload your arm muscles. To build your

---

 **SCIENCE IN ACTION: Resistance Exercise Among Youth**

Exercise scientists have developed recommendations to help youth, including preteens and teens, use PRE to build their muscle fitness. The guidelines were developed by a variety of experts—including exercise physiologists, medical doctors, and exercise professionals (such as athletic trainers and strength coaches)—who worked with the National Strength and Conditioning Association (NSCA).

Not so long ago, some experts felt that muscle fitness exercises were unsafe and inappropriate for preteens and teens. NSCA experts now provide evidence that, when done properly, PRE provides health benefits for teens similar to those for adults. These benefits include reduced risk of chronic disease, reduced risk of injury and muscle pain or soreness, improved muscle fitness and sport performance, and psychological well-being. Muscle fitness exercise also builds bone fitness, reduces the risk of osteoporosis (porous and weak bones), reduces the risk of back pain, enhances posture, and increases your ability to work and play without fatigue. In addition, well-developed muscles help you look your best. Muscle is more dense than fat, so it takes up less space. Muscle also uses more calories than fat, so increasing muscle mass helps the body to burn calories.

Keys to keeping PRE safe for youth include using proper technique and safe and appropriate equipment, following sound exercise principles, and seeking and accepting good supervision. Much of this chapter focuses on giving you the information you need in order to meet the safe exercise recommendations for PRE.

### Student Activity

PRE can be safe for teens when done properly but carries risks when done improperly. Create a list of the most important ways to make PRE safe for teens. Consider making a sign to be posted in a fitness room used by teens.

---

leg muscles, you must overload your leg muscles. Examples of types of PRE for each part of muscle fitness and the basic exercises for specific muscle groups are discussed later in this chapter.

## Principle of Rest and Recovery

The **principle of rest and recovery** holds that you need to give your muscles time to rest and recover after a workout. This is why muscle fitness exercises are typically performed on only two or three days per week. Because you need to perform exercises to build all of the important muscles of your body, some people choose to work out every day but do exercises for different muscle groups on different days. For example, they might perform upper body exercises one day and lower body exercises the next. For optimal results, you should also rest between sets of exercise (more information about rest is given throughout this chapter).

 Where there is no struggle, there is no strength. "

—Oprah Winfrey, media personality

## Muscles and Muscle Biomechanics

Your body's muscles create the movement that allows you to do the activities described in this book. There are hundreds of muscles in the human body. Some of the most frequently used muscles in physical activity are illustrated in figure 10.5. This section helps you learn more about how your muscles work.

## Muscle Contraction and Joint Movement

Your skeletal muscles are attached to your bones and make your movements possible. You use these muscles to do physical activity. They are called voluntary muscles because you consciously control them. Your muscles work together to allow your body parts to function efficiently and effectively. For example, when you contract your biceps muscle (see figure 10.6a), your arm bends at the elbow, bringing your hand closer to your shoulder. At the same time, your triceps muscle relaxes to allow your biceps to do its work.

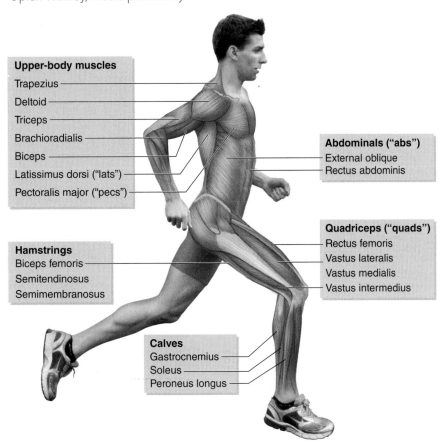

**Upper-body muscles**
Trapezius
Deltoid
Triceps
Brachioradialis
Biceps
Latissimus dorsi ("lats")
Pectoralis major ("pecs")

**Abdominals ("abs")**
External oblique
Rectus abdominis

**Hamstrings**
Biceps femoris
Semitendinosus
Semimembranosus

**Quadriceps ("quads")**
Rectus femoris
Vastus lateralis
Vastus medialis
Vastus intermedius

**Calves**
Gastrocnemius
Soleus
Peroneus longus

**FIGURE 10.5** Some of the major muscles used in physical activity.

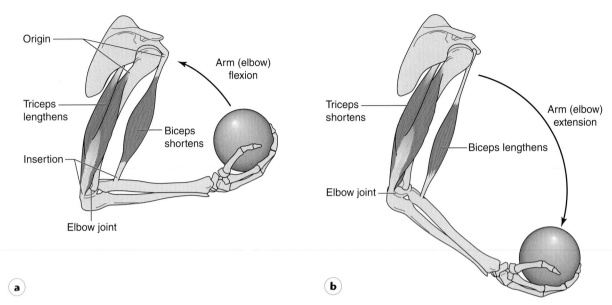

**FIGURE 10.6** The origin, insertion, and action of the arm muscles: *(a)* flexion; *(b)* extension.

The tendons of each muscle connect with bone in two places, the origin and the insertion. The origin is typically connected to the bone that is stationary during a movement, and the insertion is typically connected to the bone that moves. In figure 10.6, the origin of the biceps is at the shoulder, and the insertion is on the bone of the lower arm that moves during flexion and extension.

## Type of Muscle Fitness Exercise

As figure 10.6 shows, your skeletal muscles are attached to your bones on either side of a joint; your bones act as levers to which your muscles apply force. When stimulated by a nerve, muscle fibers are activated to apply force. Muscle contractions can be isotonic or isometric. **Isotonic contractions** pull on your bones to produce movement of your body parts. **Isotonic exercises** are those that use muscle contractions to move body parts. The two types of isotonic muscle contractions are **concentric** (shortening contraction) and **eccentric** (lengthening contraction). Figure 10.6*a* shows the biceps muscle doing a concentric contraction in which the muscle shortens to cause the elbow to flex. In figure 10.6*b*, as the arm is slowly straightened, the biceps is doing an eccentric, or lengthening, contraction that causes the elbow to extend.

In contrast, an **isometric contraction** (sometimes called a static contraction) occurs when muscles contract and pull with equal force in opposite directions so that no movement occurs. **Isometric exercises** involve isometric contractions, and body parts do not move in these exercises. One example of an isometric contraction involves pushing your hands and arms together in front of your body. You push hard with each hand, applying force against the other, but no movement occurs. You can also do isometric calisthenics, such as holding your body still in the push-up position.

**Plyometrics** is a type of muscle fitness exercise that is especially useful in building power. This type of activity involves doing isotonic muscle contractions explosively (as in jumping). You'll learn more about all forms of muscle fitness exercise later in this chapter.

## FIT FACT

An eccentric contraction is sometimes called a braking contraction because the lengthening of a muscle works against gravity to slow the lowering of a weight (see figure 10.6). For example, in a biceps curl after using a concentric contraction to flex the elbow and lift a weight, you lower the weight using an eccentric contraction. The lengthening of the biceps slows the weight down (or "puts on the brakes") so that the weight does not drop too quickly.

Isokinetic exercise is a type of isotonic exercise in which the velocity of movement is kept constant through the full range of motion. As noted in the Fitness Technology feature, isokinetic exercise requires special machines.

## Muscle Fibers

Muscle fibers are long, thin, cylindrical muscle cells. Skeletal muscles (such as those in your arms and legs) are made of many muscle fibers (figure 10.7). The strength and endurance of skeletal muscles depend on whether the muscles are made of slow, fast, or intermediate fibers and on how much exercise they get.

**Slow-twitch muscle fibers** contract slowly and are usually red because they have a lot of blood vessels delivering oxygen to the muscle. These fibers generate less force than **fast-twitch muscle fibers** but are able to resist fatigue. For this reason, a muscle with many slow-twitch fibers has good muscular endurance, and slow-twitch fibers are involved in activities such as running for distance. Fast-twitch muscle fibers contract quickly and are white because they have less blood flow delivering oxygen. They generate more force when they contract, and for this reason muscles with many fast-twitch fibers are important for strength activities.

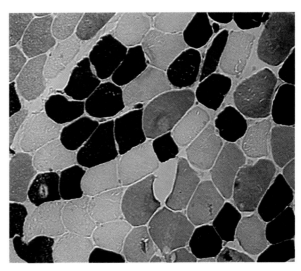

**FIGURE 10.7** This photomicrograph shows slow-twitch (black) and fast-twitch (gray and white) muscle fibers.

Reprinted, by permission, from W.L. Kenney, J.H. Wilmore and D.L. Costill, 2004, *Physiology of sport and exercise*, 5th ed. (Champaign, IL: Human Kinetics), 37.

**Intermediate muscle fibers** have characteristics of both slow- and fast-twitch fibers. You use them for activities involving both types of muscle fitness and cardiorespiratory endurance.

## ♥ FITNESS TECHNOLOGY: Isokinetic Exercise Machines

In recent years, tremendous technological advances have been made in resistance exercise machines. Innovations include adjustable benches and chairs so that machines fit people of all sizes, systems for changing resistance that make the machines easier to use, and the creation of isokinetic resistance machines. These machines use special hydraulics or electronics to regulate movement velocity and allow full exertion at all angles of joint movement during an exercise. In contrast, with traditional free weights or resistance machines, resistance is often greater during the first part of a movement than at the end of the movement, and the speed of the movement may also be greater at one point than at another. Isokinetic exercise allows the muscle to be developed equally at all joint angles and can be used to develop power by using fast (high speed) movements. Isokinetic machines are considered quite safe and are often used by researchers and people who are rehabilitating injuries. Their disadvantages include being expensive and often not allowing eccentric contractions, which are used frequently in sport performance.

### Using Technology

If your school has an isokinetic machine, ask for a demonstration and try it out. If not, see if you can find a machine locally or on the Internet (for a visual demonstration).

Your muscle capabilities are determined in part by heredity. People who inherit a large number of fast-twitch muscle fibers are especially likely to be good at activities requiring sprinting and jumping, whereas people who inherit a large number of slow-twitch muscle fibers are likely to be good at activities requiring sustained performance such as distance running and swimming. Although heredity and genes play an important role, we now know that training can also affect muscle fiber function. So, regardless of your genes, you can increase your muscle strength, endurance, and power with proper training.

## FIT FACT

Birds, like humans, have both fast-twitch and slow-twitch muscle fibers. The flying muscles (breast muscles) of a duck or goose are dark colored because they contain many slow-twitch fibers (which are typically red) that are needed for long-distance flights. In contrast, the breast of a chicken is made up of mostly fast-twitch fibers (typically white) because the chickens typically don't fly long distances.

## Muscle Hypertrophy

Muscle **hypertrophy** refers to growth in the size of muscles and muscle fibers. Hypertrophy is affected not only by overloading but also by several other factors. You've already learned that we each inherit a unique pattern of muscle fiber types and that this inheritance makes a difference in how your body responds to training. But age, maturation, and sex also play a role.

As we age, our muscles grow, as do other tissues in the body. For preteens and young teens, who are not yet fully mature, the body does not produce enough hormones to build big muscles (hypertrophy), even with PRE. These hormones are not fully present until a person reaches full maturity, which occurs at various ages for various people, though typically earlier for girls than for boys. Prior to maturity, PRE can improve strength but may not noticeably increase muscle size; in fact, the strength gains are typically due to increased skill in performing the exercises or an increase in the number of muscle fibers called upon for a movement during exercise.

In most exercises, only some of the available muscle fibers contract to cause a movement, but with regular PRE more fibers are called upon, increasing the number of exercises you can perform.

Because preteens and older teens who are late developers may not see big gains in muscle size with training, they may get discouraged and feel that PRE doesn't work. They may want to focus instead on gains in performance skills and accept the fact that noticeable muscular changes will occur when the body begins to produce more of the hormones that stimulate growth in muscle size.

Some people think that only males can build muscle fitness and increase muscle hypertrophy. This notion is false. Both males and females need strength in order to be healthy, avoid injury, look good, and be able to save themselves or others in an emergency.

Some girls and women fear that strength training will cause their body to look masculine. However, the hormones that promote muscle hypertrophy are not as prevalent in the bodies of females. In addition, females at maturity have a lower relative percent of muscle as compared with total body weight than males do. For this reason, most girls and women find it difficult to develop large, bulky muscles even when their exercise amounts are similar to those described in this book. Even so, women and girls who perform strength exercises do develop strong muscles. And both men and women look more attractive with strong muscles because they are more likely to have good posture and a firm body. Building good strength can also help build your self-confidence.

## Muscle Fitness Assessment

You can assess muscle fitness in many ways. The best test for strength is generally agreed to be the 1-repetition maximum (1RM) test (see the Self-Assessment at the end of this lesson). The 1RM test requires you to determine the amount of weight you can lift or the resistance you can overcome in 1 repetition. For example, if a person can lift 100 pounds once, but not twice, 100 pounds is the 1RM for the muscle group being tested. You can use the 1RM test for each of your major muscle groups, and you can use the results both to get a good idea of your strength and to determine how much weight or resistance to use when you perform exercises.

The true 1RM test is commonly used by athletes and adults. Done properly, it can also be safe for teens, but most experts recommend that teens use a modified self-assessment. The modified 1RM self-assessment gives you a good estimate of your true 1RM but does not require you to lift maximal weight or use maximal resistance. Teens are advised to use only a percentage of 1RM, both in testing their strength and in performing strength exercises. In the Self-Assessment feature included in this chapter, you'll estimate your 1RM by performing the modified 1RM test that uses multiple repetitions and lower than maximal weight (or resistance). This self-assessment is safe for teens when performed properly. You can do a 1RM test for many muscle groups, but two are used most often—one for the upper body (arm press) and one for the lower body (leg press).

Another 1RM test is the grip dynamometer test (figure 10.8), which tests isometric rather than isotonic strength. This grip test is easy to do but does require a grip **dynamometer**. People who score well on the isotonic 1RM test often score well on the grip test as well. This test is used in national fitness assessments in Canada, Japan, and Poland and in the ALPHA-FIT battery that is often used in Europe. Dynamometers are also available for testing other muscle groups, such as leg muscles, but they are more expensive and harder to use than grip dynamometers and thus are used less frequently.

You've already tried several self-assessments for muscular endurance and power that are used in common fitness test batteries. Muscular endurance tests typically require you to repeat the performance of **calisthenics**; examples include push-ups, curl-ups, and trunk lifts. Common tests of leg power include the long jump and vertical jump, and one common test of upper body power is the medicine ball throw. In the Self-Assessment feature in this lesson, you'll learn how to do tests of strength, muscular endurance, and power beyond those you've already tried.

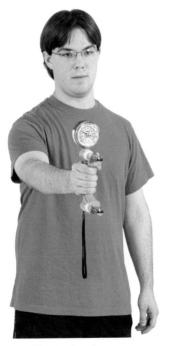

**FIGURE 10.8** The grip dynamometer test measures isometric strength.

## Absolute Versus Relative Strength

Your 1RM score is an example of **absolute strength**, which is measured by how much weight or resistance you can overcome regardless of your body size. Big people typically have more absolute strength than smaller people, and since males are generally larger than females, their average absolute strength is higher. **Relative strength**, on the other hand, is adjusted for body size. The most common method for determining relative strength is to divide your weight into your absolute strength score to get a score for your strength per pound of body weight. Relative strength scores are considered to be fairer assessments of strength for those who do not have large bodies; thus relative strength is used for the ratings in this chapter's Self-Assessment feature.

**Lesson Review**

1. What are the differences between strength, muscular endurance, and power?
2. What are the basic exercise principles of muscle fitness, and why are they important?
3. What are the types of muscle fitness exercise?
4. What are some methods for assessing muscle fitness?

Self-assessment of any part of fitness—including muscle fitness—is important because it allows you to establish your baseline level of fitness, determine your fitness needs, set goals, and determine whether you've met your goals. Certified personal trainers who know their stuff have their clients perform a baseline fitness test (a pretest) and, after they go through a fitness program, a follow-up fitness test (a post-test) to see if the program was effective. In this class, you are learning to become your own personal trainer.

Before performing these tests, consider doing a general and dynamic warm-up. If the 1RM test causes fatigue that keeps you from doing your best on the muscle fitness tests in part 3 of this sequence, repeat that assessment on another day. As directed by your instructor, record your scores and ratings for the three parts of this self-assessment. If you're working with a partner, remember that self-assessment information is personal and considered confidential. It shouldn't be shared with others without the permission of the person being tested.

# Part 1: Estimating Your 1RM

To review, 1RM means 1-repetition maximum—the maximum weight a muscle or group of muscles can lift (or the maximum resistance they can overcome) one time. Because beginners should start gradually (without heavy lifting), a modified method has been developed that allows you to determine your 1RM without overexerting. Your results indicate how strong you are.

The modified 1RM can be done with free weights or machines, but the instructions that follow are for machine use. Resistance machines are recommended for these self-assessments, especially for beginners, because they are safer. Two tests are used most often, and the ones performed in this self-assessment activity are for your upper body (arm press) and your lower body (leg press).

Use the following directions for each of the two self-assessments.

- Choose a weight (resistance) that you think you can lift (move) 5 to 10 times. Do not use a weight that you can lift fewer than 5 times or more than 10 times.

- Using correct technique, lift the weight as many times as you possibly can. Count your lifts and write the total on your record sheet. If you were able to do more than 10 lifts, wait until another day before you try a heavier weight for that assessment. Go to the next muscle group assessment.

- If you can tell that you will not be able to lift the weight at least 5 times, stop and choose a lighter weight.

- If you were able to do 5 to 10 lifts (no fewer and no more), refer to table 10.1 and find the weight you lifted. Now find the number of reps you did. Your 1RM score is the number in the box where your horizontal weight row and your vertical rep column intersect.

- Divide each of your two 1RM scores (arm press and leg press) by your body weight to get your score for strength per pound of body weight. This score adjusts for body size to indicate your relative strength. For example, a person who weighs 150 pounds and has a 1RM of 100 pounds on the arm press has a score of 0.67 pound lifted per pound of body weight. After figuring your relative strength score, use tables 10.2 and 10.3 to determine your fitness rating. Record your 1RM scores, relative strength scores, and ratings.

- Tables 10.2 and 10.3 do not show high performance ratings for the 1RM. For now, focus on getting into the good fitness zone. Athletes should consult coaches in their sport to get more information about appropriate 1RM scores.

Safety tip: Proper form is essential for safety. Before you do the 1RM test, read the descriptions of the exercises and the directions that follow. Before performing each assessment, practice the exercise and have a teacher check your form. Work with a partner to get feedback about proper lifting technique.

## TABLE 10.1  Predicted 1RM Based on Reps to Fatigue

| Weight (lb) | Repetitions | | | | | | Weight (lb) | Repetitions | | | | | |
|---|---|---|---|---|---|---|---|---|---|---|---|---|---|
| | 5 | 6 | 7 | 8 | 9 | 10 | | 5 | 6 | 7 | 8 | 9 | 10 |
| 30 | 34 | 35 | 36 | 37 | 38 | 39 | **140** | 157 | 163 | 168 | 174 | 180 | 187 |
| 35 | 40 | 41 | 42 | 43 | 44 | 45 | **145** | 163 | 168 | 174 | 180 | 186 | 193 |
| 40 | 46 | 47 | 49 | 50 | 51 | 53 | **150** | 169 | 174 | 180 | 186 | 193 | 200 |
| 45 | 51 | 53 | 55 | 56 | 58 | 60 | **155** | 174 | 180 | 186 | 192 | 199 | 207 |
| 50 | 56 | 58 | 60 | 62 | 64 | 67 | **160** | 180 | 186 | 192 | 199 | 206 | 213 |
| 55 | 62 | 64 | 66 | 68 | 71 | 73 | **165** | 186 | 192 | 198 | 205 | 212 | 220 |
| 60 | 67 | 70 | 72 | 74 | 77 | 80 | **170** | 191 | 197 | 204 | 211 | 219 | 227 |
| 65 | 73 | 75 | 78 | 81 | 84 | 87 | **175** | 197 | 203 | 210 | 217 | 225 | 233 |
| 70 | 79 | 81 | 84 | 87 | 90 | 93 | **180** | 202 | 209 | 216 | 223 | 231 | 240 |
| 75 | 84 | 87 | 90 | 93 | 96 | 100 | **185** | 208 | 215 | 222 | 230 | 238 | 247 |
| 80 | 90 | 93 | 96 | 99 | 103 | 107 | **190** | 214 | 221 | 228 | 236 | 244 | 253 |
| 85 | 96 | 99 | 102 | 106 | 109 | 113 | **195** | 219 | 226 | 234 | 242 | 251 | 260 |
| 90 | 101 | 105 | 108 | 112 | 116 | 120 | **200** | 225 | 232 | 240 | 248 | 257 | 267 |
| 95 | 107 | 110 | 114 | 118 | 122 | 127 | **205** | 231 | 238 | 246 | 254 | 264 | 273 |
| 100 | 112 | 116 | 120 | 124 | 129 | 133 | **210** | 236 | 244 | 252 | 261 | 270 | 280 |
| 105 | 118 | 122 | 126 | 130 | 135 | 140 | **215** | 242 | 250 | 258 | 267 | 276 | 287 |
| 110 | 124 | 128 | 132 | 137 | 141 | 147 | **220** | 247 | 255 | 264 | 273 | 283 | 293 |
| 115 | 129 | 134 | 138 | 143 | 148 | 153 | **225** | 253 | 261 | 270 | 279 | 289 | 300 |
| 120 | 135 | 139 | 144 | 149 | 154 | 160 | **230** | 259 | 267 | 276 | 286 | 296 | 307 |
| 125 | 141 | 145 | 150 | 155 | 161 | 167 | **235** | 264 | 273 | 282 | 292 | 302 | 313 |
| 130 | 146 | 151 | 158 | 161 | 167 | 173 | **240** | 270 | 279 | 288 | 298 | 309 | 320 |
| 135 | 152 | 157 | 162 | 168 | 174 | 180 | **245** | 276 | 285 | 294 | 304 | 315 | 327 |

To convert from pounds to kilograms, multiply by 0.45.

Adapted, by permission, from M. Brzyck, 1993, "Strength testing - predicting a one-rep max from reps-to-fatigue," *JOPERD* 64(1): 89. www.informa-world.com

## Seated Arm Press

1. Sit on the stool of a seated press machine and position yourself so that the handles are even with your shoulders. Grasp the handles with your palms facing away from you. Tighten your abdominal muscles.

2. Push upward on the handles, extending your arms until your elbows are straight.
   Caution: Do not arch your back. Do not lock your elbows.

3. Lower the handles to the starting position.

This test evaluates the strength of your triceps and pectoral muscles.

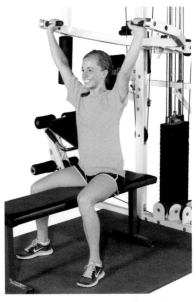

### TABLE 10.2  Rating Chart: Relative Strength for Arm Press

|  | 15 years or younger | | 16 or 17 years old | | 18 years or older | |
|---|---|---|---|---|---|---|
|  | Male | Female | Male | Female | Male | Female |
| Good fitness | ≥0.80 | ≥0.60 | ≥1.00 | ≥0.70 | ≥1.10 | ≥0.85 |
| Marginal fitness | 0.67–0.79 | 0.50–0.59 | 0.75–0.99 | 0.60–0.69 | 0.80–1.09 | 0.67–0.84 |
| Low fitness | ≤0.66 | ≤0.49 | ≤0.74 | ≤0.59 | ≤0.79 | ≤0.66 |

Relative strength is calculated by dividing 1RM by body weight.

## Seated Leg Press

1. Adjust the seat position on a leg press machine for your leg length. Sit with your feet resting on the pedal.

2. Push the pedal until your legs are straight.
   Caution: Do not lock your knees.

3. Slowly return to the starting position.

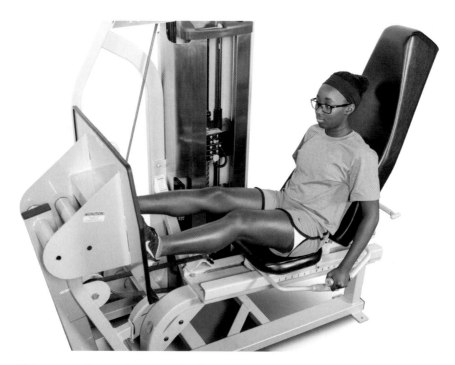

This test evaluates the strength of your quadriceps, gluteal, and calf muscles.

### TABLE 10.3  Rating Chart: Relative Strength for Leg Press

|  | 15 years or younger | | 16 or 17 years old | | 18 years or older | |
|---|---|---|---|---|---|---|
|  | Male | Female | Male | Female | Male | Female |
| Good fitness | ≥1.50 | ≥1.10 | ≥1.75 | ≥1.30 | ≥1.90 | ≥1.40 |
| Marginal fitness | 1.35–1.49 | 0.95–1.09 | 1.50–1.74 | 1.10–1.29 | 1.65–1.89 | 1.30–1.39 |
| Low fitness | ≤1.34 | ≤0.94 | ≤1.49 | ≤1.09 | ≤1.64 | ≤1.29 |

Relative strength is calculated by dividing 1RM by body weight.

# Part 2: Muscular Endurance Tests

Many tests can help you evaluate muscular endurance, but the best ones assess your body's large muscles. In this self-assessment, you'll perform several isotonic and some isometric tests. For each, check "yes" if you could do the test as long or as many times as indicated. Check "no" if you could not. Look up your rating in table 10.4. As directed by your teacher, record your results.

### TABLE 10.4 Rating Chart: Muscular Endurance

| Fitness rating | Number of tests passed |
| --- | --- |
| Good fitness | 5 |
| Marginal fitness | 3 or 4 |
| Low fitness | 0–2 |

## Side Stand (isometric)

1. Lie on your side.
2. Use both hands to get your body in position so that it is supported by your left hand and the side of your left foot. Keep your body stiff.
3. Raise your right arm and leg in the air. Hold this position. Record 1 point if you meet the standard (30 seconds if you are male or 20 seconds if you are female).
4. Return to the starting position and repeat the test on your right side.

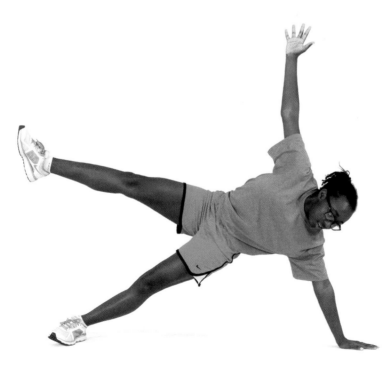

This test evaluates the isometric muscular endurance of some of your leg and arm muscles as well as your trunk-stabilizing muscles.

## Trunk Extension (isotonic)

1. Lie facedown on a stable weight bench or the end of a bleacher that is 15 to 20 inches (38 to 51 centimeters) high. The top of your hips should be even with the end of the bench, and your upper body should hang off the end of the bench. If the surface is hard, cover it with a mat or a towel.

2. Have a partner hold your calves using one hand on each leg 12 inches (30 centimeters) above your ankles. Overlap your hands and place them (palms away) in front of your chin.

3. Start with your upper body bent at the hip so that your chin is near the floor with the palm of your lower hand against the floor. Place a small mat on the floor below your hands and chin.

4. Keeping your head and neck in line with your upper body, slowly lift your head and upper body off the floor until your upper body is in line with your lower body.
   Caution: Do not to lift your upper trunk higher than horizontal (in line with your lower body).

5. Lower to the starting position so that the palm of your lower hand touches the floor.

6. Perform one lift every three seconds. You may want to have a partner say "up, down" to help you. Record 1 point if you can meet the standard (20 reps if you are male or 15 reps if you are female).

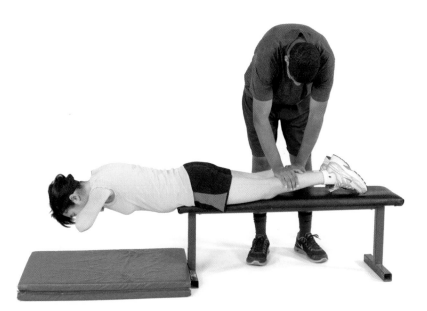

This test evaluates the isotonic muscular endurance of your upper back muscles.

## Sitting Tuck (isotonic)

1. Sit on the floor with your knees bent and your arms outstretched.
2. Lean back (to about a 45-degree angle) and balance on your buttocks. Keep your knees bent near your chest (feet off the floor).
3. Straighten your knees so your body forms a V. You may move your arms sideways for balance.
4. Bend your knees to your chest again. Repeat the exercise as many times as you can. Count each time you push your legs out. Record 1 point if you can meet the standard (25 reps if you are male or 20 reps if you are female).

Safety tip: Avoid arching your lower back repetitively.

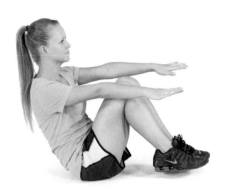

This test evaluates the isotonic muscular endurance of your abdominal muscles and some of your hip and leg muscles.

## Leg Change (isotonic)

1. Assume a push-up position with your weight on your hands and feet.
2. Pull your right knee under your chest, and keep your left leg straight.
3. Change legs by pulling your left leg forward and pushing your right leg back.
   Caution: Do not let your lower back sag.
4. Continue changing legs (about one change with each leg every 2 seconds).
5. Count the number of leg changes performed in 1 minute. Record 1 point if you can meet the standard (25 changes for both males and females).

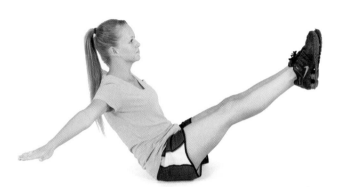

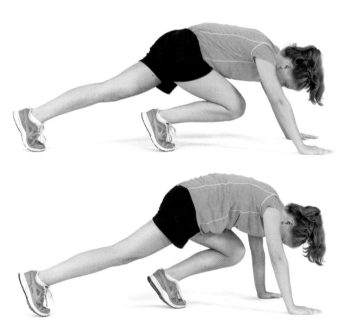

This test evaluates the isotonic muscular endurance of your hip and leg muscles.

## Flexed-Arm Hang (isometric)

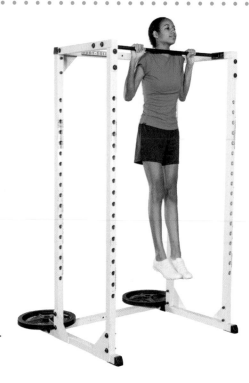

1. Hang from a chinning bar with your palms facing away from your body.

2. Standing on a chair, or with help from a partner, lift your chin above the bar.

3. At the start signal, your partner lets go or removes the chair so you are hanging by your own power. Count how long you can hang. The time count begins when the support is removed and ends when your chin touches or goes below the bar or your head tilts backward. Record 1 point if you can meet the standard (hold for 16 seconds if you are male or 12 seconds if you are female).

**This test evaluates the muscular endurance of your arm, shoulder, and chest muscles (isometric).**

# Part 3: Tests of Power

In this self-assessment, you'll test the power of your lower body by performing the standing long jump and the upper body by performing the medicine ball throw.

## Standing Long Jump

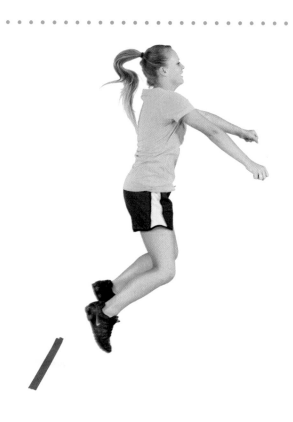

1. Use masking tape or another material to make the necessary line on the floor.

2. Stand with your feet shoulder-width apart behind the line on the floor. Bend your knees and hold your arms straight in front of your body at shoulder height.

3. Swing your arms downward and backward, then vigorously forward as you jump forward as far as possible, extending your legs.

4. Land on both feet and try to maintain your balance on landing. Do not run or hop before jumping.

5. Perform the test two times. Record the better of your two scores, then find your rating in table 10.5 and record it.

**This test evaluates the power of the lower body.**

## TABLE 10.5  Rating Chart: Standing Long Jump in Inches

|  | 13 years old | | 14 years old | | 15 years old | | 16 years old | | 17 years or older | |
|---|---|---|---|---|---|---|---|---|---|---|
|  | Male | Female | Male | Female | Male | Female | Male | Female | Male | Female |
| High performance | ≥73 | ≥59 | ≥80 | ≥60 | ≥85 | ≥61 | ≥88 | ≥62 | ≥91 | ≥68 |
| Good fitness | 67–72 | 57–58 | 73–79 | 58–59 | 78–84 | 59–60 | 82–87 | 60–61 | 86–90 | 63–67 |
| Marginal fitness | 61–66 | 54–56 | 67–72 | 55–57 | 73–77 | 56–58 | 77–81 | 57–59 | 80–85 | 58–62 |
| Low fitness | ≤60 | ≤53 | ≤66 | ≤54 | ≤72 | ≤55 | ≤76 | ≤56 | ≤79 | ≤57 |

To convert inches to centimeters, multiply by 2.54.

## Medicine Ball Throw

1. Sit on a chair positioned against a wall. Sit back as far as possible so that your lower and upper back are against the back of the chair.

2. Hold a 14-pound (about 6.5-kilogram) medicine ball with both hands so that it rests against the middle of your chest.

3. Push with both hands to throw the medicine ball as far as possible. Throw as you would in a basketball chest pass. Keep your back against the chair.

4. Measure the distance from the wall (behind the chair) to the spot on the floor where the ball landed. Measure in inches (or centimeters).

5. Measure the distance from the wall to the end of your fingers (that is, your arm length) in inches (or centimeters). Your score is the distance that the ball was thrown minus the length of your arm.

6. Perform the test two times and use the better of your two scores.

Based on your better score, use table 10.6 to determine your rating. As directed by your instructor, record your score and your rating.

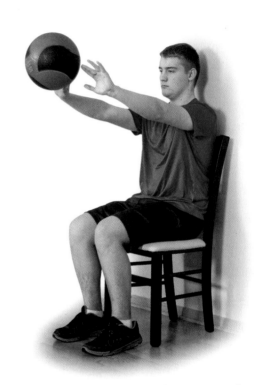

The medicine ball throw test evaluates power in your upper body.

## TABLE 10.6  Rating Chart: Medicine Ball Throw in Inches

|  | 15 years or younger | | 16 or 17 years old | | 18 years or older | |
|---|---|---|---|---|---|---|
|  | Male | Female | Male | Female | Male | Female |
| Good fitness | ≥145 | ≥98 | ≥155 | ≥102 | ≥165 | ≥108 |
| Marginal fitness | 130–144 | 90–97 | 140–154 | 94–101 | 150–164 | 98–107 |
| Low fitness | ≤129 | ≤89 | ≤139 | ≤93 | ≤149 | ≤97 |

To convert inches to centimeters, multiply by 2.54.

# Building Muscle Fitness

**Lesson Objectives**

After reading this lesson, you should be able to

1. explain the FIT formula for developing muscle fitness with isotonic PRE,
2. describe the double progressive system for using PRE,
3. describe several free weight and resistance machine exercises and their advantages and disadvantages,
4. describe several other forms of exercise for building muscle fitness,
5. describe basic guidelines for doing PRE safely, and
6. describe some myths about strength and explain why they are wrong.

**Lesson Vocabulary**

bodybuilding, body dysmorphia, double progressive system, interval training, muscle bound, powerlifting, weightlifting

**Do** you know the health benefits of PRE and muscle fitness? Have you ever wanted to increase your muscle fitness? Are you familiar with the types of resistance training? In this lesson, you'll learn some of the health benefits associated with achieving muscle fitness through PRE. You'll also learn how to apply the FIT formula for the most popular methods of building muscle fitness. And you'll learn about recommended guidelines for properly performing progressive resistance exercise (PRE) and about some common misconceptions concerning muscle fitness.

## Health Benefits of PRE and Muscle Fitness

Many of the health benefits described throughout this book are associated with doing muscle fitness exercises and achieving good muscle fitness. Most people know that muscle fitness helps reduce back problems, improves posture, reduces risk of muscle injury, and increases working capacity. They may not know that muscle fitness exercises are very important to bone health (preventing osteoporosis), prevention of heart disease and diabetes, and rehabilitation from chronic diseases such as cancer. Muscle fitness exercises can also reduce your risk of becoming overweight or obese. In addition, they provide mental health benefits such as looking and feeling your best and experiencing a high quality of

life. Among older people, muscle fitness also helps reduce the risk of falling and improves a person's ability to do tasks of daily life.

## Building Muscle Fitness With Isotonic PRE

In this section, you'll learn about the FIT formula for isotonic PRE. You'll also learn some of the advantages and disadvantages of resistance machine and free weight exercises and some general guidelines for performing isotonic PRE.

### The FIT Formula for Isotonic PRE: Resistance Machines and Free Weights

Table 10.7 provides FIT formula information for isotonic exercises using resistance machines and free weights, such as those described later in this lesson. The same FIT formula can be used for isokinetic exercises. As indicated in the table, beginners use lower resistance, do more reps, and perform fewer sets than people who are more advanced.

The American College of Sports Medicine (ACSM) recommends a two- or three-minute rest between sets. In general, you should use longer rests between high-resistance exercises and shorter rests between low-resistance exercises. To make your workout more efficient, you can alternate arm and

**TABLE 10.7  Fitness Target Zones for Muscle Fitness (Isotonic)**

| | Beginner | | Intermediate | | Advanced | |
|---|---|---|---|---|---|---|
| | Threshold | Target | Threshold | Target | Threshold | Target |
| Frequency (days per week) | 2 | 2 or 3 | 2 | 2 or 3 | 3 | 3 or 4 |
| Intensity (% of 1RM) | 50 | 50–70 | 60 | 60–80 | 70 | 70–85 |
| Time | 1 set of 10–15 reps | 1 or 2 sets of 10–15 reps | 2 sets of 8–12 reps | 2 or 3 sets of 8–12 reps | 3 sets of 6–10 reps | 3–4 sets of 6–10 reps |

leg exercises. That way, when your arms are working, your legs are resting, and vice versa.

The FIT formula for muscle fitness for teens differs somewhat from the formula for adults, especially for exercise intensity. ACSM recommends a FIT formula similar to the one shown in the table for teens. For adults, beginners can start at 60 percent of 1RM rather than 50 percent for teens, and advanced exercisers can use 80 to 90 percent of 1RM rather than 70 to 85 percent. Adult beginners can start with two sets rather than one set, which is what is recommended for teens.

## The Double Progressive System of PRE

You already know that in order to achieve optimal development of your muscle fitness, you need to progress gradually. The most commonly used method for applying the principle of progression to muscle fitness is the **double progressive system**. The first part of the system involves increasing repetitions (reps). For example, as shown in table 10.7, a beginner starts with one set of 10 reps at 50 percent of 1RM, then gradually increases the number of reps until he or she can easily perform 15 reps.

The second part of the system involves increasing resistance or weight. The number of reps is dropped back to 10, and the resistance is increased by 5 to 10 percent of 1RM; for teens, this often means an increase of about 2 to 5 pounds (0.9 to 2.3 kilograms). This double progression—increasing reps and resistance—continues until the person can do the maximum percent of 1RM in the beginner category. At that point, he or she can add a second set. It may be necessary to drop back to a lower number of reps and a lower percent of 1RM to perform two full sets of 10 to 15 reps.

When doing multiple sets, longer rest intervals between sets allow you to lift a higher percent of 1RM than shorter rest intervals. So it is important to use rest intervals of a consistent length of time.

Once a person can perform two sets of 15 reps at 70 percent of 1RM (a goal that may take several months to attain), he or she is ready to move to the intermediate stage. Here, the double progression sequence begins again. The person follows the double progressive system at the moderate stage until he or she can perform three sets of 8 to 12 reps at 80 percent of 1RM. It may take a year or longer to progress to this point.

Some exercisers choose to stay at the intermediate level because many health benefits can be achieved using the FIT formula for this stage (moderate sets and reps and moderate resistance). Because the FIT formula for advanced exercisers focuses more on low reps and higher resistance, it builds more pure strength than the FIT formula for beginners and intermediates. Therefore, the advanced FIT formula offers benefits for people who plan to do sports or jobs requiring high levels of strength and for people especially interested in muscle hypertrophy. However, the FIT formula for intermediates provides many benefits and is appropriate for regular use by most teens.

## Resistance Machines Versus Free Weights

Resistance machine and free weight exercises require considerable equipment but are among the most popular forms of isotonic PRE because they are two of the most effective methods for building muscle fitness. They allow you to build both strength and muscular endurance and isolate most of the major muscle groups in your body with specific exercises.

To help you consider these forms of PRE, compare their advantages and disadvantages as outlined in table 10.8. Some basic exercises using free weights and resistance machines are described at the end of this lesson; for each exercise, the muscles used are listed and illustrated.

> " Mens sana in corpore sano (a sound mind in a sound body). "
>
> —Juvenal, Roman poet

## FIT FACT

In addition to the National Strength and Conditioning Association (see the first lesson in this chapter), several other groups of experts have now prepared statements indicating that resistance training can be safe for teens when performed properly. These groups include the American College of Sports Medicine, the American Academy of Pediatrics (medical doctors who specialize in treating children and youth), and the American Orthopaedic Society of Sports Medicine (medical doctors who specialize in bone problems associated with sport and activity). The self-assessments and muscle fitness exercises described in this book follow the guidelines of these organizations.

## PRE

When performed correctly, resistance training is safe and improves your muscle fitness while helping you feel and look your best. Stick to the following guidelines created especially to help teens use PRE safely and effectively.

- **Warm up** with recommended dynamic exercises or perform low-resistance sets before doing your regular workout.
- **Learn proper technique.** From the beginning, get good instruction from an expert. Start with little or no weight as you're learning the fundamentals. Use the following tips for good technique.
  - **Use moderate-velocity movements**— not too slow and not too fast.
  - **Use both concentric and eccentric contractions through a full range of motion.** For example, when doing the biceps curl, lift the weight all the way up (this uses a concentric contraction) and lower the weight all the way down (this uses an eccentric contraction).
  - **Avoid sudden or quick movements.** Stop briefly at the beginning and end of each repetition. Use your muscles, not the movement of your body, to do the exercise (for example, don't rock forward and backward with the upper body during a biceps curl).

### TABLE 10.8  Resistance Machines Versus Free Weights

|  | Resistance machines | Free weights |
|---|---|---|
| Safety | Safer because weights cannot fall on lifter<br>Spotter often not needed | Greater chance of injury from falling weights<br>Easy to lose control of—spotter needed |
| Cost | Very expensive to own<br>If not owned, club membership required to use | Relatively inexpensive |
| Versatility | Easy to isolate specific muscle groups | More balance, muscle coordination, and concentration required<br>More muscles used, movements more like moving heavy loads in daily life |
| Convenience | Much floor space needed<br>Must be used where installed | Little space needed<br>Some weights small enough to carry around<br>Easily scattered, lost, or stolen |

- **Do not hold your breath when you exercise.** Holding your breath can cause you to black out. Some resistance trainers recommend exhaling when applying resistance and inhaling on the return movement.

- **Use good biomechanics.** Avoid body positions and movements that cause your joints to move in ways for which they are not intended or that put your muscles at risk of injury.

• **Make sure that your workout area is safe.** Use equipment in good working order. Keep free weights on weight racks rather than scattered on the floor. Clean the machine after you're done by wiping it with a towel—or even before you use it, if it wasn't cleaned by the previous user.

• **When working with free weights, always use spotters.** You might be tempted to work on your own, but working with a partner is much safer.

• **Progress gradually.** Young teens, and all teens with little PRE experience, should exercise with the FIT formula for beginners for several months before moving to the intermediate level. Do not let the word *beginner* be a reason for violating the principle of progression. And remember that the advanced FIT formula is typically reserved for people with at least one year of experience and for older teens who have reached physical maturity.

• **Select exercises for all major muscle groups.** Experts recommend that you perform 8 to 10 muscle fitness exercises to be sure that you build all of the major muscle groups. Performing only a few exercises can lead to unbalanced muscle development. In this book, 8 to 10 exercises are provided for many types of PRE.

• **Rest between sets.** For building pure strength, allow two to three minutes between sets; for muscular endurance, allow one to two minutes between sets.

• **Allow rest days between exercise sessions.** For best results, do not perform PRE for the same muscle group on consecutive days. You can, however, exercise daily if you alternate muscle groups to avoid exercising the same muscle group on consecutive days.

• **Vary your program to keep it interesting.** ACSM points out the importance of progression and volume when exercising. Using the double progressive method to progress gradually provides variety while helping you get optimal benefits. You can also get variety while keeping your volume (total amount of exercise) constant by varying repetitions and resistance (for example, many reps with low resistance can result in the same volume of exercise as fewer reps with higher resistance).

• **Avoid overhead lifts with free weights.** If possible, use machines for these lifts. If you must use free weights, always use a trained spotter.

• **Master single-joint exercises before attempting multiple-joint exercises or sport movements.** For example, a biceps curl is a single-joint exercise because the only joint it moves is the elbow. Most of the exercises needed to build good health, as shown in this book, are single-joint exercises. Multiple-joint lifts, such as the clean and jerk in the sport of **weightlifting**, require

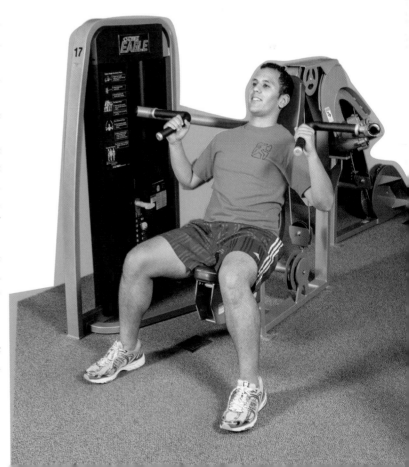

good muscle fitness that results from PRE consisting of single-joint exercises. Multiple-joint exercises also involve a high level of skill that requires special training to ensure good technique.

- **Never use weights carelessly.** Concentrate on your technique and on what you're doing. Use care when changing free weights and put them away properly when you're finished.

- **Never compete when you do resistance training.** For example, do not have a contest to see who can lift the most weight. Genetic differences have a lot to do with how strong a person can be. Concern yourself only with trying to improve your own strength gradually and enjoying the exercise—not lifting more than someone else.

## PRE Using Resistance Machines and Free Weights

Experts recommend doing 8 to 10 basic exercises to build all of your major muscle groups. At the end of this lesson, 9 free weight exercises and 10 resistance machine exercises are described. Before performing these exercises, practice each exercise and the spotting techniques described in the next section. Spotting means supporting a partner by being ready to help if he or she loses control of the weight or gets off balance. Your instructor will help you practice these techniques.

## Practicing Proper Exercise and Spotting Technique

Performing and spotting exercises properly require practice. Before you begin your PRE program, practice by moving through the four levels described in this section. Start with level 1 *for each exercise* until you achieve mastery. Then move to the next level. The specific techniques for performing exercises and spotting properly are described in this lesson in the individual descriptions of exercises using free weights and resistance machines. Some experts use the phrase "feel is not real" to emphasize that just feeling that you're doing an exercise properly does not necessarily mean that you really are. In many facilities, mirrors are provided so that you can check your form. A partner can also help you determine whether you're using correct spotting and lifting techniques (figure 10.9).

- **Level 1.** Focus on lifting technique, not weight. Perform each exercise without any weight by using a wand or stick instead of a barbell. When you're practicing a lift, concentrate on correct form (placement of your body parts). When you're watching a partner, give useful coaching.

- **Level 2.** Focus on spotting technique, not weight. While your partner performs the rep with the wand, you and another partner practice correct spotting technique. Pay particular attention to your leg and hand positions.

- **Level 3.** At this level, you combine lifting and spotting with light weights. Perform each exercise by doing five repetitions with light weight. Practice your lifting and spotting techniques and continue to give each other coaching about both lifting and spotting.

- **Level 4.** At this level, you perform a normal workout using free weights. Select the appropriate percentage of your 1RM and the appropriate number of sets and repetitions (see table 10.7). Perform each of the basic exercises.

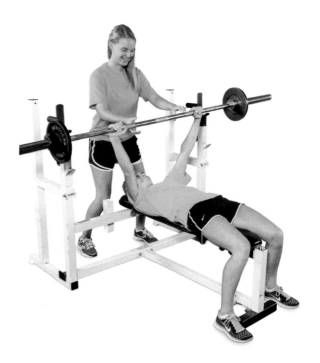

**FIGURE 10.9** Having a spotter is essential when using free weights.

## Clarifying Progressive Resistance Training Terms

As you now know, PRE is a method of building muscle fitness. It differs from three sports that use similar names or terminology.

### Olympic-Style Weightlifting

In this Olympic sport, athletes use free weights to try lifting a maximum load. The sport includes only two lifts: the snatch and the clean and jerk. For those who train with weights but do not participate in Olympic-style weightlifting, the preferred term is *weight training*.

### Powerlifting

**Powerlifting** is another competitive sport using free weights. It includes only three exercises: the bench press, the squat, and the dead lift. Athletes in this sport try to make one maximal lift for each type of lift.

### Bodybuilding

**Bodybuilding** participants are concerned primarily with the appearance of their body, and judges rate them based on how large and well defined their muscles are rather than how much they can lift. This sport can also be done competitively.

## Other Types of Isotonic PRE

Resistance machine and free weight exercises are popular and effective, but they are not the only types of isotonic PRE. The following entries describe some other frequently used forms, including calisthenics, elastic band exercises, and exercise with homemade equipment.

### FIT FACT

An electromyograph (EMG) is a machine used by researchers to determine how hard a muscle contracts. In EMG results, smaller contractions (such as those used for muscular endurance) show a low muscle action wave, whereas harder contractions (such as those used for strength) show a larger muscle action wave.

### Calisthenics

Calisthenic exercises use all or part of your body weight to provide resistance; examples include push-ups and curl-ups. Because only your body weight is used for resistance, this type of PRE is better for building muscular endurance than for building strength. The lower resistance also means that you can do calisthenics more frequently. The FIT formula for isotonic calisthenics is shown in table 10.9. Calisthenics are good for both home use and travel because you can do them almost anywhere with little equipment.

### Exercising With Elastic Bands, Homemade Weights, Partner Resistance, and Balls

These types of PRE are similar to resistance machine and free weight exercises but use various other means to provide resistance. Like calisthenics, elastic band exercises require little equipment and are easy to do both at home and when traveling. Exercises using a stability ball can also be effective in building core fitness. All of these types of PRE use the FIT formula described in table 10.7. Some exercises using partner resistance and homemade weights are described in the student section of the Fitness for Life website.

### TABLE 10.9 Target Zone for Calisthenics (Isotonic)

| | Threshold | Target zone |
|---|---|---|
| Frequency (days per week) | 3 | 3–6 |
| Intensity | Moving the weight of parts of the body | Moving the weight of parts or all of the body |
| Time | 1 set of 10 reps | 1–4 sets of 11–25 reps |

Rest for 2 minutes between sets.

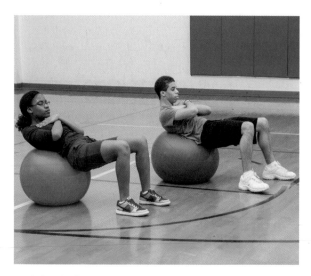

Stability ball exercises can help you build core fitness.

## Building Muscle Fitness With Isometric PRE

Isometric exercises can be done easily at home or when you travel because they require little or no equipment and can be done in a confined space—even a space as small as an airplane seat. A disadvantage of isometric PRE is that it's sometimes hard to tell when you're doing a maximum contraction, and this uncertainty can affect your motivation to work hard. In isotonic exercise, on the other hand, you can see your movement and you know how much effort you're giving. In addition, experts do not consider isometric exercise to be as effective in building muscle fitness as isotonic PRE. As with all PRE, when doing isometric exercise, breathe rather than hold your breath while you're performing exercises. The FIT formula for isometric exercises is included in table 10.10. Some basic isometric exercises are illustrated and described at the end of this lesson. The muscles used in each exercise are also listed and illustrated.

## Building Power

As you may recall, power is a combination of strength and speed. Exercise physiologists have shown that power is related to bone development in children and teens and offers health benefits similar to those provided by other parts of muscle fitness. It's also important for good performance in various sports, including track and field (as in putting the shot or throwing the discus), baseball (hitting the ball a long way), and football (rushing the passer). For this reason, athletes often want to improve their power not only for their health but also for improved performance.

One of the most frequently used methods of building power is plyometrics (plyometric exercise). Plyometrics was pioneered by Olympic track-and-field coaches from the former Soviet Union. Plyometric exercise involves a rapid eccentric contraction of a muscle followed by a concentric contraction of the muscle. For example, one common low-resistance form of plyometric exercise is rope jumping. Landing after a jump requires your calf muscle to do an eccentric, or lengthening, contraction, and the next jump into the air requires a concentric contraction of the calf muscle. Resistance is provided by body weight. Plyometrics often uses more vigorous jumping activities.

Like other forms of muscle fitness exercise, plyometrics was previously thought to be dangerous for teens. However, recent evidence suggests that when performed properly and progressively with good supervision, plyometrics can be safe for teens, enhance athletic performance, increase both power and speed, and actually reduce athletic injuries. Nevertheless, plyometric and other power-building techniques have resulted in injury when performed excessively. The FIT formula for plyometrics is described in table 10.11; the formula, developed by experts, shows a progression based on age and fitness level. Fit athletes may do advanced plyometrics or

### TABLE 10.10   Target Zone for Isometric PRE

|  | Threshold | Target zone |
|---|---|---|
| Frequency (days per week) | 3 | 3–6 |
| Intensity | Contracting muscle as tightly as possible or holding part or all of body weight | Contracting muscle as tightly as possible or holding part or all of body weight |
| Time | 3 reps (1 rep = hold for 7 sec) | 3–4 reps (1 rep = hold for 7–10 sec) |

**TABLE 10.11  Target Zone for Plyometrics**

| | Threshold | Target zone |
|---|---|---|
| Frequency (days per week) | 2 (nonconsecutive) | 2 or 3 (nonconsecutive) |
| Intensity (jumps of varying intensity based on age) | Age 12: low intensity (in place)<br>Age 13: medium intensity (moving jumps and hops)<br>Ages 14 and 15: medium intensity (box and obstacle jumps)<br>Age ≥16: high intensity (bounding—multiple jumps over distance and drop jumping) | Same as threshold |
| Time | 1 set of 6–10 repetitions<br>Rest for 1–3 minutes between sets. | 1–3 sets of 6–10 repetitions<br>Rest for 1–3 minutes between sets. |

Beginners should start at low intensity and progress to higher intensity regardless of age. Youth who have been regularly active and have high fitness may move to more advanced levels at ages lower than suggested with proper supervision by a qualified expert who has evaluated the maturational and fitness status of the exerciser.

other forms of training, but you should consult with a parent or guardian and an instructor or certified exercise leader before performing them.

# Interval Training

**Interval training** uses bouts of high-intensity exercise followed by rest periods. For example, runners and swimmers often use a series of high-intensity sprints (exercise intervals) followed by rest intervals. This type of training was developed to improve anaerobic performance in activities such as sprinting and fast swimming and in the short bursts of vigorous activity typical of soccer, hockey, football, and basketball. Now, interval training is regularly used by endurance athletes as well. For more information about interval training, check with your physical education teacher or coach.

# Myths and Misconceptions

The amount of muscle fitness you need in order to stay healthy and do what you want depends on your personal situation and interests. For example, people who do jobs requiring a lot of lifting need more strength than people who work at a desk. Despite the fact that muscle fitness exercise offers many benefits, many people still hold misconceptions about them.

## No Pain, No Gain

Some people still cling to the myth that exercise must hurt in order to be effective. Some of the worst offenders are people who are hooked on strength-building exercises. In reality, you should listen to your body. If you feel pain, your body is telling you something. When doing PRE, it's true that you'll become quite fatigued and feel a sensation sometimes called the exercise "burn," and you need to learn the difference between this feeling and pain. If in doubt, back off to avoid injury.

## Muscle Bound

Some people think that strength training will cause them to be **muscle bound**—to have tight, bulky muscles that prevent them from moving freely. However, inflexibility is caused not by resistance training but by incorrect training. Two kinds of incorrect exercise that *can* cause a muscle-bound condition are training muscles on only one side of a joint and failing to stretch muscles. Another example of incorrect training is failure to move the joints through their full range of motion when lifting weights or doing other resistance exercises. For example, your elbow joint can bend to allow your hand to reach your shoulder and to let your arm straighten completely. Therefore, when you do a biceps curl with weight, bring the weight all the way to your shoulder, then straighten your elbow each time you lower the weight. *Caution: Do not bend your elbow or any other joint backward beyond its full range of motion. You can damage a joint if you move it in a way in which it was not designed to move.* Recent research suggests that when done properly, PRE can actually enhance flexibility.

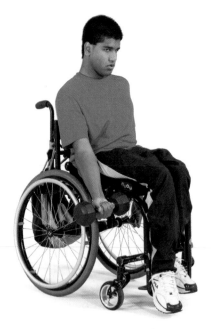 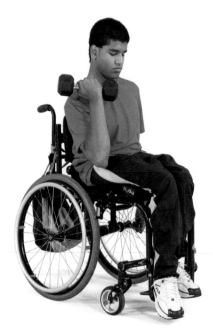

Moving a joint through the full range of motion is important for optimal functioning.

## Muscle Fitness for Females

As noted earlier, some people think that girls and women cannot build muscle fitness. Others think that PRE will cause girls and women to look masculine. Both of these statements are false.

## Muscle Tone

Advertisers often promise that a product or program can build something they call muscle tone. However, "tone" in this usage is considered to be a quack word because it does not refer to anything that can be measured in the same way as strength, muscular endurance, or power. Inspecting or feeling a muscle cannot objectively measure it; therefore, "tone" is not a good word to use to define muscle fitness, and any claim based on it is suspect.

## Body Dysmorphia

The term **body dysmorphia** refers to a condition in which a person becomes obsessed with building muscle. This psychological disorder, sometimes referred to as "reverse anorexia," often begins with a reasonable amount of exercise to build muscle fitness. At some point, however, a person with this problem gets carried away in wanting to build more and more muscle. The disorder is an obsessive-compulsive one and often requires treatment by a professional. In more than a few cases, people with this disorder have done unhealthy behaviors, such as taking drugs and doing unhealthy exercises. People with this condition experience high injury rates. Doing reasonable PRE can enhance your health. Becoming obsessed with fitness can hurt it.

## Lesson Review

1. What is the FIT formula for developing muscle fitness with isotonic PRE?
2. What is the double progressive system, and how is it helpful in using PRE?
3. What are some basic free weight and resistance machine exercises, and what are their advantages and disadvantages?
4. What are several other forms of exercise for building muscle fitness?
5. What are some of the basic guidelines for doing PRE safely?
6. What are some muscle fitness myths?

The following basic exercises use free weights to work the major muscle groups. The exercises that use barbells (bar and weights) can also be performed with dumbbells (small bar and weights or fixed weight dumbbells). The last two exercises require dumbbells. You can determine your 1RM for the various muscle groups using some of these exercises, but because resistance machines exercises are safer, they are the preferred method.

## SEATED OVERHEAD PRESS

**Weights:** barbell

This exercise requires two spotters, who stand by the lifter's shoulders on either side of the bench. If you are serving as a spotter, keep your hands under the bar with your palms up. Be ready to take the bar if the lifter loses control (especially at the top of the lift), if the barbell begins to move backward, or if the lifter begins to tremble.

1. Sit on the end of a bench in front stride (split-foot) position.
2. Hold the barbell at chest height in preparation for pushing the bar vertically. Grasp the barbell with your hands facing away from your body and positioned slightly more than shoulder-width apart.
3. Tighten your abdominal, back, and arm muscles. Tip your head back slightly.
4. Push the bar straight up, directly overhead.

Caution: Do not let the bar go forward or backward. Do not lock your elbows. Do not arch your back.

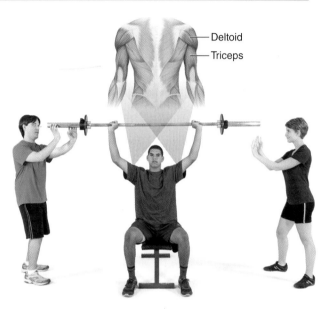

Deltoid
Triceps

This exercise uses the muscles at the top of your shoulders, between your shoulder blades, and on the back of your arms.

## BENCH PRESS

**Weights:** barbell

This exercise requires two spotters, who stand by the lifter's shoulders on either side of the bench. If you are serving as a spotter, place the bar into the lifter's hands. During the exercise, keep your hands under the bar with your palms up. Be prepared to take the bar if the lifter loses control.

1. Lie on your back on a bench with your feet on the floor and your lower back flat. Extend your arms into the up position (perpendicular to the floor).

2. Grasp the bar with a palms-up grip and your hands slightly farther than shoulder-width apart, your elbows straight, and the bar approximately over your collarbones.

3. Lower the bar until it touches your chest just below your armpits. When the bar touches your chest, your forearms should be perpendicular to the floor and your elbows should point neither toward your feet nor out to the sides but halfway between (at 45 degrees).

4. Tighten your abdominal, back, and arm muscles. Tip your head back slightly.

   Caution: Do not lock your elbows.

5. Push the bar up to the starting position with your arms perpendicular to the floor. The bar follows a slightly curved path.

   Caution: Do not lock your elbows or bounce the bar off of your chest. Do not arch your back or lift your hips. If the weight gets in front of or behind your arms, you may lose control.

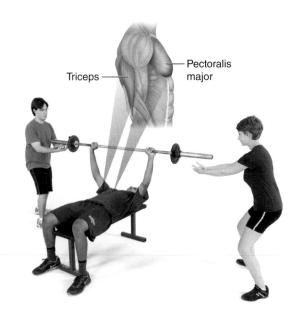

**This exercise uses the muscles on the front of your chest (pectoral) and the back of your upper arms (triceps).**

## KNEE EXTENSION

**Weights:** weighted boot or ankle weight

One person can help the lifter put on the boot or ankle weight.

1. Put the weight on one foot or ankle. Sit on a bench with your lower leg hanging over the edge. Grasp the bench with your hands.

2. Lift the weighted boot by extending your knee until your leg is straight.

   Caution: Lift slowly. Do not lock your knee when you extend and do not kick your leg upward.

3. Repeat the exercise with your other leg.

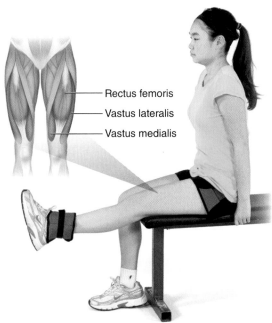

**This exercise uses the muscles at the top of your thighs (quadriceps). The fourth quadriceps muscle, the vastus intermedius, lies beneath the rectus femoris and therefore is not shown in the illustration.**

## HALF SQUAT

**Weights:** barbell

Note: This exercise can be done only if a squat rack is available.

1. Stand in a side-stride position with your feet shoulder-width or slightly farther apart. Your toes should point straight ahead or be slightly turned out. Keep your head up and your back straight.

2. Hold the barbell across the back of your shoulders at the base of your neck with your hands slightly farther than shoulder-width apart and your palms facing away from your body. Point your elbows toward the floor with your forearms perpendicular to the floor.

3. Squat until your knees are at a right angle, then rise. Keep your heels flat on the floor. Do not let your knees get in front of your toes. Focus on a spot on the wall slightly higher than your standing height. Look at this spot for the duration of the lift—when lowering and when straightening.

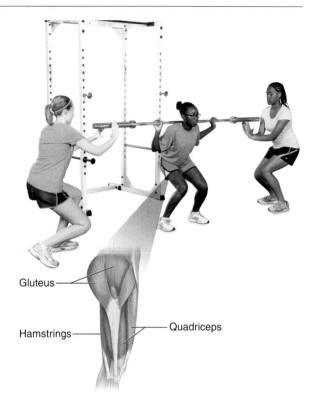

This exercise uses the muscles on the front of your thighs (quadriceps) and your buttock muscles (gluteal).

Caution: Do not round your back. Do not lean too far forward at your hips or let your knees get in front of your toes. Do not squat too deeply.

## HAMSTRING CURL

**Weights:** weighted boot or ankle weight

One person can help the lifter put on the boot or ankle weight.

1. Put the weight on one foot or ankle. Lie facedown on a bench, with your knee-caps hanging over the edge. Grasp the bench with your hands.

2. Lift the weighted boot by flexing your knee to a right angle.

    Caution: Do not lock your knee when you extend.

3. Repeat the exercise using your other leg. To determine your 1RM for this exercise, use the hamstring curl on the resistance machine.

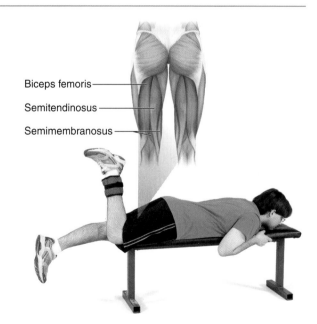

This exercise uses the muscles on the back of your thighs (hamstring).

## BICEPS CURL

**Weights:** barbell

Spotters are not required, but they can place the barbell in the lifter's palm-up hands.

1. Stand erect with your feet in side-stride position. Tighten your abdominal and back muscles.

2. Grasp the bar with your palms up and your hands slightly more than shoulder-width apart. The arms are fully extended.

3. Keep your elbows close to your sides and lift the weight by bending your elbows only. Raise the weight to near your chin, then return to the starting position.

   Caution: Do not move other joints, especially in your back.

4. You can also perform this exercise with your palms down.

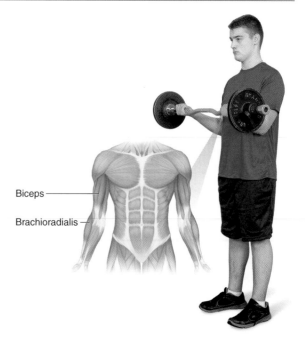

This exercise uses the muscles on the front of your upper arms (biceps) and other elbow flexor muscles.

## HEEL RAISE

**Weights:** barbell

This exercise requires two spotters, who stand by the lifter's shoulders, one on each side.

1. If weight is manageable, lift the bar above your head like you would in an overhead press (with spotters). Then lower the bar to your shoulders. If the weight is heavier than you can easily press, have spotters lift the weight to your shoulders.

2. Once the bar is on your shoulders, stand with the balls of your feet on a 2-inch (5-centimeter) board and your toes turned in slightly.

3. Rise onto your toes, then lower to the starting position.

   Caution: Keep your spine straight.

4. Advanced lifters may also try this exercise with their toes pointing straight ahead (more difficult) or with their toes turned outward (even more difficult). To determine your 1RM for this exercise, use the heel raise on the resistance machine.

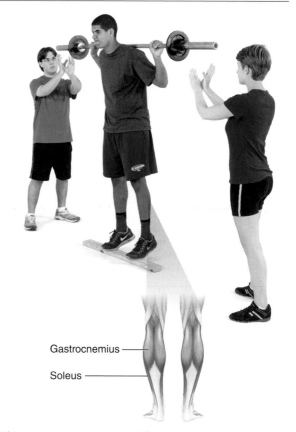

This exercise uses your calf muscles.

## SEATED FRENCH CURL

**Weights:** dumbbell

This exercise requires one spotter.

1. Sit on the end of a bench with your arms extended overhead and your palms facing up.

2. Hold one end of a dumbbell in both hands above and behind your head. Tighten your abdominal and back muscles. Slowly lower the weight toward the back of your neck until your arms are fully flexed at the elbows. Keep your elbows high.

3. Slowly return to the starting position, moving only your elbow joints. To determine your 1RM for this exercise, use the triceps press.

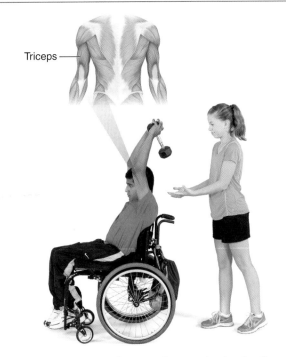

Triceps

This exercise uses the muscles on the back of your upper arms (triceps).

## BENT-OVER DUMBBELL ROW

**Weights:** dumbbell

This exercise requires no spotters.

1. Hold the dumbbell in one hand and rest your opposite hand and knee on a bench to support the weight of your trunk and protect your back.

2. Pull the dumbbell upward until it touches the side of your chest near your armpit and your upper arm is parallel to the floor.

3. Slowly lower the weight.

4. Repeat the exercise with your other arm. To determine your 1RM for this exercise, use the seated row.

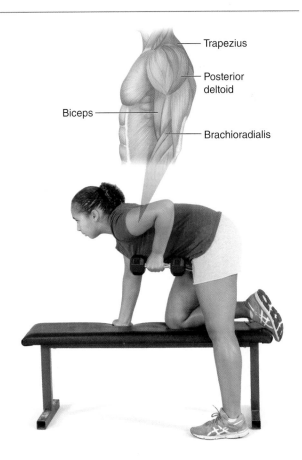

Trapezius

Posterior deltoid

Biceps

Brachioradialis

This exercise uses your biceps muscles, your shoulder muscles, and the muscles between your shoulder blades.

# RESISTANCE MACHINE EXERCISES

The following basic exercises use resistance machines to work the major muscle groups. They can be used to determine your 1RM for each muscle group just as you determined your 1RM for the seated arm press and leg press in the Self-Assessment.

## SEATED ARM PRESS

1. Sit on the stool of a seated press machine and position yourself so that the handles are even with your shoulders. Grasp the handles with your palms facing away from you. Tighten your abdominal muscles.

2. Push upward on the handles, extending your arms until your elbows are straight.
   Caution: Do not arch your back. Do not lock your elbows.

3. Lower the handles to the starting position.

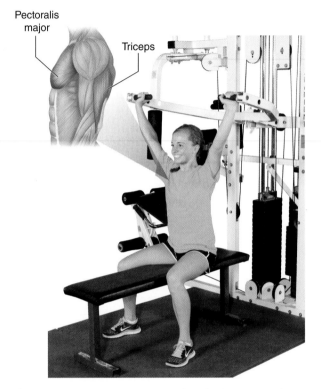

This exercise uses your pectoral and triceps muscles.

## BENCH PRESS

1. Lie on your back on the bench with your feet flat on the floor. Grasp the handles with your palms facing away from your body. Flatten your back. If possible, place your feet on the floor to help flatten your back and avoid arching it. If your feet do not reach the floor easily, bend your knees and place your feet on the bench to accomplish the same purpose.
   Caution: Do not place your feet on the bench if it so narrow that your feet might slip off the bench or if the bench is unstable.

2. Push upward on the handles, extending your arms completely.
   Caution: Do not lock your elbows. Do not arch your back.

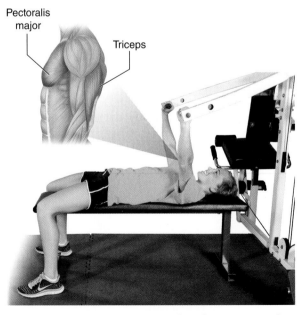

This exercise uses your pectoral and triceps muscles.

3. Return to the starting position.
4. You may choose either this exercise or the seated arm press. You may substitute this exercise in the self-assessment if you have a bench press machine and do not have a seated press machine.

## SEATED LEG PRESS

1. Adjust the seat position on a leg press machine for your leg length. Sit with your feet resting on the pedal.
2. Push the pedal until your legs are straight.
   Caution: Do not lock your knees.
3. Slowly return to the starting position.

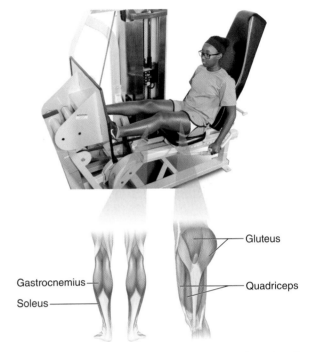

This exercise uses the quadriceps, gluteal, and calf muscles.

## KNEE EXTENSION

1. Sit on the bench and hook one of your ankles under the pad. Grasp the handles on the bench.
2. Extend your knee through its full range of motion.
3. Return to the starting position. Repeat the exercise with your other leg.
4. You may choose either this exercise or the seated leg press.

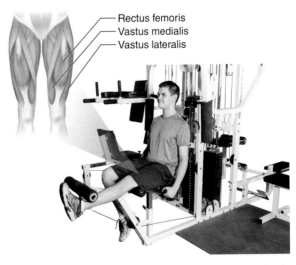

This exercise uses the muscles at the top of your thighs (quadriceps). The fourth quadriceps muscle, the vastus intermedius, lies beneath the rectus femoris and therefore is not shown in the illustration.

## HAMSTRING CURL

1. Lie facedown on the bench with your kneecaps extending over the edge of the bench. Hook your heels under the cylindrical pads. Grasp the handles on the bench.

   Caution: Do not lock your knees when putting your heels under the pads. If necessary, have a partner lift the pads so that you can avoid locking.

2. Bend your knees so that you can lift the cylindrical pads. Bend your knees through their full range of motion. At the top of the lift, the pads will almost touch your buttocks.

3. Lower to the starting position.

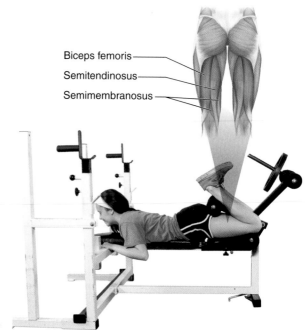

Biceps femoris
Semitendinosus
Semimembranosus

**This exercise uses your calf muscles.**

## BICEPS CURL

1. Stand in front of the station and grasp the handle of the low pulley with your palms up. Tighten your abdominal muscles and buttocks (gluteal muscles).

2. Pull the handle from thigh level to chest level. Bend your elbows but keep them close to your sides.

   Caution: Do not move other body parts.

3. Return to the starting position.

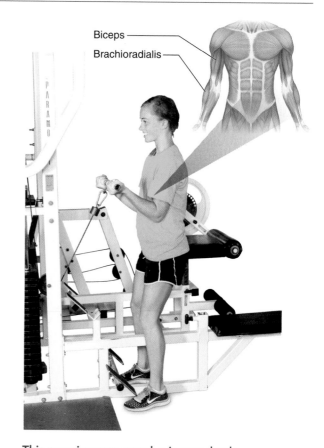

Biceps
Brachioradialis

**This exercise uses muscles in your back.**

## HEEL RAISE

1. Place a board that is 2 inches (5 centimeters) thick on the floor. Stand with the balls of your feet on the board and the handles even with your shoulders.

2. Grasp the handles with your palms facing away from your body. Keep your hands and arms stationary during the lift.

3. Rise onto the balls of your feet, then lower to the starting position.

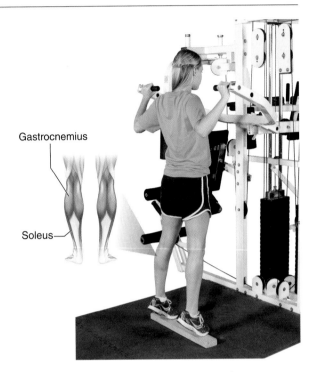

Gastrocnemius

Soleus

This exercise uses your hamstring muscles.

## LAT PULL-DOWN

1. Sit on the bench (or floor, depending on the machine). Adjust the seat height so that your arms are fully extended when you grab the bar.

2. Grab the bar with your palms facing away from you. Your arms should be at least shoulder-width apart.

3. Pull the bar down to chest level.

4. Return to the starting position.

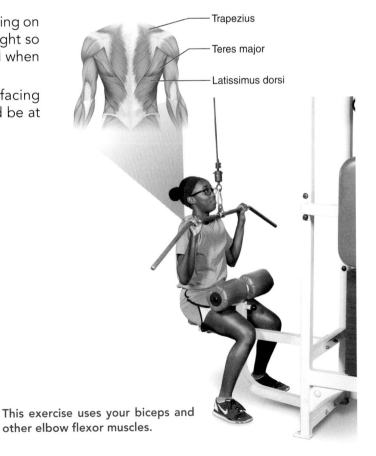

Trapezius

Teres major

Latissimus dorsi

This exercise uses your biceps and other elbow flexor muscles.

## TRICEPS PRESS

1. With your palms facing away from you, grab the handles.
   Note: If performed while sitting, adjust the seat height so that your hands are on the handles just above shoulder height.
2. Keep your elbows by your sides, and avoid leaning forward with your body.
3. Keeping your back straight, push forward and down with your arms until they are straight.
4. Return to the starting position.

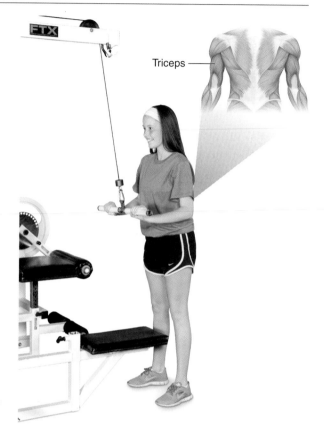

Triceps

This exercise uses the muscles on the back of your arms (triceps).

## SEATED ROW

1. Adjust the machine so that your arms are almost fully extended and are parallel to the ground.
2. Grab the handles with your thumbs up.
3. Keeping your back straight, pull straight back toward your chest.
4. Return to the starting position.

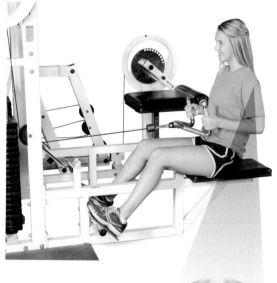

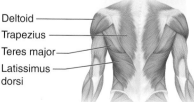

Deltoid
Trapezius
Teres major
Latissimus dorsi

This exercise uses the muscles of your back and shoulders.

# ISOMETRIC EXERCISES

The following basic isometric exercises work your major muscle groups.

## HAND PUSH

1. Sit in a sturdy chair, on a bench, or on the floor with your back straight. You may cross your legs if you prefer. Place the palms of your hands together.
2. Raise your hands and elbows to shoulder-height. Push your hands against each other as hard as you can. Hold the position for 7 seconds; rest for 30 seconds.
3. Do 2 or 3 reps as time allows.

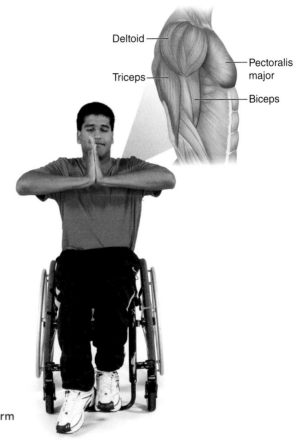

**This exercise uses your arm and shoulder muscles.**

## BACK FLATTENER

1. Lie on your back with your knees bent.
2. Pull in your abdomen by contracting your abdominal muscles as tightly as possible. Flatten your lower back against the floor. Hold the position for 7 seconds; rest for 30 seconds.
3. Do 2 or 3 reps as time allows.

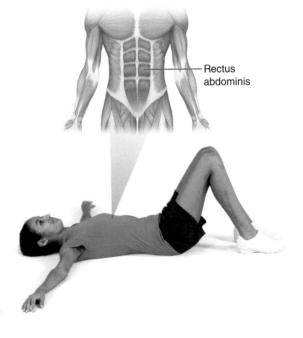

**This exercise uses your abdominal muscles.**

## KNEE EXTENDER

1. Hold onto something for support and stand on your left foot. Lift your right foot behind you, bending your knee to a 90-degree angle.

2. Loop a towel under your right ankle; hold the ends of the towel in your right hand.

3. Push downward with your foot, trying to straighten your leg against the resistance of the towel.

4. Repeat the exercise 2 or 3 times with each leg as time allows.

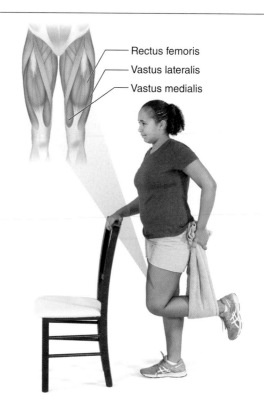

Rectus femoris
Vastus lateralis
Vastus medialis

**This exercise uses the muscles on the front of your thighs (quadriceps). The fourth quadriceps muscle, the vastus intermedius, lies beneath the rectus femoris and therefore is not shown in the illustration.**

## WALL PUSH

1. Stand with your back against a wall.

2. Move your feet out as you lower yourself into a half squat. Keep your thighs parallel to the floor.

3. Push your back against the wall by pushing with your legs as hard as you can. Hold the position for 7 seconds; rest for 30 seconds.

4. Do 2 or 3 reps as time allows.

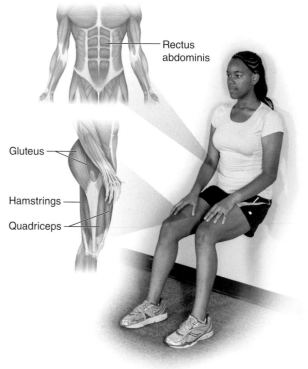

Rectus abdominis

Gluteus

Hamstrings

Quadriceps

**This exercise uses the muscles of your legs and abdomen.**

## BICEPS CURL WITH TOWEL

1. Stand with your back straight and your knees slightly bent.
2. Loop a towel under the back of your thighs.
3. Grasp the towel ends with your palms up. Keep your elbows against your sides.
4. Pull up on the towel as hard as possible. Hold the position for 7 seconds; rest for 30 seconds.
5. Do 2 or 3 reps as time allows.

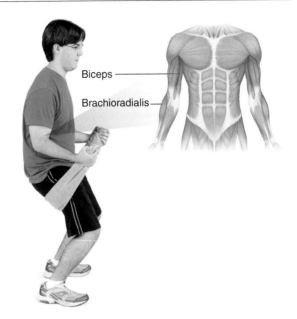

This exercise uses the muscles on the front of your upper arms (biceps).

## TOE PUSH

1. Sit on the floor using good posture.
2. Hold the end of a jump rope or towel in each hand. Loop it over the balls of your feet so that it is tight against your soles.
3. Push with the balls of your feet as you pull on the rope or towel. Keep your back straight. Hold the position for 7 seconds; rest for 30 seconds.
4. Do 2 or 3 reps as time allows.

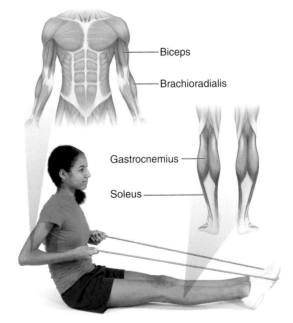

This exercise uses the muscles of your arms and lower legs.

## LEG CURL

1. Stand on your left leg. Hold on to a chair or wall for balance.

2. Loop a towel behind your right ankle and stand on the ends of the towel with your left foot.

3. Keeping your posture erect and your back straight, try to bend your knee against the resistance of the towel. Hold the position for 7 seconds; rest for 30 seconds.

4. Do 2 or 3 reps with each leg as time allows.

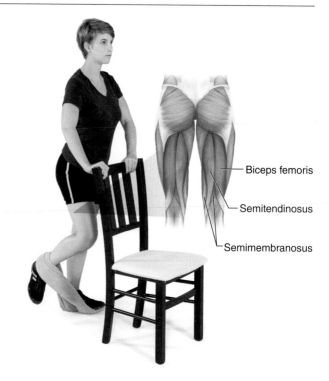

Biceps femoris

Semitendinosus

Semimembranosus

This exercise uses your hamstring muscles.

## BOW EXERCISE

1. Stand in a position that an archer would take when shooting a bow.

2. Hold a towel with your right arm as if you were holding a bow.

3. Hold the other end of the towel with your left hand near your chin as if you are holding the string of the bow.

4. Push with your right hand and pull with your left hand. Hold the position for 7 seconds; rest for 30 seconds.

5. Do 2 to 3 reps with each arm forward as time allows.

Safety tip: Breathe normally while doing these exercises. Do not hold your breath. Holding your breath can cause dizziness and possibly a blackout.

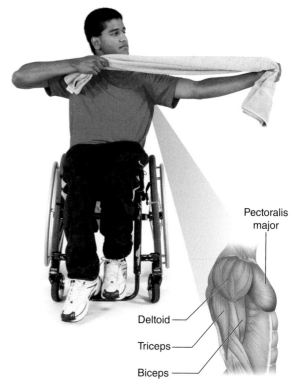

Pectoralis major

Deltoid

Triceps

Biceps

This exercise uses the muscles of your arms and shoulders.

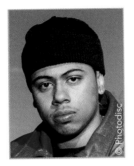

Anyone can begin a program to increase physical fitness, but just beginning a program is not enough. Some people are active for a while, then drop out for a while. This behavior is called a relapse. Those who stay active all of their lives learn how to avoid relapses that can lead to becoming sedentary.

Luis missed his old school, especially his old friends. Now he usually came straight home after school instead of heading for the neighborhood court to play a little three-on-three basketball with his buddies. For the first month after he moved, Luis ate dinner, did his homework, and then clicked on the television to fill the time.

Early one evening, his mom said, "Luis, why are you lying around? You like to be active. Get up and get moving!"

Luis yawned and said, "Where am I going to go? Who am I going to go with? I don't have any friends here."

"What about that boy who lives down the hall? I saw him leave with a gym bag the other day. He must have been going somewhere you'd like to go."

"Well, maybe," Luis said. "But maybe he was going to do weight training or something like that—something I don't know how to do."

"Maybe it wouldn't kill you to learn more about weight training. It might help you be better in basketball, right?"

Luis smiled up at his mom. "Maybe. What's his apartment number?"

"3B—and while you're there, ask his mom whether she knows about any exercise classes around here for old people like me, okay?"

## For Discussion

What caused Luis to relapse into inactivity? What could he do if it turns out that the boy down the hall hates basketball? What are some other things that cause relapse? What can be done to avoid them? What other suggestions do you have to help Luis? Consider the guidelines presented in the Self-Management feature as you answer the discussion questions.

# SELF-MANAGEMENT: Skills for Preventing Relapse

A person who relapses stops doing something that they want to keep doing or think they should keep doing. For example, you might start a PRE program but then stop doing it because you feel you can't take the time. Use the following guidelines to help you stick with something once you've started it.

- **Do a self-assessment.** It may help you see whether you're likely to stick with an activity, and it may give you ideas for how to stick with it if you've had relapse problems in the past.

- **Use the information from your self-assessment to determine areas in which you can improve.** Self-assessments help you learn about your current status (for fitness, activity, or nutrition, for example). If you are to improve, you first need to know where you need improvement.

- **Write down your goals for doing the activity.** Put them on the refrigerator or another place where you'll see them every day. You have good reasons to accomplish these goals or you would not have started to make a change in the first place. Stay focused on your goals.

- **Monitor your behavior by keeping a log or chart, then use it to reinforce or reward yourself.** Tell yourself that you've stuck with it so far and you can keep it up.

- **Tell other people what you're trying to accomplish.** Ask them to encourage you regularly.

- **Select a regular exercise time.** If you're trying to stick with exercise or another similar behavior, select a time of day and try to do the behavior at the same time every day.

- **Do not let one setback be a reason for a long-term relapse.** If you miss a day, tell yourself, "It's okay to take a day off once in a while." Repeat this saying to yourself periodically.

- **Consider a variety of activities.** Consider trying different physical activities from time to time.

If you're just starting a muscle fitness program, you may want to begin by using resistance machines at your school or local recreation center. Developing muscle fitness through resistance training will build your muscle mass and bone density and can help you develop a healthy body composition. Muscle fitness can also help you look your best and make it easier for you to perform everyday tasks, such as climbing stairs, opening food jars, and carrying your backpack. In addition, developing muscle fitness through resistance training helps you perform your best at your favorite sport and other physical activities.

**Take action** by trying some resistance machine exercises that you've learned in this chapter. Be sure to follow the guidelines for PRE described in the chapter.

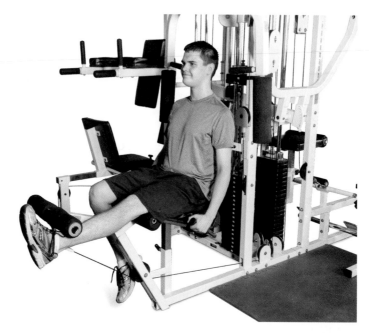

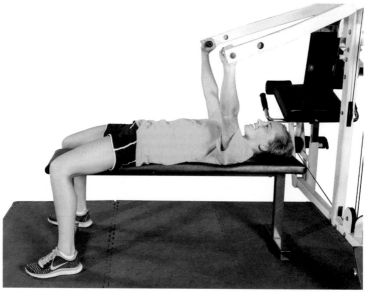

You can take action by doing PRE on resistance machines.

## Reviewing Concepts and Vocabulary

As directed by your teacher, answer items 1 through 5 by correctly completing each sentence with a word or phrase.

1. _____ is the amount of force a muscle can exert.
2. _____ refers to an increase in muscle fiber size.
3. A person can become _____ if he or she does strength training improperly by developing some muscles while ignoring others.
4. When you do calisthenics to develop strength, you use your body weight as the _____.
5. The _____ system refers to altering reps, sets, and weight as muscle fitness improves.

For items 6 through 10, as directed by your teacher, match each term in column 1 with the appropriate phrase in column 2.

6. isokinetic exercise
7. Olympic-style weightlifting
8. 1RM
9. plyometrics
10. isotonic exercise

a. sport, not an exercise program
b. the maximum weight that a person can lift once
c. exercise that requires a special machine
d. muscle fitness exercise that involves movement
e. exercise that builds power

For items 11 through 15, as directed by your teacher, respond to each statement or question.

11. How do strong muscles help you look better and prevent health problems?
12. Describe several methods for testing muscle fitness discussed in this chapter.
13. Describe two myths about muscle fitness exercise.
14. Describe several guidelines for preventing relapse.
15. Discuss the guidelines for using PRE effectively and safely.

## Thinking Critically

Go to the student section of the Fitness for Life website for this chapter. The address is on the first page of this chapter. Using information provided there and in this chapter, write a short article about muscle fitness for high school students. You can find additional information on the websites of NSCA, ACSM, and the President's Council on Fitness, Sports, and Nutrition. Share your article with your class or submit it to the school newspaper for publication.

## Project

Some schools provide wellness programs for teachers and other school employees. Typical offerings include exercise classes before and after school, fitness assessments, and classes in nutrition and stress reduction. Plan a special activity for teachers addressing one of these topics as it relates to muscle fitness. Prepare a written plan and work with other students to carry it out.

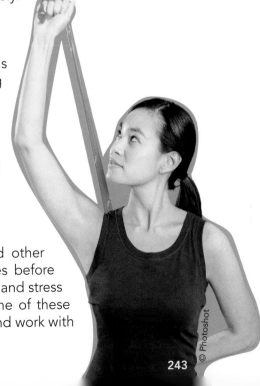

© Photoshot

# 11

# Muscle Fitness Applications

## In This Chapter

**www Student Web Resources**
www.fitnessforlife.org/student

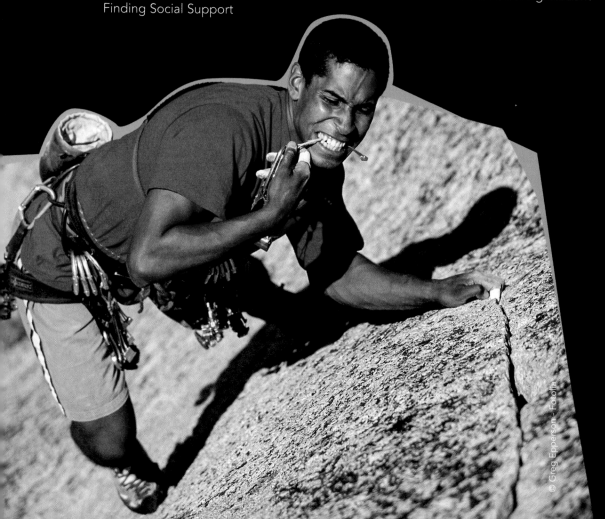

© Greg Epperson - Fotolia

# Core Fitness, Posture, and Back Care

## Lesson Objectives

After reading this lesson, you should be able to

1. name several core muscles and types of core muscle exercises and explain why they are important,
2. describe some common back and posture problems, and
3. list some biomechanical principles that can help you improve your posture and avoid back problems.

## Lesson Vocabulary

force, kyphosis, laws of motion, lordosis, Pilates, ptosis

**Do** you know what core fitness is? Do you have it? In this lesson, you'll learn about your core muscles and why they are important for good health and functioning. You'll also learn about exercises, including core muscle exercises, that you can perform to improve your posture and reduce your risk of back pain and other muscle injuries.

## Core Muscles

Your core muscles support your spine, keep your rib cage and pelvis stable, and help you maintain a healthy posture while standing, sitting, and moving in a variety of body positions. They also are the muscles that connect the upper and lower parts of your body. They include the muscles of your back, hips and pelvis, and abdominal area (see figure 11.1).

It's not uncommon for people to neglect their core muscles and focus more on muscles in their arms, legs, and shoulders because these muscles are easily seen and are considered to be important especially by young people. But you need fit core muscles—not only for healthy living and performing the tasks of daily life but also for performing sport and work-related activities and preventing injury. Core fitness allows you to keep your trunk stable while performing lifting and movements of all types. Some basic core exercises are presented at the end of this lesson.

Exercises that use resistance machines or free weights often do not build your abdominal muscles and some other core muscles. Since core exercises are an important part of a total muscle fitness program,

they are performed in addition to other progressive resistance exercises (PRE).

Many core exercises can be done without special equipment, and others can be done with inexpensive equipment. For example, you can improve core muscle fitness by exercising with large balls inflated with air. Exercises done with these balls are sometimes called stability ball exercises because physical therapists use them to help people build muscles that stabilize the body. You can also build your core muscles by doing medicine ball exercises.

## FIT FACT

Pilates is a form of training designed to build core muscle fitness that has become quite popular in recent years. It is named for Joseph Pilates, who described core exercises and developed special exercise machines for building the core muscles. However, a recent U.S. court ruling declared that the term "Pilates" is a generic name like yoga and karate, which means that anyone can call himself or herself a Pilates expert even without special training. As a result, although many Pilates instructors may be quite knowledgeable about exercises, others may not. Some Pilates programs have been modified in ways that are inconsistent with Pilates' original principles. When done properly, Pilates is a good way to build core muscles.

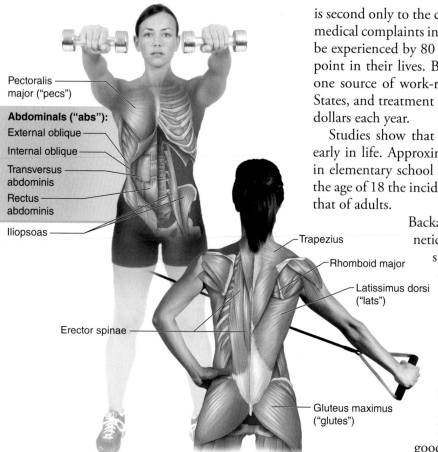

Pectoralis major ("pecs")

**Abdominals ("abs"):**
External oblique
Internal oblique
Transversus abdominis
Rectus abdominis
Iliopsoas

Trapezius
Rhomboid major
Latissimus dorsi ("lats")

Erector spinae

Gluteus maximus ("glutes")

**FIGURE 11.1** The core muscles.

## Back Problems

Have you ever had a sore back after sitting for a long time or lifting heavy objects? Each year, as many as 25 million Americans seek a doctor's care for backache. According to some experts, back pain is second only to the common cold among leading medical complaints in the United States, and it will be experienced by 80 percent of all adults at some point in their lives. Back injuries are the number one source of work-related injury in the United States, and treatment of back pain costs billions of dollars each year.

Studies show that back problems often begin early in life. Approximately one-third of children in elementary school have had back pain, and by the age of 18 the incidence rate of back pain is near that of adults.

Backache is considered a hypokinetic condition because weak and short muscles are linked to some types of back problems. Poor posture is also associated with muscles that are not strong or long enough. By building fit muscles to improve your posture, you can help reduce your risk of back pain and look your best. Even if you never experience back pain, a healthy back and good posture help you function more efficiently in your daily activities.

How does good fitness help your back operate efficiently? Good biomechanics are important. Your body parts are balanced like blocks on your legs. Your chest hangs from your spine and is balanced over your pelvis. Your head sits on top of your spine, balanced over the other blocks in the stack. Because your spine is flexible and can move back and forth, the pull of your muscles keeps your

 **FITNESS TECHNOLOGY: Exercise Machines With Memory**

Computer technology now allows exercise machines at fitness clubs to "memorize" your exercises. The machine stores your resistance amount for each exercise, making it easy to quickly prepare for each exercise. The machine also stores the number of sets and repetitions you perform for each exercise. You can also install fitness apps on a smartphone, tablet, or other personal computer to help you keep your own record of your exercises that do not require machines (for example, core exercises).

### Using Technology

Identify and describe an exercise machine or app that can be used to self-monitor muscle fitness exercise.

body parts balanced. If your muscles on one side are weak and long, but your muscles on the opposite side are strong and short, your body parts are pulled off balance.

One back problem that often occurs among teens is **lordosis**, in which the lower back has too much arch. Also called swayback, lordosis results when the core muscles, particularly the abdominal muscles, are weak and the hip flexor muscles (iliopsoas) are too short (see figure 11.2). Lordosis can lead to backache.

Even people who are relatively fit in other areas can lack fitness in the muscles related to back problems. One reason for this lack of fitness is that sports and games often overdevelop some muscles and neglect others. As a result, it is not unusual for basketball players, gymnasts, band members, and other active people to have weak back and abdominal muscles (core muscles) and short hamstrings and hip flexors.

## Posture Problems

Figure 11.2a illustrates some of the common posture problems associated with poor core fitness. Some of the most common are lordosis, **ptosis** (protruding abdomen), and **kyphosis** (rounded back and shoulders). You might recognize these problems in your own posture or that of someone you know. In figure 11.2b, you can see which muscles contribute to posture problems if they are too short or weak. Figure 11.2c shows you what good posture looks like and illustrates how it depends on long, strong muscles. Just as strong, long muscles contribute to a healthy back, they also are important for good posture.

Knowing what constitutes good posture can help you improve your own posture. And good posture helps you look good, helps prevent back problems, and helps you work and play more efficiently.

## Back and Posture Improvement and Maintenance

You can take several steps to help yourself enjoy good back health. First, you can perform self-assessments to determine your current back health and posture status. You can then identify exercises that will help you develop or maintain the muscle fitness and flexibility necessary for good back health and good posture. You can also use key principles of biomechanics to prevent back pain and injury.

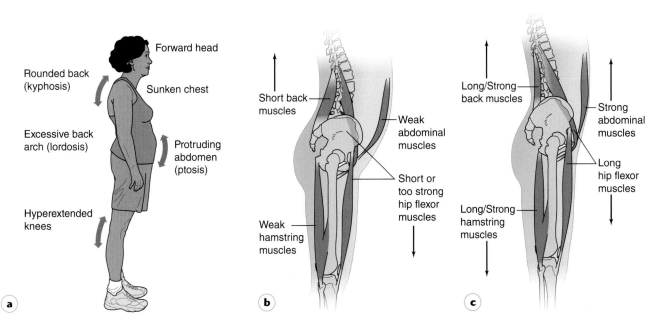

**FIGURE 11.2**  *(a)* Problems associated with poor posture; *(b)* core muscles in poor posture; *(c)* core muscles in good posture.

## FIT FACT

Many teens wear backpacks. To carry a backpack effectively, you need adequate strength and muscular endurance. In a typical year, the U.S. Consumer Product Safety Commission reports more than six thousand backpack-related injuries, mostly among youth. Improving your muscle fitness can help you reduce your risk of injury from wearing a backpack.

## Healthy Back Test

In the Self-Assessment feature at the end of this lesson, you'll get the opportunity to take the healthy back test. This will help you determine what you can do to keep your back fit and healthy. Core exercises are especially good for back health and for maintaining good posture. Stretching exercises are also commonly recommended.

 As shown in figure 11.2*c*, strong and long muscles help you avoid posture problems. The problems shown in figure 11.2*a* and 11.2*b* are not present in a healthy posture. The head is centered over the shoulders, the shoulders are back and balanced, the low back has a gentle curve, the abdomen does not protrude, and the knees do not bend backward. Working with a partner, you can evaluate posture to see whether problems exist and whether the body is in proper alignment. See the chapter titled Making Good Consumer Choices.

## Biomechanical Principles for Lifting, Carrying, and Moving Objects

For good health and safety, avoid exercises that violate the principles of biomechanics. As shown in the Science in Action feature, these principles and **laws of motion** apply when you use your body's levers—the bones of your arms and legs—to apply **force** in lifting, carrying, and moving objects. The most frequent use of these levers occurs when you walk or run or perform skills such as throwing, jumping, kicking, and striking. Using your body levers efficiently is also important in applying force when performing resistance exercises. Use the following biomechanical principles to help you avoid injury and back problems.

- **Use your large muscles when lifting.** Let your strong leg muscles—not your relatively weak back muscles—do the work.
- **Keep your weight (hips) low.** To make lifting safer, keep your weight low by squatting (bending your knees) with your back straight and your hips tucked.
- **Keep your core muscles firm when lifting.** Tighten your abdominal and back muscles to stabilize your body.
- **Use a wide base of support for balance.** Keep your feet spread about shoulder-width apart for stability when lifting.
- **Avoid a bent-over position when sitting, standing, or lifting.** Your body's levers, such as your spine, do not work efficiently when you are bent over. When sitting in a chair, sit back in the seat and lean against the backrest. Do not work for long periods of time in a bent-over position.
- **Divide a load to make it easier to carry.** For example, carrying two small suitcases, one in each hand, is easier than carrying one larger suitcase in one hand. A backpack is an efficient way to carry books. It's best to carry the backpack using both straps rather than over one shoulder. Avoid overloading your backpack or book bag. If you must carry your books in your arms, carry some in each arm. If you do carry your books in one arm, change arms from time to time.

# ⚛ SCIENCE IN ACTION: The Mechanics of Lifting

Kinesiology experts who study biomechanics have shown that lifting with your back rather than with your legs is inefficient and can be dangerous. The most efficient way to lift is to use your leg muscles and keep the weight near your body (see figure 11.3a). When you bend at your waist while lifting, you use your back muscles rather than your stronger leg muscles, and you greatly increase the amount of force necessary to lift the object (figure 11.3b). The same is true when you reach while lifting (figure 11.3c). These points are illustrated in the following example.

In figure 11.3a, a weight is held near the body. When the weight is lifted by using the leg muscles with the back straight, the force needed to do the lifting is only slightly more than the weight of the load itself because the load is held near the body. In figure 11.3b, lifting the same weight requires up to 50 times as much force because the lifter has to lift the weight of the upper body and because the necessary force is magnified when the weight is positioned at the end of a long lever. The longer the lever, the more the force is magnified. If a person reaches to lift (figure 11.3c), the necessary force is even greater because of the increased length of the lever.

The extra force needed for incorrect lifting puts unnecessary stress on the muscles and causes compression of the discs and bones, especially in the lower back. Incorrect lifting (figure 11.3, b and c) also requires the lifter to use the back muscles, rather than the stronger leg muscles, thus increasing the risk of injury. To reduce your risk of injury due to incorrect lifting, follow the principles described in the section about biomechanics.

As previously mentioned, it is best to use the stronger leg muscles rather than the weaker back muscles when lifting. It's also important to avoid bending at the waist when lifting. However, you need to improve fitness of the back muscles (back extensors) for back health and normal functioning in daily life. To build the back muscles, exercises such as the trunk lift and some forms of the leg lift are appropriate even though they use inefficient movements. The key is to perform the exercises in a controlled manner with appropriate resistance. To remind you how to perform these exercises safely, caution statements are provided for these exercises.

---

### Student Activity

What are some real-life actions that could put you at risk of injury due to movements that use your body's levers poorly?

---

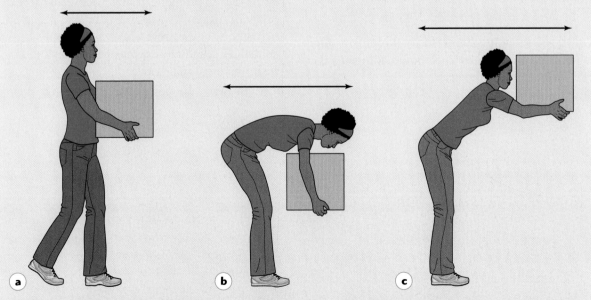

**Figure 11.3** For efficiency, *(a)* lift with the weight close to the body. *(b)* Avoid bending forward at the waist or *(c)* reaching while lifting because the longer levers increase stress on the back.

- **Avoid twisting while lifting.** If you have to turn while lifting, change the position of your feet. It's especially important to avoid twisting your spine as you are straightening or bending it.
- **Push or pull heavy objects.** Heavy lifting can cause injury. Pushing or pulling an object is more efficient than lifting it.

## Stretching

Healthy back care and good posture also depend on flexibility. Several good exercises are the knee-to-chest, the single-leg hang, the hip and thigh stretch, the back-saver sit-and-reach, and the back and hip stretch. Your instructor can show you these exercises when you study flexibility.

# Calisthenics

Calisthenics are exercises that use all or part of your body weight to provide resistance—for example, the core exercises discussed earlier in this lesson. Calisthenics for muscle fitness in your limbs are presented at the end of this lesson. Calisthenics build strength, and because they use body weight and typically involve multiple repetitions, they also build muscular endurance. The FIT formula for calisthenics is

- **F:** three to six days a week,
- **I:** lift part or all of the body weight, and
- **T:** 1 to 3 sets of 10 to 25 reps.

Calisthenics that involve explosive movement such as jumping build power and should adhere to the FIT formula for plyometrics.

# PRE and Injury

Experts have now determined that when PRE is performed properly and with good supervision, it is safe for teens. However, even when done properly, there is a risk of injury when performing both PRE and lifting sports such as weightlifting. The most frequent injury among school athletes performing PRE is back injury, especially in the low back. However, the National Strength and Conditioning Association indicates that "this risk is no greater than [the risk in] many other sports and recreational activities in which children and adolescents regularly participate." For example, studies show that the average injury rate in youth sports, especially contact sports, is much higher than for PRE. The risk of injury from PRE performed at home is much higher than the risk of PRE done in schools, primarily because of better supervision, better equipment, and required use of spotters at school.

Preventing a back injury is much easier than repairing one.

—U.S. Occupational Safety and Health Administration (OSHA)

Some injuries associated with PRE are not immediately noticeable. As a result, when cautioned about improper lifting or using incorrect biomechanics, some people might say, "I've done that before and it didn't cause a problem." But we know that repeated small injuries (microtraumas) can lead to big injuries later. Many people who ignore biomechanical guidelines eventually experience injuries and say, "I wish I hadn't done that."

## Lesson Review

1. Name some of the core muscles, describe some types of exercises for building core muscle exercises, and explain why they are important.
2. What are some common back and posture problems?
3. What are some biomechanical principles that can help you improve your posture and avoid back problems?

# CORE MUSCLE FITNESS EXERCISES

## CURL-UP

The curl-up is considered to be among the best abdominal exercises because it isn't risky like some abdominal exercises. The curl-up is sometimes referred to as the crunch, and it's a good substitute for the straight-leg sit-up and hands-behind-the-head sit-up.

1. Lie on your back with your knees bent at 90 degrees and your arms extended.
2. Curl up by rolling your head, shoulders, and upper back off the floor. Roll up only until your shoulder blades leave the floor.
   Caution: Do not hold your feet while doing a trunk curl. Do not clench your hands behind the head or neck.
3. Slowly roll back to the starting position.

### Variations

- **Arms across chest or hands by face (more difficult):** Fold your hands across your chest rather than keeping them straight, or place your hands on your

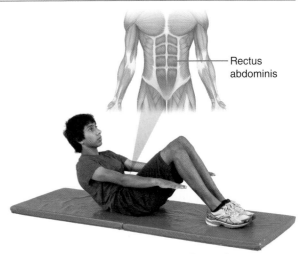

Rectus abdominis

**This exercise uses your abdominal muscles.**

face by your cheeks (not behind your head or neck).

- **Twist curl (builds oblique muscles):** Fold your arms across your chest, turn your trunk to the left, and touch your right elbow to your left hip. Repeat to the opposite side.

## TRUNK LIFT (BENCH)

1. Lie facedown on a padded bench (or a bleacher with a towel on it) that is 16 to 18 inches (41 to 46 centimeters) high. Your upper body (from your waist up) should extend off the bench.
2. Have your partner hold your calves just below the knees.
3. Place one hand over the other on your forehead with your palms facing away and your elbows held to the side at the level of your ears.
4. Start with your upper body lowered. Lift slowly until your upper body is even with the bench (in line with your legs).
   Caution: Do not lift the trunk higher than horizontal.
5. Lower to the beginning position.

Safety tip: As you do these exercises, lift slowly and move only as far as the directions specify. This exercise is appropriate when performed properly, but as noted earlier, using

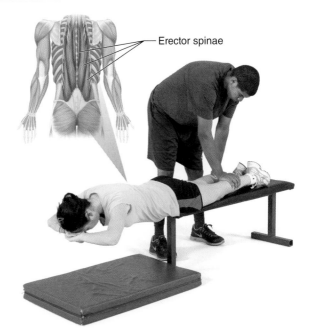

Erector spinae

**This exercise uses your back extensor muscles.**

the trunk muscles for lifting or carrying is not recommended.

## TRUNK LIFT (FLOOR)

1. Lie facedown with your hands clasped behind your neck.

2. Pull your shoulder blades together, raise your elbows off the floor, and then lift your head and chest off the floor. Arch your upper back until your breastbone (sternum) clears the floor. You may need to hook your feet under a bar or have someone hold your feet down.

   Caution: Do not lift your chin more than 12 inches (30 centimeters) off the floor. This exercise is appropriate when performed properly but as noted earlier, using the trunk muscles for lifting or carrying is not recommended.

3. Lower your trunk and repeat the exercise.

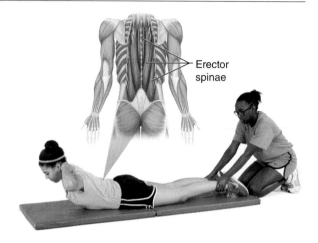

This exercise develops the muscles of your upper back and helps prevent "hump back."

## ARM-AND-LEG LIFT

1. Lie facedown with your arms stretched in front of you.

2. Raise your right arm, then lower it. Raise your left arm, then lower it. Finally, raise both arms, then lower them.

3. Raise you right leg, then lower it. Raise your left leg, then lower it.

4. Raise your right arm and right leg, then lower them. Raise your left arm and left leg, then lower them.

5. Raise your left arm and right leg, then lower them. Raise your right arm and left leg, then lower them.

Caution: Do not arch your back during this exercise.

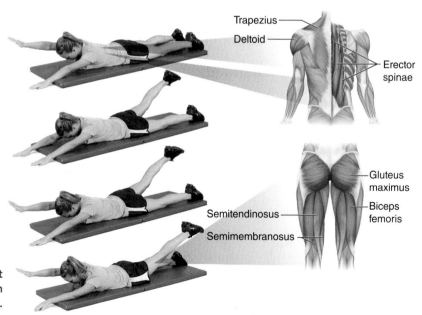

This exercise helps prevent rounded shoulders, sunken chest, and rounded upper back.

## BRIDGING

1. Lie on your back with your knees bent and your feet close to your buttocks.
2. Contract your gluteal muscles. Lift your buttocks and raise your back off the floor until your hip joint has no bend.
   Caution: Do not overarch your lower back.
3. Lower your hips to the floor and repeat the exercise.

**This exercise develops the muscles of your buttocks (gluteal) and the muscles on the back of your thighs (hamstring).**

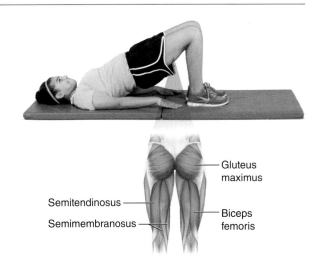

## SIDE PLANK

1. From a right-facing, side-lying position on a mat or carpet, lift your body into a side support position, supporting your body weight on your right forearm and your feet. Your left is arm bent and on your left hip. Tighten your abdominal and back muscles.
2. Keep your hips in line with your body. Hold this position for 7 to 10 seconds.
3. Repeat facing to the left.

**This exercise develops the abdominals and back muscles.**

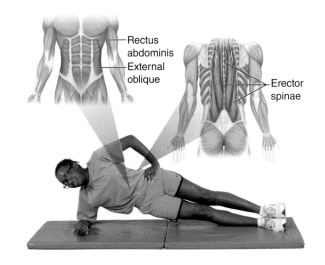

## REVERSE CURL

1. Lie on your back. Bend your knees, placing your feet flat on the floor. Place your arms at your sides.
2. Lift your knees to your chest, raising your hips off the floor.
3. Return to the starting position. Repeat the exercise up to 10 times.

**This exercise develops your abdominal muscles.**

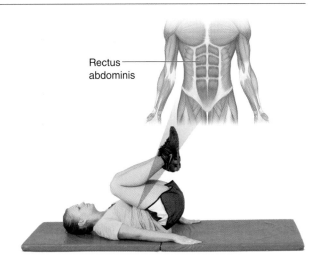

## FRONT PLANK

1. On a mat or carpet, support your body with your forearms and toes.
2. Keep your head in line with your body. Hold this position for 7 to 10 seconds.

**Variations**

- **Less difficult:** Support your body with your knees rather than your feet.
- **More difficult:** Perform the same exercise in the full push-up position.

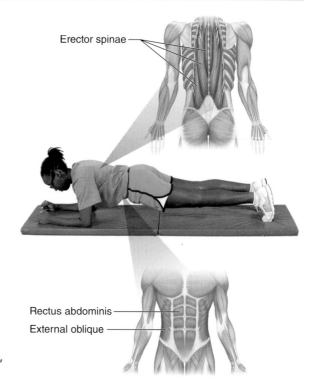

This exercise develops the abdominals, buttocks, and back muscles.

## DOUBLE-LEG LIFT (BENCH OR TABLE)

1. Lie facedown on a table (or bench) with your legs extending off the end. With a partner holding your upper body, lower your legs to the ground. If you have no partner, grasp under the edge of the table.
2. Lift your legs slowly until they are even with the top of the table.
   Caution: Do not lift any higher. If necessary, lift one leg at a time until you are able to lift both legs at once.
3. Lower to the starting position.

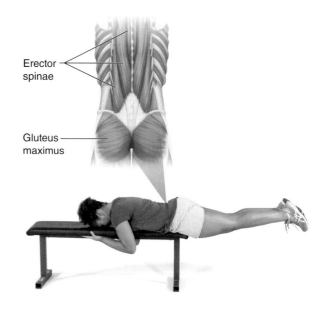

This exercise strengthens your lower back and gluteus muscles.

## PUSH-UP

1. Lie facedown on a mat or carpet with your hands under your shoulders, your fingers spread, and your legs straight. Your legs should be slightly apart and your toes should be tucked under.

2. Push up until your arms are straight. Keep your legs and back straight. Your body should form a straight line.

3. Lower your body by bending your elbows until your upper arms are parallel to the floor (elbows bent at a 90-degree angle). Then push up until your arms are fully extended. Repeat, alternating between the fully extended and the 90-degree arm positions.

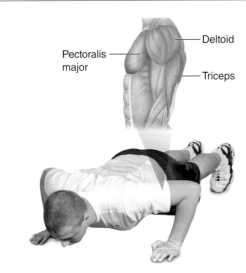

This exercise develops your chest muscles (pectorals) and the muscle (triceps) on the back of your upper arms.

## KNEE PUSH-UP

1. If you cannot complete 20 reps of the 90-degree push-up, try this version. Lie facedown with your hands placed under your shoulders.

2. Push up, keeping your body rigid, until your arms are straight, but keep your knees on the floor.

3. Keep your body rigid, and lower it until your chest touches the floor.

This exercise develops your chest muscles (pectorals) and the muscle (triceps) on the back of your upper arms.

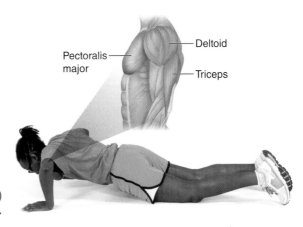

## PRONE ARM LIFT

1. Lie facedown on the floor with your arms extended and held against your ears.

2. Keep your forehead and chest on the floor and lift your arms so that your hands are 6 inches (15 centimeters) off the floor.

3. Lower your arms, then repeat the exercise. Keep your arms touching your ears and keep your elbows straight.

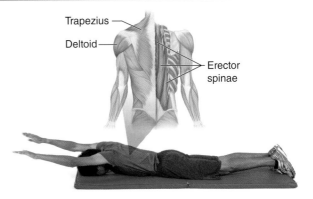

This exercise develops the muscles of your back and shoulders.

## STRIDE JUMP

1. Stand with your left leg forward and your right leg back. Hold your right arm at shoulder height straight in front of your body and your left arm straight behind you.

2. Jump and move your right foot forward and your left foot back. As your feet change places, your arms switch position. Keep your feet 18 to 24 inches (about 45 to 60 centimeters) apart.

3. Continue jumping, alternating your feet and arms. Count 1 rep each time your left foot moves forward.

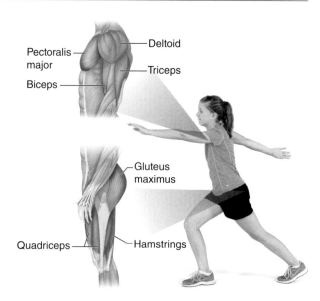

This exercise develops the muscles of your legs and arms as well as cardiorespiratory endurance and power.

## SIDE LEG LIFT

1. Lie on your right side. Use your arms for balance.

2. Lift your top (left) leg 45 degrees. Keep your kneecap pointing forward and your ankle pointing toward the ceiling. If your leg rotates so that your knee points upward, you will work the wrong muscles.

3. Lower your leg. Repeat the movement. To increase intensity, you can use an ankle weight.

4. Roll over and repeat the exercise with your right leg.

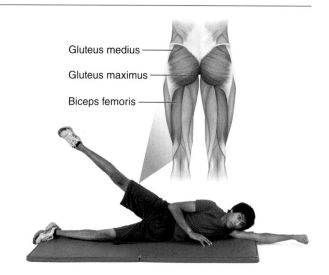

This exercise develops your hip and thigh muscles.

## KNEE-TO-NOSE

1. Kneel on all fours.
2. Pull your right knee toward your nose.
3. Extend your right leg until it is in line with the back and shoulders (parallel to the floor). Keep your head in line with the shoulders, back, and extended leg.
   Caution: Do not lift your leg higher than your hips. Do not hyperextend your neck or lower back.
4. Return to the starting position. Repeat the exercise with your left leg.

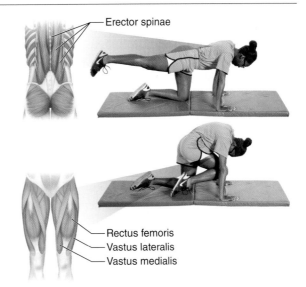

This exercise develops the gluteal, lower back, and quadriceps muscles. The fourth quadriceps muscle, the vastus intermedius, lies beneath the rectus femoris and therefore is not shown in the illustration.

## HIGH-KNEE JOG

1. Jog in place. Try to lift each knee so that your upper leg is parallel with the floor.
2. Count 1 rep each time your right foot touches the floor. Try to do one or two jog steps per second.

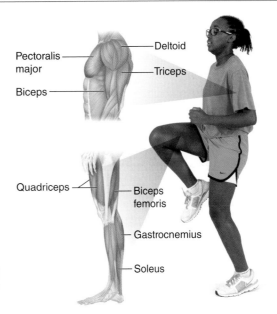

This exercise develops the muscles of your arms and legs and is also good for cardiorespiratory endurance.

Backache is often caused by weak muscles and by muscles that are too short. Test your back muscles by using the following self-assessment. Each part focuses on a certain muscle group. If you do well on this assessment, you're likely to have a healthy back. If not, it's especially important that you do exercises to improve your back health. In doing the test, work with a partner. Your partner will anchor your body for certain tests and can help in recording scores. Add your scores for the individual test item to get your total score. Then use table 11.1 to determine your risk of back problems. Record your results as directed by your instructor. Remember that self-assessment information is personal and considered confidential. It shouldn't be shared with others without the permission of the person being tested.

## Test Item 1: Single-Leg Lift (supine)

1. Lie on your back on the floor. Lift your left leg off the floor as high as possible without bending either knee.

2. Repeat using your right leg. Score 1 point if you can lift your left leg to a 90-degree angle with the floor. Score an additional point if you can lift your right leg to a 90-degree angle.

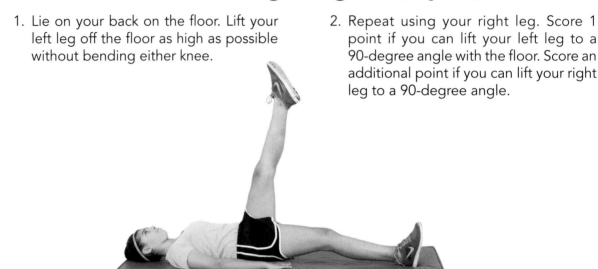

## Test Item 2: Knee-to-Chest

1. Lie on your back on the floor. Make sure your lower back is flat on the floor.

2. Grasp the back of your thigh to bring your right knee up until you can hold it tightly against your chest. Keep your left leg straight. The left leg may lift off the floor to allow the right knee to reach your chest.

3. Repeat using your left leg.

4. Score 1 point if you can keep your left leg touching the floor while holding your right leg against your chest. Score an additional point if you can keep your right leg touching the floor while holding your left leg against your chest.

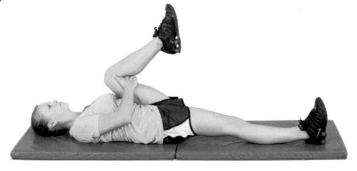

# Test Item 3: Single-Leg Lift (prone)

1. Lie facedown on the floor. Lift your straight right leg as high as possible. Hold the position for a count of 10. Then lower your leg.
2. Repeat using your left leg.
3. Score 1 point if you can hold your right leg 12 inches (30 centimeters) off the floor for a count of 10. Score an additional point if you can do the same with your left leg.

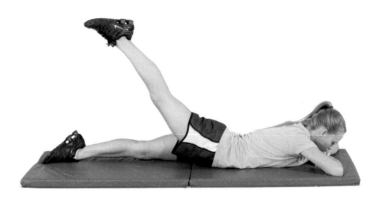

# Test Item 4: Curl-Up

1. Lie on your back with your knees bent at 90 degrees and your arms extended.
2. Curl up by rolling your head, shoulders, and upper back off the floor. Roll up only until your shoulder blades leave the floor.
3. Score 1 point if you can curl up with your arms held straight in front of you and hold the position for 10 seconds without having to lift your feet off the floor.
4. Score an additional point if you can curl up with your arms across your chest and hold the position for 10 seconds without your feet leaving the floor.

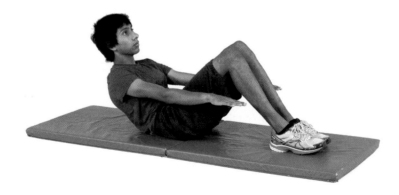

# Test Item 5: Trunk Lift and Hold

1. Lie facedown on a padded bench (or a bleacher with a towel on it) that is 16 to 18 inches (41 to 46 centimeters) high. Your upper body (from your waist up) should extend off the bench.

2. Have your partner hold your calves just below the knees.

3. Place one hand over the other on your forehead with your palms facing away and your elbows held to the side at the level of your ears.

4. Start with your upper body lowered. Lift slowly until your upper body is even with the bench. Hold the position for a count of 10.

5. Score 1 point if you can lift your trunk even with the bench. Score an additional point if you can hold your upper body even with the bench for a count of 10.

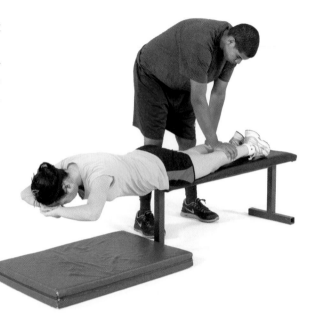

# Test Item 6: Front Plank

1. On a mat or carpet, support your body with your forearms and toes.

2. Keep your head in line with your body and hold this position for 10 seconds.

3. Score 2 points if you can hold your body straight for the full 10 seconds.

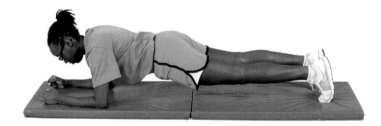

**TABLE 11.1  Rating Chart: Healthy Back Test**

| Rating | Score |
| --- | --- |
| Good fitness | 11 or 12 |
| Marginal (some risk) | 9 or 10 |
| Low (greater risk) | 6–8 |
| High risk | ≤5 |

# Lesson 11.2

# Ergogenic Aids and Muscle Fitness Exercise Planning

## Lesson Objectives

After reading this lesson, you should be able to

1. list several ergogenic aids and supplements and the risks associated with their use,
2. collect information about your personal needs and build a muscle fitness and activity profile,
3. set goals for muscle fitness exercise,
4. select muscle fitness exercises and prepare a written muscle fitness exercise plan, and
5. describe periodization and explain why it is used.

## Lesson Vocabulary

anabolic steroid, androstenedione, creatine, ergogenic aid, ergolytic, human growth hormone (HGH), periodization, rhabdomyolysis

**Do** you know someone who takes pills with the hope of finding an easy way to get muscle fitness? Do the pills really work? Would you like to improve your muscle fitness? Are you among the nearly 50 percent of teens who do no regular muscle fitness exercise? In this lesson, you'll learn about products advertised as muscle builders—and the problems associated with them. You'll also learn how to prepare a personal muscle fitness exercise plan that is safe and effective. Carrying out a good plan is the surest way to build your muscle fitness, which will help you meet national guidelines for physical activity both now and later in your life.

 Fitness—if it came in a bottle, everyone would have a great body.

—Cher, singer and actress

## Ergogenic Aids

For centuries, people, especially those interested in high-level performance, have tried to find methods of enhancing performance—including methods other than the exercise training presented in this book. *Ergo* relates to work, and *genic* relates to the word *generate*. Thus an **ergogenic aid** helps you generate work or increases your ability to do work,

including performing vigorous exercise. Some ergogenic aids, or products thought to be ergogenic aids, are classified as drugs, whereas others are classified as food supplements. In the United States, a drug must be approved by the Food and Drug Administration (FDA) before it can be sold by prescription or over the counter. Supplements, however, are not subject to FDA approval, so there is no assurance that they are what they appear to be or that they are as effective as advertisements indicate.

Many ergogenic aids can be dangerous. Others are not ergogenic at all because they do not work as advertised. Some are detrimental to health and performance and are better referred to as **ergolytic** (*ergo* again meaning work and *lytic* meaning destruction). Examples of ergolytic substances include alcohol, tobacco, and marijuana. Some of the products marketed as ergogenic aids are described in the following pages.

## Anabolic Steroids and Their Dangers

Many types of steroid are used by doctors to treat disease. **Anabolic steroids** are synthetic drugs that resemble the male hormone testosterone and produce lean body mass, weight gain, and bone maturation. For certain diseases, doctors legally prescribe anabolic steroids in small doses. However, some people illegally buy and use anabolic steroids to increase muscle size and strength. Anabolic steroids are not only illegal when used without a doctor's prescription but also dangerous. For this reason, their use is prohibited by the United States Olympic Committee (USOC) and most other athletic associations. Some of their harmful effects are illustrated in figure 11.4.

Teenagers are at high risk for harm from steroids because their bodies are still growing. Anabolic steroids can damage the growth centers of bones, causing the long bones of the body to stop growing. This condition can prevent a person from growing to his or her full height. Many side effects do not go away when use of the drug is discontinued; examples include hair loss, acne, deepening voice, and dark facial hair growth in women. For athletes, another major problem is the increased risk of injury to tendons and ligaments, which become less elastic with steroid use.

Some athletes also use certain drugs in an attempt to enhance their performance, and sport officials develop tests to detect these drugs. Like steroids, they can be dangerous, and most are banned by sport groups and may also be illegal.

## Steroid Precursors

A precursor is a substance from which another substance is formed; thus a steroid precursor is a nonsteroid substance that leads to the formation of a steroid. Some supplements are marketed as precursors,

and they can cause the body to form its own anabolic steroids. Examples are **androstenedione**, DHEA, and androstenediol.

Androstenedione, often referred to as "andro," is considered to be a steroid precursor because it is converted into anabolic steroids such as testosterone (male hormone) after it enters the body. In some countries, it is viewed as a food supplement. It was formerly considered to be a food supplement in the

## FIT FACT

**Rhabdomyolysis** is a condition in which muscle fibers break down, causing the bloodstream to absorb muscle fiber elements (such as myoglobin), which can damage the kidneys. Symptoms include muscle weakness and aching, fatigue, joint pain, and, in severe cases, seizure. Causes of this condition include exercising in the heat, lack of water replacement, and severe exertion. In several reported instances, high school and college athletes have been hospitalized for rhabdomyolysis due to excessive calisthenics and training drills. Some athletes push beyond healthy limits after taking supplements that they think will give them the ability to do extreme training. This practice can result in problems such as rhabdomyolysis.

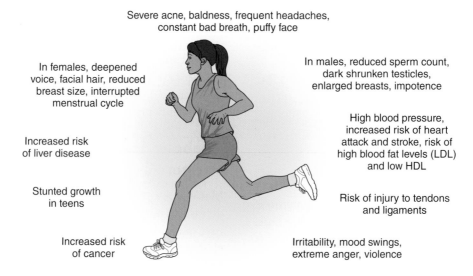

Severe acne, baldness, frequent headaches, constant bad breath, puffy face

In females, deepened voice, facial hair, reduced breast size, interrupted menstrual cycle

Increased risk of liver disease

Stunted growth in teens

Increased risk of cancer

In males, reduced sperm count, dark shrunken testicles, enlarged breasts, impotence

High blood pressure, increased risk of heart attack and stroke, risk of high blood fat levels (LDL) and low HDL

Risk of injury to tendons and ligaments

Irritability, mood swings, extreme anger, violence

**FIGURE 11.4**　The dangers of using anabolic steroids.

## CONSUMER CORNER: Health and Fitness in a Bottle

Many products sold as ergogenic aids are classified as food supplements. Most people in the United States think that the Food and Drug Administration (FDA) tests food supplements to make sure that they are safe. This assumption is false. Unlike medicines, which must be tested before they are approved for safe use, food supplements are unregulated by the government. The law does *not* require that they be tested for effectiveness or safety before they are sold. And unlike foods, which must be labeled with nutrition information, food supplements are not required to carry a label. As a result, there is great variation in the content of different products with the same name. Be aware of the following facts about food supplements.

- **Regulation.** Manufacturers are supposed to regulate their products, but many do not.
- **Claims.** Manufacturers are not supposed to make unsubstantiated health claims for their products, but many do it anyway. Although the FDA does not test products, it can investigate claims and has taken action against some companies for making false claims. However, because there are few investigators, many false claims do not get caught. Beware of health claims made for supplements.

- **Contents.** Many supplements do not contain what their makers claim they do. Some contain too little or too much of the key substance they are supposed to contain. Some have been shown to contain substances that they are *not* supposed to contain. These problems have led to health risks for some users.
- **USP.** The U.S. Pharmacopeial Convention (USP) is a nonprofit organization that tests supplements on store shelves to see whether they meet advertised standards for purity, strength, and quality. Products with the USP label are more likely than other products to be what they claim to be.
- **Recall.** Although the FDA does not regulate or test supplements, it does maintain a registry of side effects experienced from use of a supplement. You can report side effects to the FDA, and user reports have resulted in FDA bans on several supplements.
- **Dose or amount.** Because research is not required for supplements, as it is for medicines, very little is known about appropriate doses (amounts) for most supplements.

United States, but because manufacturers failed to meet marketing requirements it can no longer be sold in the country as a supplement. In fact, the FDA has sent letters to companies that sell it indicating that "enforcement action" can be taken against them. The FDA took this action after concluding that use of androstenedione "may increase the risk of serious health problems."

The use of steroid precursors such as androstenedione results in side effects similar to those associated with steroid use. As a result, just as USOC and other sport organizations banned steroid use, they now also ban the use of androstenedione, androstenediol, DHEA, and other steroid precursors.

Cautions against the use of steroid precursors have also been issued by several medical associations, including the American Medical Association and the American Academy of Pediatrics.

## Human Growth Hormone (HGH)

**Human growth hormone (HGH)** is an illegal drug that is exceptionally dangerous, especially for teens. It causes the bones to stop growing properly, and its effects can be deforming and even life threatening. Like anabolic steroids, HGH is banned by virtually all high school, college, national, and international sport groups. Testing is now possible to detect HGH, and many sport groups now do mandatory testing. Many high-profile athletes have destroyed their reputations and careers by using HGH and other substances described in this lesson.

## Creatine

**Creatine** is a natural substance manufactured in the bodies of meat-eating animals, including humans. It is needed for the body to perform anaerobic exercise, including many types of progressive resistance exercise. Creatine can also be taken as a food supplement. Taking extra creatine as a supplement allows your body to store more of it. Medical and kinesiology experts who have studied creatine indicate that it may be effective in improving performance in high-intensity exercise, such as sprinting, possibly because it allows training with shorter rest periods. It does not seem to improve aerobic or endurance performance or to improve performance among older people or highly trained athletes. Doctors use it to treat some medical conditions.

There is some evidence that creatine "loading"—using 20 grams daily for five days—may be more effective than continuous use. But remember, there is still some uncertainty about exactly who can benefit from creatine and at what dose. Studies to date have included only a small number of people (all have involved fewer than 40 participants), and it is not possible to draw firm conclusions from such small numbers.

In addition, because creatine is a supplement, it is not regulated by the FDA, and for this reason some products marketed as creatine may not be creatine or may contain substances other than creatine. Little or no information exists about potential long-term dangers of using creatine. Short-term use of appropriate amounts has not been linked with serious health effects, but the U.S.-based Institute of Medicine indicates that high doses are possibly unsafe. There is also some concern about possible increased risk of dehydration among athletes who use creatine. Experts agree that before teens consider using any supplement, including creatine, they should consult with their parents or guardians and a qualified expert such as a medical doctor.

## Other Supplements

Athletes and bodybuilders hoping to enhance their appearance or sport performance sometimes use one or more of many other supplements as well. Sport organizations and the FDA have banned more than a few of these substances due to health problems associated with them. Ephedra is one example of a substance that was included in many supplements alleged to improve athletic performance and aid in weight loss. It was shown to cause several problems, including irregular heart rate and other potentially dangerous effects on the heart and the nervous system. For this reason, it is considered to be an ergolytic substance.

Protein supplements are also used very commonly among athletes because they are legal and easy to obtain. Indeed, your body needs protein for growth and development of most tissues. Because protein is a major part of the muscles, many people believe that taking extra protein builds extra muscle. However, most people eat more protein in their regular diet than they really need. The United States government suggests that a healthy diet should contain about 12 to 15 percent of calories as protein. A more liberal recommendation of 10 to 35 percent of the diet as protein was recently presented by the Institute of Medicine to allow for dietary differences among individuals.

Athletes and very active people do need to consume more calories of protein than inactive people, but because they take in many more total calories, experts agree that 12 to 15 percent of their diet is adequate to meet their body's protein need. Taking more than 15 percent of the diet as protein does not result in greater gains in muscle. If not taken in excess, extra protein in the diet is relatively safe, but too much protein can cause kidney problems. Protein supplements in the form of pills, powders, and protein bars are very expensive, costing as much as 50 cents per gram of protein. In contrast, the

## FIT FACT

Approximately 27 percent of adults say they do muscle fitness exercise. The percentage of men who do muscle fitness exercise decreases from nearly 50 percent among young men (18 to 24 years old) to only 16 percent at age 75. The percentage of women decreases from 28 percent among young women to only 11 percent at age 75.

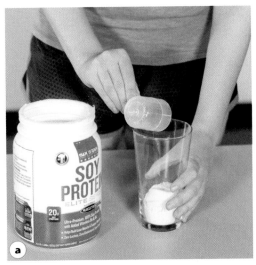 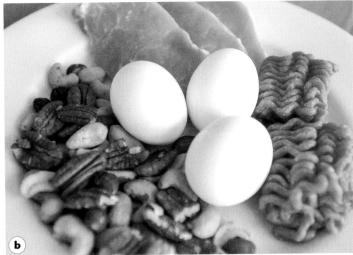

**FIGURE 11.5** *(a)* Protein supplements can be expensive; *(b)* foods with protein are generally less expensive than supplements.

protein in foods such as meat, poultry, fish, beans, and eggs is much cheaper, costing only a few cents per gram (figure 11.5). The calories in extra dietary protein (in excess of body needs) are stored as fat, as are calories from extra dietary fat and carbohydrate.

# Planning a Muscle Fitness Exercise Program

Molly is 15 years old and has used the five steps of program planning to prepare a muscle fitness exercise program. Her program is described here.

## Step 1: Determine Your Personal Needs

To get started, Molly made a list of the muscle fitness exercises and activities she had performed over the last week. She also wrote down her fitness test results that related to vigorous physical activity. Her results are shown in figure 11.6.

Molly met the national activity guideline for muscle fitness (exercising on two days a week). But when she was not in physical education class, she did no muscle fitness exercise. In addition, Molly's fitness test scores were mostly in the marginal zone, indicating that she needed improvement. Molly wanted to try out for the softball team, and she now knew that she needed to improve her fitness in order to be the best player she could be.

## Step 2: Consider Your Program Options

Molly wanted to consider all of the various types of muscle fitness exercise, so she made a list of the types of PRE that she had to choose from. Her list is included here.

- Resistance machine exercises
- Free weight exercises
- Core exercises
- Calisthenics
- Elastic band exercises
- Ball exercises
- Homemade weights
- Isometric exercises
- Isokinetic machine exercises
- Pilates
- Plyometric exercises (jump rope)

## Step 3: Set Goals

For this muscle fitness plan, Molly set a time period of two weeks—too short for long-term goals—so she developed only short-term physical activity goals. Later, she'll develop long-term goals, including some muscle fitness improvement goals, when she prepares a longer plan. For now, she wanted to

| Physical activity profile | | |
|---|---|---|
| Day | Muscle fitness exercise(s) | How much? |
| Mon. | Curl-up<br>Knee push-up | 1 set, 10 reps<br>1 set, 10 reps |
| Tues. | None | |
| Wed. | Curl-up<br>Knee push-up | 1 set, 10 reps<br>1 set, 10 reps |
| Thurs. | None | |
| Fri. | Curl-up<br>Knee push-up | 1 set, 10 reps<br>1 set, 10 reps |
| Sat. | None | |
| Sun. | None | |

| Physical fitness profile | | |
|---|---|---|
| Fitness self-assessment | Score | Rating |
| 1RM arm press<br>(score divided by body weight) | 0.55<br>(strength per pound of body weight) | Marginal |
| 1RM leg press<br>(score divided by body weight) | 1.10<br>(strength per pound of body weight) | Good fitness |
| Grip strength | 105 lb | Marginal |
| Muscle endurance test | 4 points | Marginal |
| Back test | 9 points | Marginal |
| Standing long jump | 59 in. | Marginal |
| Medicine ball throw | 95 in. | Marginal |

**FIGURE 11.6** Molly's muscle fitness exercise (physical activity) and fitness profiles.

try some new exercises to get started and improve her chances of making the softball team.

Molly used the information she put together in step 2 to help develop her short-term goals for muscle fitness exercise (PRE). She had many choices but decided on resistance machines, core exercises, and plyometrics (jump rope). Before writing down her goals, Molly made sure that she chose SMART goals. Here they are:

1. Continue to perform two calisthenics in physical education class (1 set of 10 reps).

2. Perform five resistance machine exercises two days a week (1 set of 10 reps at 50 percent of 1RM).

3. Perform four core exercises three days a week (hold 10 seconds or do 1 set of 10 reps).

4. Perform jump rope two days a week (5 minutes).

## Step 4: Structure Your Program and Write It Down

Molly's fourth step was to write down her two-week muscle fitness plan (see figure 11.7). Molly chose resistance machine exercises because she could use the school's exercise room on Tuesdays and Thursdays after school and she thought these exercises would be good for preparing for softball. She decided to do them just two days a week because she was just beginning this type of exercise. She decided to do her jump rope (plyometrics) on Tuesday and Thursday as well. She scheduled core exercises because they were good for back health and good posture and she could do them at home. She listed the exercises she did in physical education class because she expected to keep doing them for the two weeks of her plan. Molly's plan met the national guideline of performing muscle fitness exercises on at least two to three days a week.

| Day | Week 1 | | ✔ | Week 2 | | ✔ |
|---|---|---|---|---|---|---|
| | Exercises | Time, sets, reps | | Exercises | Time, sets, reps | |
| Mon. | Curl-up*<br>Knee push-up*<br>**Core exercises**<br>  Front plank<br>  Side plank (left)<br>  Side plank (right)<br>  Reverse curl | 1 set, 10 reps<br>1 set, 10 reps<br><br>Hold 10 sec<br>Hold 10 sec<br>Hold 10 sec<br>1 set, 10 reps | | Curl-up*<br>Knee push-up*<br>**Core exercises**<br>  Front plank<br>  Side plank (left)<br>  Side plank (right)<br>  Reverse curl | 1 set, 10 reps<br>1 set, 10 reps<br><br>Hold 10 sec<br>Hold 10 sec<br>Hold 10 sec<br>1 set, 10 reps | |
| Tues. | Jump rope<br>**Resistance machine**<br>  Arm press<br>  Knee extension<br>  Hamstring curl<br>  Biceps curl<br>  Heel raise | 3:30–3:35 p.m.<br>3:35–4:30 p.m.<br>1 set<br>10 reps<br>50% 1RM for<br>each exercise | | Jump rope<br>**Resistance machine**<br>  Arm press<br>  Knee extension<br>  Hamstring curl<br>  Biceps curl<br>  Heel raise | 3:30–3:35 p.m.<br>3:35–4:30 p.m.<br>1 set<br>10 reps<br>50% 1RM for<br>each exercise | |
| Wed. | Curl-up*<br>Knee push-up*<br>**Core exercises**<br>  Front plank<br>  Side plank (left)<br>  Side plank (right)<br>  Reverse curl | 1 set, 10 reps<br>1 set, 10 reps<br><br>Hold 10 sec<br>Hold 10 sec<br>Hold 10 sec<br>1 set, 10 reps | | Curl-up*<br>Knee push-up*<br>**Core exercises**<br>  Front plank<br>  Side plank (left)<br>  Side plank (right)<br>  Reverse curl | 1 set, 10 reps<br>1 set, 10 reps<br><br>Hold 10 sec<br>Hold 10 sec<br>Hold 10 sec<br>1 set, 10 reps | |
| Thurs. | Jump rope<br>**Resistance machine**<br>  Arm press<br>  Knee extension<br>  Hamstring curl<br>  Biceps curl<br>  Heel raise | 3:30–3:35 p.m.<br>3:35–4:45 p.m.<br>1 set<br>10 reps<br>50% 1RM for<br>each exercise | | Jump rope<br>**Resistance machine**<br>  Arm press<br>  Knee extension<br>  Hamstring curl<br>  Biceps curl<br>  Heel raise | 3:30–3:35 p.m.<br>3:35–4:45 p.m.<br>1 set<br>10 reps<br>50% 1RM for<br>each exercise | |
| Fri. | Curl-up*<br>Knee push-up*<br>**Core exercises**<br>  Front plank<br>  Side plank (left)<br>  Side plank (right)<br>  Reverse curl | 1 set, 10 reps<br>1 set, 10 reps<br><br>Hold 10 sec<br>Hold 10 sec<br>Hold 10 sec<br>1 set, 10 reps | | Curl-up*<br>Knee push-up*<br>**Core exercises**<br>  Front plank<br>  Side plank (left)<br>  Side plank (right)<br>  Reverse curl | 1 set, 10 reps<br>1 set, 10 reps<br><br>Hold 10 sec<br>Hold 10 sec<br>Hold 10 sec<br>1 set, 10 reps | |
| Sat. | | | | | | |
| Sun. | | | | | | |

*Performed in physical education class

**FIGURE 11.7** Molly's written plan.

## Step 5: Keep a Log and Evaluate Your Program

Over the next two weeks, Molly will self-monitor her activities and place a checkmark on her plan beside each activity she performs. Then she'll evaluate to see whether she met her goals.

## Periodization

Variety and enjoyment are important because they can help you stick with your exercise plan. Experts have found that if you change your program from time to time, you'll find it more interesting and feel more motivated to continue. **Periodization** is a systematic approach to scheduling your muscle fitness training and is used for long-term fitness programs (months to years). When you periodize a training program, you use variations in your exercise routines based on your needs for that phase of training.

For example, over 15 weeks of training, a person might do three periods of 5 weeks each. In one period, you might focus on muscular endurance exercises with relatively high repetitions and relatively low resistance. In another period, you might focus more on strength using higher resistance and fewer repetitions. Your third period might focus on combining strength and muscular endurance training or on using plyometrics to develop power. Many periodization options exist, so the three periods might look different for different people.

Periodization is used by athletes to gradually increase performance so that they peak, or reach their best performance level, at the right time. For example, an Olympic athlete would want to reach peak performance at the Olympic games, whereas a high school athlete might want peak performance for a key game or meet. Nonathletes use periodization more to provide variety and continued interest than peaking to prepare for a specific sporting event.

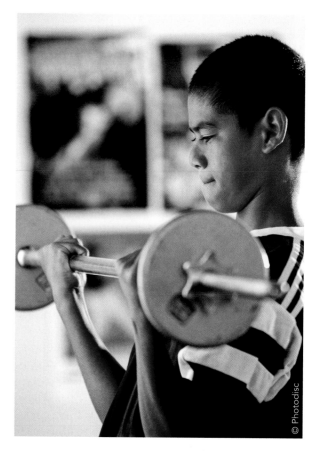

Varying your schedule for resistance training can help keep it interesting.

## Lesson Review

1. What are some ergogenic aids and supplements, and what risks are associated with using them?
2. How do you assess your personal needs and build a muscle fitness and activity profile?
3. What should you consider in setting goals for muscle fitness exercise?
4. How do you select muscle fitness exercises and prepare a written muscle fitness exercise plan?
5. What is periodization, and why is it used?

# ⚡ TAKING CHARGE: Finding Social Support

Social support involves your family members, friends, teachers, and community members encouraging your physical activities or participating with you. You're more likely to begin or continue an activity if the people you associate with also do it.

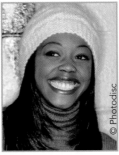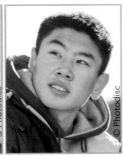

Shannon's family has always enjoyed bike riding. As a toddler, she would ride in the child's seat behind her mother. Every evening, the family would ride through the neighborhood. By the time she was in school, Shannon had her own two-wheeler. Now a teenager, Shannon still loves to ride, but school activities sometimes prevent her from riding with her family. She wants to continue riding but doesn't want to do it alone.

Jim's family has never been very active. Most of his friends tend to watch television, play video games, or just hang out rather than do anything active. Sometimes, Jim watches while a group of his classmates plays a quick game of volleyball after school. They often invite him to join the game. He has been tempted to join but has hesitated because he is not friends with any of the players. He has enjoyed the activities he has tried in the past but has never continued them for very long.

Both Shannon and Jim need social support. Shannon needs it to continue an activity she already enjoys. Jim needs it to begin an activity and then reinforce his participation.

## For Discussion

Who might Shannon ask to go riding with her? What could Jim do to become involved in physical activity? What other suggestions can you offer for finding social support? What groups might Shannon and Jim identify with to get social support? Consider the guidelines presented in the Self-Management feature when you answer the discussion questions.

# ➡ SELF-MANAGEMENT: Skills for Finding Social Support

Experts indicate that people who experience support from others are more likely to participate in regular physical activity, especially over the course of a lifetime. Social support is also helpful to people in losing weight, building muscle fitness, and improving their eating habits. Consider the following guidelines to help you gain others' support for your physical activity.

- **Do a self-assessment of your current level of social support.** Ask your teacher about the social support worksheet that can help you do this assessment. Use the self-assessment to determine areas in which you can improve your social support.

- **Birds of a feather flock together.** Find friends who are interested in the activities that interest you, or encourage your current friends to support you or join you in your participation.

- **Join a club or team.** If no club or team exists for your chosen activity, talk to a teacher, family member, or community recreation leader about starting one.

- **Discuss your interests with family and teachers.** Ask them for their support. Ask them to help you learn the activity.

- **If possible, get lessons.** In addition to formal lessons, you can also ask teachers and others to support you by helping you learn to perform an activity properly.

- **Family matters.** Encourage your family members to try the activity.

- **Get proper equipment.** Ask for equipment for your birthday or other special occasion.

Prepare an exercise plan for muscle fitness using the five steps described in the second lesson of this chapter. Like Molly, consider activities from a variety of types of PRE. The goal is to perform the exercises on at least two days per week (for beginners) and as many as three days per week for more advanced exercisers. Carry out your written plan over a two-week period. Your teacher may give you time in class to do some of the activities included in your plan. Consider the following suggestions for **taking action**.

- Before your PRE, perform a dynamic warm-up.
- Follow the tips for safe PRE.
- Progress gradually—don't try to do too much too soon.
- After your workout, perform a cool-down.

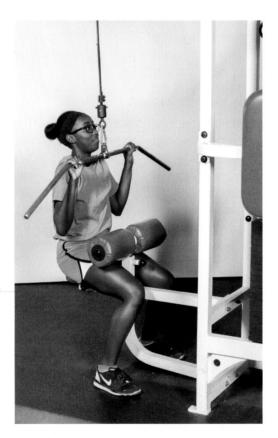

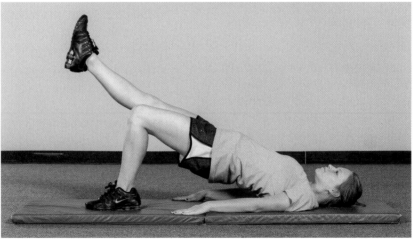

**Take action by performing your muscle fitness plan.**

# Reviewing Concepts and Vocabulary

As directed by your teacher, answer items 1 through 5 by correctly completing each sentence with a word or phrase.

1. The muscles that support your spine and keep your rib cage and spine stable are referred to as your _____ muscles.
2. About _____ percent of adults experience back pain at some point.
3. _____ are exercises that use all or part of your body weight to provide resistance.
4. _____ is the real name of the supplement sometimes called andro.
5. The full name for the substance called HGH is _____.

For items 6 through 10, as directed by your teacher, match each term in column 1 with the appropriate phrase in column 2.

6. rhabdomyolysis     a. swayback
7. periodization     b. rounded shoulders
8. lordosis     c. breakdown of muscle fiber
9. kyphosis     d. varying your program schedule for muscle fitness
10. ptosis     e. protruding abdomen

For items 11 through 15, as directed by your teacher, respond to each statement or question.

11. What are some of the best exercises for building your core muscles?
12. Describe three guidelines for properly lifting, carrying, and moving objects.
13. What self-assessments can you do to determine whether you are at risk for back pain?
14. What are some harmful effects of steroids?
15. What are some good strategies for finding social support?

# Thinking Critically

Write a paragraph to answer the following question.

A friend of yours is excited about an advertisement in a muscle magazine. The ad describes a pill that is "guaranteed to add size to your muscles in two weeks without exercise." What advice would you give your friend?

# Project

Assume that you've been hired as a reporter for a local newspaper. Write an article about preventing back pain or injury. Interview relevant people, such as a physical therapist, a physical education teacher, an athletic trainer, and a person who has experienced back pain or injury. Present your article in class or submit it to a newspaper for publication.

© Greg Epperson / Fotolia

# 12

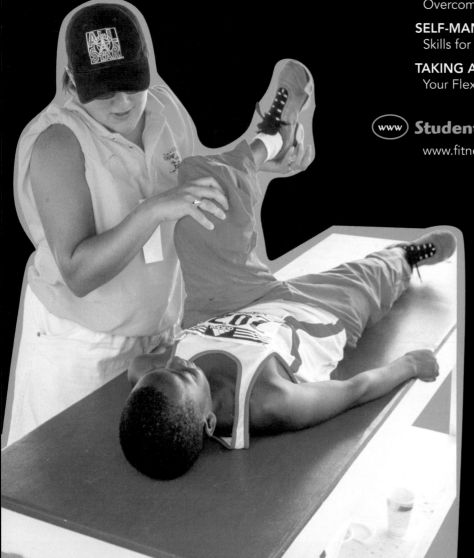

# Flexibility

## In This Chapter

**LESSON 12.1**
Flexibility Facts

**SELF-ASSESSMENT**
Arm, Leg, and Trunk Flexibility

**LESSON 12.2**
Preparing a Flexibility Exercise Plan

**TAKING CHARGE**
Overcoming Barriers

**SELF-MANAGEMENT**
Skills for Overcoming Barriers

**TAKING ACTION**
Your Flexibility Exercise Plan

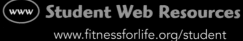 **Student Web Resources**
www.fitnessforlife.org/student

# Lesson 12.1

# Flexibility Facts

## Lesson Objectives

After reading this lesson, you should be able to

1. explain the difference between a warm-up and a flexibility workout,
2. describe flexibility and some of the factors that influence it,
3. explain the benefits of good flexibility,
4. describe types of flexibility exercise and the FIT formula for each, and
5. explain why it is important to balance strength and flexibility exercise.

## Lesson Vocabulary

active stretch, antagonist, ballistic stretch, CRAC, dynamic movement exercise, dynamic stretching, hypermobility, muscle-tendon unit (MTU), passive stretch, PNF stretch, range of motion (ROM), range-of-motion (ROM) exercise, static stretch

**Do** you have good flexibility? Do you do any regular stretching to improve your flexibility? In this lesson, you'll learn about the importance of being flexible and how to improve your flexibility by applying fitness principles. You'll also learn to evaluate your flexibility.

Sometimes people confuse a warm-up with a flexibility workout, but they are two different things. A warm-up is a group of exercises done to get ready for a specific workout or competition. A flexibility workout is a group of exercises done to build flexibility. Stretching exercises are now used less frequently in warm-ups than in the past, especially when preparing for certain types of activity, such as those involving strength, speed, and power. But this does not mean that flexibility exercises, including stretching, are not important. Flexibility is a key component of health-related physical fitness.

## What Is Flexibility?

Flexibility is the ability to move your joints through a full **range of motion (ROM)**. A joint is a place in your body where bones come together. The best-known joints include the knees, ankles, elbows, wrists, knuckles, shoulders, hips, and the joints between the vertebrae in the spine. Some joints, such as your knees and elbows, work like a hinge, permitting movement in only two directions. Other

joints, such as your hips and shoulders, work like a ball and socket, allowing movement in all directions. ROM is the amount of movement you can make in a joint (figure 12.1).

Your bones are connected at your joints by non-elastic bands called ligaments; as you'll see later, they should not be stretched. Your bones are connected to your muscles by tendons. When your muscles contract, they pull on your tendons to cause your bones to move. Unlike ligaments, muscles and tendons need to be stretched in order to maintain a healthy length. Together, muscles and tendons are called a **muscle-tendon unit (MTU)** (figure 12.1). Both parts of the MTU are stretched when performing flexibility exercises, but we frequently refer only to "stretching the muscle" for simplicity. If your muscles and tendons are too short, they restrict a joint's ROM.

## Benefits of Good Flexibility

Flexibility is sometimes referred to as the forgotten part of health-related fitness because many people focus exclusively on the other parts. We know, however, that good flexibility provides many benefits, including health benefits, especially when you grow older.

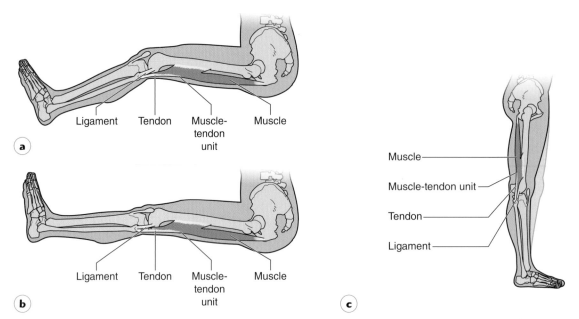

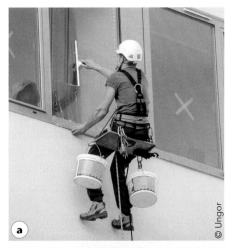

**FIGURE 12.1** *(a)* Poor joint range of motion—knee does not fully extend because of short hamstring muscles; *(b)* good range of motion—knee fully extends because of long hamstrings; *(c)* too much range of motion—knee bends backward.

## Improved Function

Everyone needs at least some flexibility in order to maintain health and mobility. The exact amount of flexibility needed for normal daily function depends on the demands of the activities that you perform. For example, plumbers, painters, and dentists often need to bend and stretch, and some musicians need very flexible fingers and wrists. As people grow older, their flexibility tends to decrease, which can limit simple movements such as looking over the shoulder while driving. Therefore, it's especially important for older people to do exercises that build and maintain a full range of motion.

Flexibility is also important to many athletes, especially in certain sports. Dancers and gymnasts must be very flexible to perform their routines. Swimmers need good flexibility to get maximum performance, as do kickers in football. Good flexibility also allows a longer backswing—and therefore a faster forward swing—in the throwing and striking movements that are crucial in golf, tennis, and baseball pitching. While some research has questioned the value of stretching right before a competition or performance, muscles of adequate length can be beneficial even in such activities as weightlifting and the shot put.

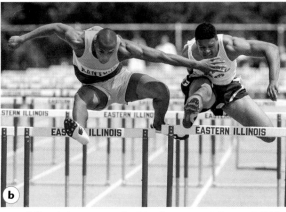

Good flexibility is needed *(a)* for some jobs and *(b)* by most athletes.

## Improved Health and Wellness

Good flexibility is important for your back health and your posture. For example, back pain and poor posture are associated with short hamstring and hip flexor muscles. More generally, very short muscles are at risk of being overstretched and injured. Stretching exercises also have a beneficial effect on a number of conditions. Flexible musicians are less likely to have pain in their joints. Stretching exercises can often alleviate menstrual cramps in women. They can prevent or provide relief from leg cramps and shin splints (pain in the front of the shins caused by overuse). Stretching a muscle can also help it relax, and some forms of stretching can help you manage stress.

## Rehabilitation From Injury and Medical Problems

Flexibility exercises are used for rehabilitation from a variety of injuries and medical problems. Both physical therapists (PTs) and athletic trainers (ATs) use a variety of techniques, including stretching and muscle fitness exercises, in their work. PTs treat patients after surgery and patients with medical conditions such as arthritis, back pain, stroke, and osteoporosis. ATs help athletes train to prevent injury and help them recover when injury does occur.

### FIT FACT

Physical therapists (PTs) are health care professionals who treat patients with medical problems or who have had surgery. They help patients manage pain and improve their mobility. They also help people perform regular exercises to prevent muscle-related problems and to maintain or regain their ability to function normally. PTs have many years of advanced education and, in the United States, must be licensed in the state in which they practice. They work in many settings, including private practices, hospitals, nursing homes, outpatient clinics, schools, and sport and fitness facilities. More than 75,000 PTs belong to the American Physical Therapy Association, a professional group whose goal is to help people improve their health and quality of life.

> " I want to get old gracefully. I want to have good posture, I want to be healthy and be an example to my children. "
>
> —Sting, musician

# Factors Influencing Flexibility

You already know that short muscles and tendons reduce flexibility and that they can be stretched to improve flexibility. Your flexibility is also influenced by the following factors.

## Heredity

Inherited anatomical differences in our bodies help determine what we can and cannot do. Some people inherit joints that do not favor a large a range of motion. These people will have to exercise regularly in order to develop a healthy range of motion. Other people have an unusually large range of motion in certain joints—a condition sometimes referred to as being double jointed but officially called **hypermobility**. People with hypermobility score better on flexibility tests and can extend the knee, elbow, thumb, or wrist joint past a straight line, as if the joint could bend backward. Some people who have hypermobile joints are prone to joint injury and may be more likely to develop arthritis, a disease in which the joints become inflamed. For the most part, however, those with hypermobile joints do not have problems, other than a slight disadvantage in some sports. For example, when doing push-ups, the elbows of a hypermobile person might lock when the arms straighten, making it difficult to unlock the elbows to begin the downward movement.

## Body Build

Can short people touch their toes more easily than tall people? In most cases, this is not true, because a shorter person tends to have not only shorter legs and trunk but also shorter arms (though there are exceptions). In contrast, a taller person tends to have longer legs and trunk and longer arms. Some people do have exceptionally long arms or legs, and these characteristics may make it easier or harder for them to score well on flexibility tests, but this is the exception rather than the rule.

## Sex and Age

Generally, females tend to be more flexible than males. About twice as many females as males are hypermobile, and at most ages more females than males meet minimum fitness standards for flexibility. Similarly, younger people tend to be more flexible than older people. As people grow older, their muscles typically grow shorter because they are used less, and their joints tend to allow less movement due to conditions such as arthritis. With this in mind, one important reason for doing regular flexibility exercises when you're young is to reduce your risk of joint problems when you're older. Good flexibility also enhances performance in a variety of tasks for people of all ages.

# Different Types of Flexibility Exercise

The following discussion presents methods of building and maintaining flexibility. For best results, perform exercises especially designed to improve your flexibility (step 5 of the Physical Activity Pyramid; figure 12.2). The four major types of exercise for building flexibility are range-of-motion exercise, static stretching, ballistic stretching, and dynamic stretching.

## Range-of-Motion (ROM) Exercise

Technically, all flexibility exercises are range-of-motion exercises because they are all designed to help allow a healthy ROM in the joints. More specifically, the term **range-of-motion (ROM) exercise** refers to exercise that requires a joint to move through a full ROM, powered either by the body's own muscles or by assistance from a partner or therapist. Such exercises are commonly used in physical therapy for people who have lost ROM or who want to avoid loss of ROM associated with an injury or medical problem. The exercise movement is typically continuous and performed at a slow to moderate pace.

Each joint has its own normal or healthy range of movement, so exercises are designed specifically for each joint. Examples include shoulder rotation exercises for people with shoulder injuries (for example, baseball pitchers) and knee flexion and extension of the fingers for people with arthritis.

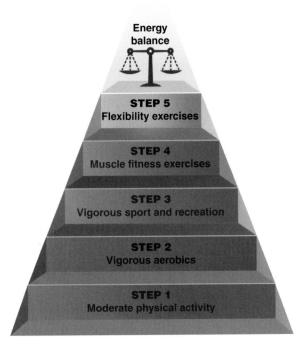

**FIGURE 12.2** Exercises for building flexibility are represented by step 5 of the Physical Activity Pyramid.

The weight of the body part and the momentum of the movement do cause some stretch in the muscles and connective tissues, but these exercises typically do not use the same intensity of stretch as those described in the next section; therefore, ROM exercises are not as good as stretching exercises for improving flexibility.

Muscles often work as **antagonists**—meaning they perform opposite functions—to allow multiple movements and full range of motion. For example, if you're lying down and contract the quadriceps muscles on the front of your thigh, they lift your leg off the floor; at the same time, the muscles on the back of your thigh, which are the antagonists, relax to allow the quadriceps to lift your leg.

## Static Stretching

A **static stretch** involves stretching slowly as far as you can without pain, until you feel a sense of pulling or tension. For best results, static stretches are held for 10 to 30 seconds. The FIT formula for static stretching is described in table 12.1. Done correctly,

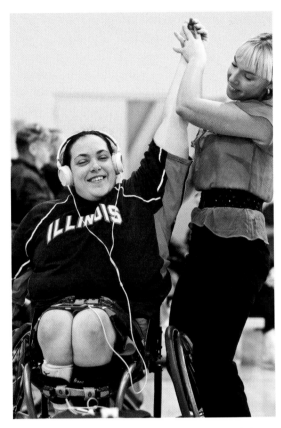

ROM exercises are commonly used in physical therapy for people who have lost range of motion associated with an injury or medical condition.

static stretching increases your flexibility and can help you relax. Some experts think that static stretching exercises are safer than ballistic stretching exercises because you're less likely to stretch too far and injure yourself.

Static stretching can be performed using either **active stretch** or **passive stretch**. A static stretch requires an assist from an external source, such as gravity, a partner (as in figure 12.3*b*), or some other source. Active static stretch is caused by contracting your own antagonist muscles—for example, contracting your shin muscle to move your toes upward, thus causing a stretch in your calf muscles (figure 12.3*a*). Passive static stretch is achieved without use of an antagonist muscle. The calf stretch, for example, can be done by having a partner push gently on your foot or by using your own arms to pull your foot upward (figure 12.3*b*).

Some experts consider active static stretch to be safer than other types of stretch because you don't have to worry about the external force overstretching your muscle (for example, if a partner pushes too hard). The advantage of passive static stretch is that makes it easier to create adequate stretch in order to improve the length of the muscle.

## PNF Stretching

**PNF stretching** (PNF stands for proprioceptive neuromuscular facilitation) is a stretching technique originally used by physical and occupational therapists to help soldiers who had been injured. It is now widely used by many people interested in improving their flexibility, including athletes. PNF stretching is a variation of static stretching. Some experts believe that it is the most effective type of exercise for improving flexibility, though it may cause more soreness than static stretching. PNF involves contracting the muscle before you stretch it to help the muscle relax so that it can be more easily stretched. Active stretch is sometimes called active isolated stretch because the contraction

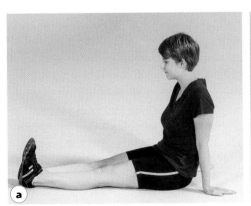
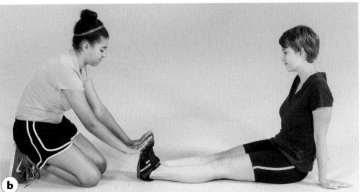

**FIGURE 12.3** Stretching the calf: *(a)* active stretch; *(b)* passive stretch (with a partner assisting).

before the stretch isolates, or identifies, the muscle to be stretched. One popular form of PNF is called **CRAC** (contract-relax-antagonist-contract). After you contract a muscle that you want to stretch, the muscle automatically relaxes. Contracting the opposing (antagonist) muscles during the stretch also makes the muscle you're stretching relax. CRAC does both of these actions.

The static stretch exercise shown in figure 12.3*b* can be made into a CRAC form of PNF exercise by contracting the calf muscles by pushing the toes against the partner's hands before doing the stretch.

The FIT formula for PNF stretch is described in table 12.1.

## Ballistic Stretching

**Ballistic stretching** involves a series of gentle bouncing or bobbing motions that are not held for a long time. The FIT formula for ballistic stretch is described in table 12.1. Like static stretching and PNF, ballistic stretching exercises are designed to use

the joints through a full range of movement and cause the muscles and tendons to stretch beyond their normal length. Most of the static stretching exercises shown in this chapter can be made into ballistic stretching exercises. For example, the hamstring stretch can be made into an active ballistic stretch by using the thigh muscles to bob the upper leg forward. It can be made into a passive ballistic stretch by having a partner alternately push forward and pull backward to produce a bobbing movement of the upper leg.

Sport movement stretching uses movements that closely mimic those of a specific sport. Examples include baseball batters who swing with a weighted bat and golfers who swing the club several times before beginning a round of golf. This type of warm-up has also been referred to as sport-specific ballistic stretching. Regardless of the name preferred, it involves using the muscles to initiate a sport-specific movement that causes the muscles to be used beyond their normal ROM. Consult with

### TABLE 12.1 FIT Formula and Fitness Target Zones for Stretching Exercise

| | Static and PNF | Ballistic |
|---|---|---|
| Frequency | **Threshold of training:** Stretch each muscle group on 2 or 3 days each week. **Target zone:** Stretch each muscle group on 2–7 days each week. | **Threshold of training:** Stretch each muscle group on 2 or 3 days each week. **Target zone:** Stretch each muscle group on 2–7 days each week. |
| Intensity | **Threshold of training:** Stretch the muscle beyond its normal length until you feel tension, then hold. **Target zone:** Stretch the muscle beyond its normal length, from first point of tension to point of mild discomfort (not pain). Hold. | **Threshold of training:** Stretch the muscle beyond its normal length until you feel tension. Use slow, gentle bounces or bobs. Use the motion of your body part to stretch the specific muscle. **Target zone:** Stretch the muscle beyond its normal length, from first point of tension to point of mild discomfort (not pain). Use the same gentle bouncing stretch as for threshold. *Caution: No stretch should cause pain, especially sharp pain. Be especially careful when doing ballistic stretching.* |
| Time | **Threshold of training:** Do 2 stretches of 10–30 sec for each muscle group. **Target zone:** Do 2–4 stretches with a goal of 60 sec (total) of stretching for each muscle group (6 × 10, 4 × 15, or 2 × 30 sec). Rest for 15 sec between stretches. | **Threshold of training:** For each muscle group, perform 2 sets. Bounce against the muscle slowly and gently. Perform 15 reps. Rest for 10 sec between sets. **Target zone:** For each muscle group, perform 2–4 sets of 15 reps. Rest for 10 sec between sets. Start with 2 sets and progress to 4. |

## ❤ FITNESS TECHNOLOGY: Goniometers

When you perform flexibility self-assessments, you use low-tech aids such as a yardstick or ruler. In some cases, you may use a flexibility box that includes a built-in measuring stick. When experts do research on flexibility, they use more sophisticated instruments, such as a goniometer, which measures joint angles. Some goniometers are electronic. Your school may have an inexpensive goniometer, such as the one shown, that you can use when assessing the range of motion in your joints.

### Using Technology

Do some investigation to learn more about goniometers and other devices for measuring flexibility.

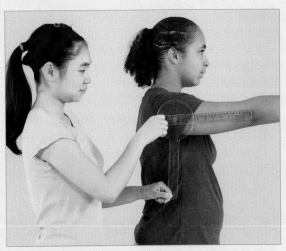

A goniometer can be used to assess range of motion and flexibility.

your instructor or coach to find out about recommended exercises for a given sport.

## FIT FACT

ACSM refers to dynamic stretching exercises as an additional way to build flexibility. They are similar to static stretching exercises, but the stretch is slow, gradual, and continuous until the muscle is fully stretched. Developmental stretching is another type of flexibility exercise recommended by some experts. It is performed slowly like dynamic stretching, and the stretch is held for 10 to 30 seconds (the same as static stretching). The difference is that in developmental stretching you stretch until you feel slight tension and then reduce the stretch for 3 to 5 seconds. The stretch is then increased slightly beyond the previous stretch. You repeat these steps (stretch, reduce stretch, stretch) until you reach a full stretch as outlined in table 12.1. Both dynamic and developmental stretching exercises are good alternatives for people who have been injured or who are just beginning a stretching program.

Some teachers and coaches have concerns about ballistic stretching because of the possibility of overstretching and injuring muscles if it is not done carefully. However, studies show that, if performed properly, ballistic stretching can be safe and does not cause as much muscular soreness as static stretching. Therapists do caution against ballistic stretching after a muscle or tendon injury, and they recommend consulting an expert to determine the best method of stretch for rehabilitation.

## Balancing Muscle Fitness and Flexibility

You should do muscle fitness and flexibility exercises together. We now know that muscle fitness exercises, when properly performed, need not limit flexibility. In fact, when done through a full range of motion, they can even help you build flexibility. But muscle fitness exercises are best for building muscle fitness, and flexibility exercises are best for building flexibility.

Therefore, a balanced exercise program includes both muscle fitness and flexibility exercises for all of your muscles so that they can apply equal force on all sides of a joint. People commonly use the flexors (muscles on the front of the body) a great

## ⚛ SCIENCE IN ACTION: Dynamic Movement Exercise

**Dynamic movement exercises** include jumping, skipping, and calisthenics such as those used in a warm-up. They move the joints beyond normal resting ROM and cause the muscles and tendons to stretch. The stretch caused by dynamic movement exercise is followed by a contraction of the stretched muscle. For example, jumping stretches the calf muscle; after the stretch caused by landing from a jump, the muscle contracts again to provide the force for the next jump. This type of exercise is also referred to as dynamic calisthenics. Dynamic movement exercises should not be confused with dynamic stretching exercises (see the Fit Fact on dynamic stretching).

Experts who pioneered the use of dynamic movement exercises point out that they are not the same as ballistic stretching exercises because they do not involve bobbing or bouncing against the muscle. Dynamic movement exercise routines use many kinds of movement, including muscle fitness calisthenics (such as push-ups, curl-ups, and half squats) and some other types of muscle fitness exercise (such as elastic band exercise).

Whereas dynamic *stretching* exercises are done primarily to build flexibility, that is not the primary intent of dynamic *movement* exercises (calisthenics). For this reason, a specific FIT formula is not provided for this type of exercise. However, it is often included in a warm-up and as part of other exercise circuits, and it does provide flexibility benefits and improve muscle fitness and power. Typically, when dynamic movement

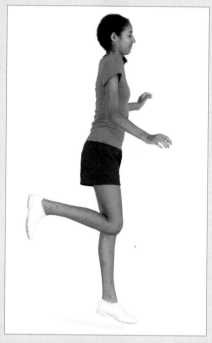

Dynamic movement exercises, such as the backward hop, stretch muscles and tendons.

exercises are included in a warm-up, exercises are chosen for different muscle groups, and the total time for the exercise is 5 to 10 minutes.

### Student Activity

Prepare a brochure explaining dynamic movement exercise and the reasons for doing it.

---

deal because many daily activities emphasize the use of those muscles. For example, the majority of people have strong biceps muscles (on the front of the arms), pectoral muscles (on the front of the chest), and quadriceps muscles (on the front of the thighs). The pull of these strong muscles results in the body hunching forward. To avoid becoming permanently hunched over, you need to make certain that these strong, short muscles on the front of your body get stretched. At the same time, you must strengthen the weak, relatively unused muscles on the back of your body. Table 12.2 lists

the muscles for which most people need the most flexibility exercise.

## Specificity of Stretching

Are there any muscles that do not need stretching? For many people, the answer is yes. For example, some people eventually begin to develop a hunched-over posture often called humpback at some point in life. Because the upper back muscles become overstretched in people with this postural problem, they should avoid further stretching of those muscles.

**TABLE 12.2   Muscles That Need the Most Stretching**

| Muscle(s) | Reason for stretching |
|---|---|
| Chest | Prevent poor posture |
| Front of shoulders | Prevent poor posture |
| Front of hip joints | Prevent swayback posture, backache, pulled muscle |
| Back of thighs (hamstring) | Prevent swayback posture, backache, pulled muscle |
| Inside of thighs | Prevent back, leg, and foot strain |
| Calf | Avoid soreness and Achilles tendon injury (may result from running and jumping) |
| Lower back | Prevent soreness, pain, back injury |

The abdominal muscles are another example. You do need to keep your abdominal muscles strong, but most people don't need to stretch them, In fact, if they're stretched, they begin to sag, and the abdomen protrudes, leading to poor posture.

Each person must evaluate his or her own needs to avoid stretching already-overstretched muscles and avoid strengthening muscles that are already so strong that they are out of balance with their opposing muscles. Keeping muscles on opposites sides of a joint in balance helps them pull with equal force in all directions. This balance helps align your body parts properly, ensuring good posture.

**Lesson Review**

1. How does a stretching warm-up differ from a flexibility (stretching) workout?
2. What is flexibility, and what factors influence it?
3. What are the benefits of good flexibility?
4. What are the types of flexibility exercise, and what is the FIT formula for each?
5. Why is it important to balance strength and flexibility exercise?

In this self-assessment, you'll evaluate the flexibility in several areas of your body. Use these general directions for the tests that follow. Then score yourself using table 12.3.

- Perform each exercise as described and illustrated here.
- Stretch and hold the position for two seconds while a partner checks your performance.
- Score one point for each test for which you meet the standard. Total your score for all tests.
- Determine your rating using table 12.3. Record your results as directed by your instructor.

You are expected to do these tests in class only once, unless your instructor tells you otherwise. However, you may want to retest yourself periodically. A retest helps you to see progress and can also be used to help set new goals. If you're working with a partner, remember that self-assessment information is personal and considered confidential. It shouldn't be shared with others without the permission of the person being tested.

Safety tip: Before taking a flexibility test, do a general warm-up and try each movement two or three times.

**TABLE 12.3  Rating Chart: Flexibility**

| Fitness rating | Score (items passed) |
| --- | --- |
| Good | 8–11 |
| Marginal | 5–7 |
| Low | 0–4 |

## Arm Lift

1. Lie facedown. Hold a ruler or stick in both hands. Keep your fists tight and your palms facing down.
2. Raise your arms and the stick as high as possible. Keep your forehead on the floor and your arms and wrists straight.
3. Hold this position while your partner uses a ruler to check the distance of the stick from the floor.
4. Record one point if you meet the standard: 10 inches (25 centimeters) or more.

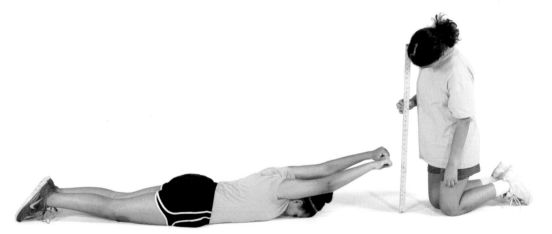

**This test evaluates your chest and shoulder flexibility.**

# Zipper

1. Reach your left arm and hand over your left shoulder and down your spine, as if you were going to pull up a zipper.

2. Hold this position while you reach your right arm and hand behind your back and up your spine to try to touch or overlap the fingers of your left hand.

3. Hold the position while your partner checks it.

4. Repeat, this time reaching your right arm and hand over your right shoulder and your left arm and hand up your spine.

5. Record one point for each side on which you meet the standard: touching or overlapping fingers.

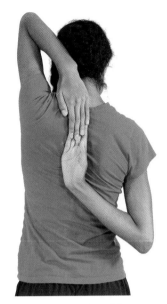

This test evaluates your shoulder, arm, and chest flexibility.

# Trunk Rotation

1. Stand with your toes on the designated line. Your left shoulder should be an arm's length (with fist closed) from the wall and directly on a line with the target spot located on the wall.

2. Drop your left arm and extend your right arm to your side at shoulder height. Make a fist with your palm down.

3. Without moving your feet, rotate your trunk to the right as far as possible. Your knees may bend slightly to permit more turn, but don't move your feet. Try to touch the target spot or beyond with a palm-down fist.

4. Hold the position while your partner checks it.

5. Repeat, rotating to the left.

6. Record one point for each side on which you meet the standard: touch the center of the target or beyond.

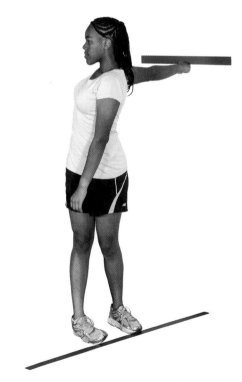

This test evaluates your spine, shoulder, and hip flexibility.

# Wrap-Around

1. Raise your right arm and reach behind your head. Try to touch the left corner of your mouth. You may turn your head and neck to the left.

2. Hold the position while your partner checks it.

3. Repeat with your left arm.

4. Record one point for each side on which you meet the standard: touching the corner of the mouth.

This test evaluates your shoulder and neck flexibility.

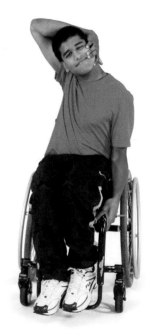

# Knee-to-Chest

1. Lie on your back and extend your right leg. Place your hands on the back of your left thigh and pull toward you to draw the knee closer to the chest. Do not place your hands on top of the knee.

2. Keep your right leg straight and on the floor if possible. Keep your lower back flat on the floor.

3. Hold the position. Have your partner check to see if your upper left thigh and knee are against your chest and your right leg is straight and on the floor.

4. Repeat with the opposite leg.

5. Record one point for each side on which you meet the standard: thigh and knee against the chest and calf on the floor.

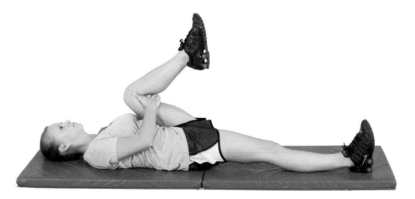

This test evaluates the flexibility of your hamstrings, your lower back, and the hip flexor muscles.

# Ankle Flex

1. Sit erect on the floor with your legs straight and together. You may lean backward slightly on your hands if necessary.

2. Start with the soles of your shoes at 90 degrees (perpendicular) to the floor.

3. Flex your ankles by pulling your toes toward your shins as far as possible. Hold this position while your partner checks whether the angle that the sole of each foot makes with the floor is 75 degrees. (You can use a protractor to make a 75-degree angle on a sheet of paper.).

4. Record one point for each ankle for which you meet the standard: soles angled 75 degrees or more.

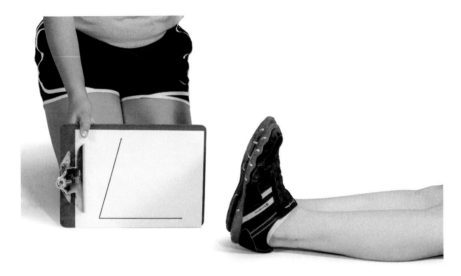

**This test evaluates the flexibility of your calf muscles and your range of ankle movement.**

# Lesson 12.2

# Preparing a Flexibility Exercise Plan

## Lesson Objectives

After reading this lesson, you should be able to

1. describe several basic flexibility (stretching) exercises,
2. describe other forms of activity that build flexibility,
3. describe and explain how to apply basic guidelines for stretching, and
4. select flexibility exercises and prepare a written flexibility exercise plan.

 **Lesson Vocabulary**

tai chi, yoga

**Do** you know which specific exercises are best for developing flexibility using the different types of stretching? Have you ever considered safety issues when performing flexibility exercise? In the previous lesson, you learned about several types of flexibility exercise. In this lesson, you'll learn some of the most common exercises used to build flexibility; you'll also learn how to plan a personal flexibility exercise program.

## Exercise Choices for Building Flexibility

The type of exercises that you choose for building flexibility depends on your personal goals. The following sections describe some of the most popular flexibility exercises.

### Basic Flexibility Exercises

The American College of Sports Medicine recommends that you perform exercises to stretch all of your major muscle groups. The 12 exercises described at the end of this lesson allow you to do so by choosing 8 to 10 exercises. As you'll see, all of these exercises can be done using static stretching, and some can also be done using PNF or ballistic stretching. The following guidelines will help you perform these exercises effectively.

- Consider the FIT formula information in table 12.1. Also consider the recommendations for the appropriate number of reps, sets, and time that accompany each of the exercises described in this lesson.

- The exercises labeled as PNF include a contraction of the muscle before stretching. To perform them as static stretches, omit the contraction phase.

- The exercises labeled as ballistic can be made ballistic by using a gentle bobbing movement rather than a static stretch.

### ROM Exercises

As noted in this chapter's first lesson, ROM exercises are commonly used in physical therapy and can be performed daily to help retain a healthy ROM. Dynamic and developmental stretching exercises can also be used by people recovering from injury and by beginners. Specific details for these types of exercises are not provided here because the static, PNF, and ballistic exercises are better choices for healthy teens. However, most of the basic exercises listed here can be done using dynamic or developmental stretching.

### Yoga, Tai Chi, and Pilates

In addition to the static, PNF, and ballistic stretching exercises described in this chapter, there are other popular activities that can be good for building flexibility. ACSM refers to these types of activities as functional fitness training because they help people (especially older people) perform tasks of daily living effectively. They also have health benefits (see Fit Fact). Tai chi and yoga are sometimes called neuromotor exercises because they build components of skill-related fitness such as agility and balance that require the nerves (neuro) and muscles to work together.

**Tai chi** is an ancient form of exercise that originated in China. It is considered to be a martial art and has many different forms. Tai chi is now practiced worldwide as a form of exercise rather than a martial art, and its basic movements have been shown to increase flexibility and reduce symptoms of arthritis in some people. When practiced regularly, it can help in developing muscle fitness, preventing back pain, and improving posture and balance.

## FIT FACT

Research studies show that tai chi provides a variety of benefits, including improved bone health, improved functional fitness, better quality of life, and, among older people, reduced risk of falls.

**Yoga** was introduced centuries ago in India. Traditional forms include meditation as well as the exercises and breathing techniques that are common in modern forms. Yoga poses, called asanas, are similar to many flexibility exercises and can contribute to improved flexibility and provide other health benefits similar to those for tai chi. Yoga is practiced by millions of young adults as a method of relaxing and training, and many schools now have yoga clubs. However, yoga should be undertaken with care. Physical therapists and other health experts caution against performing certain yoga poses because they are considered to be risky exercises. In addition, beginners are cautioned to progress gradually; it can be more harmful than helpful to try advanced poses without weeks or even months of practice.

Pilates was originally developed as a form of therapy but is now practiced as a method of building muscle fitness and flexibility. It focuses on core muscle fitness but also includes exercises for building flexibility. When practiced properly, it helps prevent back pain, improves posture, and aids functional capacity in daily life.

If you're considering tai chi, yoga, or Pilates, you should seek qualified instruction and follow the guidelines outlined in this chapter for building flexibility.

# Guidelines for Flexibility Exercise

To get the most benefit and enjoyment from your exercise program, perform the exercises correctly and exercise caution to avoid injury. Before you begin stretching, follow these guidelines and cautions to help you safely achieve and maintain flexibility.

- **Before stretching, do a general warm-up.** Warm muscles respond better than cold ones, and ACSM recommends doing a general warm-up of 5 to 10 minutes before performing stretching exercise.

- **Make flexibility exercises part of your workout.** Don't rely on warm-up exercises to build flexibility. Select an appropriate type of exercise and follow the FIT formula for that type.

- **Choose exercises for all major muscle groups.** Twelve different exercises for all muscle groups are described later in this lesson.

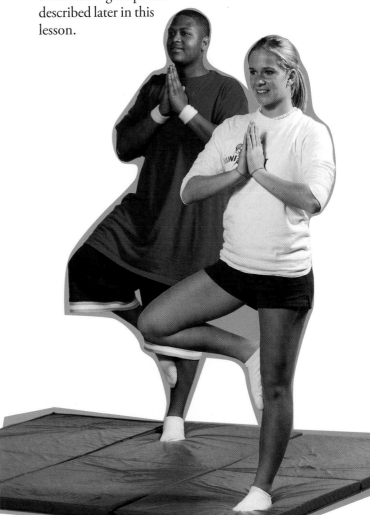

- **When beginning (or for general health), use static stretching or PNF.** Consider ballistic stretching after achieving the good fitness zone. Dynamic and developmental stretching may also be beneficial.

- **Progress gradually.** Regardless of the type of flexibility exercise you choose, progress gradually. Some flexibility exercises may seem easy, but, as with muscular endurance exercise, it does not take much to make your muscles sore. Gradually increase the time and number of repetitions and sets.

- **Avoid risky exercises.** Exercises that hyperflex or hyperextend a joint should be avoided as should exercises that cause joint twisting and compression.

- **Do not stretch joints that are hypermobile, unstable, swollen, or infected.** People with these conditions or symptoms are at risk of injury from overstretching.

- **Do not stretch to the point of feeling pain.** The old saying "no pain, no gain" is wrong. Stretch only until your muscle feels tight and a little uncomfortable.

- **Avoid stretching muscles that are already overstretched from poor posture.** The abdominal muscles, for example, typically do not need to be stretched.

- **Avoid stretches that last 30 seconds or more before performing strength and power activities.** Research suggests that stretches lasting longer than 30 seconds may have a negative effect on performances of strength and power in sport and other activities. As a result, some experts recommend doing dynamic movement exercises rather than stretching before strength and power performances.

> " I never struggled with injury problems because of my preparation—in particular my stretching. "
>
> —Edwin Moses, Olympic gold medalist

### FIT FACT

Once you've reached an acceptable level of muscle flexibility, you must continue to move all of your joints and muscles through this new and improved range of motion on a regular basis. If you don't, your muscles will begin to shorten again, and you'll lose that flexibility. All types of exercise described in this lesson help maintain flexibility.

## Planning a Flexibility Exercise Program

Elijah is a 16-year-old who used the five steps of program planning to prepare a flexibility exercise program. His program is described here.

### Step 1: Determine Your Personal Needs

To get started, Elijah prepared a table summarizing his flexibility activity (or lack thereof) over the past two weeks and his flexibility scores. (He wrote his plan during the summer when he was not in school.) As you can see in figure 12.4, he did no flexibility exercise during that two-week period. He also had

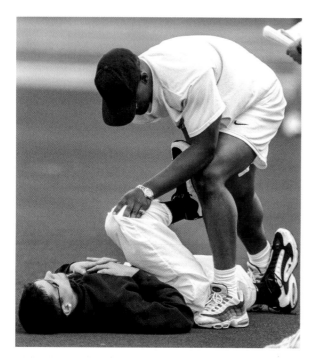

Stretching works best after a 5- to 10-minute general warm-up.

| Day | Flexibility exercises | Amount |
|---|---|---|
| Mon. | None | None |
| Tues. | None | None |
| Wed. | None | None |
| Thurs. | None | None |
| Fri. | None | None |
| Sat. | None | None |
| Sun. | None | None |

| Fitness self-assessments | Score | Rating |
|---|---|---|
| Arm lift | 8 in. (20 cm) | Need improvement |
| **Zipper**<br>Right<br>Left | Fingers touch<br>Fingers do not touch | Met standard<br>Need improvement |
| **Trunk rotation**<br>Right<br>Left | Reached target<br>Did not reach target | Met standard<br>Need improvement |
| **Wrap-around**<br>Right<br>Left | Touched mouth<br>Touched mouth | Met standard<br>Met standard |
| **Knee-to-chest**<br>Right<br>Left | Calf lifted >1 in. (2.5 cm)<br>Calf lifted >1 in. (2.5 cm) | Need improvement<br>Need improvement |
| **Ankle flex**<br>Right<br>Left | 75 degrees<br>80 degrees | Met standard<br>Need improvement |
| Total score | 6 items passed | Marginal fitness |
| Back-saver sit-and-reach | 5 in. (13 cm) | Low fitness |

**FIGURE 12.4**  Elijah's flexibility exercise (physical activity) and fitness profiles.

not done any recent flexibility tests, but he did have scores from tests he had done in school during the previous semester.

Elijah obviously did not meet the ACSM recommendation of performing flexibility exercise for the major muscle groups on at least two days a week. Even so, he had passed several of his recent flexibility tests (and he had been doing some flexibility exercises at that time).

## Step 2: Consider Your Program Options

Elijah listed seven types of flexibility exercise that he wanted to consider. He reviewed many types of exercises before preparing a list of exercises that he thought would be good for him and that he would be most likely to perform.

- Static stretching exercises
- PNF exercises
- Ballistic stretching exercises
- Yoga
- Tai chi
- Pilates
- Dynamic movement exercises (for warm-up)

## Step 3: Set Goals

For his flexibility exercise plan (see figure 12.5), Elijah chose a time period of two weeks. This was too short a time for setting long-term goals, so he developed only short-term physical activity goals for this plan. Later, he'll develop long-term goals, including some flexibility improvement goals, when he prepares a longer plan. For now, he just wanted

| Day | Exercise type | ✔ | Time, sets, reps |
|-----|---------------|---|------------------|
| Mon. | **Static Stretch**<br>Back-saver sit-and-reach<br>Knee-to-chest<br>Side stretch<br>Sitting stretch<br>Zipper<br>Hip stretch<br>Chest stretch<br>Calf stretch | | 3:00 p.m. after daily jog<br>One set of two repetitions for each exercise. Hold each exercise 15 seconds. |
| Tues. | **Dynamic Movement Exercise Warm-Up**<br>High-knee march<br>Standing flutter<br>Quarter-turn cha-cha<br>Shutter<br>Grapevine<br>Frankenstein<br>Knee-high skip<br>Jump-and-tuck<br>Slow jog, fast sprint | | 1:00 p.m. before soccer<br>Approximately 10 minutes. Perform each exercise five times, then continue on to the next exercise. Exercises followed by a slow jog for 30 seconds and a fast sprint for 10 seconds repeated three times. |
| Wed. | **Static Stretch**<br>Back-saver sit-and-reach<br>Knee-to-chest<br>Side stretch<br>Sitting stretch<br>Zipper<br>Hip stretch<br>Chest stretch<br>Calf stretch | | 3:00 p.m. after daily jog<br>One set of two repetitions for each exercise. Hold each exercise 15 seconds. |
| Thurs. | **Dynamic Movement Exercise Warm-Up**<br>High-knee march<br>Standing flutter<br>Quarter-turn cha-cha<br>Shutter<br>Grapevine<br>Frankenstein<br>Knee-high skip<br>Jump-and-tuck<br>Slow jog, fast sprint | | 1:00 p.m. before soccer<br>Approximately 10 minutes. Perform each exercise five times, then continue on to the next exercise. Exercises followed by a slow jog for 30 seconds and a fast sprint for 10 seconds repeated three times. |
| Fri. | **Static Stretch**<br>Back-saver sit-and-reach<br>Knee-to-chest<br>Side stretch<br>Sitting stretch<br>Zipper<br>Hip stretch<br>Chest stretch<br>Calf stretch | | 3:00 p.m. after daily jog<br>One set of two repetitions for each exercise. Hold each exercise 15 seconds. |
| Sat. | Yoga class | | 10:00–10:30 a.m. with sister |
| Sun. | None | | None |

**FIGURE 12.5**  Elijah's written flexibility exercise plan.

to get started by trying some new exercises. Besides, it was summer, and he didn't have access to school facilities, nor was he a member of a fitness club. So he chose SMART goals for his specific situation and wrote them down.

1. Perform one set of eight static stretching exercises on three days a week, including back-saver sit-and-reach, knee-to-chest, side stretch, sitting stretch, zipper, hip stretch, chest stretch, and calf stretch.

2. Perform a dynamic movement exercise warm-up for 10 minutes including nine basic exercises before playing sports.

3. Perform yoga for 30 minutes on one day a week.

## Step 4: Structure Your Program and Write It Down

Elijah's next step was to write down his two-week flexibility exercise plan (see figure 12.5). He chose

static stretching that he could do at home three days a week. Since he played soccer two days a week, he also decided to do a dynamic movement exercise warm-up prior to his matches. He didn't expect the warm-up to be his main source of flexibility development, but he thought it would supplement his other flexibility exercise. He also agreed to go to yoga class with his sister Nicole, who was allowed to bring a guest for two free sessions.

## Step 5: Keep a Log and Evaluate Your Program

Over the next two weeks, Elijah will self-monitor his activities and place a checkmark beside each activity he actually performs. At the end of the two weeks, Elijah will evaluate his activity to see whether he met his goals. He can then use the evaluation to help him write a future activity plan.

### Lesson Review

1. Describe several basic flexibility (stretching) exercises.
2. What are some other forms of activity that build flexibility?
3. What are the basic guidelines for stretching?
4. What flexibility exercises should you include in your written flexibility exercise plan? Why?

## BACK-SAVER SIT-AND-REACH (PNF OR STATIC)

1. Assume the back-saver sit-and-reach position with your right knee bent and your left leg straight.

2. Bend your left knee slightly and push your heel into the floor as you contract your hamstrings hard for 3 seconds. Relax.

    Note: For static stretch, omit step 2.

3. Immediately grasp your ankle with both hands and gently pull your chest toward your knee. Hold the position for 15 seconds.

4. Repeat the exercise on the other leg.

**This exercise stretches your hamstrings and lower back muscles.**

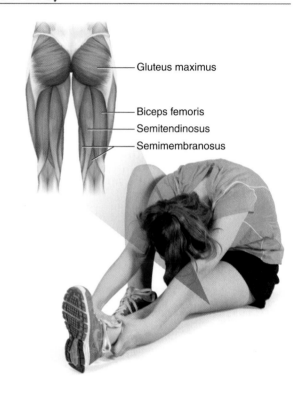

## KNEE-TO-CHEST

1. Lie on your back and extend your right leg. Place your hands on the back of your left thigh and pull toward you to draw the knee closer to the chest. Do not place your hands on top of the knee.

2. Keep your right leg straight and on the floor if possible. Keep your lower back flat on the floor.

3. Hold the position for 15 seconds.

4. Repeat with the opposite leg.

**This exercise stretches your hamstrings, your lower back, and the hip flexor muscles.**

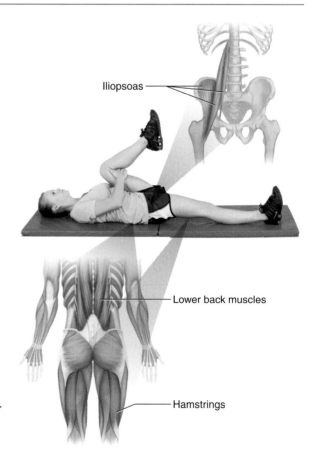

## BACK AND HIP STRETCH (PNF OR STATIC)

1. Lie on your back with your knees bent and your arms at your sides.
2. Lift your hips until there is no bend at the hip joint. Squeeze the buttocks muscles hard for 3 seconds. Relax by lowering your hips to the floor.
   Note: For a static stretch, omit step 2.
3. Immediately place your hands under your knees and gently pull your knees to your chest. Hold the position for 15 seconds or more.

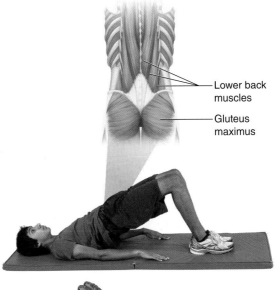

**This exercise stretches your lower back and gluteal muscles.**

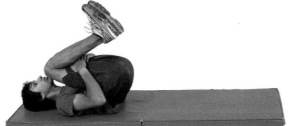

## SIDE STRETCH (STATIC OR BALLISTIC)

1. Stand with your feet slightly wider than shoulder-width apart.
2. Lean to your left.
3. Reach down to your left foot with your left hand. Reach over your head with your right arm. Hold for a count of 10 to 30 seconds.
   Caution: Do not twist or lean your body forward.
4. Repeat the exercise on your right side.
   Note: For a ballistic stretch, do a gentle bouncing stretch.

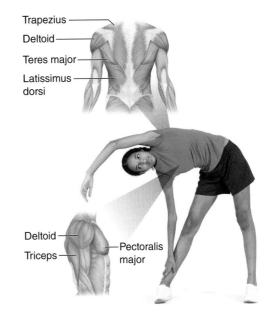

**This exercise stretches the muscles of your arms and shoulders and the sides of your body.**

## TRUNK AND HIP STRETCH (STATIC)

1. Lie on your back with your knees bent and your arms extended at shoulder level.

2. Cross your left leg over your right leg.

3. Keep your shoulders and arms on the floor as you rotate your lower body to the left and touch your right knee to the floor. Stretch and hold the position for 10 to 30 seconds.

4. At the end of the stretch, reverse the position of your legs (cross your right leg over your left), then rotate to the right and hold the position.

**This exercise stretches the muscles of your hips and lower back.**

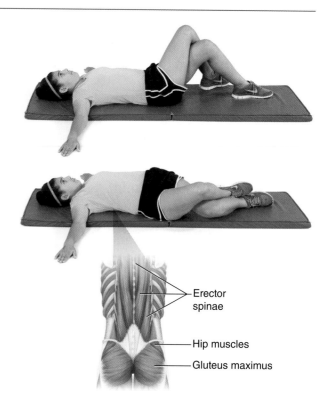

Erector spinae

Hip muscles

Gluteus maximus

## SITTING STRETCH (PNF OR STATIC)

1. Sit with the soles of your feet together and your elbows or hands resting on your knees.

2. Contract the muscles on the inside of your thighs, pulling up as you resist with your arms pushing down. Hold the position for 3 seconds. Relax your legs.
   Note: For a static stretch, omit step 2.

3. Immediately lean your trunk forward and push down on your knees with your arms to stretch your thighs. Hold the position for 10 to 30 seconds.

**This exercise stretches the muscles of the inside of your thighs.**

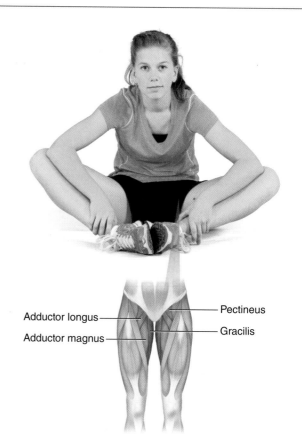

Adductor longus

Adductor magnus

Pectineus

Gracilis

## ZIPPER (PNF OR STATIC)

1. Stand or sit. Lift your right arm over your right shoulder and reach down your spine.

2. With your left hand, press down on your right elbow. Resist the pressure by trying to raise that elbow, contracting the opposing muscles. Hold the position for 3 seconds. Relax.

   Note: For a static stretch, omit step 2.

3. Immediately stretch by reaching down your spine with your right arm as your left arm assists by pressing on your elbow. Hold the position for 10 to 30 seconds.

4. Repeat the exercise with your other arm.

**This exercise stretches your triceps and latissimus muscles.**

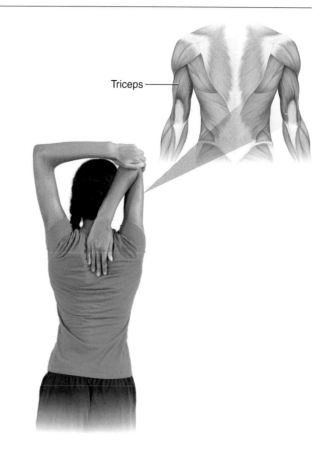

Triceps

## ARM PRETZEL (STATIC OR BALLISTIC)

1. Stand or sit. Bend your elbows and hold both hands as if shaking hands. Cross your right hand over your left so that the backs of the two hands are facing each other about two inches apart. Turn your right palm upward and point your thumb down over the left hand.

2. Grasp your right thumb with your left hand and pull down gently. Stretch and hold the position for 10 to 30 seconds.

3. Reverse arm positions and stretch your left shoulder.

   Note: For a ballistic stretch, do a gentle bouncing stretch.

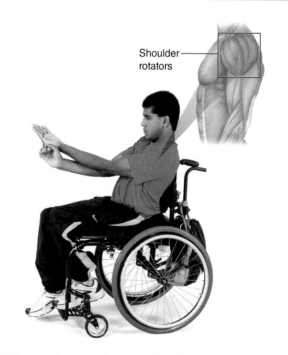

Shoulder rotators

**This exercise stretches your shoulder rotator muscles.**

## HIP STRETCH (STATIC OR BALLISTIC)

1. Take a long step forward on your right foot and kneel on your left knee. Your right knee should be directly over your ankle and bent at a right angle.

2. You should feel a stretch across the front of your left hip joint and in the front of your thigh muscles.

3. Place your hands on your right knee for balance. Stretch by shifting your weight forward as you tilt your pelvis and trunk backward slightly. Keep your back knee in the same spot to stretch your hip and thigh muscles. Hold the position for 10 to 30 seconds.

4. Repeat the exercise with your other leg.
   Note: For a ballistic stretch, do a gentle bouncing motion forward as you tilt your pelvis back.

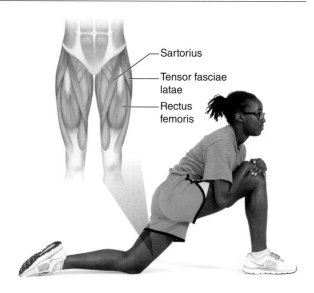

This exercise stretches the quadriceps muscles on the front of your thighs and the muscles on the front of your hips.

## ARM STRETCH (STATIC)

1. Sit or stand and cross your right arm over your left (just above your head) with your palms facing. Lace your fingers together.

2. Straighten your elbows to raise your arms overhead as high as possible (your upper arms should touch your ears). Hold the position 10 to 30 seconds.

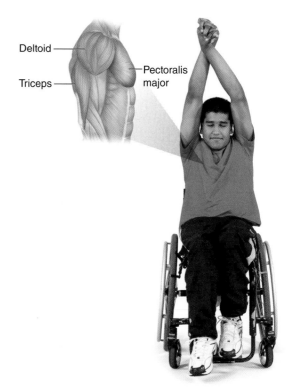

This exercise stretches the muscles of your shoulders, arms, and chest.

## CHEST STRETCH (PNF, STATIC, OR BALLISTIC)

1. Stand in a forward stride position in a doorway. Raise your arms slightly above shoulder-height. Place your hands on either side of the doorway.

2. Lean your body into the doorway. Resist by contracting your arm and chest muscles. Hold the position for 3 seconds. Relax.

3. Immediately lean further forward, letting your body weight stretch your muscles. Hold the position for 10 to 30 seconds.

4. For a ballistic stretch, gently bounce your body forward.
     Note: For a static stretch, omit steps 2 and 4.

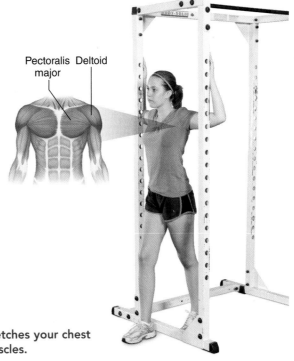

This exercise stretches your chest and shoulder muscles.

## CALF STRETCH (STATIC OR BALLISTIC)

1. Step forward with your right leg in a lunge position. Keep both feet pointed straight ahead and your front knee directly over your front foot. Place your hands on your right leg for balance.

2. Keep your left leg straight and the heel on the floor. Adjust the length of your lunge until you feel a good stretch in your left calf and Achilles tendon. Hold the position for 10 to 30 seconds.

3. Repeat the exercise with your other leg.
     Note: For a ballistic stretch, gently bounce your heel toward the floor.

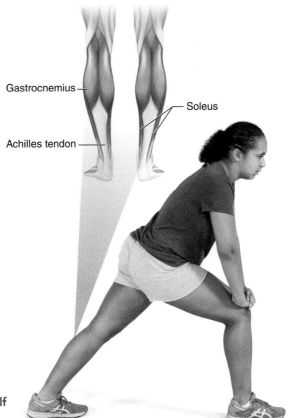

This exercise stretches your calf muscles and Achilles tendons.

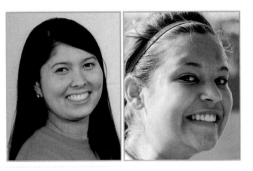

When some people face a problem beyond their control, they use it as an excuse for not being physically active. Someone might say, "I'm too short to be a basketball player, so I'm not going to try out for any sports." To be physically active, focus not on what you can't change but on what you *can* do.

Connie stood at the window. "It's pouring out there! How can we go hiking?"

Bridgette sighed. "I guess we're stuck spending the afternoon here."

Yesterday it was too hot to go hiking; now it was too rainy. It seemed as if they were never going to have good weather. But the weather was not the only problem. The last time they tried hiking at the state park, it was sunny, but the paths were too crowded.

"I bet Alanzo is at the athletic club right now," Bridgette said. "He can exercise no matter what the weather is. I wish we could afford to go there!"

Connie glanced down at her sweats. "I'd need to buy more than a membership to go there. They wear really expensive exercise clothes at that club. I'd get laughed out of the place in these clothes."

Bridgette smiled. "You don't look so bad—and the rain's starting to let up now. What if we put on older clothes, take rain gear, and hike around the park for a while?"

"You're right! So what if we get a little damp?"

## For Discussion

What reasons do Connie and Bridgette give for not being active? Which of these problems can they control? They eventually decide not to let the weather stop them; what other strategies could they use to cope with the problems they've identified? Consider the guidelines in the Self-Management feature when answering the discussion questions.

# SELF-MANAGEMENT: Skills for Overcoming Barriers

People face many barriers to becoming and staying active. Some barriers involve the environment (such as areas unsafe for exercise, lack of nearby exercise facilities, bad weather, expense), some involve personal physical characteristics (lack of physical size or skill), and some are psychological (low self-confidence, perceived lack of time). People who are active throughout life overcome such barriers, and programs have been developed to help people overcome barriers. Use the following strategies to overcome the barriers you face.

- **Find a way to exercise at home or at school.** If parks, fitness clubs, and other places for exercise are too expensive, too far away, or unsafe, find another way to exercise. Buy some equipment that you can use at home. If possible, use school facilities to exercise before or after school. Start a fitness club at school and ask school officials to help you find facilities and equipment.

- **Develop alternate plans.** Make multiple plans for activity. That way, for example, if

you plan to play tennis and it rains, you can switch to your alternate plan, which might be an indoor activity. If something interferes with your planned exercise time, find another time.

- **Get active in community or school affairs.** Many communities have developed community centers; trails for biking, walking, and jogging; and other recreational facilities, such as tennis courts, basketball courts, and sport fields. If these options are not available in your community, write to your city or county officials or contact school officials and see what you can help create.

- **Use self-management skills to develop realistic plans that you will stick with.** Practice skills such as goal setting, program planning, self-monitoring, and time management.

- **Develop a new way of thinking.** Accept yourself as you are. If negative self-talk is an issue, use the strategies presented in this book to adjust your self-perceptions and boost your self-confidence.

Prepare a two-week muscle fitness flexibility exercise plan. As directed by your teacher, prepare tables similar to those used by Elijah and use the five steps of program planning. Try out your program and see if you can meet your goals. The goal is to perform flexibility exercises three days a week. Carry out it over a two-week period. Your teacher may give you time in class to do some of the activities in your plan. Consider the following suggestions for **taking action**.

- Before performing stretching exercises, do a general warm-up.
- Consider the guidelines for flexibility exercise presented in lesson 2 of this chapter.
- If you're already participating in organized sport or physical activity, consider doing your flexibility exercise during the cool-down portion of your workout.

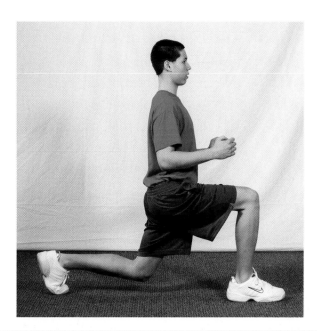

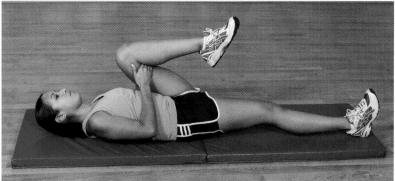

Take action by performing your flexibility exercise plan.

## Reviewing Concepts and Vocabulary

As directed by your teacher, answer items 1 through 5 by correctly completing each sentence with a word or phrase.

1. The amount of movement you can make in a joint is called your _____.
2. Exercises including jumping, skipping, and calisthenics (such as those used in a warm-up) are called _____ exercises.
3. Being able to move beyond a typical healthy range of motion is called _____.
4. _____ is an ancient form of exercise that originated in China.
5. Gentle bouncing motions are part of _____.

For items 6 through 10, as directed by your teacher, match each term in column 1 with the appropriate phrase in column 2.

6. zipper
7. passive stretch
8. active stretch
9. PNF
10. yoga

a. stretch created by gravity or an outside force
b. form of exercise from India
c. stretch created by an antagonist muscle
d. stretch after muscle contraction
e. arm stretching exercise

For items 11 through 15, as directed by your teacher, respond to each statement or question.

11. What are some benefits of good flexibility?
12. What are some factors that influence flexibility other than stretching?
13. What are some good tests of flexibility described in this chapter?
14. What are some good basic flexibility (static stretching) exercises for the major muscle groups?
15. What are some guidelines for overcoming barriers?

## Thinking Critically

Write a paragraph to answer the following question.

Sean's father went to a physical therapist to get treatment after a hip injury. The therapist recommended static stretching with a passive assist. Sean's dad asked him to help with the exercises. What safety concerns should Sean have in helping his father?

## Project

Young people typically have better flexibility than older people. For this reason, parents and grandparents are likely to be less flexible than their children or grandchildren. Interview a parent or grandparent. Prepare a list of five questions related to current flexibility, past flexibility (at an earlier age), steps taken to maintain flexibility, and future plans for flexibility exercise. Prepare a report presenting your findings.

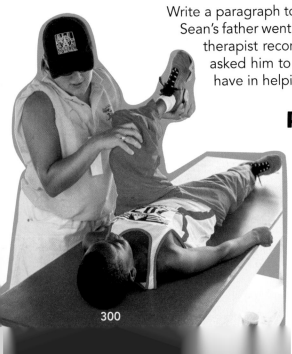

# UNIT V

# Healthy Choices

● ● ● ● ● ● ● ● ● ● ● ● ● ● ● ● ● ● ● ● ●

**Healthy People 2020 Goals**

- Reduce teen overweight and obesity.
- Prevent inappropriate weight gain among teens.
- Increase body mass index (BMI) measurement by physicians.
- Reduce disordered eating among adolescents.
- Reduce the percentage of teens who do no leisure-time physical activity.
- Increase the percentage of adults who meet guidelines for aerobic and muscle fitness activity.
- Increase teen participation in daily physical education.
- Increase participation in adolescent extracurricular and out-of-school activities.
- Increase number of schools with activity spaces that can be used during nonschool hours.
- Increase the number of trips made by walking and biking.
- Reduce the percentage of teens who get too much screen time.
- Improve health literacy.
- Increase web access and wise use of health information available on the web.
- Increase the number of high-quality websites presenting health-related information.
- Increase the percentage of teens who have had a wellness checkup in the past 12 months.
- Increase the percentage of people who have good social support.

**Self-Assessment Features in This Unit**

- Body Measurements
- Your Personal Fitness Test Battery
- Assessing Your Posture

**Taking Charge Features in This Unit**

- Improving Physical Self-Perception
- Changing Attitudes
- Learning to Think Critically

**Self-Management Features in This Unit**

- Skills for Self-Perception
- Skills for Building Positive Attitudes
- Skills for Thinking Critically

**Taking Action Features in This Unit**

- Elastic Band Workout
- Your Physical Activity Plan
- My Health and Fitness Club

# 13

# Body Composition

## In This Chapter

**LESSON 13.1**
Body Composition Facts

**SELF-ASSESSMENT**
Body Measurements

**LESSON 13.2**
Energy Balance

**TAKING CHARGE**
Improving Physical Self-Perception

**SELF-MANAGEMENT**
Skills for Self-Perception

**TAKING ACTION**
Elastic Band Workout

 **Student Web Resources**
www.fitnessforlife.org/student

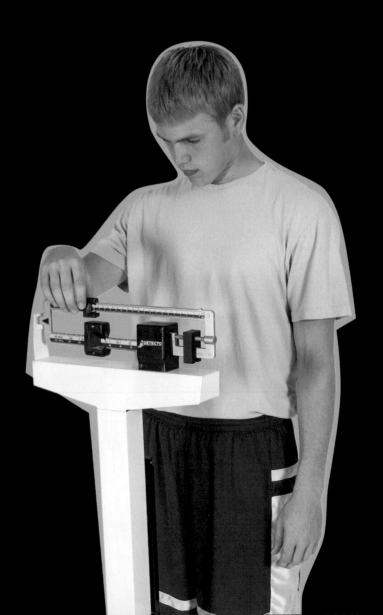

# Lesson 13.1
# Body Composition Facts

## Lesson Objectives

After reading this lesson, you should be able to

1. define *body composition*, *overweight*, and *obesity*;
2. describe some factors that influence body composition;
3. define *anorexia nervosa*, *bulimia*, and *anorexia athletica*;
4. explain how body composition and body fat level are related to good health; and
5. describe several laboratory and nonlaboratory tests for measuring body composition.

## Lesson Vocabulary

anorexia athletica, anorexia nervosa, basal metabolism, body composition, body fat level, bulimia, essential body fat, lean body tissue, metabolic syndrome, obesity, overweight, skinfold, underweight

**Body** composition is a part of health-related physical fitness. It refers to all the tissues that make up your body. In this lesson, you'll learn about the types of tissue that make up your body and about key terms related to body composition. You'll also learn how to assess your current body composition and determine whether it is optimal for good health.

## Body Composition Definitions

Your body is made up of two major types of tissue. In a healthy person, the great majority of the body consists of **lean body tissue**, including muscle, bone, skin, and body organs such as the heart, liver, kidneys, and lungs. All of the types of physical activity included in the Physical Activity Pyramid build lean body tissue, but muscle fitness exercises are especially good because they both build muscle and enhance bone development.

The other major type of body tissue is fat. Your **body fat level** refers to the percentage of your body that is fat tissue. A fit person has the right amount of body fat—neither too much nor too little.

About half of your body fat is located deep within your body. The remaining fat is located between your skin and your muscles. People who do regular physical activity typically have a larger percentage of lean body weight (especially from muscle and bone) and less body fat than people who do not do such activity. It's good if fat accounts for a relatively low percentage of your total body weight. However, for good health, you do need some body fat. Determining your body fatness requires special equipment and expertise. Later, you'll learn how to measure the fat between your skin and muscles to estimate your total body fatness.

The terms **underweight** and **overweight** are commonly used to describe a body weight that is outside the healthy weight range—either below the range or above it. These terms have limitations because weight, or the combination of weight and height, does not always accurately reflect the amount of fat and lean tissue in the body. You'll learn more about underweight and overweight later in this chapter. The term **obesity** refers to the condition of being especially overweight or high in body fat.

## FIT FACT

More than two-thirds of all American adults are considered overweight or obese. Fewer children and teens are considered overweight or obese, and the percentage varies by age, sex, and ethnic group. Obesity is high among Hispanic, African American, and Native American youth. For all ethnic groups combined, about 18 percent of youth and teens are considered obese. This is more than three times the rate of 30 years ago.

# Factors Influencing Body Fatness

Many factors influence a person's level of body fat. Some are described in the following sections.

## Heredity

You inherit your body type from your parents. Some people are born with a tendency to be lean, or muscular, or heavy. Inherited tendencies make it easier for some people and harder for others to keep their body fat level in the good fitness zone. You can't control your heredity, but you can be aware of tendencies in your family.

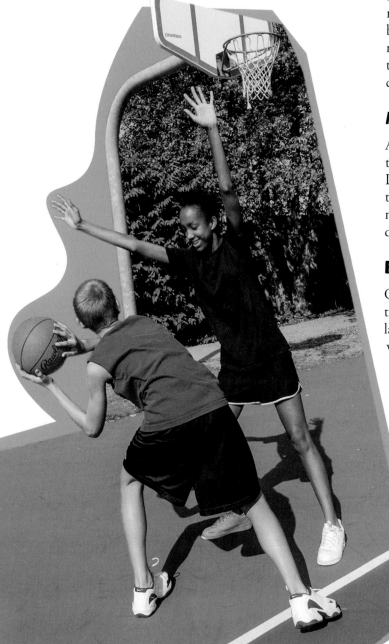

## Metabolism

Your **basal metabolism** is the amount of energy (calories) your body uses just to keep you living. Your basal metabolism does not include the calories you burn while working, enjoying recreation, studying, or even sitting and watching television. Some people have a higher basal metabolism than others. This means that their bodies, at complete rest, burn more calories than the bodies of people with a lower metabolism. People with more muscle mass have a higher metabolism than people with less muscle mass. People with a higher metabolism can consume more calories than others can without increasing their level of body fat.

Your metabolism is affected by your heredity, age, and maturation. Most young people have a high metabolism because their bodies are growing and building muscle. As you grow older and lose muscle mass, your metabolism typically slows, which means that most people need to reduce the number of calories in their diet in order to avoid gaining fat.

## Maturation

As you grow older and your hormone levels begin to change, your level of body fat also changes. During the teen years, female hormones cause girls to develop more body fat than boys. Because of male hormones, teenage boys have greater muscle development than girls.

## Body Fat Levels Early in Life

Children who are too fat develop extra fat cells that make it more difficult to control their fat level later in life. Therefore, keeping your body fat level within the good fitness zone during your childhood and teen years will help you keep it in check throughout life.

## Diet

The amount of energy contained in foods is measured in calories. Teens typically need more calories than adults. A typical teen male needs to consume about 2,500 to 3,000 calories a day to maintain an ideal level of body fat. A typical teenage female needs about 2,000 to 2,500 calories a day. Most males need more calories than most females because they are larger and have more muscle mass.

## Physical Activity

Your body burns calories for energy. Therefore, the more vigorous activity you do (the more energy your body uses), the more calories you need. An inactive person uses less energy each day than an active person and thus needs to consume fewer calories. As a result, teens who participate in sports need to consume more calories than less active teens.

## Body Fatness, Health, and Wellness

Having too much fat can be unhealthy. Scientists report that people who are high in body fat have a higher risk of heart disease, high blood pressure, diabetes, cancer, and other diseases. Until recently, type 2 diabetes was considered to be an adult disease, but it has become more common among youth primarily because of increases in body fat levels among youth. High levels of body fat are also associated with a condition called **metabolic syndrome**. This syndrome occurs when a person has a high level of body fat, large waist girth, and other health risks, such as high blood pressure, high blood fat, and high blood sugar.

In addition, health costs for obese people total thousands of dollars a year more than for people with healthy levels of body fat, and being high in body fat reduces a person's chances of successful surgery. A person with too much body fat also tires more quickly and easily than a lean person and therefore might be less efficient in both work and recreation. Many experts believe that the reason so many adults have too much body fat is that they try to achieve an unrealistic weight or fat level. For example, many people try to be as lean as a movie star or an athlete shown in a commercial. When they cannot attain or maintain such an exceptionally low level of body fat, they give up and gain body fat. Instead, experts recommend setting less extreme goals that are achievable, which helps people maintain a healthy level of body fat throughout life.

> " We have to make sure that our kids still feel good about themselves no matter what their weight, no matter how they feel. We need to make sure that our kids know that we love them no matter who they are, what they look like. "
>
> —Michelle Obama,
> First Lady of the United States

## Too Little Body Fat

Having too little body fat is also a health risk. Eating disorders such as **anorexia nervosa**, **anorexia athletica**, and **bulimia** have many negative health consequences and can even be fatal. It is extremely important to identify the symptoms of an eating disorder as early as possible. An excessive desire to lose fat or maintain a very low fat level can lead to serious health problems.

The minimum amount of body fat required for healthy body functioning is called **essential body fat**. Having too little body fat can cause abnormal functioning of various organs. In fact, exceptionally low body fat can result in serious health problems, particularly among teenagers. Females with especially low body fat experience health problems related to their reproductive system and risk losing bone density. The following list summarizes several reasons your body needs some fat.

### The Importance of Body Fat

- Fat is an insulator; it helps your body adapt to heat and cold.

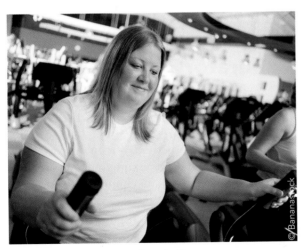

**Regular exercise expends calories.**

- Fat acts as a shock absorber; it can help protect your organs and bones from injury.
- Fat helps your body use vitamins effectively.
- Fat is stored energy that is available when your body needs it.
- In reasonable amounts, fat helps you look your best, thus increasing your feelings of well-being.

## Anorexia Nervosa

Anorexia nervosa is a serious eating disorder. A person who has this disorder severely restricts the amount of food that he or she eats in an attempt to be exceptionally low in body fat. In addition, many people with anorexia do extensive physical activity, thus further lowering their body fat to extremely dangerous levels.

Anorexia is most common among teenage girls, but it is becoming increasingly common among teenage boys. People with this disorder are usually very hard workers and high achievers. They have a distorted view of their body and see themselves as being too fat even when they are extremely thin. Persons with this disorder often fear maturity and the weight gain associated with adulthood. They often try to hide their condition by wearing baggy clothing, pretending to eat, and exercising in private. Anorexia is a life-threatening condition, and people who have it need immediate professional help.

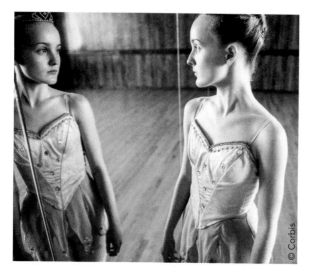

**People with eating disorders may be obsessed with their body weight even if they're already thin.**

## Anorexia Athletica

Anorexia athletica has many symptoms similar to those of anorexia nervosa. It is most common among athletes involved in sports—such as gymnastics, wrestling, and cheerleading—in which low body weight is desirable. This disorder can lead to anorexia nervosa. It is thought to be related to the pressure to maintain low weight and an excessive preoccupation with dieting and exercising for weight loss.

## Bulimia

Bulimia is an eating disorder in which a person engages in binge eating—eating a very large amount of food in a short time. Bingeing is followed by purging, perhaps by vomiting or by the use of laxatives to rid the body of food and prevent its digestion. Bulimia can result in severe digestive problems and other health problems such as tooth loss and gum disease.

### FIT FACT

Studies show that the number of teens who think they are overweight is four to five times the number who really are. At the same time, interviews with teens who actually are overweight show that 44 percent either have been or currently are teased about their body weight. Getting teased for being overweight—or just feeling like one is overweight—can result in low physical self-perceptions. Teens can help other teens improve their self-perceptions by being supportive rather than critical.

## Laboratory Measurements for Assessing Body Composition

The most accurate methods for measuring body composition require special equipment and trained people. They are typically done in a laboratory. Three of the best methods are DXA, underwater weighing, and the Bod Pod (figure 13.1). All three are useful in determining how much of the body weight is fat and how much is lean tissue.

## SCIENCE IN ACTION: Media Misrepresentation

Over the years, both exercise psychologists and nutrition scientists have conducted research about physical self-perceptions. They have found that people of all ages are self-conscious about the way they look. In fact, most people are far more critical of their own body than other people are. One reason is that we often compare ourselves with movie stars and other celebrities. Experts point out that the pictures we see of these people have been designed specifically to make them look as glamorous as possible and are touched up to enhance appearance. For example, computer programs can be used to make a female movie star's waist smaller and a male star's muscles larger. Some magazines have promised to limit changes in photos, but there are no regulations, and each magazine can do as it pleases.

Websites also use fake or altered pictures. Advertisements frequently show supposed before-and-after pictures to promote a product. The "before" photos often are taken with bad lighting and in unflattering conditions. The "after" photos are taken with better lighting and are sometimes altered. Video games also present unrealistic images of the human body. For example, body proportions for some male and female video game figures are literally impossible for real-life people.

Many experts believe that the misrepresentation of the human body in the media results in an obsession with leanness. Statistics indicate that many teens, especially girls, set unrealistic standards in judging their body composition. Many feel that they have more fat than they really do, and they try to lose weight unnecessarily.

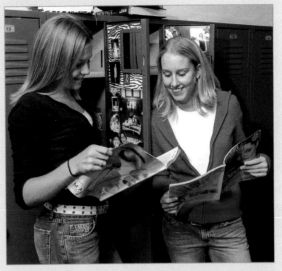

Magazines and websites often alter photos of models and celebrities to make their bodies look unrealistically thin.

Because we are all a bit self-conscious, it is easy to overreact when others make comments about the way we look. For this reason, experts point out the importance of not making critical comments about others. It is also important to keep personal information, such as self-assessment results, confidential. You'll learn more about self-perceptions in the Taking Charge feature in the next lesson of this chapter.

---

**Student Activity**

Explore a variety of media sources to find examples of misrepresentation of the human body.

---

## Dual-Energy X-Ray Absorptiometry

Dual-energy X-ray absorptiometry (DXA) is now considered the best method of assessing body composition (figure 13.1a) because it can accurately detect body fat, bone, muscle, and other body tissues. First, a high-tech X-ray machine takes a three-dimensional picture of the entire body. Then a computer analyzes the picture to determine the amounts of different kinds of tissue, including fat, bone, and muscle.

## Underwater Weighing

Until recently, underwater weighing was considered the best way to assess body fat level, and it is still a very good laboratory method. With this technique, you are weighed on land, then immersed in a tank of water and weighed again (figure 13.1b).

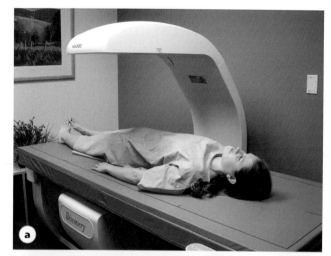

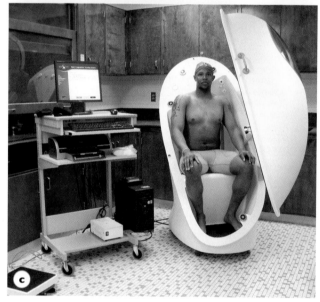

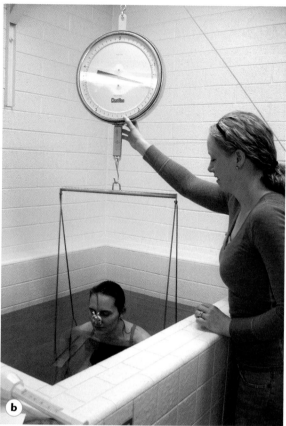

**FIGURE 13.1** Laboratory methods for assessing body composition: *(a)* DXA; *(b)* underwater weighing; *(c)* Bod Pod.

Measurements of your lung capacity are also taken because the amount of air in your lungs influences your weight in water. A formula is then applied to determine your body fat level based on your land weight, your underwater weight, and your lung capacity.

### Bod Pod

A third type of laboratory assessment of body composition uses a machine called the Bod Pod. In this method, the person being tested sits in an egg-shaped chamber or pod (figure 13.1c). The person's body, of course, takes up space in the pod, thus causing air to be moved from the pod. Information gained from changes in the pod's air

is then plugged into a special formula to determine the person's body fatness.

## Nonlaboratory Measures

Because laboratory measures require special equipment and special training, they are rarely used in schools. For school and home use, nonlaboratory measures are available. Several practical methods of assessment are described here. However, not all of these measures accurately predict the amount of fat and lean body tissue; for this reason, they are typically referred to as body measurements. Body measurements are easier to use than laboratory measures and can be performed at school and often at home. Because you will probably encounter all of these measures at some time in your life, you should try each one of them.

## Skinfold Measurements

Your body fat level can also be determined by measuring **skinfold** thickness (the amount of fat under your skin). Skinfold thickness is measured by means of a special instrument called a caliper (see figure 13.2). Skinfold measurements can be used to provide an estimate of the total amount of fat in the body. As noted earlier, a high level of body fat is associated with a variety of health problems, including diabetes, heart disease, and other chronic diseases. You'll learn to do skinfold measurements in this chapter's Self-Assessment feature.

## Height–Weight and BMI

Height and weight are commonly used in two ways. One method uses height–weight tables that show "normal" weight ranges for people according to age, height, and sex. These tables indicate what the average person of a given sex weighs at a given height. However, because nearly two-thirds of adults in the United States are overweight or obese, many people who are classified as "normal" or "average" are still overweight or obese. For this reason, height–weight tables are considered less useful than some other methods presented in this chapter. You'll get a chance to use height–weight charts in the self-assessment that follows this lesson.

Height and weight are also used to calculate a person's body mass index (BMI). This index is considered to be a better measure than height and weight alone, but it still does not give as accurate an assessment of body fatness as DXA, underwater weighing, Bod Pod analysis, or skinfold measurement. Both the BMI and the height–weight charts can provide inaccurate measurements for people who have a lot of muscle (athletes, for example) because muscle weighs a lot more than fat. As a result, a very muscular person could be high in weight but not too fat. Similarly, a person who appears normal according to height–weight and BMI charts could actually have an unhealthy level of body fat. This is why skinfolds and laboratory techniques are often considered to be better measures.

In spite of the BMI index's limitations, however, high BMI has been associated with a variety

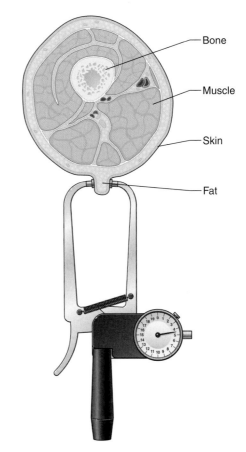

Bone

Muscle

Skin

Fat

**FIGURE 13.2**   A caliper measures skinfolds.

of health problems among both teens and adults. In addition, BMI is often used because it's easy to measure, especially in large groups.

## Body Measurements: Waist-to-Hip Ratio

The waist-to-hip ratio is used not to determine body fatness but to assess health risk. Scientists now know that people who carry more weight in the middle of the body have a higher risk of disease than people who carry more weight in the lower body (legs and hips). People who carry too much weight in their midsection are said to have an apple body type, whereas people who carry more weight in their hips are said to have a pear body type. In general, women are more likely to be the pear type, and men are more likely to be the apple type.

The waist-to-hip ratio is a simple method for assessing the risk associated with body type. As you'll see when you do the self-assessment for this chapter,

**FITNESS TECHNOLOGY: Bioelectrical Impedance Analysis**

Computers and other machines have been developed to test body fat levels. For example, bioelectrical impedance analysis (BIA) requires a special machine and expertise in using the machine, but in recent years BIA machines have become more common in schools because of lower prices and improved ease of use. Used properly, they can provide reliable and accurate estimates of body fatness. One limitation is that different machines can give different results, so it is important to use the same machine and to be sure that the machine is properly calibrated (tested for accuracy). In addition, testing should be done under similar conditions each time you are tested—for example, at the same time of day and not at times when you might be dehydrated. Some health and fitness clubs and doctors' offices now have BIA machines. Results of a BIA test can help determine the accuracy of measurements made using other techniques described in this chapter.

> **Using Technology**
>
> If possible, arrange to have a BIA test done. Compare your BIA results with the results of other self-assessments performed in this chapter. If a BIA test is not available, do some research about BIA testing and report your findings.

this ratio is determined by using a tape to measure your waist circumference and your hip circumference. It is desirable to have a waist circumference smaller than your hip circumference.

## Body Measurements: Waist Girth (Circumference)

Waist girth (also called waist circumference) can be used by itself as an indicator of health risk. Evidence indicates that people with a very large waist are at risk for health problems. As people grow older, their waist size often increases, thus exposing them to greater health risk. Thus waist girth is a useful health risk indicator that you can use throughout your life.

# What Is My Ideal Body Weight?

Even after learning about the various forms of assessment, many people wonder what their ideal body weight is. Experts agree that there is no such thing as one ideal body weight for all people; that is, there is no single table or test that provides a best number for everyone. The best advice is to set a long-term goal of achieving a body fat level in the good fitness zone. Once you have achieved a body fat level that you are comfortable with and that puts you in the good fitness zone, weigh yourself and maintain that weight (this is sometimes referred to as target weight). It's a desirable lifetime goal to maintain this weight and a fat level in the good fitness zone.

If you're in the marginal or low fitness zone, develop a plan that will gradually move you to the next zone. Trying to achieve the good fitness zone when you're too far from it is unrealistic. Instead, people in the low fitness zone should try to move to the marginal zone. Those in the marginal zone should try to move to the good fitness zone. If you're already in the good fitness zone, a reasonable goal for you is simply to stay there.

Some athletes and people in careers that require high levels of fitness may be in the very lean zone, and some people can be very lean because of hereditary factors. While it is possible to be fit and healthy and be in the very lean zone, exceptional leanness is not necessarily a sign of good health and may not be a realistic goal for all people. As noted earlier in this chapter, your body needs a certain amount of body fat (essential body fat), and having too little can cause health problems. Too little body fat can also indicate an eating disorder. If you already have too little fat, increase your weight by gaining body fat. People with eating disorders often try to reduce body fat even when they already have too little for good health. It is important for all people to eat well, especially people who want to be athletes or perform jobs that require high levels of fitness.

As part of a lifelong self-assessment plan, you may choose to monitor your hip-to-waist ratio and your waist girth, especially if you find it difficult to get a good assessment of your body fat level. These measurements are good indicators of health risk. You may also choose to track your BMI over time because physicians often use this measure. High scores are associated with health risks, but because BMI does not estimate body fat levels or lean body mass, it may misclassify some people as overweight or obese when they are not. Similarly BMI may classify a person as "normal" in weight when the person has a higher than healthy level of body fat. The same is true for height–weight charts.

## Assessment Confidentiality

Self-assessments are done to gain information that will help the person build an accurate personal profile and plan for healthy active living. The results of self-assessments are personal information. In many assessments, you'll work with a partner, and you and your partner must agree to keep test results private. Information may be submitted to an instructor or a parent or guardian but always with the expectation that the information is private. Assessment-related information should not be shared with others without permission from the person being tested.

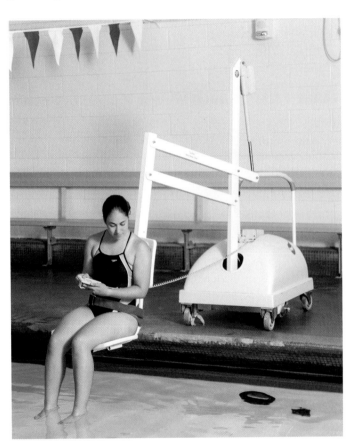

**Body fat helps buoyancy in water, so people with disabilities can do exercises in water that they can't do on land.**

## Lesson Review

1. What do the terms *body composition*, *overweight*, and *obesity* mean?
2. What are some factors that influence body composition?
3. What do the terms *anorexia nervosa*, *bulimia*, and *anorexia athletica* mean?
4. How are body composition and body fat level related to good health?
5. What are some laboratory and nonlaboratory tests for measuring body composition?

**SELF-ASSESSMENT: Body Measurements**

Earlier in this chapter, you learned about ways to determine body composition. Laboratory measures are the most accurate, but they typically require expensive equipment and people who know how to use the equipment correctly. Height and weight are the most commonly used nonlaboratory measures because they can be determined easily and do not require a lot of equipment.

In addition, body circumferences (such as waist-to-hip ratio and waist girth) can be used to determine health risks, and skinfold measurements can be used both to estimate body fat and to assess health risk. Your fitness scores are your personal information and should be kept confidential. You should also be sensitive to the feelings of others when body fat measurements are being taken; it may be appropriate to take measurements privately. Record your results as directed by your instructor.

## Height–Weight Charts

1. Locate the appropriate part of table 13.1 for your sex. Next, find your height (to the nearest inch) at the left and your age at the top of the table. The "normal" weight range for your sex, height, and age is shown in the box where your height row and your age column intersect.

2. Record the weight range for your sex, age, and height.

### TABLE 13.1  Normal Weight Ranges in Pounds

| Male | | | | | Female | | | | |
|---|---|---|---|---|---|---|---|---|---|
| Height | | Age (years) | | | Height | | Age (years) | | |
| Ft | In. | 13 or 14 | 15 or 16 | 17–20 | Ft | In. | 13 or 14 | 15 or 16 | 17–20 |
| 4 | 6 | 69–72 | | | 4 | 6 | 73–76 | | |
| 4 | 7 | 73–76 | | | 4 | 7 | 76–79 | | |
| 4 | 8 | 78–81 | | | 4 | 8 | 79–82 | | |
| 4 | 9 | 82–85 | 82–85 | | 4 | 9 | 86–89 | 91–94 | |
| 4 | 10 | 87–90 | 87–90 | | 4 | 10 | 91–94 | 98–101 | 99–102 |
| 4 | 11 | 88–91 | 88–91 | | 4 | 11 | 96–99 | 102–105 | 104–107 |
| 5 | 0 | 89–92 | 97–100 | 101–104 | 5 | 0 | 104–107 | 106–109 | 109–112 |
| 5 | 1 | 97–100 | 101–104 | 106–109 | 5 | 1 | 105–108 | 109–112 | 113–116 |
| 5 | 2 | 100–103 | 106–109 | 114–117 | 5 | 2 | 106–109 | 112–115 | 116–119 |
| 5 | 3 | 106–109 | 111–114 | 121–124 | 5 | 3 | 110–113 | 115–118 | 120–123 |
| 5 | 4 | 113–116 | 115–118 | 124–127 | 5 | 4 | 115–118 | 120–123 | 125–128 |
| 5 | 5 | 116–119 | 120–123 | 129–132 | 5 | 5 | 119–122 | 124–127 | 129–132 |
| 5 | 6 | 120–123 | 126–129 | 134–137 | 5 | 6 | 126–129 | 128–131 | 134–137 |
| 5 | 7 | 126–129 | 132–135 | 137–140 | 5 | 7 | 127–130 | 131–134 | 137–140 |
| 5 | 8 | 130–133 | 135–138 | 140–143 | 5 | 8 | 128–131 | 135–138 | 143–146 |
| 5 | 9 | 135–138 | 139–142 | 147–150 | 5 | 9 | 129–132 | 137–140 | 148–151 |
| 5 | 10 | 141–144 | 142–145 | 149–152 | 5 | 10 | 130–133 | 139–142 | 153–156 |
| 5 | 11 | 146–149 | 149–152 | 152–155 | 5 | 11 | | 142–145 | 158–161 |
| 6 | 0 | 151–154 | 152–155 | 156–159 | 6 | 0 | | 146–149 | 163–166 |
| 6 | 1 | | 158–161 | 162–165 | | | | | |
| 6 | 2 | | 160–163 | 167–170 | | | | | |
| 6 | 3 | | | 177–180 | | | | | |

To convert inches to centimeters, multiply by 2.54 (1 ft = 12 in.). To convert pounds to kilograms, multiply by 0.45.

# Waist-to-Hip Ratio (Male and Female)

1. Measure your hips at the largest point (the largest circumference of your buttocks). Make sure that the tape is at the same level (horizontal to ground) in the front, in the back, and on your sides. The tape should be snug but not so tight as to cause indentations in your skin (do not use an elastic tape). Stand with your feet together when making the measurement.

2. Measure your waist at the smallest circumference (called the natural waist). If there is no natural waist, measure at the level of the umbilicus. Measure at the end of a normal inspiration (just after a normal in-breath). Do not suck in to make your waist smaller. This measurement is slightly different from the one used to measure waist girth by itself.

3. To calculate your waist-to-hip ratio, divide your waist girth by your hip girth.

4. Find your ratio in table 13.2 to determine your rating.

5. Record your hip and waist measurements and rating.

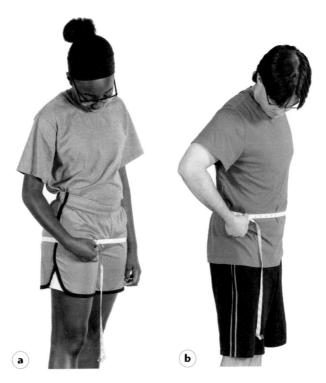

**To determine your waist-to-hip ratio, measure (a) your hips and (b) your waist.**

## TABLE 13.2 Rating Chart: Waist-to-Hip Ratio

|  | Male | Female |
|---|---|---|
| Good fitness zone | ≤0.90 | ≤0.79 |
| Marginal | 0.91–1.0 | 0.80–0.85 |
| Low fitness zone | ≥1.1 | ≥0.86 |

# Waist Girth (Circumference)

1. Measure your waist at a level just above the top of your hipbones. Mark the top of your hipbone on each side and hold the tape just above the marks.
2. Measure after a normal inspiration (at the end of a normal in-breath). Do not suck in to make your waist smaller. Keep the tape horizontal to the ground when making the measurement.
3. Use table 13.3 to determine your rating.
4. Record your waist girth and rating.

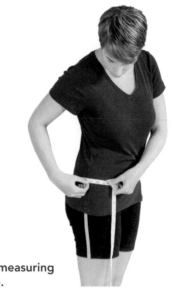

Waist girth is determined by measuring your waist above the hipbone.

**TABLE 13.3   Rating Chart: Waist Girth in Inches**

| Age (years) | 12 | 13 | 14 | 15 | 16 | 17 | ≥18 |
|---|---|---|---|---|---|---|---|
| **Male** | | | | | | | |
| Good fitness zone | ≤28.9 | ≤29.9 | ≤30.9 | ≤31.9 | ≤32.9 | ≤33.9 | ≤34.9 |
| Marginal | 29.0–33.4 | 30.0–34.4 | 31.0–35.9 | 32.0–37.4 | 33.0–38.4 | 34.0–39.9 | 35.0–41.4 |
| Low fitness zone | ≥33.5 | ≥34.5 | ≥36.0 | ≥37.5 | ≥38.5 | ≥40.0 | ≥41.5 |
| **Female** | | | | | | | |
| Good fitness zone | ≤28.9 | ≤29.9 | ≤30.9 | ≤31.9 | ≤32.4 | ≤33.4 | ≤34.4 |
| Marginal | 29.0–32.4 | 30.0–33.9 | 31.0–34.9 | 32.0–35.9 | 32.5–38.4 | 33.5–38.4 | 34.5–39.9 |
| Low fitness zone | ≥32.5 | ≥34.0 | ≥35.0 | ≥36.0 | ≥38.5 | ≥38.5 | ≥40.0 |

To convert inches to centimeters, multiply by 2.54 (1 ft = 12 in.).

# Skinfold Measurements

Skinfold measurements require a special caliper, and using the caliper requires special training. But when done properly by a trained expert, skinfold measurements can provide a good estimate of body fatness. For best results, an expensive caliper is used, but research has shown that inexpensive plastic calipers, such as those shown in the photos here, can be quite accurate if used properly by a trained person who practices the measurement technique. Various measurements can be used; in this book, the calf and triceps are used because of their ease of measurement.

Use the following procedures to complete the various measurements and determine your ratings for each assessment. You can use skinfold measurements to estimate your body fat percentage and determine your target weight. For teenagers, upper arm (triceps) and calf measurements provide a good estimate of body fat percentage. If possible, have the measurements done by an expert. If not, work with a partner to take each other's measurements. With practice, you and your partner will improve your measurement skills. Comparing your measurements to those done by an expert will help you determine the accuracy of the measurements. If you're working with a partner, remember that self-assessment information is personal and considered confidential. It shouldn't be shared with others without the permission of the person being tested.

For the triceps skinfold, pick up a skinfold on the middle of the back of the right arm, halfway between the elbow and the shoulder. The arm should hang loose and relaxed at the side.

For the calf skinfold, the person being tested should stand and place his or her right foot on a chair. Pick up a skinfold on the inside of the right calf, halfway between the shin and the back of the calf, where the calf is largest.

1. Use your left thumb and index finger to pick up the skinfold. Do not pinch or squeeze the skinfold.

2. Hold the skinfold with your left hand while you pick up and use the caliper with your right hand to get a reading.

3. Place the caliper over the skinfold about 0.5 inch (1.3 centimeter) below your finger and thumb. Hold the caliper on the skinfold for 3 seconds, then note

the measurement. If possible, read the caliper measurement to the nearest half-millimeter.

4. Make three measurements each for the triceps and the calf skinfolds. Allow at least 10 seconds between measurements. Use the middle of the three measures as the score. For example, an 8, 9, and 10 give a score of 9. If your three measurements differ by more than 2 millimeters, take a second, or even third, set of three measurements.

5. Now determine your percent body fat and your body fatness rating. Add your triceps and calf scores to get your sum in millimeters, then use table 13.4 to estimate your body fat percentage based on your sum. Use the appropriate table for your sex and find your skinfold sum. Your percent body fat is the number just to the right. For example, if you're male and your skinfold sum is 26, your percent body fat is 21.

6. Once you have determined your percent body fat, use table 13.5 to determine your body fatness rating.

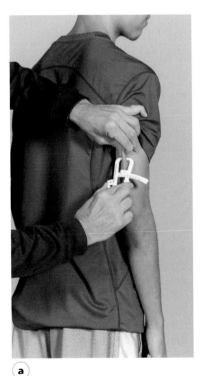 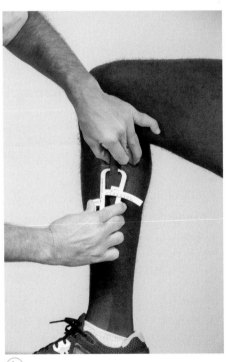

(a)  (b)

Skinfold measurements: *(a)* triceps; *(b)* calf.

## TABLE 13.4   Percent Body Fat From Skinfolds

| Sum (mm) | % fat | Sum (mm) | % fat | Sum (mm) | % fat | Sum (mm) | % fat | Sum (mm) | % fat | Sum (mm) | % fat | Sum (mm) | % fat |
|---|---|---|---|---|---|---|---|---|---|---|---|---|---|
| | | | | | | **Male** | | | | | | | |
| 5 | 6 | 15 | 13 | 25 | 20 | 35 | 28 | 45 | 35 | 55 | 42 | | |
| 6 | 7 | 16 | 14 | 26 | 21 | 36 | 28.5 | 46 | 36 | 56 | 43 | | |
| 7 | 7.5 | 17 | 14.5 | 27 | 21.5 | 37 | 29 | 47 | 36.5 | 57 | 43.5 | | |
| 8 | 8 | 18 | 15 | 28 | 22 | 38 | 30 | 48 | 37 | 58 | 44 | | |
| 9 | 9 | 19 | 16 | 29 | 23 | 39 | 30.5 | 49 | 37.5 | 59 | 44.5 | | |
| 10 | 10 | 20 | 17 | 30 | 24 | 40 | 31 | 50 | 38 | 60 | 45 | | |
| 11 | 10.5 | 21 | 17.5 | 31 | 25 | 41 | 32 | 51 | 39 | | | | |
| 12 | 11 | 22 | 18 | 32 | 26 | 42 | 33 | 52 | 39.5 | | | | |
| 13 | 11.5 | 23 | 18.5 | 33 | 26.5 | 43 | 33.5 | 53 | 40 | | | | |
| 14 | 12 | 24 | 19 | 34 | 27 | 44 | 34 | 54 | 41 | | | | |
| | | | | | | **Female** | | | | | | | |
| 5 | 7 | 15 | 14 | 25 | 21 | 35 | 29 | 45 | 36 | 55 | 43 | | |
| 6 | 8 | 16 | 15 | 26 | 22 | 36 | 29.5 | 46 | 37 | 56 | 44 | | |
| 7 | 8.5 | 17 | 15.5 | 27 | 22.5 | 37 | 30 | 47 | 37.5 | 57 | 44.5 | | |
| 8 | 9 | 18 | 16 | 28 | 23 | 38 | 30.5 | 48 | 38 | 58 | 45 | | |
| 9 | 10 | 19 | 17 | 29 | 24 | 39 | 31 | 49 | 38.5 | 59 | 45.5 | | |
| 10 | 11 | 20 | 18 | 30 | 24.5 | 40 | 32 | 50 | 39 | 60 | 46 | | |
| 11 | 12 | 21 | 18.5 | 31 | 25 | 41 | 33 | 51 | 40 | | | | |
| 12 | 12.5 | 22 | 19 | 32 | 26 | 42 | 34 | 52 | 40.5 | | | | |
| 13 | 13 | 23 | 19.5 | 33 | 27 | 43 | 34.5 | 53 | 41 | | | | |
| 14 | 13.5 | 24 | 20 | 34 | 28 | 44 | 35 | 54 | 42 | | | | |

Reprinted by permission, from Dr. Tim G. Lohman, Department of Exercise and Sport Sciences, University of Arizona.

## TABLE 13.5   Rating Chart: Body Fatness

| | Age (years) | | | | | |
|---|---|---|---|---|---|---|
| Rating | 13 | 14 | 15 | 16 | 17 | 18 or older |
| | | | **Male** | | | |
| Very lean | ≤7.7 | ≤7.0 | ≤6.5 | ≤6.4 | ≤6.6 | ≤6.9 |
| Good fitness | 7.8–22.8 | 7.1–21.3 | 6.6–20.1 | 6.5–20.1 | 6.7–20.9 | 7.0–22.2 |
| Marginal | 22.9–34.9 | 21.4–33.1 | 20.2–31.4 | 20.2–31.5 | 21.0–32.9 | 22.3–35.0 |
| Low fitness | ≥35.0 | ≥33.2 | ≥31.5 | ≥31.6 | ≥33.0 | ≥35.1 |
| | | | **Female** | | | |
| Very lean | ≤13.3 | ≤13.9 | ≤14.5 | ≤15.2 | ≤15.8 | ≤16.5 |
| Good fitness | 13.4–27.7 | 14.0–28.5 | 14.6–29.1 | 15.3–29.7 | 15.9–30.4 | 16.6–31.3 |
| Marginal | 27.8–36.2 | 28.6–36.7 | 29.2–37.0 | 29.8–37.3 | 30.5–37.8 | 31.4–38.5 |
| Low fitness | ≥36.3 | ≥36.8 | ≥37.1 | ≥37.4 | ≥37.9 | ≥38.6 |

# Lesson 13.2

# Energy Balance

## Lesson Objectives

After reading this lesson, you should be able to
1. explain how to use the FIT formula for fat control,
2. describe how many calories are expended in doing various physical activities,
3. explain how physical activity helps a person maintain a healthy body fat level, and
4. describe some common myths about fat control.

## Lesson Vocabulary

calorie, calorie expenditure, calorie intake, energy balance

**Do** you know how many **calories** you expend in a typical day? Do you know how many calories you consume in a typical day? One major health goal is to achieve and maintain an acceptable level of body fat throughout your life. To do this, you must balance the calories you consume and the calories you expend. In this lesson, you'll learn the FIT formula for fat control and appropriate activities for gaining weight and losing body fat.

## Balancing Calories

The term *calorie* is commonly used to describe the amount of energy in a food. The true term is *kilocalorie* (a unit of energy or heat), but when talking about diet and nutrition, *calorie* is typically used. **Energy balance** refers to balancing **calorie intake** and **calorie expenditure** (figure 13.3; also see figure

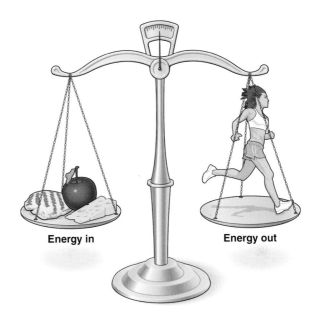

**Energy in**          **Energy out**

**FIGURE 13.3** Balancing energy (calorie) intake with energy (calorie) output is essential for healthy weight maintenance.

### FIT FACT

One pound of fat contains 3,500 calories. Therefore, you can lose 1 pound (about 0.5 kilogram) of fat by eating 3,500 calories fewer than you normally eat in a given time or by burning 3,500 calories more than normal in physical activity. Eating food that provides more calories than your body uses will cause you to gain weight. Therefore, you can gain a pound of fat by eating 3,500 calories more than you usually eat within a given time or by expending 3,500 calories fewer than usual in physical activity within a given time.

13.4 and notice the energy balance scale at the top of the Physical Activity Pyramid). Calorie intake is the number of calories or total energy in the foods you eat. Calorie expenditure is the number of calories (energy) you expend in physical activity. If you take in (eat) more calories than you expend (in activity), you will gain weight because extra energy is stored in the body as fat. If you expend more calories than you take in, you will lose weight. If you balance the calories you consume and expend, you will maintain your current weight.

# The FIT Formula

Both diet and physical activity are important for fat control. For this reason, each has a target zone, as shown in table 13.6.

# Gaining Weight

Combining proper physical activity and diet is the best way to gain weight. In terms of activity, strength and muscular endurance exercises can help you gain weight. Resistance exercises that help build muscle are especially effective because muscle weighs more than fat.

Remember that every physical activity burns calories. Therefore, when you're active, you need to increase your intake of calories in order to gain weight. You do not, however, need to eat a special diet or take protein supplements; you need only eat a well-balanced diet that contains more calories.

# Physical Activity and Calories

You might wonder how many calories are burned by different activities. Table 13.7 shows the approximate number of calories burned each hour during

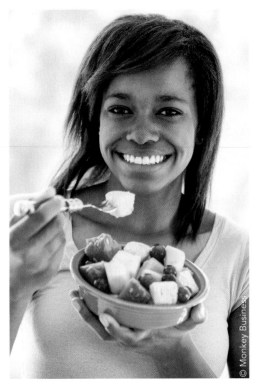

Eating a healthy diet is an essential component of maintaining a healthy weight.

selected vigorous recreational activities. To use the table, find the weight value nearest to your own weight. If you weigh more than the nearest weight,

## TABLE 13.6 FIT Formula for Fat Control

| | Diet* | Physical activity** |
|---|---|---|
| Frequency | Eat three regular meals or four or five small meals daily. Regular, controlled eating is best for losing fat. Skipping meals and snacking is usually not effective. | Participate in physical activity daily. Regular physical activity is best for losing fat. Short or irregular physical activity does little to control body fat. |
| Intensity | To lose 1 pound (about 0.5 kg) of fat, you must eat 3,500 fewer calories than normal over a given span of time. To gain 1 pound (0.5 kg) of fat, you must eat 3,500 more calories than normal over a given span of time. To maintain your weight, you must keep eating the same number of calories over a given span of time. | To lose 1 pound (0.5 kg) of fat, you must use 3,500 more calories than normal over a given span of time. To gain 1 pound (0.5 kg) of fat, you must use 3,500 fewer calories than normal over a given span of time. To maintain your weight, you must keep your level of physical activity the same over a given span of time. |
| Time | Neither dietary change nor physical activity results in quick fat loss. Medical experts recommend that a person lose no more than 2 pounds (1 kg) per week without medical supervision. | Together diet and physical activity can be used to safely lose 1 or 2 pounds (0.5–1.0 kg) per week. |

*Assumes physical activity is constant.

**Assumes that diet is constant.

### TABLE 13.7 Energy Expenditure

| | Calories used per hr based on weight | | | | |
| --- | --- | --- | --- | --- | --- |
| | 100 lb (45 kg) | 120 lb (54 kg) | 150 lb (68 kg) | 180 lb (82 kg) | 200 lb (91 kg) |
| Backpacking/Hiking | 307 | 348 | 410 | 472 | 513 |
| Badminton | 255 | 289 | 340 | 391 | 425 |
| Baseball | 210 | 238 | 280 | 322 | 350 |
| Basketball (half-court) | 225 | 240 | 300 | 345 | 375 |
| Bicycling (normal speed) | 157 | 178 | 210 | 242 | 263 |
| Bowling | 155 | 176 | 208 | 240 | 261 |
| Canoeing (4 mph [6.5 kph]) | 276 | 344 | 414 | 504 | 558 |
| Circuit training | 247 | 280 | 330 | 380 | 413 |
| Dance (ballet/modern) | 240 | 300 | 360 | 432 | 480 |
| Dance (aerobic) | 300 | 360 | 450 | 540 | 600 |
| Dance (social) | 174 | 222 | 264 | 318 | 348 |
| Fitness calisthenics | 232 | 263 | 310 | 357 | 388 |
| Football | 225 | 255 | 300 | 345 | 375 |
| Golf (walking) | 187 | 212 | 250 | 288 | 313 |
| Gymnastics | 232 | 263 | 310 | 357 | 388 |
| Horseback riding | 180 | 204 | 240 | 276 | 300 |
| Interval training | 487 | 552 | 650 | 748 | 833 |
| Jogging (5.5 mph [9 kph]) | 487 | 552 | 650 | 748 | 833 |
| Judo/Karate | 232 | 263 | 310 | 357 | 388 |
| Racquetball/Handball | 450 | 510 | 600 | 690 | 750 |
| Rope jumping (continuous) | 525 | 595 | 700 | 805 | 875 |
| Running (10 mph [16 kph]) | 625 | 765 | 900 | 1,035 | 1,125 |
| Skating (ice or roller) | 262 | 297 | 350 | 403 | 438 |
| Skiing (cross-country) | 525 | 595 | 700 | 805 | 875 |
| Skiing (downhill) | 450 | 510 | 600 | 690 | 750 |
| Soccer | 405 | 459 | 540 | 575 | 621 |
| Softball (fastpitch) | 210 | 238 | 280 | 322 | 350 |
| Swimming (slow laps) | 240 | 272 | 320 | 368 | 400 |
| Swimming (fast laps) | 420 | 530 | 630 | 768 | 846 |
| Tennis | 315 | 357 | 420 | 483 | 525 |
| Volleyball | 262 | 297 | 350 | 403 | 483 |
| Walking | 204 | 258 | 318 | 372 | 426 |
| Weight training | 352 | 399 | 470 | 541 | 558 |

add 5 percent to the number of calories for each 10 pounds (4.5 kilograms) you weigh above the listed weight value. If you weigh less than the nearest weight, subtract 5 percent from the number of calories for each 10 pounds you weigh below the listed weight value. Use this table to determine which physical activities are best for burning calories, then see which activities appeal to you.

> **"** Choice, not chance, determines your destiny. **"**
>
> —Aristotle, Greek philosopher

# Physical Activity and Fat Loss

The best way to lose fat is to combine regular physical activity with a healthy diet. Research shows that a person who reduces calorie intake without increasing activity will lose both fat and muscle tissue, whereas a person who increases physical activity and reduces calorie consumption loses mostly body fat. Notice that physical activities from all steps of the Physical Activity Pyramid (figure 13.4) are appropriate for helping to control body fat level and provide energy balance.

## Moderate Physical Activity

Moderate physical activity is especially effective in long-term fat control. In fact, studies indicate that moderate activity is just as effective as organized sports and games for losing fat—and more effective for permanent fat loss. You can do moderate activities for relatively long periods of time, thus burning many calories.

## Vigorous Aerobics

Because vigorous aerobic activity is more intense than moderate activity, you can burn more calories in a shorter time with this type of activity. It is most often continuous, thus allowing you to expend calories for the full duration of the activity. Vigorous aerobic activities can be sustained for a relatively long time and therefore have potential for considerable calorie expenditure.

## Vigorous Sport and Recreation

Like vigorous aerobics, vigorous sport and recreational activities are more intense than moderate activities. Therefore more calories are expended per unit of time than in moderate activities. The way you perform these activities makes a difference in the number of calories you expend. For example, shooting baskets typically expends fewer calories than playing a game of full-court basketball. The greater the intensity of the activity, the greater the number of calories expended over a similar length of time.

## Muscle Fitness Exercises

Muscle fitness exercise expends considerable calories and is therefore beneficial in maintaining a healthy level of body fat. In addition, the extra muscle tissue you build with these exercises provides a second benefit by helping you expend more calories even when you're resting.

## Flexibility Exercises

Flexibility exercises do not expend as many calories as the other four types of activity represented in the Physical Activity Pyramid. They do, however, expend more calories than resting, and any calories expended above normal can help you control body fatness.

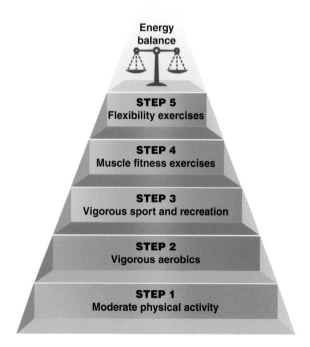

**FIGURE 13.4** All activities in the Physical Activity Pyramid result in calorie expenditure and aid in energy balance.

## Calculating Your Daily Calorie Expenditure

If you keep a record of all the activities you perform in a day, you can determine the total calories you expended. As directed by your teacher, keep a daily record. After recording your activities for a full day, you can calculate your daily calorie expenditure and compare it with your daily calorie intake. To maintain weight, you must expend as much energy as you take in. To lose weight, you must expend more energy than you take in. To gain weight, you must take in more calories than you expend.

## Myths About Fat Loss

Some people hold incorrect ideas about physical activity and fat loss. Read table 13.8 to identify some mistaken ideas and learn some facts about

### FIT FACT

If you maintain your normal calorie intake and increase your activity by playing 30 minutes of tennis daily, you will lose 16 pounds (about 7 kilograms) in a year. If you walk briskly for 15 minutes a day instead of watching TV, you will lose 5 or 6 pounds (about 2.5 kilograms) in a year. On the other hand, if you sit for 15 minutes instead of taking a regular 15-minute walk each day, you will gain 5 to 6 pounds in a year.

losing body fat. No matter what your body is like now, regular physical activity and proper diet will help you control body fatness. When you're fit, you look better, feel better, and have fewer health problems than people who have a high level of body fat and are unfit.

### TABLE 13.8 Myths and Facts About Fat Loss

| Myth | Fact |
|------|------|
| Exercise cannot be effective for fat loss because it takes many hours of exercise to lose even 1 pound (0.5 kg) of fat. | You can lose body fat over time with regular physical activity if your calorie intake remains the same. Fat lost through physical activity tends to stay off longer than fat lost through dieting alone. |
| Exercise does not help you lose fat because it increases your hunger and encourages you to overeat. | If you are moderately active instead of inactive, your hunger should not increase. Even moderate to vigorous activity will not cause hunger to increase so much that you overeat. People who overeat usually do so for other reasons (habit, anxiousness, presence of empty calories, large portion sizes, and so on). |
| Most people with too much body fat have glandular problems. | While some people do have glandular problems, most people who are high in body fat eat too much, do too little physical activity, or both. |
| You can spot-reduce by exercising a specific body part to lose fat in that area. | Any exercise that burns calories will cause the body's general fat deposits to decrease. A given exercise does not cause one area of fat to decrease more than another. |

### Lesson Review

1. How can you use the FIT formula to control your body fat level?
2. How many calories are expended in the five most common physical activities that you perform?
3. How can physical activity help you maintain a healthy body fat level?
4. What are some common myths and facts about fat control?

Each person has a mental picture of himself or herself. If you think you do well in a certain activity, you'll probably take part in that type of activity. If you feel embarrassed about your appearance or ability level while doing an activity, you'll probably avoid that activity. Here are two very different examples of physical self-perception.

Michael was not sure that he wanted to go back to school after the summer break. It seemed as if all of his friends had grown taller in the last few months, but he had stayed the same height. Michael felt embarrassed and a little jealous, even though none of his friends seemed to notice. His height certainly did not alter his ability to play tennis. In fact, his friends still called him "King of the Court" because he usually won.

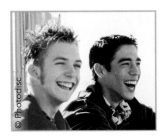

© Photodisc

Raul was one of the shortest people in his class, but his height did not stop him from being involved in activities. He realized that he had never been a great basketball player, but he still liked to play with his friends from school. He also discovered that height had nothing to do with his ability to go hiking, nor did it prevent him from being a good wrestler.

## For Discussion

Michael had a negative self-perception because of his height. What can he do to change his negative perception? How does Raul keep a positive self-perception? What else can a person do to develop a positive self-perception? Consider the guidelines presented in the Self-Management feature as you answer the discussion questions.

## SELF-MANAGEMENT: Skills for Self-Perception

A self-perception is an idea you have about your own thoughts, actions, or appearance. It is influenced by how you think other people view you. Some of the many kinds of self-perception are academic, social, and artistic. In this book, the focus is on physical self-perceptions—the way you view your physical self.

Four aspects of physical self-perception are strength, fitness, skill, and physical attractiveness. People with good physical self-perceptions are happy with their current strength and fitness levels; they also feel that their skills are adequate to meet their needs, and they like the way they look. We know that people who have positive physical self-perceptions are more likely to be physically active than those who do not. The following list provides guidelines you can use to maintain or improve your physical self-perceptions.

- **Assess your physical self-perceptions.** You may use the worksheet provided by your teacher.

- **Consider your self-assessment results.** Use the self-assessment worksheet to determine whether you have any areas in which your physical self-perceptions are especially low (strength, fitness, skill, or physical attractiveness).

- **Perform regular physical activity to improve your physical fitness or practice regularly to improve your physical skills.** Regular physical activity can help you look your best, and learning skills can help you perform your best.

- **Consider a new way of thinking about yourself.** People often set unrealistic standards for themselves, such as looking like someone they see on television or in the movies. Understand that in real life these people do not look the way they look on the screen. In fact, their appearance is often enhanced by special cameras and computers programs. You also do not know whether a movie star has an eating disorder or practices healthy habits. Consider your heredity and set realistic standards for yourself.

- **Think positively.** Almost all people have a physical characteristic that they would like to change. But studies show that the things people don't like about themselves are rarely seen as problems by other people. You're often your own worst critic, and thinking positively can help you present yourself in a positive way.

- **Do not let the actions of a few insensitive people cause you to feel negatively about yourself.** There will always be some people who are insensitive to others' feelings. These people often have low self-perceptions and try to build themselves up by tearing other people down. Recognize that criticism from these people is their problem, not yours.

- **Consider how your behavior and actions influence the way other people view you.** Acting cheerful and friendly has as much to do with how others perceive you as your physical characteristics.

- **Realize that all people have some imperfections.** Try to build on your strengths and improve your areas of weakness.

- **Find a realistic role model and be a role model for others.** Instead of trying to be like someone who is totally unlike you, find someone you admire who has characteristics you can realistically achieve. And, just as you look to others for models, remember that others may look to you as a model. Providing a positive model for others can help you think positively about yourself.

 ## Academic Connection: Quartiles

Various statistics can be used to describe scores for a group of people. The term *quartile* is used to describe the scores for each quarter of a distribution. In the following example, each number represents a score (in inches) on the waist girth test for 36 15-year-old females. The distribution is divided into quartiles (25 percent of scores per quartile, listed in different colors).

A good fitness rating for waist girth for 15-year-old females is 32 inches or less. Which color of quartile includes scores for the good fitness range? What percentage of girls were in the good fitness zone for waist girth? What percentage of girls had scores that did not qualify them to be in the good fitness zone?

### Distribution of Waist Girth Scores (Inches) for 15-Year-Old Females

|    |    |    |    |    |    |    | 34 |    |    |    |    |    |    |    |    |    |
|----|----|----|----|----|----|----|----|----|----|----|----|----|----|----|----|----|
|    |    |    |    |    |    | 33 | 34 | 35 |    |    |    |    |    |    |    |    |
|    |    |    |    |    | 32 | 33 | 34 | 35 | 36 |    |    |    |    |    |    |    |
|    | 28 |    | 30 |    | 32 | 33 | 34 | 35 | 36 | 37 | 38 | 39 | 40 |    |    |    |
| 27 | 28 | 29 | 30 |    | 32 | 33 | 34 | 35 | 36 | 37 | 38 | 39 | 40 | 41 | 42 | 43 |

### Check Your Answers

The red quartile includes scores in the good fitness range, so 25 percent of the girls were in the good fitness zone. That also means that 75 percent, or three quartiles, of the girls were not in the good fitness zone.

Muscle fitness exercises provide a triple benefit in helping you maintain a healthy body composition. First, they build muscles that help you look your best. Second, they expend energy, thus helping you to achieve a good energy balance. Finally, the extra muscle that you build through resistance exercise causes you to burn extra calories even at rest.

You can **take action** by completing an elastic band resistance circuit. Elastic bands are beneficial because they are affordable, travel well, and allow you to easily exercise many muscles. They are appropriate for people of all fitness levels, and they will help you improve your overall coordination and your muscular fitness. Consider the following guidelines for performing resistance band (elastic band) exercises.

- When choosing bands, make sure they are the right length for you and that they do not have cracks or other signs of wear.
- Choose a band that provides the proper resistance that allows you to perform the recommended number of sets and reps.
- You can also do resistance exercises that use your body weight to add variation and create a good workout circuit.

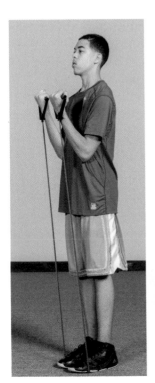
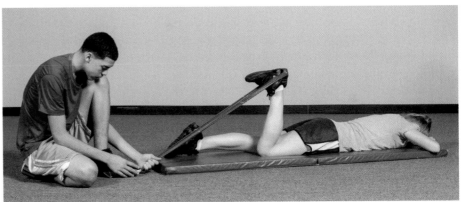

**Take action by performing elastic band exercises.**

# CHAPTER REVIEW

## Reviewing Concepts and Vocabulary

As directed by your teacher, answer items 1 through 5 by correctly completing each sentence with a word or phrase.

1. A term used to describe a person who has a high body fat level is _____.
2. An eating disorder characterized by bingeing and purging is called _____.
3. The minimum amount of body fat needed for good health is _____.
4. People with _____ see themselves as too fat even when they are extremely thin.
5. Keeping your calories consumed equal to your calories expended is called _____.

For items 6 through 10, as directed by your teacher, match each term in column 1 with the appropriate phrase in column 2.

6. metabolic syndrome
7. caliper
8. DXA
9. anorexia athletica
10. basal metabolism

a. best measure of body composition
b. used to measure skinfolds
c. condition associated with health risk factors
d. energy your body uses just to keep you living
e. eating disorder most common among performers

For items 11 through 15, as directed by your teacher, respond to each statement or question.

11. Discuss why 3,500 calories is an important number for maintaining a healthy body composition.
12. Why is confidentiality so important when making body composition assessments?
13. Why is it important to maintain essential body fat?
14. Describe one myth about fat loss and explain how it is incorrect or misleading.
15. What are some guidelines for improving physical self-perceptions?

## Thinking Critically

Each year, people spend billions of dollars on weight loss and muscle-building products that do not work. Look at a newspaper, popular magazine, or website and find an advertisement for a weight loss product. Read the ad and make a list of its claims. Place a checkmark by the claims that are consistent with the information presented in this chapter. Place an X by those that appear to be false or questionable. Write a paragraph evaluating the advertisement.

## Project

The U.S. government provides annual ratings of obesity for each state and for some cities. Prepare a poster showing how your city or state compares with the U.S. average obesity rate. List five factors that you think may cause your state to rank as it does.

# 14

# Physical Activity Program Planning

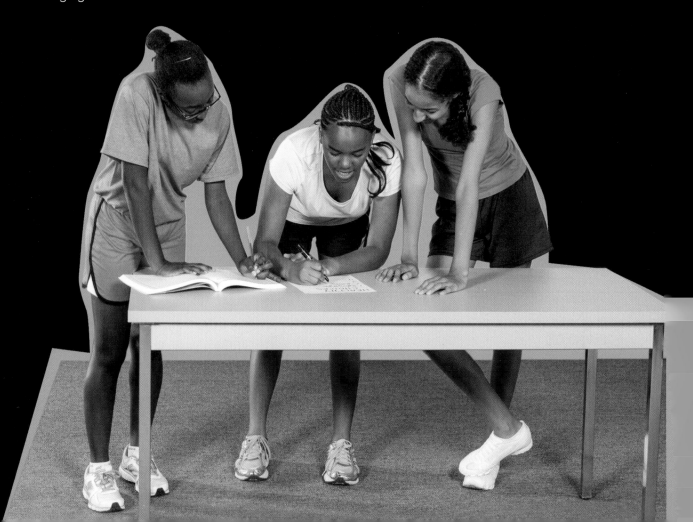

# Lesson 14.1

# Physical Activity and Fitness Assessment

**Lesson Objectives**

After reading this lesson, you should be able to
1. explain how to use a fitness profile to plan a personal fitness program,
2. describe the five steps in planning a comprehensive personal fitness program, and
3. describe some ways in which physical activity enhances academic performance.

**Lesson Vocabulary**

cognitive skills, fitness profile

**Do** you have a personal fitness and physical activity plan? In other chapters, you've been introduced to the five steps of program planning, learned which types of activity are most appropriate for building each part of health-related physical fitness, and planned a program for each of the five types of activity included in the Physical Activity Pyramid. In the first part of this chapter, you'll use the plans you've previously developed to create a comprehensive personal physical activity program. First, read about the comprehensive program that Alicia developed, then plan your own program. To help you create your plan, your teacher will provide you with worksheets.

## Step 1: Determine Your Personal Needs

As you know from your previous program planning, collecting information is the first step toward making good decisions and preparing a good plan. In this case, construct a comprehensive fitness profile and an activity profile to help you determine your needs and interests. Use the many self-assessments that you've performed throughout this class.

A **fitness profile** is a brief summary of your self-assessment results that helps you determine your areas of personal need. You can see a sample for Alicia, a 15-year-old, in figure 14.1. To create a fitness profile, first make a list of all of the fitness self-assessments that you have performed. Then record your scores and ratings for each of the self-assessments. Your profile should look similar to the one that Alicia prepared.

She determined that she met the national physical activity goals for moderate and vigorous physical activity and placed a checkmark by those goals (figure 14.2). Her walks to school and jogs on two days a week helped her meet these goals. Alicia did not do any exercises for muscle fitness and flexibility on a regular basis and did none for the last week. Alicia did not meet the national goals for muscle fitness and flexibility exercises, so she did not place a check by those. Alicia was not enrolled in physical education class, so she did not get any physical activity at school that lasted at least 10 minutes at a time. Prepare a written activity profile using a chart similar to the one used by Alicia. List the activities that you regularly perform and answer the questions related to national physical activity goals.

### FIT FACT

Each year high school students are surveyed to determine their activity levels. Teens are asked if they meet national goals for moderate activity, vigorous activity, and muscle fitness. The questions are similar to those that you ask yourself when you prepare a physical activity profile.

## Step 2: Consider Your Program Options

Alicia prepared a list of several activities to consider for her activity plan. She was already doing some walking and jogging, but she was not doing any muscle fitness or flexibility exercise. She prepared

| Self-assessment | Rating |
|---|---|
| **Cardiorespiratory endurance** | |
| PACER | Good fitness |
| Step test | Good fitness |
| Walking test | Good fitness |
| One-mile run | Marginal |
| **Muscle fitness** | |
| Curl-up | Good fitness |
| Push-up | Marginal |
| 1RM arm press (per lb of body weight) | Good fitness |
| 1RM leg press (per lb of body weight) | Marginal |
| **Muscular endurance** | |
| Grip strength (left) | Marginal |
| Grip strength (right) | Good fitness |
| Standing long jump | Marginal |
| Medicine ball throw | Good fitness |
| **Body composition** | |
| Body mass index (BMI) | Good fitness |
| Height–weight | Good fitness |
| Skinfold measures | Good fitness |
| Waist-to-hip ratio | Good fitness |
| Waist girth | Good fitness |
| **Flexibility** | |
| Back-saver sit-and-reach | Low fitness |
| Trunk lift | Marginal |
| Arm, leg, and trunk flexibility | Marginal |

**FIGURE 14.1**   Alicia's fitness profile.

the following list that included her current activities and additional activities from the Physical Activity Pyramid that she thought she might enjoy and was likely to perform regularly.

**Moderate Physical Activity**

- Walking to and from school
- Additional walking
- Yardwork
- Biking

**Vigorous Aerobics**

- Continue her current jogging
- Additional jogging
- Aerobic dance class

**Vigorous Sport and Recreation**

- Volleyball club
- Tennis

**Muscle Fitness Exercise**

- Elastic band exercises
- Jump rope

**Flexibility Exercises**

- Static stretching exercises
- Yoga

Make a list similar to the one that Alicia made. Consider activities that you currently perform, as well as other types of moderate activity, vigorous activity (including vigorous aerobics, sports, and recreation), muscle fitness exercise, and flexibility exercise. As you choose activities, consider the health benefits and health-related fitness benefits provided by each.

# Step 3: Set Goals

Setting SMART goals can help you build a complete fitness and physical activity program that meets your personal needs. First, consider the reasons for doing your program. Are you primarily interested in fitness and physical activity for health and wellness, or are you interested in building a higher level of fitness necessary for playing a sport?

For example, Alicia is interested in health but also wants to try out for the volleyball team. First, however, she's going to participate in the volleyball club to develop skills that will help her make the team when volleyball season comes.

Next, consider your fitness and activity profiles. If you're low in one part of physical fitness, you may want to work on it. If you did not meet national activity guidelines for one type of physical activity, you might want to do more of that type. Alicia had marginal ratings in flexibility and muscle fitness and did not meet the national guidelines for muscle fitness and flexibility exercises.

In your earlier plans, you've focused only on physical activity goals because you were just learning to plan and were doing a short-term plan with short-term goals. Now that you're more experienced

in planning, you can build a plan for a longer time that addresses long-term goals, including physical *fitness* goals.

As you can see in figure 14.3, Alicia chose physical activity (process) and fitness (product) goals designed to improve her weaknesses—specifically, flexibility exercise to improve her flexibility and muscle fitness exercise to improve her muscle fitness and volleyball performance. Alicia wanted to keep walking to school because she wanted to do a moderate activity that she can continue to do later in life. She decided to drop her jogging two days a week so that she could attend volleyball club on Tuesdays and Thursdays. She felt that the vigorous activity in volleyball club would serve the same purpose. She decided to include tennis just for fun. She also included jump rope as a warm-up before her muscle fitness exercise and to build power in her legs.

Alicia set some of her activity goals for eight weeks (long-term). She did this because she had been walking to school on a regular basis so she felt confident that she could continue to do it regularly. She also set eight weeks for her volleyball club meetings. She felt that she could stick with it for eight weeks

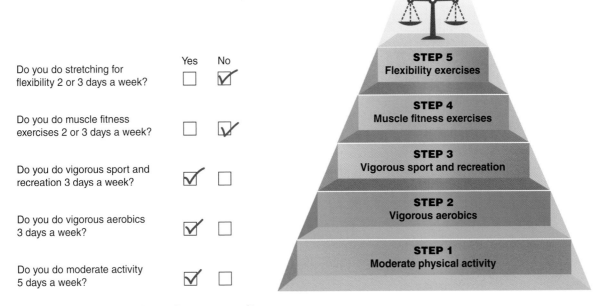

| | Yes | No |
|---|---|---|
| Do you do stretching for flexibility 2 or 3 days a week? | ☐ | ☑ |
| Do you do muscle fitness exercises 2 or 3 days a week? | ☐ | ☑ |
| Do you do vigorous sport and recreation 3 days a week? | ☑ | ☐ |
| Do you do vigorous aerobics 3 days a week? | ☑ | ☐ |
| Do you do moderate activity 5 days a week? | ☑ | ☐ |

**FIGURE 14.2** Alicia's physical activity profile.

| Physical activity goals | Days | Amount | | Weeks |
|---|---|---|---|---|
| | | **Long-term goals** | | |
| 1. Brisk walk to and from school | 3 | 30 minutes a day (15 minutes each way) | | 8 |
| 2. Volleyball club | 2 | 60 minutes after school | | 8 |
| 3. Stretching exercises | 2 | 2 sets of 2 reps of each exercise, hold stretch 30 seconds (performed after volleyball club when the muscles are warm) | | 8 |
| | | **Short-term goals** | | |
| 1. Jump rope warm-up | 3 | 5 minutes, alternate jumping 30 seconds, walking 15 seconds | | 2 |
| 2. Resistance machine exercises | 3 | 2 sets of 10 reps, 60% of 1RM | | 2 |
| 3. Cool-down | 3 | 5-minute walk | | 2 |
| 4. Jump rope warm-up | 1 | 5 minutes, alternate jumping 30 seconds, walking 30 seconds | | 2 |
| 5. Tennis | 1 | 60 minutes | | 2 |
| 6. Cool-down | 1 | 5-minute walk | | 2 |
| **Physical fitness component** | | **Goal** | | **Completion date** |
| 1. Improve push-up score. | | 8 reps | | Nov. 15 (8 weeks) |
| 2. Improve leg press score. | | 1.75 lb (0.8 kg) per lb (kg) of body weight | | Nov. 15 (8 weeks) |
| 3. Improve back-saver sit-and-reach score. | | 12 in. (30 cm) | | Nov. 15 (8 weeks) |
| 4. Improve arm, leg, and trunk flexibility score. | | Score of 8 points | | Nov. 15 (8 weeks) |

**FIGURE 14.3** Alicia's activity and fitness goals.

because it was important for improving her skills for making the volleyball team. She set two-week goals (short-term) for her muscle fitness, flexibility, and tennis goals. She wanted to try her plan for these new activities to see if it was reasonable. If necessary, she planned to modify her short-term activity goals after two weeks. She added jump rope to her plan as a warm-up for her muscle fitness exercises. Alicia did not use all of the activities from her list of possible activities because she wanted to be realistic. She set fitness goals for two muscle fitness self-assessments and two flexibility self-assessments. She hoped to achieve these fitness goals in eight weeks (long-term goals) because she knew that improving fitness takes weeks to achieve. Using a chart similar to Alicia's (figure 14.3), prepare your own SMART physical activity and physical fitness goals, including both short-term and long-term goals.

> " A good plan is like a road map: it shows the final destination and usually the best way to get there. "
>
> —H. Stanley Judd, author

# Step 4: Structure Your Program and Write It Down

Once Alicia had established her goals, she built a schedule. Her schedule included all of the activities that she listed as goals in step 3 (figure 14.4). Alicia chose the days of the week that made exercise most convenient for her. She chose Monday, Wednesday, and Friday for her jump rope and muscle fitness exercise because the school fitness center was open after school on those days. Volleyball club met on Tuesdays and Thursdays and she planned to do her flexibility exercises after volleyball club when the muscles were warm. The flexibility exercises also served as a good cool-down after volleyball club. She chose to do tennis on Saturday morning and planned no activities on Sunday.

In a separate chart, she listed her flexibility and muscle fitness exercises (see figure 14.5). Since they were the same exercises each time, she needed to list them only once to help her remember them.

## FIT FACT

Walking or biking to school increases the amount of activity that teens accumulate by an average of 16 minutes a day. According to a report by the Surgeon General of the United States, approximately 200,000 lives could be saved each year if adults were more physically active.

# Step 5: Keep a Log and Evaluate Your Program

The Taking Action feature in this chapter allows you to perform your plan, but you won't have time to complete your entire plan in this class. Therefore, you'll need to put your program into action on your own. In the weeks ahead, try out your plan and use a log to keep a record of your activities. A log will help you see if you met your goals.

After you've tried your program for some time (the specific time depends on your goals), evaluate

| Day | Activity | Time of day | How long? |
|---|---|---|---|
| Mon. | Walk to school<br>Jump rope warm-up<br>Muscle fitness exercises<br>Walking cool-down | 7:15–7:30 a.m.<br>3:35–3:40 p.m.<br>3:40–4:25 p.m.<br>4:25–4:30 p.m. | 15 min<br>5 min<br>45 min<br>5 min |
| Tues. | Walk to school<br>Volleyball club<br>Cool-down and flexibility exercises | 7:15–7:30 a.m.<br>3:45–4:45 p.m.<br>4:45–5:00 p.m. | 15 min<br>60 min<br>15 min |
| Wed. | Walk to school<br>Jump rope warm-up<br>Muscle fitness exercises<br>Walking cool-down | 7:15–7:30 a.m.<br>3:35–3:40 p.m.<br>3:40–4:25 p.m.<br>4:25–4:30 p.m. | 15 min<br>5 min<br>45 min<br>5 min |
| Thurs. | Walk to school<br>Volleyball club<br>Cool-down and flexibility exercises | 7:15–7:30 a.m.<br>3:45–4:45 p.m.<br>4:45–5:00 p.m. | 15 min<br>60 min<br>15 min |
| Fri. | Walk to school<br>Jump rope warm-up<br>Muscle fitness exercises<br>Walking cool-down | 7:15–7:30 a.m.<br>3:35–3:40 p.m.<br>3:40–4:25 p.m.<br>4:25–4:30 p.m. | 15 min<br>5 min<br>45 min<br>5 min |
| Sat. | Jump rope warm-up<br>Tennis<br>Walking cool-down | 9:00–9:05 a.m.<br>9:05–10:05 a.m.<br>10:05–10:10 a.m. | 5 min<br>60 min<br>5 min |
| Sun. | None | | |

**FIGURE 14.4** Alicia's schedule for her physical activity plan.

| Cool-down and flexibility exercises | Repetitions | Time |
|---|---|---|
| Back-saver sit-and-reach | 2 sets of 2 reps | 15 sec |
| Knee-to-chest | 2 sets of 2 reps | 15 sec |
| Sitting stretch | 2 sets of 2 reps | 15 sec |
| Zipper | 2 sets of 2 reps | 15 sec |
| Hip stretch | 2 sets of 2 reps | 15 sec |
| Calf stretch | 2 sets of 2 reps | 15 sec |
| **Muscle fitness exercises** | **Repetitions** | **Resistance** |
| Bench press | 2 sets of 2 reps | 60% of 1RM |
| Knee extension | 2 sets of 2 reps | 60% of 1RM |
| Hamstring curl | 2 sets of 2 reps | 60% of 1RM |
| Biceps curl | 2 sets of 2 reps | 60% of 1RM |
| Triceps press | 2 sets of 2 reps | 60% of 1RM |

**FIGURE 14.5**   Alicia's muscle fitness and flexibility exercises.

## ⚛ SCIENCE IN ACTION: Exercise and Academics

The U.S. Centers for Disease Control and Prevention (CDC) is a government agency created to help people and communities "protect their health through health promotion; prevention of disease, injury, and disability; and preparedness for new health threats." The CDC recognizes the importance of regular physical activity as one means of achieving its goal of good health for all people and all communities. CDC scientists reviewed more than 400 studies and found that in addition to providing health benefits, regular physical activity can "help improve academic achievement, including grades and standardized test scores." The CDC also concluded that physical activity improves **cognitive skills** such as concentration and attention, as well as academic behavior (including classroom behavior).

The conclusion that physical activity helps students concentrate on academic tasks is supported by research conducted by kinesiologists at the University of Illinois. They found, for example, that walking stimulates brain areas that increase concentration and attention in the

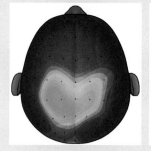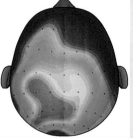

**Brain activation:** *(a)* after 20 minutes of sitting; *(b)* after 20 minutes of walking.

Reprinted from *Neuroscience*, Vol. 159, C.H. Hillman et al., "The Effect of acute treadmill walking on cognitive control and academic achievement in preadolescent children," pgs. 1044-1054, copyright 2009, with permission of Elsevier.

classroom. The images show brain activation after 20 minutes of sitting and 20 minutes of walking. The red and yellow areas (after exercise) indicate activation of the brain.

The CDC report and the University of Illinois research suggest that classroom-based physical activity, including exercise breaks, can help students perform well both on tests and in academics in general.

### Student Activity

Given the evidence concerning physical activity and academic achievement, create a plan for introducing physical activity in your high school classrooms.

#  FITNESS TECHNOLOGY: Swim Watches

One good option for your personal physical activity program is swimming, which is an excellent total body activity. It can also be done by most people, including those who have joint problems, who are recovering from an injury, or who are high in body fat and have a hard time with other forms of exercise. To help you self-monitor your swimming activity, consider using a swim watch. These waterproof devices are worn on the wrist and have a built-in accelerometer similar to the technology used in activity watches to monitor steps in walking or running. Most swim watches provide information about total time for a swim session, laps completed, pace and total time per lap, total distance covered, stroke type, and stroke length. You can download the information

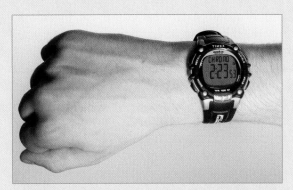

**A waterproof swim watch can help you self-monitor swimming activity.**

to your computer and store or print records of each workout. The watch can also estimate the number of calories you expend in a swim session.

---

### Using Technology

Investigate different types of swim watches and prepare a review. Submit your review to the school newspaper or a school blog.

---

it. List the activities in your plan that you did complete and those that you didn't complete. For the part of your plan that you didn't complete, list your reasons why not (for example, bad weather or homework). Perform tests of fitness to see if you met your fitness goals. Next, prepare a written evaluation of your program. To help you with this evaluation, answer the following questions.

- Do you think your daily plan is one you can regularly complete?

- Do you think you need to make any changes in your program?
- What changes would you make in your program and why?

Evaluating your program will help you determine how well it's working for you. If you're not meeting your goals, revise your program so that you can perform activities that will meet them.

## Lesson Review

1. How do you build a fitness and physical activity profile?
2. What are the five steps in planning a personal fitness program? Describe each step.
3. How does physical activity enhance academic performance?

As you've worked your way through this book, you've had the opportunity to take many physical fitness tests. The tests available to you are listed in table 14.1. After you finish this class, you would be wise to continue assessing your fitness, but it's not reasonable to perform all the tests you've done here. To simplify things, you can prepare your own fitness test battery that includes tests from each of the four categories (cardiorespiratory endurance, body composition, muscle fitness, and flexibility) listed in table 14.1. A test battery refers to several tests designed to measure all parts of fitness. Use the following guidelines in choosing tests for your test battery.

- For cardiorespiratory endurance choose at least one test.
- For flexibility choose at least two of the three tests available.
- For body composition choose at least one test.

- For muscle fitness choose at least one test for the arms and upper body, one test for the trunk and abdominals, and one test for the lower body. Consider including tests for different parts of muscle fitness (muscular endurance, strength, power).
- Choose tests for which you have adequate equipment.
- Choose tests that you think you're likely to actually do.
- Use a chart similar to table 14.1 to select tests for your battery.

Perform the tests in class, then retest yourself from time to time to see how you're doing and to help you set future fitness and physical activity goals. If you're working with a partner, remember that self-assessment information is personal and considered confidential. It shouldn't be shared with others without the permission of the person being tested.

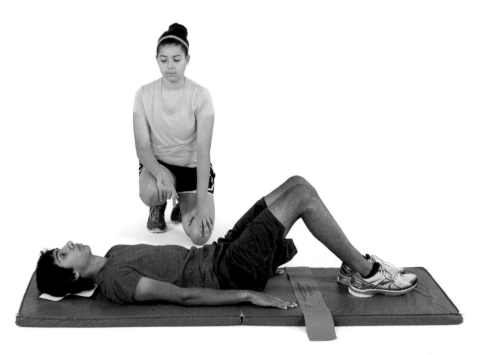

Create your own fitness test battery to track your fitness over time and help you prepare future personal plans.

**TABLE 14.1   Choices for Your Personal Fitness Test Battery**

| Self-assessment | Place a ✔ to select a test |
|---|---|
| **Cardiorespiratory endurance** | |
| PACER | |
| Step test | |
| Walking test | |
| One-mile run | |
| **Muscle fitness** | |
| Curl-up | |
| Push-up | |
| Side stand | |
| Sitting tuck | |
| Arm press 1RM (per lb of body weight) | |
| Leg press 1RM (per lb of body weight) | |
| Grip strength (right) | |
| Grip strength (left) | |
| Standing long jump | |
| Medicine ball throw | |
| **Body composition** | |
| Height–weight (based on BMI) | |
| Skinfold measures | |
| Waist-to-hip ratio | |
| Waist girth | |
| **Flexibility** | |
| Back-saver sit-and-reach | |
| Trunk lift | |
| Arm, leg, and trunk flexibility tests | |

# Lesson 14.2

# Maintaining Active Lifestyles

## Lesson Objectives

After reading this lesson, you should be able to

1. list and describe several self-management skills that help you maintain physical activity throughout life,
2. define *attitude* and describe several positive and negative attitudes about physical activity, and
3. explain ways to create positive attitudes about physical activity and reduce negative ones.

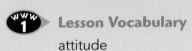 **Lesson Vocabulary**

attitude

**Now** that you have learned how to plan your comprehensive physical activity program, do you think you will be able to perform your plan on a regular basis? Consider the information that follows to help you stick with your plan.

## Stages of Change and Self-Management Skills

As you learned earlier, there are five stages of change that people go through in adopting healthy lifestyles such as being regularly active. By now, you have probably moved well past the first three stages of change (see table 14.2) and are either at the stage of action or maintenance. The goal is to reach the stage of maintenance and stay there. There are several things that you can do to increase the likelihood that you will maintain your active lifestyle throughout life. One thing that you can do is use the self-management skills that you learned about in each

of the chapters of this book. Table 14.3 provides a review of the different self-management skills. Research shows that people who use self-management skills are more active and stay in the top stage of change (maintenance) over the long haul.

## Strengthening Positive Attitudes and Avoiding Negative Attitudes

Another important thing that you can do is to adopt positive attitudes about physical activity. A physical activity plan is worthwhile only if you carry it out, and that is determined in large part by your attitudes. The word **attitude** refers to your feelings about something. We all have attitudes about food, subjects of study, music, clothing, and many other topics—including physical activity. Active people have more positive attitudes toward physical activity

**TABLE 14.2  Five Stages of Physical Activity**

| Stage of physical activity | Description |
| --- | --- |
| 5. Active exerciser (maintenance) | Active on a regular basis. Can overcome obstacles that may discourage others. |
| 4. Activator (action) | Active but participates inconsistently. |
| 3. Planner (planning to change) | Has taken steps to get ready to be active, such as buying special clothing or equipment. |
| 2. Contemplation (thinking about change) | Not active but thinking about becoming active. |
| 1. Precontemplation (not thinking about change) | Sedentary living; does no regular activity. |

### TABLE 14.3 Self-Management Skills for Fitness, Health, and Wellness

| Skill | Description |
|---|---|
| Self-assessment | This skill helps you see where you are and what to change in order to get where you want to be. |
| Building knowledge and understanding | You can use a modified form of the scientific method to solve problems—such as how to make healthy changes in your life. |
| Identifying risk factors | Identifying your health risks enables you to assess and then reduce them. |
| Positive attitude | This skill helps position you to succeed in adopting healthy lifestyles. |
| Self-confidence | This skill helps you build the feeling that you're capable of making healthy changes in your lifestyles. |
| Goal setting and self-planning | These skills create a foundation for developing your personal plan by setting goals that are SMART (specific, measurable, attainable, realistic, and timely) and preparing a written schedule. |
| Time management | This skill helps you be efficient so that you have time for the important things in your life. |
| Choosing good activities | This skill involves selecting the activities that are best for you personally so that you will enjoy and benefit from doing them. |
| Learning performance skills | This skill helps you perform well and with confidence. For example, learning motor skills helps you become active, learning stress-management skills helps you avoid or reduce stress, and learning nutrition skills helps you eat well. |
| Improving self-perception | This skill helps you think positively about yourself so that you're more likely to make healthy lifestyle choices and feel that they will make a difference in your life. |
| Stress management | This skill involves preventing or coping with the stresses of daily life. |
| Self-monitoring | This skill involves keeping records (logs) to see whether you are in fact doing what you think you're doing. |
| Overcoming barriers | This skill helps you find ways to stay active despite barriers, such as lack of time, temporary injury, lack of safe places to be active, inclement weather, and difficulty in selecting healthy foods. |
| Finding social support | This skill enables you to get help and support from others (such as your friends and family) as you adopt healthy behaviors and work to stick with them. |
| Saying "no" | This skill helps keep you from doing things you don't want to do, especially when you're under pressure from friends or other people. |
| Preventing relapse | This skill helps you stick with healthy behaviors even when you have problems getting motivated. |
| Thinking critically | This skill enables you to find and interpret information that helps you make good decisions and solve problems in living a healthy lifestyle. |
| Resolving conflicts | This skill helps you solve problems and avoid stress. |
| Positive self-talk | This skill helps you perform your best and make healthy lifestyle choices such as being active by thinking good thoughts rather than negative ones that detract from success. |
| Developing good strategy and tactics | This skill helps you focus on a specific plan of action and successfully execute the plan. |
| Finding success | Finding success is technically not a skill. Finding success is something that comes from using a variety of self-management skills to change behavior. If you use the self-management skills described in this table, and believe that they will help you to succeed, your chances of success improve dramatically. |

than negative ones. If you follow certain guidelines, you can strengthen your positive attitudes and get rid of any negative ones (see the Self-Management feature later in this chapter).

## FIT FACT

Active teens have more positive attitudes than negative attitudes. This state of mind is called a positive balance of attitudes.

Active people have more positive than negative attitudes. Here's a list of reasons that people like to be physically active. Think about these attitudes and how you might make some of them your own.

- **"Physical activities are a great way to meet people."** Many activities provide opportunities to meet people and strengthen friendships. For example, aerobic dance and team sports are good social activities.

- **"I think physical activity is really fun."** Many teenagers do activities simply because they're fun. Participating in activities you enjoy also helps you reduce stress.

- **"I enjoy the challenge."** When the famous mountain climber George Mallory was asked why he climbed Mount Everest, he replied, "Because it's there." Helen Keller was deaf and blind but became a famous author. She said in one of her books that "life is either a daring adventure or nothing at all." Some people just enjoy a challenge. Are you one of them?

- **"I like the rigor of training."** Some people enjoy intense training. For these people, competition and winning can be secondary to training.

- **"I like competition."** If you enjoy competition, sport and other physical activities provide ways to test yourself against others. You can even compete against yourself by trying to improve your score or time in an activity.

- **"Physical activity is my way of relaxing."** Physical activity can help you relax mentally and emotionally after a difficult day—for example, a day of demanding schoolwork.

- **"I think physical activity improves my appearance."** Physical activity can help you build muscle and control body fat. Remember, however, that regular activity cannot completely change your appearance.

- **"Physical activity is a good way to improve my health and wellness."** As you are learning from this book, regular physical activity helps you resist illness and improves your general sense of well-being.

- **"Physical activity just makes me feel good."** Many people just feel better when they exercise, and many have a sense of loss or discomfort when they don't exercise.

> " The greatest discovery of my generation is that human beings can alter their lives by altering their attitudes. "
>
> —William James, American philosopher

## Changing Negative Attitudes

The following list shows you some negative attitudes, along with suggestions for turning them into positive ones. To decrease any negative attitudes you may have, give some thought to the suggested alternative.

**Negative:** "I don't have the time."

**Positive:** "I will plan a time for physical activity." If you planned time for physical activity, you would feel better, function more efficiently, and therefore have more time to do other things that you want to do.

**Negative:** "I don't want to get all sweaty."

**Positive:** "I'll allow time to clean up afterward." Sweating is a natural by-product of a good workout. Allow yourself time to change before exercising and to shower and change afterward. Focus on how good you will feel.

**Negative:** "People might laugh at me."

**Positive:** "When they see how fit I get, they'll wish they were exercising too." Find friends who are interested in getting fit. Anyone who does laugh may simply be jealous of your efforts and results.

**Negative:** "None of my friends work out, so neither do I."

**Positive:** "I'll ask my friends to join me, and maybe we'll work out together." Talk with your friends. Some of them may be interested in working out or doing lifestyle activities together.

**Negative:** "I get nervous and feel tense when I play sports and games."

**Positive:** "Everyone gets nervous. I'll stay as calm as I can and do the best I can." Many athletes learn techniques to reduce their stress levels. You can learn them too.

**Negative:** "I'm already in good condition."

**Positive:** "Physical activity will help me stay in good condition." Use the self-assessments in this book, then take an honest look at yourself. Are you as fit as you thought? Physical activity can help you get in shape and stay in shape.

**Negative:** "I'm too tired."

**Positive:** "I'll just do a little to get started, then as I get more fit I'll do more." You'll probably find that once you get started, physical exertion gives you *more* energy. Begin realistically, then gradually increase the amount of activity you do.

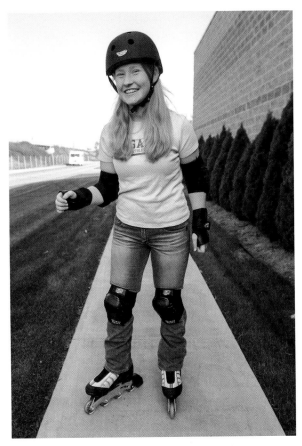

Physical activity can be fun and challenging.

## FIT FACT

The U.S. guideline for teens calls for doing 60 minutes of physical activity on each day of the week. This goal is met by only 29 percent of high school students, and 14 percent don't do 60 minutes of physical activity on any day of the week.

## Lesson Review

1. What are some self-management skills that you can use to maintain physical activity throughout life?
2. What is an attitude, and what are some common positive and negative attitudes about physical activity?
3. What are some things you can do to build positive attitudes and reduce negative ones?

Allen and Matt are friends who often do things together, including sport activities. Sometimes they play tennis together on the weekend. Lately, Allen has been winning most of their matches.

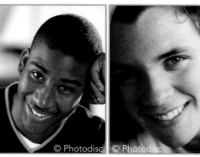
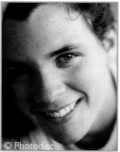

© Photodisc © Photodisc

"You ready to hit the court?" Allen asked Matt as he grabbed his tennis racket.

"I don't feel like playing today," Matt said. "Anyway, there's a good show on TV." He walked into the family room and sat on the couch.

Allen followed him. "I think you just don't want to lose again."

"You're right," Matt admitted. "I hate losing."

"You win sometimes, Matt. The competition is what makes tennis fun."

"Not when I lose," Matt replied.

Allen thought for a minute. "How about taking a jog around the block?" he asked.

"There'll be no winner or loser that way."

"I don't want to get all sweaty," Matt replied. "I'd rather relax watching TV."

"Oh, come on, Matt. Jogging will help you relax. We need to stay in shape."

Matt looked at Allen and said, "I'm thinking about it."

## For Discussion

What does Allen like about being physically active? What does Matt like—and not like—about physical activity? How could Matt change his negative attitudes and become more active? What are some other negative attitudes that keep people from being active, and how can they be changed? What are some positive attitudes that help people stay active? Consider the information in the Self-Management section when answering the discussion questions.

# SELF-MANAGEMENT: Skills for Building Positive Attitudes

Most of us have had both positive and negative attitudes about physical activity at one time or another. Experts have shown that people with more positive attitudes toward physical activity than negative ones are likely to be active. Use the following guidelines to build positive attitudes and get rid of negative ones.

- **Assess your attitudes.** Make a list of your positive and negative attitudes. You can use the attitudes listed in this lesson to help you.

- **Identify your reasons for any negative attitudes.** Your self-assessment will help you identify any negative attitudes you hold. Ask yourself why you feel negative about physical activity. If you can find the reason, it may help you change. For example, you may not have liked playing a sport when you were young because you didn't like a particular coach or player. Maybe you can now

find a situation that will make an activity more fun. Consider the alternatives to negative attitudes described earlier in this chapter.

- **Find activities that bring out fewer negative attitudes.** People have different attitudes and feelings about different activities. For example, maybe you don't like team sports but you do enjoy recreational activities. List your negative attitudes, then ask yourself whether there are activities you don't dislike. If so, consider trying them.

- **Choose activities that accentuate the positive.** If you really like certain activities and feel good about them, focus on these activities rather than ones you don't like as much.

- **Change the situation.** You may feel negatively about an activity because of things unrelated to the activity. For example, if you hated playing basketball because you had too little time to get dressed and groomed after participating, maybe you can find a situation in which you can do the activity and also have more time to shower and dress.

- **Be active with friends.** Activities are often more fun when you do them with friends. Sometimes participating with other people you like is enough to change your feelings about an activity.

- **Discuss your attitudes.** Just talking about your attitudes can sometimes help. People sometimes think they're the only ones who have problems in certain situations. Talking about it with others can help you change the situation to make it more fun for everyone concerned.

- **Help others build positive attitudes.** The ways in which others react can affect a person's feelings about physical activity. Your positive reactions can help others change negative feelings about physical activity. Consider the following suggestions when you interact with others in physical activity.

  - **Instead of laughing, provide encouragement.** Do you remember how difficult it is to start something new or different? You can encourage others by making statements such as, "Good to see you exercising. Way to go!"

  - **Try to make new friends through participation in physical activities.** Introduce yourself to others and offer to help others when appropriate.

  - **Don't hesitate to ask for help from others.** Start or join a sport or exercise club at school. An activity club can be a great way for you and your friends to combine socializing with physical activity. If you're thinking about starting a club, check with your school's activity coordinator first.

  - **Be sensitive to people with special needs.** Some people need certain accommodations or modifications when performing physical activity. People with no special needs can help by participating with those who do have special challenges and by being sensitive to their needs.

  - **Be considerate of differences.** The popularity of physical activities varies from culture to culture. What is popular in one culture is not necessarily popular in another. For example, field hockey and curling are not popular in the United States but are very popular in other countries. Similarly, what one person enjoys may not be so enjoyable to another. Learning to accept cultural and personal differences helps all people enjoy activity and contributes to better interpersonal understanding.

You've learned how to prepare a physical activity plan and have already done some planning for certain types of activity included in the Physical Activity Pyramid. Now you'll prepare a comprehensive written plan for personal physical activity that includes many types of physical activity. You will not be able to perform your full program in class, but you can start trying it out in class. **Take action** by performing one day of your personal physical activity plan in class. Choose a day from your program that includes enough activities to fill a full class period. If no single day's activities last as long as one class period, supplement your program for that day with activity planned for another day. If needed equipment is not available for your chosen activity, select a different activity that offers similar benefits and is one that you're likely to enjoy.

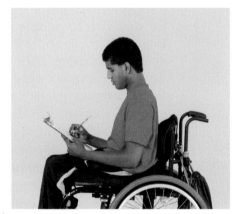

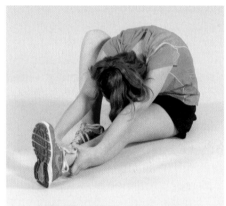

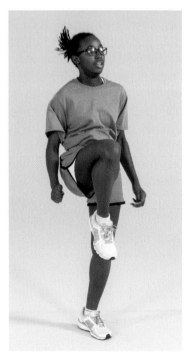

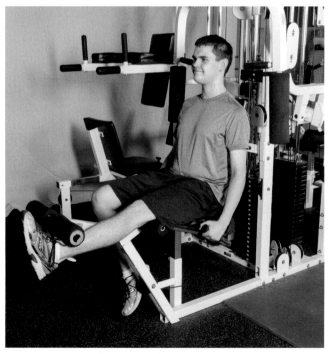

**Take action by performing your physical activity plan.**

# CHAPTER REVIEW

## Reviewing Concepts and Vocabulary

As directed by your teacher, answer items 1 through 5 by correctly completing each sentence with a word or phrase.

1. A _____ is a brief summary of your fitness self-assessment results.
2. _____ is an acronym used to characterize good goals for your program.
3. A device that can be used in the water to monitor physical activity is called a _____.
4. A self-management skill that helps you see where you are and what you need to change is called _____.
5. A/An _____ refers to how you feel about something.

For items 6 through 10, as directed by your teacher, match each term in column 1 with the appropriate word or phrase in column 2.

6. Stage of change 1 for physical activity
7. Stage of change 2 for physical activity
8. Stage of change 3 for physical activity
9. Stage of change 4 for physical activity
10. Stage of change 5 for physical activity

a. sometimes active
b. sedentary
c. thinking about it
d. maintenance
e. planner

For items 11 through 15, as directed by your teacher, respond to each statement or question.

11. Explain why constructing a fitness profile is an important part of collecting information for program planning.
12. Explain the link between academic performance and regular physical activity.
13. Describe the steps in preparing a personal physical fitness test battery.
14. Describe some of the most common positive attitudes about physical activity.
15. Describe several guidelines for turning negative attitudes into positive attitudes.

## Thinking Critically

Write a paragraph to answer the following question.

Why is it important to develop your own fitness program and not just use one developed for someone else?

## Project

Fitnessgram is the national youth fitness test for the President's Youth Fitness Program. Many of the self-assessments you performed in this book are derived from Fitnessgram.

Build a fitness profile by summarizing your results on all of the Fitnessgram self-assessments. Use the worksheet provided by your teacher or enter your results on the Fitnessgram website (your school must be enrolled for you to use the site). If you choose, you can share your fitness profile with your parents or guardians. You may also want to encourage them to perform health-related fitness assessments of their own.

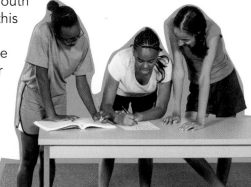

# 15

# Making Good Consumer Choices

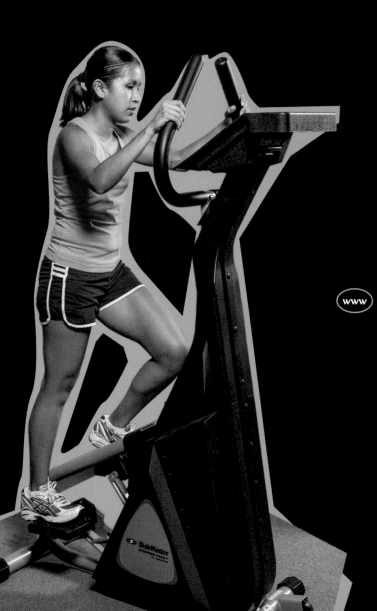

### In This Chapter

**LESSON 15.1**
Health and Fitness Quackery

**SELF-ASSESSMENT**
Assessing Your Posture

**LESSON 15.2**
Evaluating Health Clubs, Equipment, Media, and Internet Materials

**TAKING CHARGE**
Learning to Think Critically

**SELF-MANAGEMENT**
Skills for Thinking Critically

**TAKING ACTION**
My Health and Fitness Club

**www Student Web Resources**
www.fitnessforlife.org/student

# Lesson 15.1

## Health and Fitness Quackery

**Lesson Objectives**

After reading this lesson, you should be able to

1. explain the difference between quackery and fraud;
2. explain the importance of being an informed consumer in the area of fitness, health, and wellness;
3. name some reliable sources of health- and fitness-related information; and
4. describe some examples of health and fitness misconceptions and quackery.

**Lesson Vocabulary**

con artist, electrolyte, fraud, passive exercise, quack, quackery

**You've** probably come across ads for health and fitness products and services in newspapers and magazines and on radio, television, and the web. Is a product or service effective simply because it is advertised? Would you buy the product advertised in figure 15.1? In this lesson, you'll learn how to become a wise consumer (purchaser) of health and fitness products.

### What Is Quackery?

Some people are in a hurry to lose body fat or gain muscle. Often, people who want quick results are persuaded to purchase useless health or fitness products or services. In other words, they become victims of **quackery**—a method of advertising or selling that uses false claims to lure people into buying products that are worthless or even harmful. Some people who practice quackery actually believe their products work; thus they may have good intentions but still do harm. A person who practices quackery is sometimes referred to as a **quack**.

Some people who practice quackery are guilty of **fraud**. People who practice fraud try to deceive you and get you to buy products or services that they *know* are ineffective or harmful. A person who practices fraud is called a **con artist**. Because what they do is often illegal, con artists may be convicted of a crime.

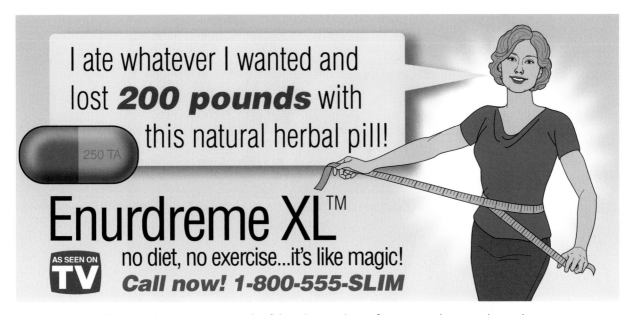

**FIGURE 15.1** Some advertisements make false claims about fitness products and supplements.

The common saying, "If it seems too good to be true, it's probably untrue!" cautions buyers that con artists are good at making you believe they're offering you a good deal. But deals that seem exceptionally good are often not as good as the con artist makes them seem.

> " Modern health quacks are super-salesmen. They play on fear. They cater to hope. And once they have you, they'll keep you coming back for more . . . and more . . . and more. "
>
> —Stephen Barrett and William T. Jarvis of the Quackwatch website

# Detecting Quackery and Fraud

People who commit quackery and fraud use a variety of deceptive practices to get you to buy their products or services or use products they endorse. Separating fact from fiction can be difficult. Use the guidelines presented in the following sections to help you spot health and fitness quackery and fraud.

## Check Credentials

Be sure that the person you think is an expert really is an expert. A con artist might claim to be a doctor or to have a college or university degree. However, the degree might be in a subject unrelated to health and physical fitness. It might also come from a nonaccredited school; it might even be falsified. You can verify credentials by checking with your local or state health authorities or with professional organizations.

If you have questions about health or fitness, ask a real expert's advice. For example, physical education teachers have a college degree that requires them to study all branches of kinesiology. Some other fitness leaders are certified by a group such as the American College of Sports Medicine. For medical advice, talk to a physician (MD or DO) or a registered nurse (RN). For questions about general health, ask a certified health education teacher. For questions about using exercise to rehabilitate from injury, consult a registered physical therapist (RPT). All of these experts have college degrees and relevant training in their area of specialization.

For questions about diet, food, and nutrition, consult a registered dietitian (RD). Be aware that a person who uses the title of nutritionist is not necessarily an expert. Similarly, staff members in health clubs are often not required to hold college degrees. Practitioners certified by a well-respected organization are more qualified than those without certification, but certification without a degree is not adequate to be considered an expert. Neither nutritionists nor health club employees are considered

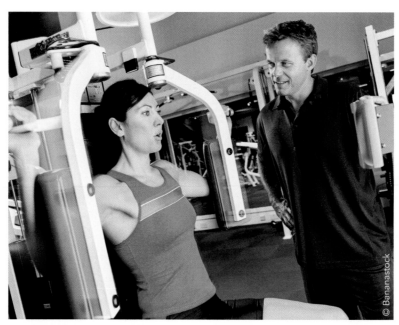

© Bananastock

Check credentials to make sure that "experts" are really experts.

reliable sources of health or fitness information unless they hold the credentials described here.

## FIT FACT

*Caveat emptor* is a Latin phrase that means "let the buyer beware." People who commit fraud make promises that they know they cannot or will not keep, and buyers must beware of people trying to sell fraudulent products. However, if a seller makes a promise (warranty) for a product, it must be fulfilled.

## Check the Organizations of the Experts You Consult

Quacks and con artists sometimes try to get you to believe that they know more than experts from well-known organizations such as those listed in the Consumer Corner feature. Be wary of people who claim they know more than well-known experts or who try to discredit respected organizations.

Quacks and con artists also use names and initials of phony organizations with important-sounding names that are similar to the names of well-known organizations. But anyone can form an organization and use it to try to impress you. Check the background of anyone who claims to be a member of an organization whose name you've never heard.

As a consumer, you need to be informed about the products and services you use. Do not assume that every advertised product is safe and effective.

Corporations do not always live up to their claims for their products. For example, the Federal Trade Commission (FTC) recently stopped two famous shoe companies from making untrue claims (for details, see the relevant Fit Fact in the second lesson of this chapter). In another example, a study by the American Council on Exercise found so-called "hologram bracelets," commonly worn by many famous athletes, to be ineffective. The bracelets' maker falsely claimed that they improved fitness in areas such as strength, flexibility, and balance.

So remember: The fact that a famous person uses a product does not mean that it is safe or effective. Agencies such as the ones named in the Consumer Corner feature can provide accurate information, but they do not police all products. In many cases, *you* are the one who has to make the final decision about buying a product or service. Being informed can help you stay safe and avoid spending money on worthless products.

# Guidelines for Preventing Quackery and Fraud

Consider the following guidelines before purchasing a product or service.

## Be Wary of Advisors Who Sell Products

People who sell products make money by selling them, and salespeople often have little training in

## CONSUMER CORNER: Reliable Consumer Groups

Many organizations work to protect consumers from misleading advertising and quackery. U.S. governmental agencies that do this type of work include the Centers for Disease Control and Prevention, the Consumer Product Safety Commission, the Federal Trade Commission, the Food and Drug Administration, the Department of Agriculture, and the U.S. Postal Service. Some reputable private organizations include the Society of Health and Physical Educators, the American College of Sports Medicine, the American Medical Association, the American

Dental Association, the Academy of Nutrition and Dietetics, the Better Business Bureau, Consumer Reports, the Cooper Institute, the Mayo Clinic, and the National Council Against Health Fraud.

The groups listed here maintain websites that provide reliable health information. However, some other popular websites are unreliable. As a consumer, you need to be able to accurately evaluate potential sources of health and fitness information, as well as the quality of products and services offered for purchase.

health, fitness, and wellness. For example, people who sell exercise equipment or food supplements may know less about their products than their customers do. In addition, salespeople are often willing to stretch the truth in order to make a sale. With this in mind, consult a true expert before you make a purchase.

## Be Suspicious of Sales Pitches That Promise Results Too Good to Be True

Look for words and phrases such as *miracle*, *secret remedy*, *scientific breakthrough*, and *endorsed by movie stars*. A quack or con artist is likely to use these or similar terms in a sales pitch for an item that is useless. Be suspicious if a salesperson promises immediate, effortless, or guaranteed results.

## Be Cautious About Mail-Order and Internet Sales

You cannot examine mail-order and Internet-marketed products before buying them. Money-back guarantees may seem to protect you, but a guarantee is only as good as the company that backs it. Unlike a brick-and-mortar store, where you can take a product back and talk to someone in person, mail-order and Internet-based companies may not offer this opportunity. Some have staff members to help you with returns and questions, but many do not. Some also require you to pay return mail costs. Before buying from any source, know the company's return policy. Internet-based companies are usually rated for reliability and quality of service, and you should check a company's rating before buying from it.

 ## SCIENCE IN ACTION: Sport and Energy Drinks

Exercise physiologists, dietitians, and medical scientists work together to investigate heat-related conditions that can result from physical activity, especially during hot weather. In fact, regardless of the weather, you need to keep your body hydrated during exercise to prevent conditions such as heat stress and heatstroke. To replenish the body, researchers have developed flavored "sport drinks" that contain important minerals called **electrolytes**. When appropriate ingredients are used, these drinks can help adults keep their body hydrated during exercise. "Energy drinks" are also popular, but they are not intended primarily to replace fluids lost during exercise. They may contain ingredients similar to those in sport drinks, but they often also contain large amounts of sugar and relatively large amounts of caffeine.

The American Academy of Pediatrics (AAP) has expressed concern about sport and energy drinks because they are often marketed to children and teens via TV, magazines, and the web. The AAP discourages use of these drinks by children and teens and notes that high-caffeine energy drinks have "no place in the diet of children and adolescents." The group further states that sugars in these drinks may be linked to increases in

weight and even obesity. The AAP indicate that sport drinks (not energy drinks with caffeine) can be helpful to young athletes who are engaged in "prolonged, vigorous physical activity, but in most cases they are unnecessary on the sport field or in the school lunch room." For most teens who perform the amount of activity recommended by national guidelines, plain water is best.

A separate group of medical doctors has asked the U.S. Food and Drug Administration (FDA) to restrict the amount of caffeine in energy drinks to protect youth from medical problems. Indeed, each year more than 20,000 ER visits involve health problems in which energy drink consumption was a contributing factor. Common problems caused by too much caffeine include fast heart rate, inability to sleep, stomach upset, anxiety, and headache. The FDA has issued warnings indicating that mixing alcohol and caffeine is especially dangerous.

### Student Activity

Research a sport or energy drink. Find out about its key ingredients and prepare a report about the possible benefits and dangers associated with the drink.

## Be Wary of Product Claims

A favorite trick of some con artists is to claim that a product is "brand new" or is just now being offered for the first time. Others may claim to be "available in the United States for the first time." They try to make you think that you're getting something special. Quacks and con artists may also try to get you to believe their product is popular in Europe, Asia, or some other location. This technique is usually used to impress you. It does not provide any useful information.

## Be Wary of Untested Products

Using untested products can be risky. Quacks do not subject their products to thorough scientific testing. Their products are often rushed to market in order to make money as quickly as possible. One way to tell whether a product or service is a good one is to see whether information about it has been published in a respected journal. If so, the study was conducted by a qualified expert.

# Health Quackery

The market is flooded with health products, many of which are useless. Although some of these products may not be harmful, false advertising claims give people unrealistic expectations about the benefits they can provide. Indeed, many advertisers promote myths about health and fitness.

## FIT FACT

*Cellulite* is a term often used for fat that causes the skin to look rippled or bumpy. Con artists would have you believe that cellulite is a special kind of fat that can be eliminated with creams or other special products. In fact, cellulite occurs when fat cells become enlarged. It is best reduced by expending more calories than you consume.

## Food Supplements

A food supplement is a product that is not part of the typical diet. Supplements are often produced as syrups, powders, or tablets (figure 15.2). Generally, they are sold in health food stores or through the mail. Common supplements include protein (amino acids), vitamins, minerals, and herbs. Packaged food—such as canned goods, boxed goods, and frozen foods—must carry a label that informs you of the product's ingredients. Such labels are *not* required on food supplements.

Most Americans believe that food supplements are regulated by the government in the same way as drugs and foods. This is not true. A law passed in 1994 changed the regulation of supplements from government control to manufacturer control. Manufacturers do not have to prove that a supplement works before they sell it, and the law does not regulate the contents of a supplement. For

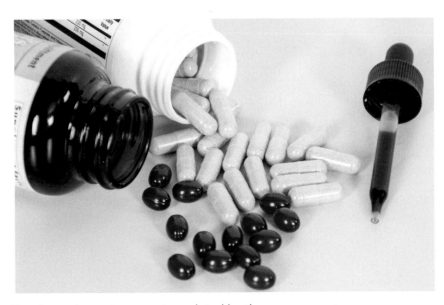

**FIGURE 15.2** Food supplements are not regulated by the government.

this reason, you cannot be sure that you're buying what you think you are buying when you purchase a supplement. More than a few people have died from taking supplements that were contaminated or contained ingredients that were not supposed to be in the supplement. Many people have also suffered illness and even death as the result of taking supplements marketed as causing fat loss or enhancing performance. While food supplements are not regulated, the FDA will investigate if enough complaints are received for a specific supplement. The supplement ephedra, for example, has been implicated in several deaths. After an FDA investigation, ephedra was banned by the U.S. Food and Drug Administration.

Some other supplements are not harmful but simply do not provide the benefits promised by those who sell them. Since the regulation of supplements was changed in 1994, the sale of supplements has increased dramatically. Many people are wasting money on products that don't work.

Some supplements can be beneficial if used according to a physician's recommendation. For example, a vitamin $B_{12}$ supplement is recommended for strict vegetarians (vegans), and a folic acid supplement is recommended for expectant mothers. But even vitamins can be dangerous if taken in amounts that are too large. Before you take any supplement, consult with your parent or guardian, as well as your family physician.

## Sport Supplements

One current fad involves the use of sport supplements or sport vitamins—products sold to enhance athletic performance. These supplements are also called ergogenic aids. Many supplements sold as ergogenic aids are actually quack products. Many supplements can also be harmful to your health.

## Fad Diets

"Lose pounds a day on the ice cream diet!" "The rice diet works wonders!" "Fruit diet dissolves fat!" How many similar weight-loss claims have you seen? Each of these claims is false and serves as an example of a fad diet. Although fad diets are popular because they usually promise fast results, nearly all are nutritionally unbalanced. They often restrict eating to only one or two food groups, or even one specific food. As you've learned, the only safe and effective way to reduce body fatness and lose weight is to combine physical activity with eating fewer calories. Eating healthy, low-calorie foods can help you control your calorie intake.

## Restricting Fluids

It is possible to lose weight in a short time as a result of dehydration. If you do not drink enough fluid, or if you lose excessive water through sweating, you will become dehydrated, thus losing water weight. Some people think this weight loss is permanent. It is not! Restricting fluid intake and taking products that cause water loss do *not* help you lose body fat, and as soon as you replace the fluids, your weight will return to normal. In addition, these practices can be dangerous to your health. Dehydration can lead to physical problems such as headache and fatigue, mental problems such as lack of concentration and mood changes, and heat illnesses such as heat exhaustion and heatstroke.

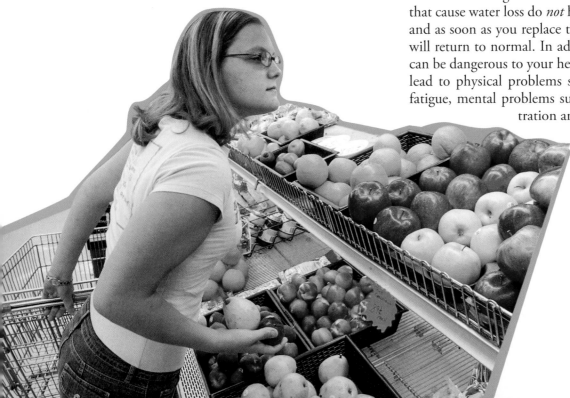

**FITNESS TECHNOLOGY: Quack Machines**

You've learned in other chapters about many technological innovations that can make our lives better. However, not all technological devices are safe and effective. Some unscrupulous people sell devices that not only are ineffective but also can be quite dangerous.

One example is a device with electrodes that are placed on the abdominal muscles. Electrical current is sent through the electrodes, thus stimulating the muscles. People who advertise these devices claim that you can use them to build strong abdominal muscles without doing any regular abdominal exercises, such as crunches or curl-ups. But studies show that these devices do not build fitness. In addition, because the electrodes are placed on the abdomen, they can cause the heart to beat irregularly and result in serious health problems.

Physical therapists do use muscle stimulators to help restore normal muscle function in people who have been injured or who are recovering from illness. These machines can be effective when used by experts for very specific therapeutic purposes. They are not the same as muscle stimulators sold with claims of building abdominal muscle. Be wary of sellers who promise fitness without exercise.

---

**Using Technology**

Check with a physical therapist to see how a muscle stimulator works and how it helps people with injury or illness. Also ask for more information about the dangers of using an abdominal muscle stimulator.

---

## Fitness Quackery

Many useless products claim to improve fitness and reduce body fat. Claims for these products are false. Be alert for the following worthless fitness devices and methods.

### Passive Exercise Machines

**Passive exercise** refers to the use of machines or devices that move your body for you and supposedly promote fat reduction and weight loss. Examples include machines with rollers that roll along your hips or legs; vibrating machines that shake certain body areas and are said to "break up" fat cells; and motorized belts, cycles, tables, and rowing machines. The claims made for these products are false. These passive exercise programs are ineffective because your body is moved by outside forces rather than your own muscles.

### Figure Wrapping

Figure wrapping involves the use of bandages or nonporous garments to compress body parts. The wraps are sometimes soaked in fluid, or the person may soak in a bath after being wrapped. The wraps are advertised for weight loss or as a method of losing "inches" from the body. In reality, they are not effective for either fat loss or size reduction. They can, however, cause overheating and dehydration and can be extremely dangerous to your health.

An unqualified fitness instructor might recommend that you perform "spot" fat loss exercises. Those who promote spot fat loss claim that fat can be removed from specific spots in the body by performing exercises in a specific location. Research shows, however, that no type of exercise causes fat loss at one specific location.

**Lesson Review**

1. What are quackery and fraud, and how do they differ?
2. Why is it important to be an informed consumer in the area of fitness, health, and wellness?
3. What are some of the more reliable sources of health-related and fitness-related information?
4. What are some examples of health and fitness misconceptions and quackery?

# SELF-ASSESSMENT: Assessing Your Posture

Assessing your posture can help you achieve and maintain good posture and prevent problems that could make you susceptible to quackery.

You can use the following self-assessment to determine whether your posture is as good as it should be. If you find that improvements are needed, you can work at applying proper biomechanics when sitting, standing, and walking.

For this self-assessment, wear exercise clothing or a swimsuit. Work with a partner to determine each other's scores. Record your results as directed by your instructor.

1. Stand sideways next to a string hanging from a point at least 12 inches (30 centimeters) above your head. The string should be weighted at the bottom so that it hangs straight and reaches nearly to the floor. Position yourself so that the string aligns with the side of your ankle bone.
   - Head: Is the ear in front of the line?

- Shoulders: Are the shoulders rounded? Are the tips of the shoulders in front of the chest?
- Upper back: Does the upper back stick out in a hump?
- Lower back: Does the lower back have excessive arch?
- Abdomen: Does the abdomen protrude beyond the pelvic bone?
- Knees: Do the knees appear to be locked or bent backward?

2. Now stand with your back to the string so that the string is aligned with the middle of your back.
   - Head: Is more than half of the head on one side of the string?
   - Shoulders: Is one shoulder higher than the other?
   - Hips: Is one hip higher than the other?

3. Add the number of yes answers to get a total score. Then determine your rating on table 15.1.

**TABLE 15.1 Rating Chart: Posture Test**

| Score (yes answers) | Rating |
|---|---|
| 0 or 1 | Good posture |
| 2–4 | Can use some improvement |
| ≥5 | Needs considerable improvement |

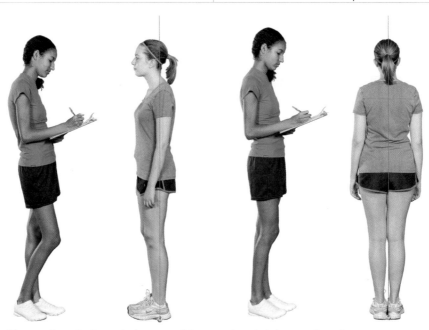

**The posture test can help you achieve and maintain good posture.**

# Lesson 15.2

# Evaluating Health Clubs, Equipment, Media, and Internet Materials

## Lesson Objectives

After reading this lesson, you should be able to

1. evaluate health-related and fitness-related facilities,
2. describe the proper clothing and equipment for physical activity,
3. evaluate printed materials and video resources related to health and fitness, and
4. describe the guidelines for choosing a good website for health and fitness information.

## Lesson Vocabulary

spa, web extension

**Where** do you get your health, fitness, and wellness information? Have you ever considered how that information is created? People in developed countries are more interested in health and fitness now than at any other time in history, and they look to many sources to get it. As a result, many magazines are now totally dedicated to health and fitness, but the leading source of health information throughout the world is the web. In fact, there has been an explosion of health and fitness information, but not all of it is accurate. In this lesson, you'll learn how to evaluate printed material and web resources. First, however, you will learn about health and fitness clubs, where many people seek information delivered in person, as well as exercise clothing and equipment.

## Evaluating Health Clubs

You do not need to join a health club, **spa**, or gym to attain or maintain fitness. Health clubs do offer their members special equipment and personnel, and modern spas offer saunas, whirlpool baths, and other services such as massage and hair and skin care. In addition, some people find that joining a club helps motivate them to exercise and remain physically active. But these services are expensive, and well-educated people can save money and still get the benefits of regular exercise by designing their own fitness and activity programs without using special facilities or equipment.

Many low-cost programs are offered through community centers, universities, churches, and other groups. In addition, your school may be among the many that have built their own fitness centers, sometimes called wellness centers. Such programs can give you the same benefits and motivation as more expensive clubs. Still, if you feel that it would help you stay active, you may be interested in joining a commercial club, spa, or gym at some point. Some schools have made cooperative arrangements with fitness clubs that allow their students to work out at special rates or allow school classes to use club facilities. Use the following guidelines when deciding whether to join a health club.

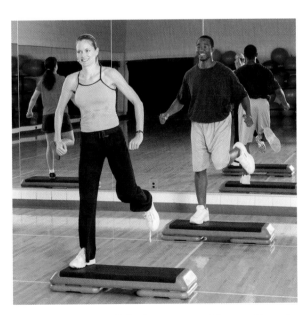

When choosing a club, be sure to pick a well-established club that includes activities you enjoy.

• **If possible, join on a pay-as-you-go basis.** If you sign a contract, make it a short-term one. Read the fine print carefully. Do not sign a contract right away. Too often, people pay a lot for a long-term contract, then stop using the facility. It's best to pay for a short membership until you're sure that you'll stick with it. The fine print may contain special clauses that will cost you money. For example, do you still have to pay if you move? Often, the salesperson pressures you to sign a contract on your first visit, but it's best to think about it for a while before signing.

• **Choose a well-established club.** Such a club is less likely to go out of business. Make sure the facility employs qualified fitness experts such as those described in this chapter. Be alert for signs of fitness quackery; if you see them, consider choosing a different club.

• **Make a trial visit to the club.** Visit at a time when you would normally use the club. Make sure you feel comfortable with the employees and other patrons. Also make sure that the equipment and facilities are available for you to use at that time.

• **Choose a club that meets your personal needs.** For example, a person with joint pain might prefer to avoid harsher activities such as jogging and decide instead to swim for cardiorespiratory endurance. Such a person, of course, should choose a facility that includes a swimming pool.

• **Avoid clubs that cater primarily to bodybuilding for adults.** Research shows that clubs frequented mostly by adults interested in bodybuilding are more likely to sell unproven supplements and even illegal products. Some people who frequent these places subscribe to their own theories and reject scientific evidence developed by experts. Furthermore, practices that may be acceptable for adults are often not appropriate for teens. Find a club that is appropriate for families and teens and employs qualified experts on its staff. Avoid advice from so-called experts with theories that are not consistent with the information provided in this book.

• **Consider any medical needs.** If weight loss is your primary goal, consider joining a program recommended by your physician or sponsored by a hospital rather than joining a health club. If you have a special medical need, you may need the help of a physical therapist.

## FIT FACT

The U.S. Federal Trade Commission (FTC) reached settlements with two major shoe companies after it was determined that they deceived consumers with their advertisements. The FTC required Reebok and Skechers to refund money to customers because of unsupported claims. Reebok made unsupported claims for its "toning shoes," and Skechers made unsupported claims for its "shape-up" and "tone-up" shoes.

## Exercise Equipment

Some people choose not to join a club but to buy home exercise equipment instead. If you're considering home exercise equipment, use the following guidelines.

• **Consider inexpensive home equipment.** For resistance exercise, you can use homemade weights, inner tubes, or rubber or latex bands. To build cardiorespiratory endurance, you can use jump ropes, stepping benches, or stairs. If you're interested in fitness for health and wellness, this equipment may be all you need.

• **Consider your personal needs before buying equipment.** If you're interested in a higher level of fitness for sport or a high-performance job, you might choose to purchase machines or other equipment for use at home. For building muscle fitness, you can use free weights and home exercise machines. For cardiorespiratory endurance, you can use home exercise machines such as treadmills, bicycles, and stair steppers. A regular bicycle is also a good choice if you have a safe place to ride. Exercise equipment is often quite expensive, so it's important to choose well. Rather than depending on the advice of a salesperson, consult an expert, the website of the American College of Sports Medicine, or Consumer Reports. Buy from a well-established company that honors the warranty, services the product, and sells replacement parts.

• **Be sure before you buy.** Avoid investing money in exercise equipment until you're sure you'll use it. Many people buy equipment, then don't use it after the first few months. You can see evidence of this behavior in the many ads for slightly used equipment. Some of the high-tech equipment described in this book, such as pedometers and heart rate watches, can be useful. However, some equipment can be quite expensive, and you may find that you won't use it regularly. See if you can try equipment owned by a friend or by your school before deciding to buy the product. In addition, some high-tech products simply are not worth the cost. For example, expensive electrical devices for measuring body fat level are not worth the personal investment when an inexpensive caliper can give you accurate fat measurements.

• **Make sure you have enough space for the equipment.** One of the main reasons people fail to use the exercise equipment they buy is that they don't have a good place to keep it. If you have to get the equipment out each time you use it or move it from place to place, you're less likely to use it than if you have a room or a place where you can set it up permanently.

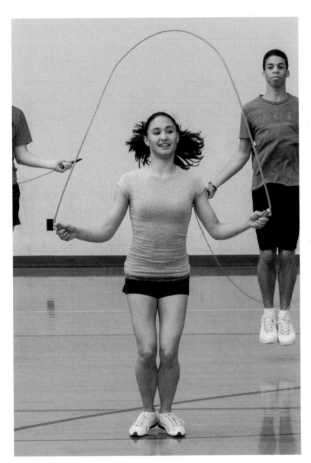

Equipment does not need to be expensive to be helpful in promoting fitness.

> " Spending money is easy. Spending money wisely is another thing altogether. "
>
> —U.S. Federal Trade Commission

## Evaluating Books and Articles

The growing emphasis on health and fitness has led to the publication of many books and articles on weight control and exercise. Unfortunately, much of the information presented through the media is misleading or incorrect. How can you evaluate health and fitness information that you read, view, or hear? Use the following guidelines to help you decide which information sources are worthwhile.

• **Consider the author's credentials.** The author or consultant should be a registered dietitian, should have completed advanced study in nutrition, or should hold an advanced degree in an exercise-related field such as exercise science, kinesiology, or physical education.

• **Check for sound information.** The book or article should provide information about a balanced diet and physical activity that is consistent with the information presented in this book. Books that promise quick and easy fitness or fat loss are not good sources. The information in the book or article should not support techniques used by quacks and con artists (see the first lesson in this chapter). Exercise discussions should address the principles of overload, progression, and specificity, in addition to the FIT formula for each type of physical fitness.

• **Recommended exercises should be safe and effective.** The exercises should require you to use your own muscles (they should not recommend effortless devices). Make sure that the exercises are performed with proper biomechanics.

## Evaluating Exercise Videos

You've probably noticed exercise videos for sale and television shows featuring exercises you can perform. Exercise videos are also available for web viewing. Use the following guidelines to help you evaluate an exercise video or show.

• **Check the creator's credentials.** The creator is the person who prepares the exercises, which may then be performed by someone other than the creator. Check to see that the creator has a degree or certification from a reputable institution or organization. Check to see that the person performing the exercises is doing them properly.

• **Choose a video that includes appropriate warm-up and cool-down exercises.** The warm-up and cool-down should be consistent with guidelines provided in this book.

• **Make sure the video contains only safe exercises.** This book provides you with information about safe exercises, as well as dangerous exercises to avoid.

• **Choose a video that rotates muscle groups and addresses all parts of fitness.** For example, use arms, then legs, then back, then abdominal muscles, and so on. If the video claims to be a total fitness program, make sure it includes activities for all parts of fitness and rotates them appropriately.

• **Choose a video that is appropriate for you.** Make sure that the activities on the video are appropriate for your skill and fitness level. For example, if it says it is for beginners, are the exercises really for beginners?

• **Make sure the exercises start gradually and progress in intensity.** If the first part of the exercise program is moderate in intensity, it may serve as the warm-up.

• **Choose a video with a fun and interesting routine.** Review the video to see if it includes exercises that you would enjoy doing on a regular basis.

• **If the video does not meet all of these guidelines, modify it.** For example, change the order of the routine to make it better.

# Evaluating Internet Resources

We depend on the web more than any other source for health and fitness information. Yet research shows that many web sources provide incorrect information. If you use the web to locate information about health, fitness, and wellness, ask yourself the following questions.

• **Who developed the website?** Websites with the best information are developed by government agencies, professional organizations, and educational institutions. Governmental health agencies' web addresses end with .gov, professional organizations' web addresses end with .org, and education institutions' web addresses end with .edu. Choose websites presented by well-known agencies, organizations, and institutions such as those listed in the Consumer Corner feature in this chapter or the student section of the Fitness for Life website. Sites with an address ending in .gov, .org, or .edu often provide you with more reliable information

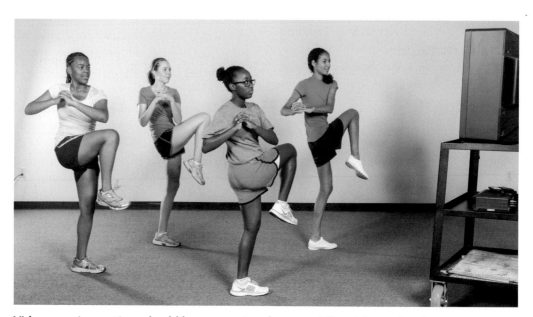

Video exercise routines should be appropriate for your skill and fitness level.

than sites with an address ending in .com or .net. Remember, however, that any organization can now obtain a .org web address, so that alone does not guarantee that the information on the site is reliable. At the same time, some websites with an address ending in .com or .net do provide good information.

• **Did you reach the website you intended to reach?** In 2013, the Internet Corporation for Assigned Names and Numbers was authorized to offer new **web extensions** (web address endings). As a result, extensions other than the most common ones (.gov, .org, and .com) are now available. Some examples of the newer extensions are .book, .movie, and .app. These are only a few of the 2,000 new extensions that will ultimately be developed. This variety makes it even more difficult to know which websites offer good information. An unscrupulous company may use a web address similar to that of a legitimate company but with a different extension. For example, the website for Fitness for Life is www.fitnessforlife.org, and another organization could set up a site with a similar address but a different extension (for example, www.fitnessforlife.xyz) and thus pretend to be the Fitness for Life website. Some quacks or con artists use websites with names very similar to legitimate ones in hopes that some people will reach them by accident if they type the intended web address incorrectly. Make sure that you avoid errors when typing health-related web addresses. For more information about good web sources for health and fitness, visit the student section of the Fitness for Life website.

• **Is the web article a research document, or is it really an advertisement?** The U.S. Federal Trade Commission has cracked down on companies that post web articles falsely appearing to be scientific research. These "fake news" articles are really advertisements. They are not based on real science, and they advertise products that do not work as claimed. Examples include dietary supplements, products that supposedly provide fitness without exercise, and weight loss products. Several compa-

## FIT FACT

Be wary of advertisements for lotions or creams to improve muscle tone. *Tone* is a term created by advertisers and cannot be easily measured. For this reason, it's easy to claim that creams or lotions can improve tone, but it's very hard to prove. There are no creams or lotions that can improve muscle fitness as measured by legitimate tests of muscle fitness. Place your trust in experts who help you build muscle fitness using sound exercises programs rather than quack products.

nies have paid fines for deceptive practices and have been banned from mounting future promotions. Unfortunately, such companies often make a lot of money before they are caught, and the fines they pay are much smaller than their profits. In light of these practices, you need to make sure that you use information from reliable news sources and scientific journals rather than the fake news articles that often appear in ads and pop-up screens on your computer. You can also visit the FTC's website to see which companies have been caught posting fake news.

To reduce your chances of being deceived by a website, ask yourself the following questions.

• **Does the website sell products?** Websites that sell products are more likely to provide false information than those that do not.

• **Do you recognize any techniques that seem suspicious?** Be wary of websites using the techniques associated with quacks and con artists as described in this chapter.

• **Do experts find the website credible?**  The site should be recommended or highly regarded by genuine health and fitness experts.

## Lesson Review

1. What are some guidelines for evaluating health and fitness clubs?
2. What should you consider before buying exercise equipment?
3. What are the guidelines for evaluating exercise videos and books and articles about health and fitness?
4. What are the guidelines for choosing a good website for health and fitness information?

# ⚡ TAKING CHARGE: Learning to Think Critically

A misconception is a belief based on incorrect or misunderstood information or lack of facts. The best way to counter a misconception is to increase your knowledge so that you can recognize and interpret facts correctly. Here's an example.

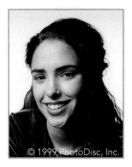

© 1999 PhotoDisc, Inc.

Mary Lou had tried several exercise programs but had not found one that she felt would help her meet her goal of developing muscle fitness. She had never even considered progressive resistance exercise (PRE) because she believed it would cause her to develop big, bulky muscles.

One day, Mary Lou's physical education teacher took her class to the fitness room. There, the teacher explained how to use the free weights and resistance machines for the best benefit. Over the next several weeks, the class practiced the correct use of the PRE equipment. As a class assignment, Mary Lou's teacher had each member of the class find one news article about PRE and write a report on it. In doing her report, Mary Lou learned that muscles do not become bulky if weight training is done properly.

With this new knowledge, Mary Lou realized that the correct PRE program would give her exactly what she was looking for. She began working out with PRE on three days each week. The knowledge she gained about PRE dispelled her original misconceptions. Now Mary Lou is trying to help others change their irrational beliefs about PRE. When friends ask her why she is trying to build big muscles, she tells them, "If muscle fitness is what you're after, you should give resistance training a try."

## For Discussion

What misconception did Mary Lou have? How was she able to build knowledge to dispel her misconception? What are some other misconceptions people have about physical activity? Why do you think people have misconceptions about PRE? Consider the guidelines provided in the Self-Management feature when answering the discussion questions.

# ➡ SELF-MANAGEMENT: Skills for Thinking Critically

Thinking critically means using a problem-solving process before making important decisions. You can use several steps to solve problems and make good choices. These steps are similar to those used in applying the scientific method. The steps are listed here with examples for using each one to help you select exercise equipment. You can use the same steps to solve problems and make decisions about other important topics.

- **Step 1: Identify the problem to be solved or clarify the decision that must be made.** If you know that you want to improve your muscle fitness but are not sure how to do it, you have to define the problem more clearly. Do you want to do your exercises at school, join a health and fitness club, buy exercise equipment, or use inexpensive equipment? You also need to clarify your reasons for

wanting to build muscle fitness. Do you want to improve your health, improve your appearance, or get fit for sport performance? For this discussion, let's assume that you want to decide what equipment to use in order to build your muscle fitness for good health. Thus the problem has been clearly defined.

- **Step 2: Collect information and investigate.** One way to collect information relevant to the defined problem is to perform self-assessments for muscle fitness. Knowing your current status will help you to know about areas of personal need so that you can select exercises to meet your needs. You can also consult experts and explore reliable websites, such as those described in this chapter's Consumer Corner feature or in the student section of the Fitness for Life website. In this case, you would also want to try out several equipment options, perhaps by using the school exercise room, visiting local health and fitness clubs, or trying out machines on display at a sporting goods store. You could also try several of the inexpensive equipment options you've learned about in this book. Focus on finding information that will help you solve the specific problem you've identified in step 1.

- **Step 3: Develop a plan of action.** Use the information gained from your investigation to formulate a plan. For example, your results from step 2 might indicate that the school exercise room is not open when you are free to use it, and perhaps the health and fitness clubs are too far from your home and cost too much. In addition, exercise equipment available in stores can be quite expensive. After rejecting these options, then, you might decide to do elastic band exercises. The equipment is inexpensive, and you can do all the exercises necessary to meet

your goal. You might decide to choose several of the exercises described in this book. You could then make a written plan specifying the days of the week on which you'll do each exercise and how many sets and reps you'll do each day.

- **Step 4. Put your plan into action.** For a plan to be effective, you must use it. The sooner you begin to act after preparing your plan, the more likely you are to change your behavior. In this example, you would use the plan developed in step 3 to get started with the elastic band exercises.

- **Step 5. Evaluate the effectiveness of your plan.** Use self-monitoring to keep records and use self-assessments (reassessments) to chart your progress. As you go forward, you can continue using the five critical thinking steps presented here to solve problems that arise and make effective decisions about your health, fitness, and wellness.

## ACADEMIC CONNECTION: Critical Thinking Skills

Preparing for a career or for college requires critical thinking skills. Education experts have described learning standards for the English language arts that help you prepare. Following are some of the skills needed for success in the workplace and in college:

- **Demonstrating independence.** In addition to being able to understand ideas presented by others, independence requires a person to add to others' ideas and express his or her own thoughts and views.

- **Building strong knowledge of subject matter.** Research and study are required to develop knowledge in different subject matter areas, including health and physical education. This requires extensive reading and attentive listening.

- **Comprehending as well as knowing facts.** Knowing refers to possessing infor-

mation or facts. Comprehending refers to grasping the significance of information or facts.

- **Valuing evidence.** Evidence refers to something tangible or visible. One step in the scientific method is collecting data (tangible evidence). This evidence can be used to help make decisions or solve problems.

- **Using technology capably.** Modern technology makes a considerable amount of information available in an instant. Capable use of technology requires the ability to evaluate the quality of information acquired from online and other technical sources and the thoughtful use of that information.

Practice the self-management skills in this chapter to help you meet these important standards.

You've learned how to plan a personal physical activity program, and by now you're performing it regularly on your own. But you may also enjoy being active with others. Using school facilities and equipment, you can create your own health and fitness club for use during class time. Work with the other students in class to survey the types of activity that class members enjoy.

When putting together a workout for others, consider their current fitness, their skill levels, and their interests. Prepare several exercise stations for which equipment is available. Balance the workout so that a variety of activities are offered and all the parts of health-related fitness are addressed. Have a class member describe the purpose of each exercise station to the rest of the class in a way similar to what a fitness instructor would do at a commercial health or fitness club. **Take action** by having all class members use the health and fitness club to perform a physical activity workout that meets their personal goals. Evaluate the effectiveness of your health and fitness club.

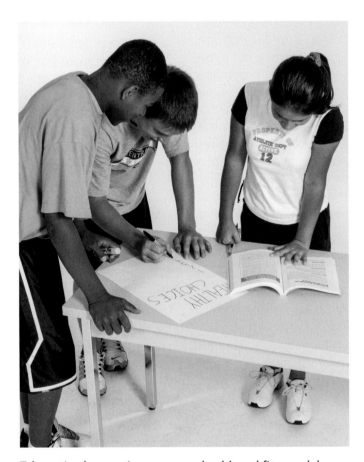

Take action by creating your own health and fitness club.

# CHAPTER REVIEW

## Reviewing Concepts and Vocabulary

As directed by your teacher, answer items 1 through 5 by correctly completing each sentence with a word or phrase.

1. A method of advertising or selling a health product or service that uses false claims is called _____.
2. Selling a health product you know to be worthless is called _____.
3. A _____ is a product added to the diet rather than being part of the regular diet.
4. _____ exercise uses machines or outside forces to move your muscles.
5. The extension .gov indicates that a website is associated with the _____.

For items 6 through 10, as directed by your teacher, match each term in column 1 with the appropriate phrase in column 2.

6. medical doctor
7. certified health education teacher
8. registered physical therapist
9. dietitian
10. nutritionist

a. may not be an expert
b. provides medical advice
c. offers advice about diet and nutrition
d. has information about exercises
e. provides general health information

For items 11 through 15, as directed by your teacher, respond to each statement or question.

11. Describe three ways to recognize quackery.
12. Describe the posture test and why it is important.
13. Describe three guidelines for selecting a fitness or health club.
14. Describe three guidelines for finding good health information on the web.
15. Describe the five steps for critical thinking that you can use to solve problems and make decisions about physical activity and good health.

## Thinking Critically

Write a paragraph to answer the following question.

Your friend Lee visited a health food store and got interested in taking a supplement. He says that he can make his own decision because the products must be safe and must work or they wouldn't be on the shelves of the store. What advice would you give your friend? Explain your reasons.

## Project

Choose one of the following: Visit a local health club, choose an article about exercise from a popular magazine, view an exercise video, or visit a health or fitness website. Use the guidelines presented in this chapter to evaluate its quality. Write a brief report of your evaluation.

# UNIT VI

# Wellness Perspective

• • • • • • • • • • • • • • • • • • • • • • •

## Healthy People 2020 Goals

- Increase consumption of fruits, vegetables, and whole grains.
- Reduce salt, saturated fat, and added sugar in the diet.
- Reduce sales of candy and sweetened beverages in schools.
- Increase the percentage of people who get adequate calcium in their daily diet.
- Increase the availability of healthy snacks.
- Increase mental health services and stress reduction programs.
- Decrease suicide and attempted suicide among teens.
- Increase the availability of treatment for depression and anxiety.
- Increase nutrition counseling and wellness check-ups.
- Increase health literacy and comprehensive school health education.
- Reduce student harassment (bullying).
- Increase recycling.
- Increase the percentage of schools with policies promoting a healthy school environment.
- Achieve high-quality, longer lives by reducing preventable disease, injury, and early death.

## Self-Assessment Features in This Unit

- Energy Balance
- Identifying Signs of Stress
- Healthy Lifestyle Questionnaire

## Taking Charge Features in This Unit

- Saying No
- Managing Competitive Stress
- Thinking Success

## Self-Management Features in This Unit

- Skills for Saying No
- Skills to Manage Competitive Stress
- Skills for Thinking Success

## Taking Action Features in This Unit

- Burn It Up Workout
- Relaxation Exercises
- Your Healthy Lifestyle Plan

# 16

# Choosing Nutritious Food

## In This Chapter

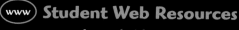
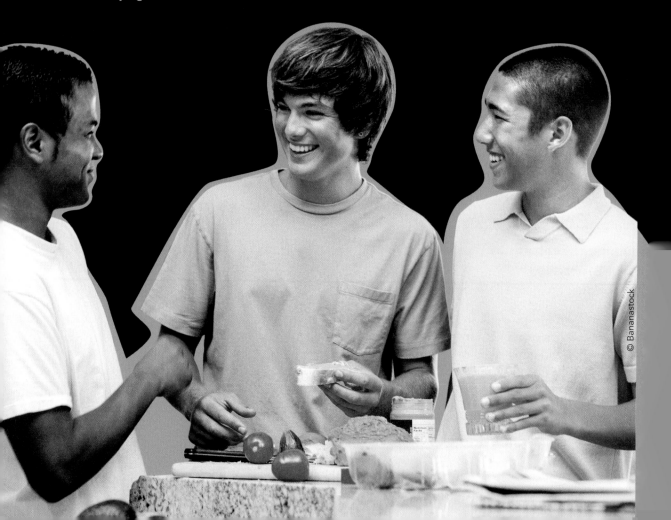

© Bananastock

# Lesson 16.1

# A Healthy Diet

## Lesson Objectives

After reading this lesson, you should be able to

1. describe the three types of nutrients that provide energy and the amount of each that is needed for good health,
2. explain why vitamins, minerals, and water are necessary for good health, and
3. describe the five food groups and explain how knowledge of these groups can help you plan for healthy eating.

## Lesson Vocabulary

Adequate Intake (AI), amino acids, basal metabolism, carbohydrate, complete protein, creeping obesity, Dietary Reference Intake (DRI), dietitian, empty calories, fat, fiber, incomplete protein, macronutrient, micronutrient, protein, Recommended Dietary Allowance (RDA), resting metabolism, saturated fat, Tolerable Upper Intake Level (UL), trans-fatty acid, unsaturated fat

**What** kinds of food are important to your health? How much food do you need to eat? In this lesson, you'll learn about healthful foods and learn how to select foods for a balanced diet.

## Nutrients Your Body Needs

Scientists have identified 45 to 50 nutrients—food substances required for the growth and maintenance of your cells. These nutrients have been divided into six groups—carbohydrate, protein, fat, vitamin, mineral, and water—each of which is discussed in this chapter.

## Nutrients That Provide Energy

Three types of nutrient supply the energy that your body needs in order to perform its daily tasks: **fat**, **carbohydrate**, and **protein**. They are referred to as **macronutrients**. Fat contains more calories than protein or carbohydrate per unit of weight. One gram of fat contains nine calories, whereas one gram of carbohydrate or protein contains four calories. The United States Department of Agriculture (USDA) and the U.S.-based Institute of Medicine recommend that most of the calories in your diet come from carbohydrate. Fewer of your calories typically come from fat and protein. Figure 16.1

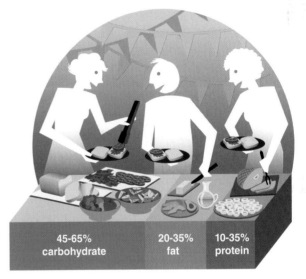

**FIGURE 16.1** Percentage of calories recommended by the Institute of Medicine's Food and Nutrition Board for carbohydrate, protein, and fat.

shows the recommended percentage of calories from each of the three types of energy-providing nutrient.

### Carbohydrate

Carbohydrate is your main source of energy, and it comes in two types: simple and complex. Simple carbohydrate includes sugars such as table sugar, fructose, and sucrose. Fructose and sucrose are commonly found in soft drinks and other sweetened foods. Simple carbohydrate provides a quick source of energy but contains few nutrients (figure 16.2*a*). Most of your carbohydrate calories should come from complex carbohydrate. Complex carbohydrate has a more complex chemical structure, so it takes longer to digest (figure 16.2*b*). It contains more nutrients than simple carbohydrate and is often rich in **fiber**. Fiber is found in foods such as whole grains and vegetables. You should minimize your intake of simple carbohydrate, although some simple carbohydrate sources are better than others. For example, bananas and oranges contain simple carbohydrate but also contain essential nutrients such as vitamins, minerals, and fiber. Foods containing simple carbohydrate—such as candy, pastry, and sugared soft drinks—contain **empty calories**, which provide energy but few if any other nutrients such as vitamins and minerals.

Fiber is a type of complex carbohydrate that your body cannot digest. It supplies no energy. Fiber sources include the leaves, stems, roots, and seed coverings of fruits, vegetables, and grains (figure 16.2*c*). Examples of foods high in fiber include whole-grain bread and cereal, the skin of fresh fruits, raw vegetables, nuts, and seeds. Fiber helps you avoid intestinal problems and might reduce your chances of developing some forms of cancer.

## Protein

Protein is the group of nutrients that builds, repairs, and maintains body cells; they are the building blocks of your body. Protein is contained in animal products (such as milk, eggs, meat, and fish) and in some plants (such as beans and grains). Protein provides energy but not as many calories as fat. If you consume more protein than is needed to build

your body tissue, the additional calories will be either used to produce energy for daily activity or stored as body fat.

During digestion, your body breaks protein down into simpler substances called **amino acids**, which your small intestine can absorb. Your body can manufacture 11 of the 20 known amino acids; you need to get the other 9—known as the essential amino acids—from food.

Foods containing all nine essential amino acids are said to provide **complete protein**. Animal sources such as meat, milk products, and fish provide complete protein. A grain called quinoa (pronounced keen' wah) and some forms of soy contain all nine essential amino acids. Quinoa can be served hot, like rice, or cold in a salad.

Foods that contain some, but not all, essential amino acids are said to contain **incomplete protein**. Examples include beans, nuts, rice, and certain other plants. You can usually get enough essential amino acids from a daily diet that includes some foods with complete protein and some with incomplete protein. People who do not eat meat need to eat a variety of foods that contain incomplete protein and, taken together, provide all the essential amino acids.

## Fat

Fat is contained in animal products and some plant products, such as nuts and vegetable oils. Fat is necessary to grow and repair your cells; it dissolves certain vitamins and carries them to your cells. In addition, fat enhances the flavor and texture of many foods. Fat is classified as either saturated or

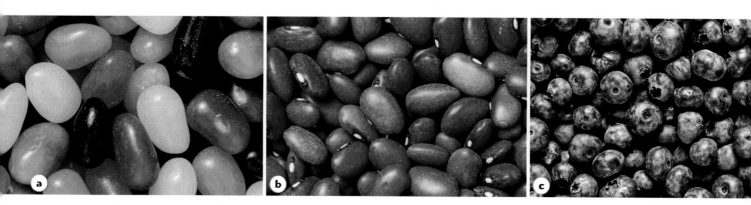

**FIGURE 16.2** Types of carbohydrate: *(a)* Simple carbohydrate (such as in candy) contains empty calories, but *(b* and *c)* complex carbohydrate (such as in vegetables and fruit) contains more nutrients and fiber.
© 1999 PhotoDisc, Inc.

unsaturated. In general, **saturated fat** is solid at room temperature, and **unsaturated fat** is liquid. Saturated fat comes mostly from animal products, such as lard, butter, milk, and meat fat. Unsaturated fat comes mostly from plants, such as sunflower, corn, soybean, olive, almond, and peanut. In addition, fish produce unsaturated fat in their cells.

At most, fewer than 35 percent of the total calories you consume should come from fat, and many experts recommend a level closer to 20 percent. The bulk of the fat in your diet should come from unsaturated fats, including fish oils. You should minimize your intake of calories from saturated fat. **Trans-fatty acids** (also called trans fat) should not be included in the diet. Trans fat is created through a process that makes unsaturated fat solid at room temperature—as, for example, in solid margarine. The U.S. Food and Drug Administration (FDA) indicates that trans fat is not "recognized as safe," so they can no longer be included in foods.

## FIT FACT

Years before the FDA banned the use of trans fat in foods, New York City passed a regulation restricting its use in restaurants. Health and nutrition scientists studied the regulation's effects and found that it reduced trans fat in food purchases without increasing saturated fat in food. According to the scientists, "Both high- and low-poverty neighborhoods benefitted equally." The biggest drop in trans fat was found in restaurants featuring burgers.

Cholesterol is a waxy, fatlike substance found in the saturated fat of animal cells, including those of humans. You consume cholesterol in foods that are high in saturated fat, such as meat. Because you are an animal, you also produce your own cholesterol. People who eat a lot of saturated fat produce more cholesterol than those who limit their consumption of saturated fat. A high level of blood cholesterol can contribute to atherosclerosis (clogged arteries) and other heart diseases. Medical experts recommend eating foods that are low in cholesterol and saturated fat. Trans-fatty acids also affect cholesterol, which was the primary reason they were banned in foods. Some kinds of fat, such as fish oil, are considered to be healthier than others.

# Nutrients That Do Not Provide Energy

Minerals, vitamins, and water have no calories and provide no energy, but they all play a vital role in your staying fit and healthy. Minerals and vitamins are called **micronutrients** because the body needs them in relatively small amounts as compared with carbohydrate, protein, and fat.

The **Dietary Reference Intake (DRI)** is a system used by the Food and Nutrition Board of the Institute of Medicine to describe recommended amounts of each micronutrient. Three types of DRI help you know how much of each vitamin or mineral you should consume. The first, **Recommended Dietary Allowance (RDA)**, is the minimum amount of a nutrient necessary to meet the health needs of most people. The second, **Adequate Intake (AI)**, is used when there is not sufficient evidence to establish an RDA for a given micronutrient. And the third, the **Tolerable Upper Intake Level (UL)**, refers to the maximum amount of a vitamin or mineral that can be consumed without posing a health risk.

## Minerals

Minerals are essential nutrients that help regulate the activity of your cells. They come from elements in the earth's crust and are present in all plants and animals. You need 25 minerals in varying amounts. Table 16.1 shows some major functions and food sources of the most important minerals.

Some minerals are especially important for young people—for example calcium, which builds and maintains bones. During your teen years, your body needs calcium to build your bones. During young adulthood, your bones become less efficient in getting calcium from food and begin to lose calcium. Later, typically around age 55, women experience a change in hormones that leads them to experience much more bone loss than men do. In fact, a large percentage of older women develop osteoporosis, a condition in which their bones become porous and break easily. Men can also have this disease, but they get it less often and much later in life. You can reduce your risk for osteoporosis by getting enough calcium and doing weight-bearing exercise (such as walking and jogging) and resistance exercise throughout your life.

## TABLE 16.1  Functions and Sources of Minerals

| Mineral | Function in the body | Food sources |
| --- | --- | --- |
| Calcium | Builds and maintains teeth and bones; helps blood clot; helps nerves and muscles function | Cheese, milk, dark green vegetables, sardines, legumes |
| Iron | Helps transfer oxygen in red blood cells and other cells | Liver, red meat, dark green vegetables, shellfish, whole-grain cereals |
| Magnesium | Aids breakdown of glucose and proteins; regulates body fluids | Green vegetables, grains, nuts, beans, yeast |
| Phosphorus | Builds and maintains teeth and bones; helps release energy from nutrients | Meat, poultry, fish, eggs, legumes, milk products |
| Potassium | Regulates fluid balance in cells; helps nerves function | Oranges, bananas, meat, bran, potatoes, dried beans |
| Sodium | Regulates internal water balance; helps nerves function | Most foods, table salt |
| Zinc | Aids transport of carbon dioxide; aids healing of wounds | Meat, shellfish, whole grains, milk, legumes |

Another important mineral is iron, which is needed for proper formation and functioning of your red blood cells. These cells carry oxygen to your muscles and other body tissues. Iron deficiency is especially common among girls and women. If your body has insufficient iron, you have a condition called iron-deficiency anemia, which causes you to feel tired all the time. Iron from animal foods is more easily absorbed than iron from plants. The best sources of iron are meat (especially red meat), poultry, and fish. You can also help your body absorb iron by getting an adequate amount of vitamin C.

Sodium is a mineral that helps your body cells function properly. It's present in many foods and is especially high in certain foods, such as snack foods, processed foods, fast foods, and cured meats (for example, ham). For many people, dietary sodium comes primarily from table salt (sodium chloride). Most people eat more sodium than they need, and recent U.S. nutrition guidelines recommend limiting the amount of sodium in your diet. People with high blood pressure, or hypertension, need to be especially careful to limit sodium because it can cause their body to retain water, thus helping keep their blood pressure high.

## Vitamins

You need vitamins for the growth and repair of your body cells. Vitamin C and the B vitamins are water soluble, so they dissolve in your blood and are carried to cells throughout your body. Because your body cannot store excess B and C vitamins, you need to eat foods containing these vitamins every day. In contrast, vitamins A, D, E, and K dissolve in fat, and excess amounts of these vitamins are stored in fat cells in your liver and other body parts. Folacin, or folic acid, is especially important for girls and young women. Research shows that children born to women low in folacin are at risk of birth defects. Table 16.2 gives you more information about specific vitamins.

## Water

Dietitians usually say that water is the single most important nutrient. It carries the other nutrients to your cells, carries away waste, and helps regulate your body temperature. Most foods contain water. In fact, 50 to 60 percent of your own body weight comes from water. Your body loses 2 to 3 quarts (1.9 to 2.8 liters) of water a day through breathing, perspiring, and eliminating waste from your bowels and bladder. You lose even more water than usual in very hot weather and when you exercise vigorously. As a result, you need to drink plenty of extra fluid.

The best beverages for this purpose are water, fruit juice, and milk. The type of juice or milk makes a difference. Pure fruit juices contain vitamins and minerals, and some contain fiber (for example, orange juice pulp). Some juice drinks contain small amounts of real juice and are supplemented with

### TABLE 16.2 Functions and Sources of Vitamins

| Vitamin | Function in the body | Food sources |
|---|---|---|
| A (retinol) | Helps produce normal mucus; part of the chemical necessary for vision | Butter, margarine, liver, eggs, green or yellow vegetables |
| $B_1$ (thiamin) | Helps release energy from carbohydrate | Pork, organ meat, legumes, greens |
| $B_2$ (riboflavin) | Helps break down carbohydrate and protein | Meat, milk products, eggs, green and yellow vegetables |
| $B_6$ (pyridoxine) | Helps break down protein and glucose | Yeast, nuts, beans, liver, fish, rice |
| $B_{12}$ (cobalamin) | Aids formation of nucleic and amino acids | Meat, milk products, eggs, fish |
| Biotin | Aids formation of amino, nucleic, and fatty acids and glycogen | Eggs, liver, yeast |
| C (ascorbic acid) | Aids formation of hormones, bone tissue, and collagen | Fruits, tomatoes, potatoes, green leafy vegetables |
| D | Aids absorption of calcium and phosphorus | Liver, fortified milk, fatty fish |
| E (tocopherol) | Prevents damage to cell membranes and vitamin A | Vegetable oils |
| Folacin | Helps build DNA and protein | Yeast, wheat germ, liver, greens |
| K | Aids blood clotting | Leafy vegetables |
| Niacin | Helps release energy from carbohydrate and protein | Milk, meat, whole-grain or enriched cereals, legumes |
| Pantothenic acid | Necessary for converting food fuel for producing energy and helps nervous system function properly | Most unprocessed foods |

 **SCIENCE IN ACTION: Vitamin and Mineral Supplements**

Scientists who study nutrition and medicine have researched the value of vitamin and mineral supplements. The most common type of supplement is taken daily and contains the amounts of vitamins and minerals recommended for daily intake. If you eat a balanced diet, however, you will most likely get the proper amounts without a supplement. **Dietitians** worry that people might think a supplement can take the place of eating well. Some medical and nutrition experts, however, recommend a multivitamin for people who do not eat regular meals and thus may not get the vitamins and minerals they need. Other experts, including scientists from the U.S. Centers for Disease Control and Prevention, say there is not enough evidence to indicate that a daily supplement is beneficial for most people.

With all this in mind, the decision to take a vitamin or mineral supplement should be done only with the advice of a nutrition or medical expert based on your medical history and personal nutrition habits. Unless advised otherwise by an expert, a supplement should contain no more than the RDA or AI value for each mineral and vitamin. Excessive amounts can lead to health problems.

**Student Activity**

Investigate a multivitamin supplement. Determine whether it contains more than 100 percent of the recommended amount of each vitamin.

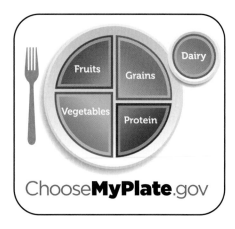

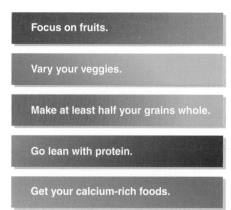

**FIGURE 16.3** MyPlate shows the five basic food groups that make up a healthy diet, and the tips to the right help remind you to think about what goes on your plate.
USDA's Center for Nutrition Policy and Promotion.

simple sugar. Skim milk provides the same basic nutrients as whole milk but without the fat.

Soft drinks that contain caffeine are not as effective as water. Sport drinks usually contain sodium and other ingredients that you don't need unless you exercise for several hours.

## Food Groups

The USDA uses a method called MyPlate to illustrate the five basic food groups (see figure 16.3). MyPlate looks like a plate and contains colored areas representing the basic types of food—grains, vegetables, fruits, and protein sources—that you typically put on your plate. Accompanying the plate is a circle that looks like a drinking glass. It represents the dairy group—for example, a glass of milk.

Foods from each of the groups contain macronutrients (carbohydrate, protein, and fat), micronutrients (vitamins and minerals), and water. Some foods are richer in nutrients than others. The goal is to eat more foods that are high in nutritional value and fewer foods containing empty calories. Foods with empty calories are typically high in fat, simple sugar, or both.

The orange area on the plate represents grains; it is relatively large because grains make up a large part of a healthy diet. At least half of your grain choices should be whole grain. Look for the whole-grain label on bread, cereal, and other grain products. The plate's green area represents vegetables, and the red area represents fruits. Together, vegetables and fruits should constitute approximately half of your total diet. There are five vegetable groups: dark green, orange, dried peas and beans, starchy, and

## FIT FACT

Periodically, the United States Department of Agriculture issues nutrition guidelines that provide easy-to-use information about eating for good health. In the past, the guidelines used a pyramid (called MyPyramid) that was similar to the Physical Activity Pyramid to provide a graphic illustration of the basic food groups. The current guidelines use a method called MyPlate.

other. The guidelines emphasize getting most of your vegetable servings from dark green and orange vegetables. Fruits can be fresh, canned, frozen, or dried. Fruit juices that are 100 percent juice are a legitimate source of fruit consumption, but the guidelines suggest that you not consume too much juice because of its high simple-sugar content.

The purple area on the plate represents the protein group. You don't need to eat as much of these foods as other foods (indicated by the smaller size on MyPlate), but they are essential to good health. This group includes meats (such as beef, poultry, and pork), seafood (fresh and canned), beans and peas, and nuts and seeds. You should limit your intake of processed meats such as hot dogs and some lunch meats, which contain very high levels of salt. Recommended foods in the protein group include lean meat cuts, poultry (without skin), and fish high in omega-3 fatty acids (such as salmon and trout). You should also use cooking methods that do not add fat to your food. For example, broiling lets fat drip away, whereas frying, especially deep-fat frying, adds many extra calories and extra fat, even to vegetables (as in French fries).

> " An apple a day keeps the doctor away. "
>
> —Anonymous proverb

Some foods—beans, peas, nuts, and seeds—are included in the protein group and the vegetable group because they are vegetables that are high in protein. These foods are especially important for vegetarians or people who do not eat a lot of meat.

The blue circle near the plate represents the dairy group. The circle looks like a glass of milk, but foods in this group can appear on your plate as well. The group includes milk, cheese, milk-based desserts, and yogurt. These foods are good sources of calcium. When choosing foods from this group, consider low-fat and fat-free options.

## The Ideal Diet?

Dietary guidelines emphasize that no single diet is best for all people. The exact amount of food that should be consumed from each food group depends on factors such as age, sex, and activity level. Alternative guidelines for eating have been developed by groups such as the American Heart Association and the American Diabetes Association for people with heart problems and those who wish to reduce their risk of heart problems. Ethnic food pyramids are also available.

Here are some general guidelines for healthy eating from the USDA and MyPlate and from the national nutrition goals for the nation (Healthy People 2020).

- Make half of your plate fruits and vegetables.
- Increase dietary complex carbohydrate.
- Make at least half your grains whole.
- Reduce consumption of calories from added sugar.
- Drink water instead of sugary drinks.
- Switch to skim or 1-percent milk.
- Reduce dietary fat, especially saturated fat. Consume no trans fat.
- Reduce daily salt (sodium) intake.
- Consume adequate dietary calcium.
- Avoid oversized portions.

Some of the guidelines described previously deserve elaboration because of their importance to a healthy diet. Consider the following strategies.

## Avoid Empty Calories

Minimize your consumption of foods high in empty calories. Examples include cake, candy, donuts, drinks with added sugar (including soda and many energy and sport drinks), processed meats (such as hot dogs, bacon, and sausage), ice cream made with real cream and added sugar, and condiments (such as ketchup and mayonnaise). Nutrition scientists have shown that from age 20 through age 40, the average American gains a pound a year; this increase is sometimes referred to as "**creeping obesity**" because the weight gain is gradual—it creeps up on you. Consumption of empty calories is a principal reason for gradual weight gain in early adulthood.

## Choose Oils Carefully

Oil is fat that is liquid at room temperature. Oils do not constitute a separate food group, but they do provide important nutrients. Because

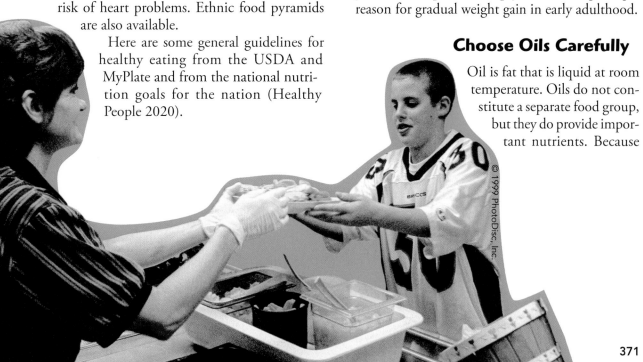

© 1999 PhotoDisc, Inc.

oil is fat, you should limit consumption of it, but some oils are better than others. For example, fish oils containing omega-3 fatty acids are considered to be a healthy part of your diet. When considering other oils, choose monounsaturated oils (such as canola oil). Polyunsaturated oils (such as corn oil) are preferred over the saturated fat in butter, lard, and margarine. Even some oils made from plants (for example, coconut and palm) contain saturated fat and therefore are not healthy diet options.

## Watch Servings and Serving Sizes

You now know that you need to eat appropriate amounts of macro- and micronutrients from the five food groups. But how much do you need from each group? Table 16.3 shows the recommended number of servings from each food group, as well as the appropriate serving size. The recommended number of servings from a given food group depends on your daily calorie intake. In general, boys require more servings than girls because they are larger and have more muscle mass. Most teen girls need about 2,000 to 2,500 calories per day, whereas teen boys typically need 2,500 to 3,000. The lower calorie amounts are appropriate for more sedentary teens, and the higher amounts are appropriate for active teens. Sedentary adults need fewer calories (2,000 or below).

## Be Active to Balance Calories

To maintain a healthy body composition throughout your life, you must balance the calories you take in with the calories you expend. Nutrition guidelines now acknowledge that both physical activity and healthy eating are important. Studies show, however, that most people overestimate their activity and underestimate how many calories they eat each day. Over time, this misperception can lead to unnecessary weight gain. The self-assessment in this chapter helps you determine how many calories you consume and how many you expend each day.

### TABLE 16.3 Recommended Number and Size of Servings

| Food group | Calorie range <2,200 | 2,200–2,800 | >2,800 | Serving size examples |
|---|---|---|---|---|
| Grain | 6 servings | 9 servings | 11 servings | 1 slice bread; 1/2 cup cooked cereal, rice, or pasta; 1 cup cold cereal; 1/4 cup wheat germ; 1 6-in. (15 cm) tortilla |
| Vegetable | 3 servings | 4 servings | 5 servings | 1 cup raw leafy vegetables, 1/2 cup other vegetables (chopped or cooked), 3/4 cup vegetable juice, 1/2 cup cooked vegetables |
| Fruit | 2 servings | 2 or 3 servings | 3 or 4 servings | 1 orange, 3/4 cup fruit juice, 1 cup cooked fruit |
| Dairy | 2 or 3 servings | 2 or 3 servings | 2 or 3 servings | 1 cup milk or yogurt, 1 1/2 cups ice cream, 1 1/2 oz. (43 g) cheese |
| Protein | 2 servings | 3 servings | 3 servings | 2–3 oz. (57–85 g) cooked meat, poultry, or fish; 1/2 cup cooked dried beans; 2 tbsp. peanut butter; 1/4 cup nuts or seeds; 1 whole egg |

More information about servings of specific foods is available in the student section of the Fitness for Life website.

## Lesson Review

1. How much dietary carbohydrate, protein, and fat are desirable for good health?
2. Why are vitamins, minerals, and water necessary for good health?
3. Describe the five basic food groups and why each is important.

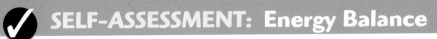

This self-assessment helps determine how many calories you take in (your calorie intake) and how many calories you expend each day. As directed, record the required information on worksheets provided by your instructor.

Remember that self-assessment information is personal and considered confidential. It shouldn't be shared with others without the permission of the person being tested.

## Step 1: Determine Your Calorie Intake

Prepare a chart indicating food types, foods, and food amounts for your consumption on one day. Figure 16.4 shows a sample food log prepared by Sandy, a 15-year-old boy in the ninth grade. Sandy kept a food log for one day to see how many calories he consumed and how many servings he ate from each food group. He recorded the number of servings for each food and made a check by the food group it came from to help him see if he was eating from each group. To help him determine serving sizes, he used table 16.3. Then he used a food calculator to determine the number of calories in each food. Finally, he added the calories and the number of servings of each food to determine his total calorie intake and see if he had met the recommended guidelines for each food group. Sandy's total calorie intake for Wednesday was 2,551, which falls in the recommended range for a male teen.

Prepare a one-day food log similar to Sandy's for your own consumption. Check to see if all food groups were represented. Use a food calculator to determine the number of calories in the foods you ate. Sandy used the FoodTracker on the MyPlate website (part of MyPlate SuperTracker).

## Step 2: Estimate Your Calorie Expenditure

First, determine your **resting metabolism**—the number of calories expended by your body for its basic functions and the typical light activities done during the day. In other words, resting metabolism includes your **basal metabolism** (the calories required for sleeping, digesting food, and other nonactive behavior) plus the calories you use for light daily activities such as teeth brushing, eating, reading, and typing. Sandy used table 16.4 to determine his resting metabolism based on his sex, age (15 years), weight (150 pounds, or 68 kilograms), and height (70 inches, or 1.8 meters). The chart indicated a resting metabolism of 1,800 calories each day. Sandy recorded this figure in his activity log.

Determine your resting metabolism using the appropriate table. For boys, use table 16.4 (ages 12 through 15) or table 16.5 (age 16 or older). For girls, use table 16.6 (ages 12 through 15) or table 16.7 (ages 16 or older). Record your resting metabolism.

Next, prepare a log of your physical activity for one day. Like Sandy, record each activity you perform and its length. Here are Sandy's calculations.

- Sandy looked at a physical activity compendium (see the student section of the Fitness for Life website) and found that a person weighing 150 pounds (68 kilograms) expends 318 calories in one hour of walking. For each minute of walking, then, Sandy expends 5.3 calories (318 calories ÷ 60 minutes = 5.3 calories per minute). Therefore, he expends 53 calories in a 10-minute walk (5.3 × 10 = 53).

- Sandy also did 30 minutes of the Burn It Up workout in physical education class. This activity causes a 150-pound person to expend 340 calories per hour, or 5.7 calories per minute (340 ÷ 60 = 5.7). Therefore, in 30 minutes, Sandy expended about 170 calories (5.7 × 30 = 170).

| Food | Servings | Calories | Grain | Vegetables | Fruit | Protein | Milk | Other |
|---|---|---|---|---|---|---|---|---|
| **Breakfast** | | | | | | | | |
| Scrambled egg | 1 | 104 | | | | ✔ | | |
| Fried ham slice | 1 | 82 | | | | ✔ | | |
| Whole wheat toast slice | 2 | 138 (69 × 2) | ✔ | | | | | |
| 8 oz. glass of orange juice | 1 | 112 | | | ✔ | | | |
| **Breakfast total** | | **436** | | | | | | |
| **Lunch** | | | | | | | | |
| Cheese pizza slice | 3 | 693 (231 × 3) | ✔ | | | ✔ | ✔ | |
| Small salad | 1 | 33 | | ✔ | | | | |
| Salad dressing | 1 | 71 | | | | | | ✔ |
| 12 oz. soda | 1 | 150 | | | | | | ✔ |
| **Lunch total** | | **947** | | | | | | |
| **Dinner** | | | | | | | | |
| Green beans | 2 | 88 (44 × 2) | | ✔ | | | | |
| Baked potato | 2 | 242 (121 × 2) | | ✔ | | | | |
| Sour cream for potato | 1 | 62 | | | | | ✔ | |
| Broiled chicken breast | 2 | 282 (141 × 2) | | | | ✔ | | |
| 16 oz. glass of fat-free milk (two 8 oz. servings) | 2 | 166 (83 × 2) | | | | | ✔ | |
| Salad | 1 | 33 | | ✔ | | | | |
| Salad dressing | 1 | 71 | | | | | | ✔ |
| **Dinner total** | | **944** | | | | | | |
| **Snack** | | | | | | | | |
| Bag of chips | 1 | 152 | | ✔ | | | | ✔ |
| Apple | 1 | 72 | | | ✔ | | | |
| Snack total | | 224 | | | | | | |
| **Daily total** | | **2,551** | | | | | | |

Figure 16.4  Sandy's food log for Wednesday.

## TABLE 16.4  Resting Metabolism (Calories) for Males Aged 12 to 15

| Height (in.) | Weight (lb) | | | | | |
|---|---|---|---|---|---|---|
| | 100 | 120 | 150 | 180 | 200 | ≥220 |
| 60–64 | 1,380 | 1,500 | 1,700 | 1,900 | 2,000 | 2,100 |
| 65–68 | 1,430 | 1,550 | 1,750 | 1,950 | 2,050 | 2,200 |
| 69–72 | 1,480 | 1,600 | 1,800 | 2,000 | 2,100 | 2,230 |
| ≥73 | 1,500 | 1,630 | 1,820 | 2,010 | 2,130 | 2,240 |

To convert inches to centimeters, multiply by 2.54. To convert pounds to kilograms, multiply by 0.45.

## TABLE 16.5   Resting Metabolism (Calories) for Males Aged 16 or Older

| Height (in.) | Weight (lb) | | | | | |
|---|---|---|---|---|---|---|
| | 100 | 120 | 150 | 180 | 200 | ≥220 |
| 60–64 | 1,360 | 1,480 | 1,670 | 1,860 | 1,980 | 2,110 |
| 65–68 | 1,410 | 1,540 | 1,720 | 1,910 | 2,035 | 2,160 |
| 69–72 | 1,460 | 1,590 | 1,770 | 1,960 | 2,085 | 2,210 |
| ≥73 | 1,490 | 1,610 | 1,800 | 1,985 | 2,110 | 2,235 |

To convert inches to centimeters, multiply by 2.54. To convert pounds to kilograms, multiply by 0.45.

## TABLE 16.6   Resting Metabolism (Calories) for Females Aged 12 to 15

| Height (in.) | Weight (lb) | | | | | |
|---|---|---|---|---|---|---|
| | 90 | 100 | 120 | 150 | 180 | ≥200 |
| 60–64 | 1,275 | 1,320 | 1,410 | 1,540 | 1,670 | 1,755 |
| 65–68 | 1,295 | 1,340 | 1,425 | 1,560 | 1,690 | 1,775 |
| 69–72 | 1,315 | 1,360 | 1,445 | 1,575 | 1,705 | 1,795 |
| ≥73 | 1,325 | 1,370 | 1,455 | 1,585 | 1,715 | 1,800 |

To convert inches to centimeters, multiply by 2.54. To convert pounds to kilograms, multiply by 0.45.

## TABLE 16.7   Resting Metabolism (Calories) for Females Aged 16 or Older

| Height (in.) | Weight (lb) | | | | | |
|---|---|---|---|---|---|---|
| | 90 | 100 | 120 | 150 | 180 | ≥200 |
| 60–64 | 1,260 | 1,300 | 1,390 | 1,520 | 1,650 | 1,740 |
| 65–68 | 1,275 | 1,320 | 1,405 | 1,540 | 1,670 | 1,755 |
| 69–72 | 1,295 | 1,340 | 1,425 | 1,555 | 1,685 | 1,775 |
| ≥73 | 1,305 | 1,350 | 1,440 | 1,565 | 1,700 | 1,785 |

To convert inches to centimeters, multiply by 2.54. To convert pounds to kilograms, multiply by 0.45.

- Mowing the lawn expends 316 calories per hour for a person of Sandy's size, or about 5.25 calories per minute (316 ÷ 60 = about 5.25). Thus in mowing the lawn for 15 minutes, he expended about 79 calories (5.25 × 15 = 79).

Sandy recorded his calories expended in his activity log (see figure 16.5). His calories expended in physical activity totaled 355. He added this number to his resting metabolism of 1,800 to determine that his total energy expenditure for the day was 2,155 calories (355 + 1,800 = 2,155).

Prepare an activity log similar to the one that Sandy prepared. Record each activity you performed on the day of your log. Use the compendium for physical activity or a physical activity calculator to determine the number of calories you expended in each activity that you performed. Total the calories expended in these activities. Then add this calorie total to your resting metabolism calories to determine your total calories expended for the day.

| Activity | Minutes | Calories per hour | Calories |
|---|---|---|---|
| **Morning** | | | |
| Physical education: Burn It Up workout | 30 | 340 | 170 |
| Walk to and from classes | 10 | 318 | 53 |
| **Afternoon** | | | |
| Walk to and from classes | 10 | 318 | 53 |
| **Evening** | | | |
| Mow lawn | 15 | 316 | 79 |
| **Daily activity total** | 65 | | 355 |
| **Resting metabolism** | | | 1,800 |
| **Total daily calories expended** | | | 2,155 |

Figure 16.5　Sandy's activities for Wednesday.

# Step 3: Evaluate Your Calorie Balance

Compare your calorie expenditure to your calorie intake to see if your calories balance for the day. Sandy expended 2,155 calories for the day but consumed 2,551, so he consumed 396 calories more than he expended (2,551 − 2,155 = 396). It's not unusual to consume more calories than expended on one day, then consume less than expended on another. However, if Sandy regularly consumed 396 calories a day more than he expended, he would gain body fat over time.

Determine if you have energy balance (calorie intake equals calorie expenditure) or if you have imbalance. Subtract the smaller number (whether calorie intake or calorie expenditure) from the larger number.

# Lesson 16.2
## Making Healthy Food Choices

### Lesson Objectives

After reading this lesson, you should be able to

1. describe the FIT formula for meeting nutritional needs,
2. identify several important elements of food labels and describe the information they provide,
3. identify some nutrients that should be limited in your diet, and
4. describe some common myths about nutrition and explain why they are not true.

### Lesson Vocabulary

calorimeter, food label, food supplement

**Do** you know how to read a nutrition label? Have you ever wondered if your portion sizes are the same as the serving size listed on a nutrition label? In the previous lesson, you learned how to choose foods from different food groups in order to build a nutritious diet. You also learned how following dietary guidelines can help you attain and maintain good health. In this lesson, you'll learn more about choosing healthy foods for a balanced diet.

### The FIT Formula and Nutrition

Table 16.8 shows how you can use the FIT formula as a guideline for nutritional fitness. Too often, teens in particular violate the FIT formula. For example, some skip breakfast or lunch, which often leads them to overeat later in the day. Skipping meals can make you feel tired during the day and can make it difficult to concentrate, thus contributing to poor school performance. If you play on a sports team, skipping meals can negatively affect your performance.

In addition, many people don't know how many calories they should consume each day. This number, however, can easily be determined (see this chapter's self-assessment). As you learned earlier, a person's nutrient needs vary according to age, sex, height, weight, and daily physical activity. Young people who are going through puberty or are still growing have special nutritional needs; specifically, they need to eat foods high in minerals (potassium, calcium, iron) that aid in the development of bones and blood. If you eat the recommended number of servings from each of the food groups, you're well on your way to consuming a diet that meets your nutritional needs.

### Servings and Portions

A serving of food and a portion of food are not necessarily the same thing. As described in table 16.3, a serving is a recommended amount. A portion, on the other hand, is the amount of food you put on your plate (or, at a restaurant, the amount put there for you). Therefore, a portion can be large or small. A large portion can contain much more than

**TABLE 16.8  Fitness Target Zones and Nutrition**

| | Nutrition target zone |
|---|---|
| Frequency | Eat three meals a day. Healthy planned snacks can be part of a healthy diet. |
| Intensity | The number of calories you consume daily should fall within the range determined by factors described in this chapter's self-assessment. Calories should come from recommended servings for each food group (see table 16.3). |
| Time | Eat meals at regular intervals, such as morning, noon, and evening. |

a recommended serving, and a small portion can contain less than a recommended serving. Use the following strategies to control your portion sizes so that you eat an appropriate amount of food.

- Know the size of a recommended serving (see table 16.3).

- Choose portions equal to recommended servings.

- Eat only part of large portions; save extra food for another meal.

- Read food labels carefully. Calorie totals listed on food labels (see figure 16.6) typically show the number of calories in one serving, but a package often contains several servings. To consume the number of calories on the label, choose only an amount from the package that is equal to a recommended serving.

## FIT FACT

One reason for Americans' increase in portion sizes in recent years is the marketing of larger meals sometimes referred to as "super sized." For example, the original size of most French fry orders contained 450 calories, but the size of a large order currently promoted by many fast food outlets contains more than 600 calories. Another example is the all-you-can-eat buffet offered at a set price, which can motivate people to eat large portions in order to get their money's worth. Use the information presented in table 16.3 in the previous lesson to help you determine how much you eat. You may find that one portion is equal to several servings.

You can also get an idea of appropriate serving sizes by referring to certain common objects typically found around the house. The following list provides some examples of single servings.

- Baked potato: computer mouse
- Bagel: can of tuna
- Apple: baseball
- Hard cheese: three game dice
- Lean beef: deck of cards

# Food Labels

Many teenagers do not shop for groceries, plan meals, or cook for a family. But it's important for you to start learning how to do these things now because you'll need these skills at some point in your life. Reading and understanding **food labels** can help you plan your diet and shop for healthy foods. By law, manufacturers must now use a standard format for food labels. Be aware that the food labels required by the government are not the same as the food labels sometimes provided by manufacturers on the front of food packages (for example, cereal boxes). Front-of-box labels are not regulated and may not be accurate. In fact, nutrition experts criticize these labels because they are often deceptive and are really part of a strategy to sell the food rather than provide nutrition information. Experts worry that consumers will look at the front-of-box label rather than the regulated side-of-box label that provides scientifically sound information.

You've probably already used side-of-box nutrition labels at one time or another, but you may not know how to use them most effectively. When reading a food label, start at the top and use the following six steps, which refer to the sample label

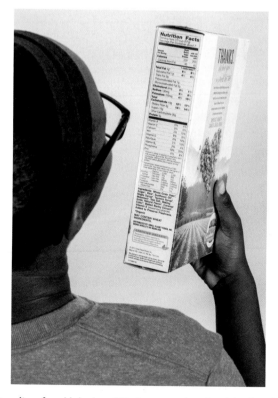

Reading food labels will help you select healthy foods.

from a package of macaroni and cheese presented in figure 16.6. (Food labels are typically all white on food containers, but colors are used in this example to help you easily find each area on the label.)

## Step 1: Servings

The number of servings in the container is shown in the green area. In this case, two servings are listed, and the size of each serving is 1 cup, thus making a total of 2 cups in the package.

## Step 2: Calories

The white area shows the number of calories per serving—in this case, 250 calories. Therefore, the total calorie content of the food package is 500 (250 calories × 2 servings = 500 calories). Some food labels include both total calories in the package and calories per serving. However, many labels only include calories per serving, which may lead some people to think that the calorie number listed (250) is the amount in the total package. The real calorie content is 500 (2 servings × 250 = 500 calories).

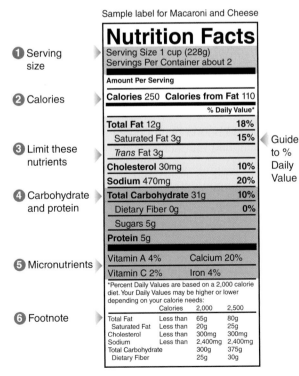

**FIGURE 16.6** Sample food label.

From USDA.

## Step 3: Nutrients That Should Be Limited

The yellow area presents information about some nutrients that should be limited in your diet, such as fat and salt. The number beside each nutrient indicates the amount in grams (g) or milligrams (mg) and the percentage of that nutrient's daily amount provided by one serving. In this case, one serving of the macaroni and cheese provides 18 percent of the total fat and 20 percent of the salt you should consume each day. If you eat two servings, you need to double the listed numbers to know how much fat and salt you're consuming. Trans fat amounts are shown in figure 16.6 even though they will be excluded from foods in the future. Until the FDA ban is fully implemented, the grams of trans fat in foods must still be included on food labels.

## Step 4: Carbohydrate and Protein

Carbohydrate and protein are two of the three macronutrients that provide your body with energy. Two types of carbohydrate are listed on the label (in blue): dietary fiber and sugars. As shown in pink, 10 percent of the daily requirement of carbohydrate is provided by one serving. Dietary fiber, a type of carbohydrate, is desirable in the diet, and the label helps you determine if you eat enough of it. Sugars should be limited in the diet like fat and sodium. The number of grams of protein is shown on the label in pink. The FDA recommends a minimum of 0.3 grams of protein per pound of body weight each day (45 grams for a person weighing 150 pounds).

## Step 5: Micronutrients

Micronutrients, such as vitamins and minerals, are especially important to your diet. You need to get 100 percent of these each day. Four types of micronutrients, two vitamins and two minerals, are highlighted in blue on the label. As you can see from the label in figure 16.6, one serving of the macaroni and cheese provides 20 percent of daily calcium, but only 2 to 4 percent of the other micronutrients.

## Step 6: Footnote

Use the information in the white area at the bottom of the label to make adjustments for the total number of calories you consume. The total number of calories needed each day varies from person to person depending on age and body size. People who require more calories need to adjust the nutrient amounts, and the information presented at the bottom of the label helps you make these adjustments. For example, a person requiring 2,200 calories per day is allowed more fat, and needs more fiber, than a person requiring 2,000 calories per day.

## FIT FACT

Calories from soda add up fast. Most soft drinks contain about 150 calories in a 12-ounce (about 0.4-liter) can—that's 450 calories in three cans—and many teens drink multiple cans per day. A 64-ounce (about 1.8-liter) drink, such as those sold at many fast food and convenience stores, contains almost 800 calories. Not surprisingly, studies show that excessive consumption of soft drinks may be one reason for the high incidence of over-weight in developed countries. In fact, if all other aspects of your diet stayed the same, adding one soft drink a day would cause you to gain 15 pounds (about 7 kilograms) of fat in a year. The solution? Water quenches your thirst and contains zero calories.

## Other Food Labels

You've learned that side-of-box labels provide useful information and that some front-of-box labels can be deceiving. But there are also other food labels you should know about. One type of label refers to a food's fat content. In the United States, labels such as "fat free" can be displayed on food containers only if the food meets legal standards set by the government. The terms, presented in table 16.9, were developed to prevent false advertising. Even with these standardized terms, however, you can still be fooled by advertisements relating to a food's fat content. Some foods, such as milk and packaged meats, are advertised as 2 percent fat—that is, 98 percent fat free. This is true if fat is measured by the product's weight, but it is not true if fat is measured by the total number of calories in the food. For example, only 2 percent of the weight of a glass of 2 percent milk is fat, but more than 30 percent of the calories come from fat.

You can calculate the true percentage of fat calories in food for yourself. Simply divide the calorie total per serving into the calorie total for fat per serving. For the food label shown in figure 16.6, the calorie total per serving is 250 and the calorie total for fat per serving is 110, so the percentage of fat calories in this food is 44 percent (110 calories ÷ 250 calories = 0.44).

You also might see health claims such as "good for heart health" on some food labels. Manufacturers must comply with government regulations regarding such labeling. For example, if it is advertised that a product's fat content is good for your heart, the product must be low in fat, saturated fat, and cholesterol. Fruits, vegetables, and grain products for which such claims are made must not only be low in fat, saturated fat, and cholesterol but also contain at least the minimum amount of fiber per serving. Foods that display health claims related to blood pressure must be low in sodium.

## Common Food Myths

You may have heard a number of incorrect or mis-leading statements about nutrition. Some common nutrition myths are exposed in the following list.

### TABLE 16.9    Key Words on Food Labels and What They Mean

| Key words | What they mean |
| --- | --- |
| Fat free | Equal to or less than 0.5 g of fat |
| Low fat | Equal to or less than 3 g of fat per serving |
| Lean | Equal to or less than 10 g of fat, 4 g of saturated fat, and 95 mg of cholesterol |
| Light (or "lite") | 1/3 fewer calories or no more than 1/2 the fat of the higher-calorie or higher-fat version; or no more than 1/2 the sodium of the higher-sodium version |
| Cholesterol free | Equal to or less than 2 mg of cholesterol and 2 or less g of saturated fat per serving |

# FITNESS TECHNOLOGY: What's in Your Food?

A **calorimeter** is an apparatus designed to determine the amount of heat generated by a chemical reaction. In Latin, *calor* means heat and *metron* means measure; thus a calorimeter measures heat. A special type of calorimeter is used to determine the amount of heat created when different types of food are burned. In this way, nutrition scientists have determined the calorie counts of various foods. You can find these amounts listed on many websites, including the USDA's Food Tracker, a part of the SuperTracker found at the MyPlate website.

The web has also made it relatively easy for you to find other information about food content. For example, some nutrition websites list the specific nutrient content (carbohydrate, protein, fat, vitamins, and minerals) of various foods. Some address foods of all kinds, and others provide information specifically about fast food. The Cooper Institute has developed nutrition software called NutriGram as a companion to Fitnessgram.

---

**Student Activity**

Find the SuperTracker at the MyPlate website (www.ChooseMyPlate.gov). Notice that it includes six different online tracking tools, including FoodTracker and Physical Activity Tracker. Try one of the tools and write an evaluation of it that is several paragraphs long. Explain how the tool would or would not be useful.

---

**Myth:** Skipping meals is a good way to lose weight.

**Fact:** Studies show that people who skip meals typically eat more than those who eat regular meals. Skipping meals stimulates the appetite, so eating fewer meals can lead to eating more food at each meal, whereas eating more meals usually means eating less at each meal. Skipping breakfast or lunch is common but is ineffective in weight loss and results in lower work and school performance.

**Myth:** A **food supplement** is tested to ensure that it is safe and that it meets the claims advertised by the seller.

**Fact:** Since 1994, food supplements have been unregulated in the United States. This means that they are not tested by the government either for safety or to ensure that they meet the claims made for them. Beware of food supplements that make claims that are too good to be true.

**Myth:** A high-protein diet is best for losing weight, building muscle, and maintaining good health.

**Fact:** A review of a large number of studies shows that a balanced diet—based on the nutrient percentages listed in this chapter's first lesson—is most effective in both fat loss and weight maintenance. Popular high-protein diets cause quick loss of body water, but a diet is effective in fat loss only if it results in consumption of fewer calories. Because these diets are high in fat, experts fear that they can result in increased health problems if used for a long time. Active people need more protein than inactive people, but because active people consume more calories they also get the protein they need through a balanced diet.

**Myth:** If you limit the amount of fat in your food, you do not need to be concerned with how many calories a food contains.

**Fact:** It's the total number of calories you consume that makes a difference in weight maintenance. Fat does contain more calories per gram than carbohydrate and protein, but many foods advertised as low in fat actually contain more calories than foods higher in fat.

> “ You are what you eat. ”
>
> —Ludwig Feuerbach, philosopher

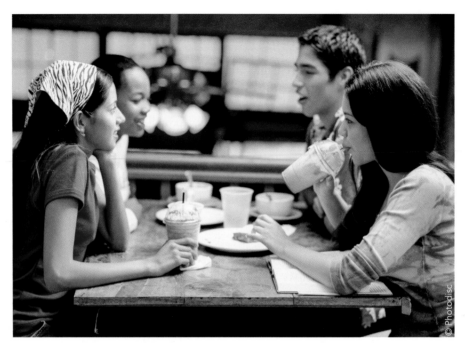

Snacks with friends can be all right if they are low in empty calories and included as part of a total dietary plan.

**Myth:** Diets very low in calories are effective for weight loss.

**Fact:** Your body needs calories in order to function. Eating too few calories in a day (800 or less) causes the body to conserve calories to keep the body functioning, which means your body uses fewer calories than it normally would. Therefore, eating too few calories is not an effective way to reduce body fat. In fact, it can be dangerous because very low calorie diets typically do not provide the basic nutrients (such as vitamins and minerals) that your body needs.

Because health and nutrition quackery is so common, many other myths also exist. When making choices about your nutrition, follow the USDA dietary guidelines. Use information that comes from reliable sources, such as the USDA, the U.S. Food and Drug Administration (FDA), the American Dietetic Association, the American Medical Association, the American Heart Association, the American Cancer Society, and the Center for Science in the Public Interest. You can find more information in the student section of the Fitness for Life website.

# Nutrition Advertising Strategies and Tactics

You might know about strategy and tactics in games and sport. A strategy is a general plan of action for reaching a specific goal; in sport, a strategy is an overall plan to help win a game, match, or other competition. After the first level of planning—outlining a strategy—tactics are devised to help reach a goal. Tactics are specific actions taken to implement the strategy and reach the goal. Some food manufacturers have adopted a strategy of selling to the youth market (children and teens). This strategy is designed not to sell foods that are healthy but simply to sell more food. One tactic used by marketers is to concentrate television advertisements for sugared cereals at times when children are out of school and shows are directed at children. Another tactic is to include toys with meals in fast food restaurants to boost interest in fast food among children.

Today, teens represent one of the largest groups of consumers in the United States. Using the "merchants of cool" strategy is one way companies target the teen market. In this approach, companies (merchants) try to make their products seem cool to teens. This strategy is used to sell, among other things, clothing, electronics, energy drinks, sport drinks, and soda. One specific tactic used to carry out this strategy is to feature movie stars and entertainers promoting a brand. Nutrition scientists and dietitians want to make you aware of these strategies and tactics so you can make informed decisions when you choose foods and drinks.

# Eating Before Physical Activity

Most people can do moderate activity after a meal if they wait about 30 minutes to an hour. People who have problems doing activity after eating may have to wait longer or modify when and what they eat. You may also have to modify your eating pattern if you plan to do vigorous physical activity or participate in a highly competitive athletic event. Use the following guidelines for eating before physical activity.

- **A special diet is usually not necessary before an athletic competition.** Some athletes think they need a steak before they compete. Steak, however, is high in protein and fat, both of which are digested slowly. As a result, eating steak within two hours of the event might interfere with your performance. In general, you can eat what you like as long as it doesn't disagree with you.

- **Allow extra time between eating and a vigorous competitive event.** Eat one to three hours before competing. Allow more time if you're eating food that's difficult to

digest (for example, large servings of meat, spicy foods, and high-fiber foods).

- **Before competition, reduce meal size.** Small meals are easier to digest than large ones. If you get very nervous or often have an upset stomach before competition, limiting meal size can be helpful.

- **Before competition, avoid snacks that are high in simple carbohydrate (simple sugar).** Some people think that having a candy bar or drink that's high in simple carbohydrate before competition will provide quick energy. In fact, taking a big dose of simple carbohydrate right before an event causes blood sugar to go up, but a drop in blood sugar level often follows after exertion. This can cause lack of energy and even dizziness, and it may negatively affect performance and increase risk of injury.

- **Drink before, during, and after activity.** Whether you're competing or not, it's important to drink water. You don't usually need added salt or sugar, except for during especially long events and events occurring in high heat and humidity. Using drinks with too much sugar can even detract from your performance for reasons described in the previous bulleted item. Drinking too much before activity can cause a side stitch in some people. These people should drink fluids well before the activity and in several small amounts. They should not drink a large amount right before the activity.

## Lesson Review

1. How can the FIT formula help people meet their nutritional needs?
2. What are three examples of information you can find on a food label?
3. What are some nutrients that should be limited in your diet?
4. What are two common food myths? How are they incorrect or misleading?

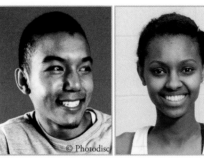 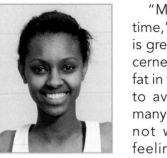
© Photodisc

Sometimes the simple act of saying no is the best way to avoid a potentially harmful situation. However, while it may seem easy, saying no can actually be very difficult to carry out successfully. Here's an example.

Many cultures celebrate holidays with special meals and foods. On one such occasion, Manny was invited to spend the Cinco de Mayo holiday with his girlfriend's family. Plans were made to spend the afternoon water-skiing at a nearby lake, then have a big party. Manny's girlfriend Rita warned him that her mother always prepared huge amounts of food for this special day. The family did not normally eat so much, but on this special day it was their tradition to feast on traditional foods. She told him to make sure he came with a big appetite. Unfortunately, Manny's doctor had just instructed him to restrict his intake of salt, fat, and calories.

Manny arrived at the party just as Rita's mother was setting out the food. The table was loaded with tortilla chips, guacamole, beef and bean burritos, chiles rellenos, and fresh corn, as well as cakes, pies, and cookies. Manny knew that he faced a difficult situation as Rita came forward with a plate piled with high cookies.

"Manny, you're just in time," she said. "The food is great!" Manny was concerned about the salt and fat in the food and wanted to avoid consuming too many calories, but he did not want to hurt Rita's feelings. So he replied, "Everything looks good, but I have to watch my diet."

Rita offered him a cookie, knowing they were Manny's favorite. "But you've got to try my mother's cookies. Everyone says they're the best. You'll hurt my mother's feelings if you don't eat one." Manny felt pressured to eat something he didn't really want.

## For Discussion

In what way does the party put Manny in a difficult situation? How can Manny say no to Rita without embarrassing her or hurting her feelings? What can he do so that his refusal won't hurt Rita's mother's feelings? What could he have done to prepare for the situation before going to the party? What are some other situations in which saying no would be the best response? Consider the guidelines presented in the Self-Management feature when answering the discussion questions.

Most of us try to eat well, do regular physical activity, and live a healthy lifestyle. But sometimes the situation we're in or the people we're around make it difficult to stick with healthy behaviors. We're tempted to do things that we wouldn't normally do. You can take steps to make it easier to say no when you're in situations that encourage you to engage in behaviors you know are not best for you. The following guidelines will help you say no to eating food that you don't want or need. You may also be able to use these strategies to help you say no in other situations involving choices about health-related behavior.

- **Say no to food offered on special occasions.** Eat a light meal before a holiday event so that you don't arrive hungry. Practice ways to refuse food so that you don't hurt the host's feelings. For example, talk to the host or hostess ahead of time to explain why you may limit your food intake. Prepare statements ahead of time that you can use if you're pressured to eat.

- **Use strategies to avoid temptation.** Avoid standing near food. If you feel the urge to eat, talk to someone or find something else to do.

- **Say no to extra food when eating out.** Plan in advance what you will eat. Resist ordering foods that are advertised or that others eat. Choose small servings—avoid big orders such as large burgers and fries. Say no to special deals that include foods you don't want; instead, order single items you do want. Say no to extra sauces, toppings, and condiments such as mayonnaise.

- **Shop with a strategy.** Prepare a list ahead of time and stick with it to help you say no to foods that are high in empty calories. Use food labels and avoid foods that are high in calories per serving. Look for better choices. Eat before you shop so that you're not hungry while making choices.

- **Consume healthy snacks.** Eating vegetables and fruits for snacks can help you say no to snacks that are high in empty calories, such as potato chips, cookies, and candy. Avoid sugared soft drinks and sport drinks; instead, carry a water bottle.

- **Eat healthy foods at school.** Prepare your own lunch and snacks for school to help you say no to unhealthy food offered in snack machines. If you have free time, find a way to be active to avoid thinking about eating things you don't really want or need. If you eat school food, ask for small servings to avoid eating too much. If you have free time with friends, bring healthy snacks to share.

- **Say no to large servings and seconds.** Tell family members and friends not to offer seconds. Limit dessert servings.

- **Eat slowly and avoid eating while studying or watching television.** Some experts recommend that you limit your eating to the kitchen or dining room to help you say no to unwanted food.

All types of activity included in the Physical Activity Pyramid use calories and therefore help you balance your calorie expenditure with your calorie intake. Moderate activity can be beneficial because it can be performed over a long span of time. Vigorous activity is also good because it uses more calories in the same amount of time. For example, a 120-pound (54-kilogram) person burns about 85 calories by walking for 20 minutes (a moderate activity) but 125 calories by jogging for 20 minutes (a vigorous activity). You can also boost your energy expenditure fairly easily by adding bursts of higher-intensity effort to your exercise routine. Muscle fitness exercises also expend calories, as well as build muscle mass that causes you to expend more calories even at rest.

**Take action** by trying the Burn It Up workout. This workout includes activities of various types and intensities. During the workout, monitor your overall effort to see if the intensity is moderate or keeps you in the target heart rate zone for vigorous physical activity.

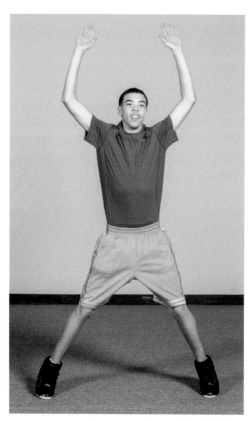 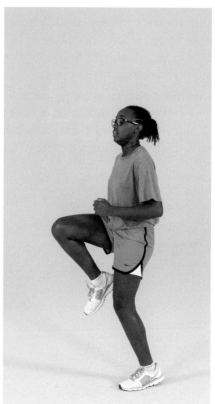

Take action with the Burn It Up workout.

## Reviewing Concepts and Vocabulary

As directed by your teacher, answer items 1 through 5 by correctly completing each sentence with a word or phrase.

1. _____ are nutrients that provide energy.
2. Foods that are high in calories but low in nutrients are said to contain _____ calories.
3. _____ are food substances that make up protein.
4. A portion of food is the amount of a specific food on your plate; it differs from a _____, which is the recommended amount for a specific food.
5. _____ obesity refers to gradual weight gain as a person grows older.

For items 6 through 10, as directed by your teacher, match each term in column 1 with the appropriate phrase in column 2.

6. carbohydrate
7. protein
8. fiber
9. saturated fat
10. mineral

a. major source of energy
b. regulates cell activity
c. solid at room temperature
d. cannot be digested by the body
e. building block for your body

For items 11 through 15, as directed by your teacher, respond to each statement or question.

11. Describe your body's need for fat and the best types to include in your diet.
12. Describe the five groups depicted in MyPlate.
13. Explain how side-of-box food labels can help you eat well.
14. Describe several guidelines about eating before physical activity.
15. Describe several guidelines for saying no in situations when you might feel pressured to do something you don't want to do.

## Thinking Critically

Your friend asks for your advice about her diet. She wonders whether the food choices she makes are important or whether she only needs to count calories. She has also started to increase her physical activity and wonders how that will affect her caloric and nutritional needs. Write a paragraph explaining the advice you would give her.

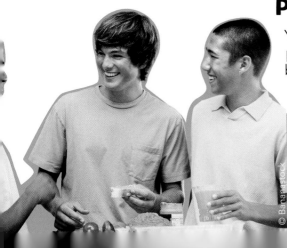

## Project

You learned about MyPlate in this chapter. MyPlate was preceded by a similar diagram called MyPyramid and, before that, the Food Guide Pyramid. Other diagrams, including the rainbow-themed Canada's Food Guide, have been developed to help people make sound nutrition decisions. Create a poster that compares MyPlate to another diagram, or create a poster with a new nutrition diagram to help people better understand the types of food in a healthy diet.

© Bananastock

# 17

# Stress Management

## In This Chapter

 **Student Web Resources**
www.fitnessforlife.org/student

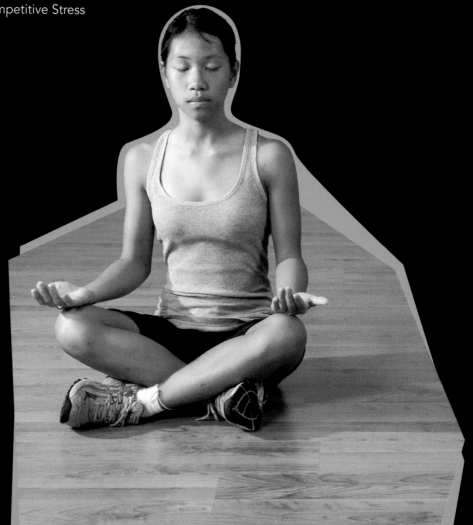

# Lesson 17.1

# Facts About Stress

## Lesson Objectives

After reading this lesson, you should be able to

1. define *stress* and *stressor*,
2. explain the three stages of general adaptation syndrome,
3. describe the five steps in the Stress Management Pyramid, and
4. discuss some causes and effects of stress.

 ## Lesson Vocabulary

alarm reaction, coping, coping skills, distress, eustress, general adaptation syndrome, stage of exhaustion, stage of resistance, stress, stressor

**Have** you ever given a speech or performance in front of a lot of people? Did it make you anxious? If so, your heart rate may have increased and your muscles may have gotten tense. Stressful situations can bring these changes about by causing your body to release a chemical called adrenaline. The changes are part of what is called the stress response—your body's way of preparing you to deal with a demanding situation.

You probably face stressful situations every day that affect you both physically and emotionally. In fact, two-thirds of Americans report feeling "stressed out" at least once a week. In this lesson, you'll read more about stress, how your body responds to it, and stress management. Along with regular physical activity and good nutrition, stress management should be a priority in your healthy lifestyle. This lesson will teach you about the Stress Management Pyramid and its five steps (figure 17.1).

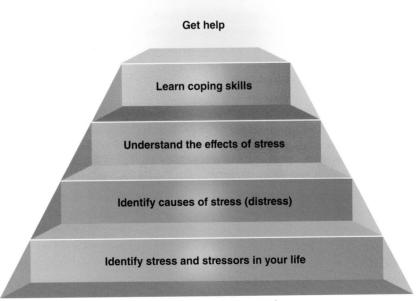

Get help

Learn coping skills

Understand the effects of stress

Identify causes of stress (distress)

Identify stress and stressors in your life

**FIGURE 17.1** The five steps of the Stress Management Pyramid.

# The Stress Management Pyramid

Just as the Physical Activity Pyramid depicts types of physical activity to help you get fit and build health and wellness, the Stress Management Pyramid helps you deal effectively with stress. The pyramid's five steps are described in the following pages.

## Step 1: Identify Stress and Stressors in Your Life

**Stress** is the body's reaction to a demanding situation. A **stressor** is something that causes or contributes to stress. The first step in managing stress is to identify stress when you have it.

When you're in a highly stressful situation, a series of physical changes takes place automatically. As researcher Hans Selye showed, when people are exposed to stressors, they adapt through what is called **general adaptation syndrome**, which includes three stages (see figure 17.2). In responding to a stressor, the body first initiates an **alarm reaction**. Anything that causes you to worry, get excited, or experience other emotional and physical changes can be a stressor and thus can start your body's alarm reaction. For adults, common stressors include bills, vacation plans, work responsibilities, and family conflicts. Common stressors for teenagers include grades and schoolwork, family arguments, peer pressure, moving to a new home, serious illness or death in the family, poor eating habits, lack of physical activity, feelings of loneliness, a change or loss of friends, substance abuse, bullying, and trouble with school or legal authorities.

Some of the physical changes that occur when your body starts its alarm reaction to a stressor are shown in figure 17.3. The alarm reaction causes your heart rate to increase and initiates other physical changes. After your body has had a chance to adjust, it enters the second stage of general adaptation syndrome—the **stage of resistance**—in which your body systems start to resist or fight the stressor. In the case of an illness, antibodies are sent out to fight. In the case of a physical stressor, such as doing heavy exercise, the heart rate increases to supply more blood and oxygen to various parts of your body. In most cases, your resistance is enough to overcome the stressor, and you adapt by returning to your normal state of being.

In extreme cases, however, the body is not able to resist well enough and thus enters the third stage of the syndrome—the **stage of exhaustion**. In this case, various medical treatments may be necessary to help the body resist and overcome the stressor. If the stressor is too great, as in the case of a disease that the body and medicine cannot fight, death can occur.

> " One person's stress is another's pleasure. "
>
> —Ruth Lindsey, fitness author

## Step 2: Identify Causes of Stress (Distress)

Not all stressful experiences are harmful. Scientists use the term **eustress** to describe positive stress (figure 17.4a). Situations that can produce eustress

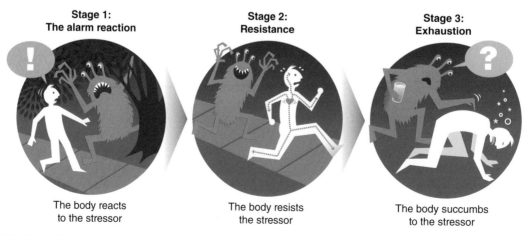

| Stage 1: The alarm reaction | Stage 2: Resistance | Stage 3: Exhaustion |
|---|---|---|
| The body reacts to the stressor | The body resists the stressor | The body succumbs to the stressor |

**FIGURE 17.2** General adaptation syndrome.

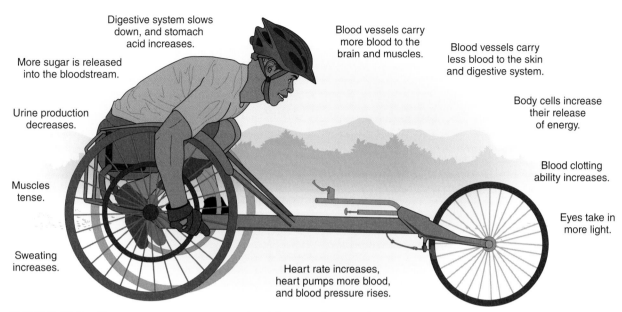

**FIGURE 17.3** The stress response: your body's way of preparing.

include riding a roller coaster, successfully competing in an activity, passing a driving test, playing in the school band, and meeting new people. Eustress helps make your life more enjoyable by helping you meet challenges and do your best.

Negative stress is sometimes called **distress**, which is produced by situations that cause worry, sorrow, anger, or pain (figure 17.4b). A situation that causes eustress for one person can cause distress for another. For example, an outgoing person might look forward to joining extracurricular activities at school or attending social events, whereas a shy person might dread the same situations. In addition,

### FIT FACT

The prefix *eu* in the word *eustress* is taken from the word *euphoria*, which means a feeling of well-being.

the same experience can be eustressful for you at one time and distressful at another. For example, taking a test for which you're well prepared can cause eustress, but taking a test for which you are not prepared might cause distress. You'll learn more about identifying stressors in your own life in the Self-Assessment feature that follows this lesson.

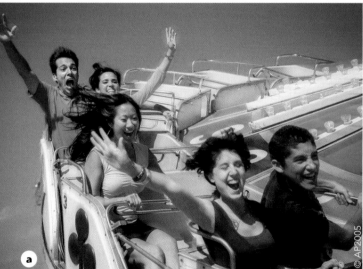

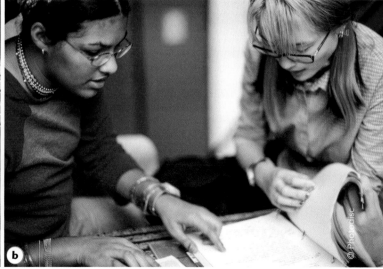

**FIGURE 17.4** Stress can be positive or negative: *(a)* Eustress is positive stress; *(b)* distress is negative stress.

## FIT FACT

Sometimes being in controlled stressful situations can help you prepare for more stressful situations in the future. For example, doing physical activity may be a stressor, but regular physical activity can help you become fit, healthy, and better able to handle stress in the future.

Distress can negatively affect your total health and fitness (more on this in the section describing step 3 of the Stress Management Pyramid). To control stress in your life, you need to understand the cause of the stress you're experiencing. Some causes of stress are described in the following sections.

## Physical Stressors

Physical stressors are conditions in your body or environment that affect your physical well-being. Examples include thirst, hunger, overexposure to heat or cold, lack of sleep, illness, pollution, noise, accident, and catastrophe (such as a flood or fire). Even excessive exercise can be a stressor, as in the case of athletes who overtrain. However, healthy people who follow good exercise principles and achieve good fitness are better able to adapt to the changes produced by physical stressors.

## Emotional Stressors

Emotions such as fear, anger, grief, depression, worry, and even falling in love are powerful stressors that can strongly affect your physical and emotional well-being. Another cause of emotional stress is overload—taking on more tasks than you can accomplish in the time available. To prevent or correct overload, learn to say no and develop your time management skills.

## Social Stressors

Social stressors arise from your relationships with other people. Each day, you have experiences that involve your family members, friends, teachers, employers, and others. As a teenager, you're probably exposed to many social stressors. Think about the stressors you experience in social situations in your life; these stressors can cause much of the stress you experience.

# Step 3: Understand the Effects of Stress

Stress—particularly high levels or prolonged periods of stress—can lead to both physical and emotional changes. Physical effects include increased stomach acid, which can aggravate ulcers. High blood pressure can also be related to stress and can lead to serious cardiovascular diseases and disorders. Prolonged stress can also lower the effectiveness of your body's immune system, making you more susceptible to certain diseases. These and other physical signs of stress include the following:

- Acne flare-ups
- Allergy flare-ups
- Backaches
- Blurred vision
- Constipation
- Diarrhea
- Difficulty sleeping
- Extreme fatigue
- Headaches
- Hyperventilation
- Increased blood pressure
- Indigestion
- Irregular heartbeat
- Light-headedness
- Muscle spasms
- Muscle tension
- Neckaches
- Perspiring
- Shortness of breath
- Tightness in throat or chest
- Trembling
- Upset stomach
- Vomiting

Some doctors think that many health problems in the United States requiring medical attention are stress related, which should give us all the motivation we need to deal effectively with stress, especially distress.

Emotional effects of stress include feelings of nervousness; anger, anxiety, or fear; frequent criticism

# SCIENCE IN ACTION: Depression Among Teens

Psychologists and public health scientists have done considerable research about depression among teens. As many as one in four teens report feeling sad for as long as two weeks at some time during the high school years. While feeling sad is something that we all feel from time to time, extended bouts of sadness can be a sign of depression. Other feelings that we all experience such as anxiousness, restlessness, guilt, and irritability can also be signs of depression when experienced in excess. Other more serious signs of depression include feelings of emptiness and hopelessness. The risk of teen suicide is higher among depressed teens than among those who are not. The U.S. National Institute of Mental

Health offers the following suggestions for helping a friend who shows signs of depression.

- Encourage your friend to talk to an adult and get evaluated by a doctor.
- Offer emotional support, understanding, patience, and encouragement.
- Talk with your friend—not necessarily about depression—and listen carefully.
- Never discount the feelings your friend expresses, but point out realities and offer hope.
- Never ignore comments about suicide.
- Report comments about suicide (see step 5 about getting help).

**Student Activity**

Interview a school guidance counselor or school nurse. Ask what help your school offers to help reduce stress and depression among teens. Ask what students can do to help. Write a summary of the interview.

of others; frustration; forgetfulness; difficulty paying attention; difficulty making decisions; irritability; lack of motivation; boredom, depression, or withdrawal; and change in appetite.

## Step 4: Learn Coping Skills

Once you've learned about the causes and effects of stress, you can move to the next level in the pyramid—learning **coping skills**. **Coping** means attempting to deal with problems, and coping skills are techniques that you can use to manage stress and address problems. The next lesson describes five types of coping skills.

## Step 5: Get Help

Social support is important. People often need help with managing their stress. Good sources of help and support can include parents, other family members, teachers, clergy, and friends. In addition, experts such as school counselors, guidance counselors, nurses, and physicians can provide advice about stress management and dealing with depression. Many communities also make health professionals available to help people manage stress, and you can find out about such resources in your community by asking a doctor, school counselor, or hospital referral service. Special hotlines are also available for assistance.

**Lesson Review**

1. What is meant by the terms *stress* and *stressor*?
2. What are the three stages of general adaptation syndrome?
3. What are the five steps in the Stress Management Pyramid?
4. What are some causes and effects of stress?

All people experience some negative stress in their lives, and when you experience distress, your body sends off certain signals. You'll learn to identify some of these signals in this self-assessment.

Table 17.1 lists some common signs of stress. You may notice some of these signs when you are not under excessive stress, but they're often especially apparent in times of great stress.

One way to determine whether an activity is stressful to you is to self-assess for signs of stress before and after the activity. Working with a partner, use the following steps to look for the signs of stress included in table 17.1. Record results as directed by your instructor. Remember that self-assessment information is personal and considered confidential. It shouldn't be shared with others without the permission of the person being tested.

1. Lie on the floor, close your eyes, and try to relax. Have your partner count your pulse and your breathing rate. Ask your partner to observe you for irregular breathing and unusual mannerisms. Then ask your partner to evaluate how tense your muscles seem using the list in table 17.1. Report any feeling of butterflies in your stomach or other indicators of stress to your partner. Record your results. Then have your partner lie down while you make the same assessments for him or her.

2. When directed by your instructor, all members of the class should write their names on a piece of paper and place the papers in a hat or box. The teacher will then draw names until only three remain in the container. The students whose names remain will each give a one-minute speech about the effects of stress. During and after the name drawing, observe your partner. Look for signs of stress. Also, notice your own feelings during the drawing. Finally, observe the people who were required to make a speech. Write down your observations about stress symptoms in you, your partner, and other class members. Refer to table 17.1 as needed.

3. Finally, walk or jog for five minutes after your second stress assessment. Then, once again, work with a partner to assess your signs of stress. Notice that the exercise causes your heart rate and breathing rate to increase. At the same time, however, it may help reduce earlier signs of the emotional stress related to the possibility of performing in front of the class. Record your observations.

### TABLE 17.1 Signs of Stress

| | |
|---|---|
| Heart rate | Is it higher than normal? |
| Muscle tension | Are your muscles tighter than usual?<br>Arms and shoulders<br>Back and neck<br>Legs |
| Mannerisms | Are unusual mannerisms present?<br>Frowning or twitching<br>Hands to face (nail biting) |
| Nervous feelings | Do you feel different than you normally do?<br>Feeling of butterflies in stomach<br>Tense or anxious feelings |
| Breathing | Is your breathing different than usual?<br>Irregular<br>Rapid or shallow |

# Lesson 17.2
## Managing Stress

**Lesson Objectives**

After reading this lesson, you should be able to
1. describe five types of coping strategies,
2. describe some guidelines for using the five coping strategies, and
3. explain why avoidance is often an ineffective method of coping.

**Lesson Vocabulary**

competitive stress, runner's high

**We** all get "stressed out" at times. What stresses you? How do you react to stress? Do you have strategies for dealing with your stress? Are they healthy strategies? Distress in life is unavoidable. Perhaps you feel overwhelmed by the many causes of distress and its effects. The first three steps in the Stress Management Pyramid require you to know and understand stress and the stressors that cause it. The fourth step refers to coping skills that you can use to manage stress. As described in the previous lesson, coping means attempting to overcome problems. Table 17.2 presents five types of coping skills.

## Physical Coping

As shown in table 17.2, the first type of coping skill involves taking physical steps to deal with stress. Here are some examples.

- **Do regular physical activity.** Regular physical activity can help you reduce your stress. Noncompetitive physical activity can help you get your mind off of stressful situations. For example, people who jog regularly report experiencing a **runner's high**. The runner's high refers to feelings of eustress experienced during or after a run. Similar feelings of eustress are experienced during or after other forms of vigorous aerobic exercise. Certain specific exercises, such as those described at the end of this lesson, are especially useful in helping you to relax. Yoga, tai chi, stretching exercises, and deep breathing exercises also can be useful in managing stress.

- **Reduce your breathing rate.** Sit down or lie quietly. Take a long slow breath, breathing in through your nose for 4 to 6 seconds. Exhale

### TABLE 17.2 Five Types of Coping Skills

| Coping skill | Description and examples |
|---|---|
| Physical coping | Using physical techniques: exercising, reducing muscle tension, eating well, and getting enough sleep |
| Intellectual coping | Using your thought processes: using problem-solving techniques, establishing priorities, managing time effectively |
| Emotional coping | Altering your emotions, especially in stress-producing situations: laughing and seeking fun activities, using intellectual coping skills such as thinking positive thoughts (thinking that you will do well) and avoiding negative thoughts, being flexible and having a willingness to adjust to the situation |
| Social and spiritual coping | Using positive social and spiritual situations and guidance: seeking social support, seeking spiritual support, seeking professional help |
| Coping by avoidance | Pretending the problem doesn't exist or putting off taking action to solve it: ignoring, avoiding, and escaping |

slowly through your mouth, again for 4 to 6 seconds. Repeat several times.

- **Reduce muscle tension.** Relaxing your muscles can help you reduce distress. You'll learn helpful relaxation techniques for reducing muscle tension in this chapter's Taking Action feature.

- **Rest in a quiet place.** Relax indoors or outdoors. Read. Listen to peaceful music. Take time out to relax in a quiet place.

- **Eat a nutritious, well-balanced diet.** Good nutrition contributes to good health, which can help you handle stress better. On the other hand, foods or drinks high in caffeine may cause you to be irritable and restless.

- **Get enough sleep.** Lack of sleep can lead to distress; in fact, lack of sleep is itself a stressor. Some problems might be easier to handle when you feel rested. Try to sleep at least 8 hours a night.

- **Pay attention to your body.** Notice how your body reacts in different situations. If you experience physical signs of distress, use some of the stress-management techniques described in this lesson.

## Intellectual Coping

The second type of coping skill, intellectual coping, involves using your thought processes to manage stress. Here are some examples.

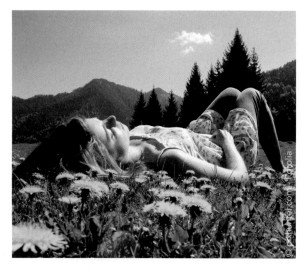

**Sometimes taking a moment to rest in a quiet place can help you manage stress.**

- **Use problem solving.** Use the scientific method to solve problems that cause stress. Rather than worrying about a problem, try to solve it. Make decisions and carry them out. When making a decision, look at several choices, consider the likely results of each, and choose the best one.

- **Establish your priorities and tackle one thing at a time.** If several problems pile up, ask yourself which is most important and which can wait.

- **Manage your time effectively.** Prioritize your activities so that you have time for the most important things. Learn to say no to new responsibilities and activities if you can't give them the time required.

- **Reduce your mental activity.** In stressful situations, imagining pleasant circumstances can help you relax. Try imagining a pleasant outdoor scene before a test or when you have thoughts that make you feel anxious. Some athletes listen to relaxing music before a competition to help reduce mental activity.

### FIT FACT

Bullying is a major source of stress among teens. The U.S. government's website Stopbullying.gov defines bullying as "unwanted, aggressive behavior among school aged children that involves a real or perceived power imbalance. The behavior is repeated, or has the potential to be repeated, over time. Bullying includes actions such as making threats, spreading rumors, attacking someone physically or verbally, and excluding someone from a group on purpose."

## Emotional Coping

The third way to manage stress is to use emotional coping skills. Here are some examples.

- **Have fun.** Laughter can help reduce distress. Take time to laugh and do things that are fun for you. Enjoy your life!

- **Change the way you think.** Not all problems can be solved as you would like, but

##  FITNESS TECHNOLOGY: Prevention of Cyberbullying

Many websites, including some developed by the U.S. government, have been designed to prevent bullying. In addition to defining bullying, these websites discuss who is at risk of bullying, how to prevent bullying, methods of responding to bullies, and how to get help regarding bullying. Teens more likely to be targeted for bullying include those who are perceived as different from their peers, as weak or unable to defend themselves, or as having few friends, but all teens can be subjected to bullying at one time or another. Others who face higher risk for bullying include teens who are lesbian, gay, bisexual, or transgender and those with a disability.

Many of the websites discuss cyberbullying—bullying that involves electronic technology. Cyberbullying includes bullying using devices such as cell phones, computers, and tablets. This type of bullying often uses social media, text messages, and chatrooms. Cyberbullying is different from other forms of bullying because it can be done 24-7, it often reaches teens when they are alone and without social support, and messages can be posted anonymously and distributed to many people very quickly. New technology also makes it relatively easy to take and post embarrassing photos to be used in cyberbullying.

Some of the better websites, including those described on the student section of the Fitness for Life website, offer content designed to help schools assess bullying and create effective anti-bullying rules and policies.

---

### Using Technology

Investigate your school to see if it has anti-bullying policies. Assess the extent of bullying and cyberbullying in your school. Assessment tools are available on anti-bullying websites.

---

you can still deal with them effectively. For example, suppose you're asked to trim the hedges at home. You do the job, then find that you did it incorrectly. You can't change what you've already done, but you can deal with the stress by recognizing that all people make mistakes. You can also learn from your mistake and make sure you understand the directions next time so that you can do a better job.

- **Think positively.** Positive thoughts can help you reduce distress. For example, try thinking that you *will* get a hit in the softball game instead of worrying about striking out. In softball, and all activities of life, success does not come with every attempt you make. Even the best hitters only get a hit about 30 percent of the time. A positive thinker would have confidence that she or he will get a hit the next time at bat. Making an effort to perceive a stressor as a challenge rather than as a problem can help you think positively.

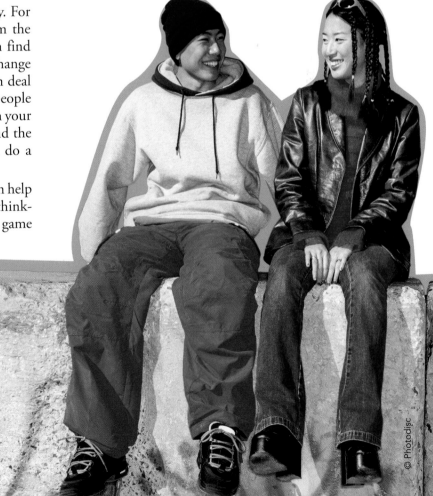

© Photodisc

- **Try not to let little things bother you.** Many events in life are simply not worth stressing over. For example, if you're disappointed, remind yourself that a situation might be better the next time.
- **Be flexible.** In stressful situations, be willing to bend a little, or adjust to changes as the situation demands.

> " Adopting the right attitude can convert a negative stress into a positive one. "
>
> —Hans Selye, stress researcher

# Social and Spiritual Coping

You can also manage stress by using social and spiritual coping skills. The following list gives some examples, all of which relate to getting help—the top step in the Stress Management Pyramid.

- **Seek help from friends and family.** When you feel down, don't keep it to yourself. Talk to family members and friends you trust. Just talking about problems can often help reduce distress.
- **Seek spiritual guidance.** Again, just talking to others often helps reduce stress, and trusted spiritual advisors may be able to offer additional help.
- **Seek professional help.** Sometimes it's necessary to seek professional help from a school official (such as a guidance counselor)

or, after consulting a parent or guardian, an outside professional (such as a counselor or psychiatrist).

## FIT FACT

When faced with a stressor, your body initiates a process called the fight-or-flight response. In earlier times, when people were hunter-gatherers, they had to fight wild animals or flee from them. We don't typically have that problem today, but when faced with a stressor our bodies still engage in the same fight-or-flight response, which results in the stress symptoms described in this chapter.

# Coping by Avoidance

The final type of coping is called avoidance, which involves pretending that the problem doesn't exist or putting off action to solve it. In some cases, avoidance can work; sometimes, if you know a situation will be stressful, you can avoid it. For example, you can choose to avoid an event at which alcohol might be served. However, avoiding or ignoring a problem often just lets it get more serious, and the other coping strategies described in this chapter are typically much more effective.

Similarly, trying to escape a problem is rarely effective. For example, using drugs may be a method of trying to cope by escaping, but it is both ineffective and comes with serious long-term consequences.

**Lesson Review**

1. What are the five types of coping strategies?
2. What are some guidelines for using the five coping strategies?
3. Why is avoidance often an ineffective method of coping?

Did your self-assessment indicate that you have a high level of stress? Most people need to deal with stress at one time or another. In this activity, you will get the opportunity to perform several exercises that are useful in reducing stress. You will also get the opportunity to practice a muscle relaxation procedure called contract-relax.

You can do some of these exercises at almost any time and almost any place. You might do them when you are sitting and studying or while you are riding or waiting for a bus. You can do most of them lying down or from a sitting position. You can even adapt some of these exercises to do them while standing.

## RAG DOLL

1. Sit in a chair (or stand) with your feet apart. Stretch your arms and trunk upward as you inhale.

2. Then exhale and drop your body forward. Let your trunk, head, and arms dangle between your legs. Keep your neck and trunk muscles relaxed. Remain relaxed like a rag doll for 10 to 15 seconds.

3. Slowly roll up, one vertebra at a time. Repeat the stretch and drop.

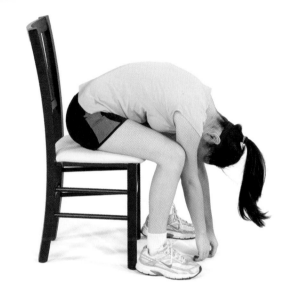

## NECK ROLL

1. Sit in a chair or on the floor with your legs crossed.

2. Keeping your head and chin tucked, inhale as you slowly rotate your head to the left as far as possible. Exhale and slowly return your head to the center.

3. Repeat the movement to the right.

4. Rotate three times in each direction, trying to rotate farther each time so that you feel a stretch in the neck.

5. Now drop your chin to your chest. Inhale as you slowly roll your head in a half circle to the left shoulder, and then exhale as you roll it back to the center. Repeat the movement to the right shoulder.

    Caution: Do not roll your head backward or in a full circle.

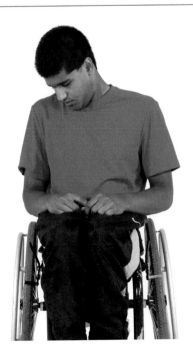

## BODY BOARD

1. Lie on your right side. Hold your arms over your head.
2. Inhale and stiffen your body as if you were a wooden board. Then exhale as you relax your muscles and collapse completely.
3. Let your body fall without controlling whether you tip forward or backward.
4. Lie still as you continue letting the tension go out of your muscles for 10 seconds. Then repeat the exercise starting on your left side.

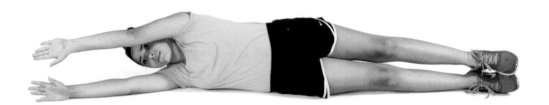

## JAW STRETCH

1. Sit in a chair or on the floor with your head erect and your arms and shoulders relaxed.
2. Open your mouth as wide as possible and inhale. (This may make you yawn.) Relax and exhale slowly.
3. Open your mouth and shift your jaw to the right as far as possible; hold for 3 counts.
4. Repeat the movement to the left. Repeat it on both sides 10 times.

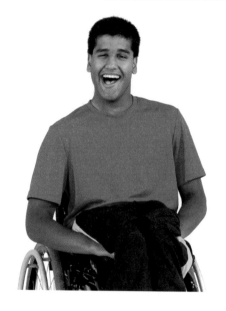

# CONTRACT-RELAX METHOD OF MUSCLE RELAXATION

Lie on your back with a rolled-up towel placed under your knees. Contract your muscles in the order that they are named in the following instructions. Hold each contraction for 3 counts. Then relax the muscles and keep relaxing for 10 counts. Each time you contract, inhale; each time you relax, exhale.

Do each exercise twice. Try this routine at home for a few weeks. With practice, you should eventually progress to a combination of muscle groups and gradually eliminate the contracting phase of the program.

1. Hand and forearm—Contract your right hand, making a fist. Relax and continue relaxing. Repeat the exercise with your left hand. Repeat it with both hands simultaneously.

2. Biceps—Bend both elbows and contract the muscles on the front of your upper arms. Relax and continue relaxing. Repeat the exercise.

3. Triceps—Bend both elbows, keeping your palms up. Straighten both elbows and contract the muscles on the back of the arm by pushing the back of your hand into the floor. Relax.

4. Hands, forearms, and upper arms—Concentrate on relaxing these body parts all together.

5. Forehead—Make a frown and wrinkle your forehead. Relax and continue relaxing. Repeat the exercise.

6. Jaws—Clench your teeth. Relax. Repeat the exercise.

7. Lips and tongue—With your teeth apart, press your lips together and press your tongue to the roof of your mouth. Relax. Repeat the exercise.

8. Neck and throat—Push your head backward while tucking your chin. Relax. Repeat the exercise.

9. Relax your forehead, jaws, lips, tongue, neck, and throat. Relax your hands, forearms, and upper arms. Keep relaxing all of these muscles.

10. Shoulders and upper back—Hunch your shoulders to your ears. Relax. Repeat the exercise.

11. Relax your lips, tongue, neck, throat, shoulders, and upper back. Keep relaxing these muscles all together.

12. Abdomen—Suck in your abdomen, flattening your lower back to the floor. Relax. Repeat the exercise.

13. Lower back—Contract and arch your lower back. Relax. Repeat the exercise.

14. Thighs and buttocks—Squeeze your buttocks together and push your heels into the floor. Relax. Repeat the exercise.

15. Relax your shoulders, upper back, abdomen, lower back, thighs, and buttocks. Keep relaxing these muscles all together.

16. Shins—Pull your toes toward your shins. Relax. Repeat the exercise.

17. Toes—Curl your toes. Relax. Repeat the exercise.

18. Relax every muscle in your body all together and keep relaxing.

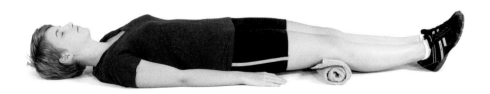

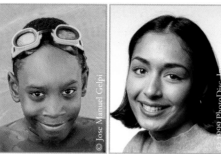

A little stress can give you more energy and help you meet a challenge. However, the effects of too much stress can interfere with your performance, especially during a competition. To do your best, you need to recognize the symptoms of **competitive stress** and know how to manage them. Here's an example.

Shelly watched from the bottom row of the bleachers as Willie shook his shoulders and arms. Shelly knew that swimmers do that to help them stay relaxed.

"You're the best, Willie! You're going to win!" Shelly had to yell so that Willie would hear her because the crowd was cheering so loudly.

Willie thought to himself, *I'm not so sure.* He shook his shoulders and legs again.

"You can do it!" Shelly screamed. "You're faster than anyone! We're all behind you!" She wasn't sure whether Willie heard her.

Willie had heard, and he thought, *That's the problem! The whole school is watching! My parents, too! If I don't get at least second place, our team might not make it to the regionals.*

*The way my stomach feels, these people are more likely to see me throw up than win the 200.*

Willie knew it was just stress. He'd felt the same way at the last meet. And Shelly had told him she felt the same kind of stress during a debate last week. The debate coach had shown her how to slow down her breathing to help her relax, and she had shown Willie how to do it.

Shelly stood up and took a deep breath. Willie saw her and did the same thing, and then he grinned to let her know he felt better. Willie was ready.

## For Discussion

How were Willie's muscles affected by the stress he felt? What were his other symptoms? How was Willie's stress similar to the stress Shelly had felt before her debate? What advice would you give Willie and Shelly (or anyone who is in a similar situation)? Consider the guidelines presented in the Self-Management feature when answering the discussion questions.

## SELF-MANAGEMENT: Skills to Manage Competitive Stress

In lesson 2 of this chapter, you learned that doing regular, noncompetitive physical activity can help you reduce stress. On the other hand, stress can be caused or increased by competitive sports and other competitive activities, such as performing a music solo or giving a speech. Factors that can make these activities stressful include competition, being evaluated by others, performing in front of a crowd, and feeling that the outcome is important. If you get involved in situations that cause competitive stress, use the following guidelines to help you manage your stress.

- **Learn to identify signs of stress.** You can learn this skill by using the self-assessment included in this chapter.
- **Avoid competitive stress.** One way to prevent competitive stress is to avoid

competitive and other situations in which you perform for others. This approach could, however, cause you to miss participating in activities that are fun. You might also fail to accomplish things that you're capable of doing.

- **Use muscle relaxation techniques.** Use the muscle relaxation techniques presented in this chapter's Taking Action feature.
- **Get experience.** Remember that most people feel stressed the first few times they compete or perform in public. With experience, competing and performing become easier.
- **Practice and prepare.** Practice and preparation help you experience eustress when competing and performing, thus

helping you achieve your full potential. When you practice, try to simulate the real event. Competitive practices with an audience can help you prepare.

- **Use mental imagery.** Some people do well in practice but not in actual competition. One method used by experienced competitors to address this issue is mental imagery. During the real event, they imagine themselves as they are in practice—relaxed and confident.

- **Use a routine.** For example, golfers find a regular putting routine very helpful. Following a routine before and during

a competitive event can help you stay focused and avoid being affected by factors around you.

- **Take a deep breath and slow your breathing.** For example, take a deep breath before shooting a free throw or performing a solo. If you find yourself becoming tense, slow down your breathing—it can help.

- **Use other effective methods of managing stress.** Use the effective ways of managing stress discussed earlier in this lesson.

 # ACADEMIC CONNECTION: Literacy

*Literacy* refers to being educated or cultured. In addition to physical literacy, it includes literacy in language (ability to read, write, and speak effectively), mathematics, science, humanities (including art and music), health, and technology. But how can you find reliable sources of information to increase your understanding in these various areas?

If you're like most teens today, you probably use the Internet to search for information. But you need to make sure the information you find on the Internet is from a reliable source. (See the Making Good Consumer Choices chapter for more on this subject.) Even with all the easily accessible information on the Internet, it's still important for you to know how to find information in print resources. People who have studied

library and information science (LIS) can assist you in finding information that will help you in all areas of study. Your school librarian is one such person. One indicator of college and career readiness is the ability to gather information from a variety of print and digital resources and integrate them in order to answer questions. In this book, you are asked to use a simplified form of the scientific method to make decisions, solve problems, and plan programs. School libraries have print materials (books, magazines, journals, and other documents) and extensive digital materials (online journals, documents, and resources) to help you in your studies. Explore your school library and consult with the school librarian to learn about the best methods for gathering information.

# TAKING ACTION: Relaxation Exercises

Did your self-assessment indicate that you have a high level of stress? Even if it didn't, you will have to deal with stressful situations from time to time. One way to manage the effects of stress on your body is to learn how to perform relaxation exercises, such as deep breathing, meditation, guided imagery exercises, and simple stretching techniques. Relaxation exercises may not seem beneficial the first time you try them because they may be unfamiliar or even uncomfortable. But as with any skill, you can learn to use them effectively if you perform them properly and practice them regularly. The more you practice using the techniques, the more successful you'll become in using them to manage your stress. **Take action** by performing relaxation exercises and trying the muscle relaxation procedures such as the contract-relax method.

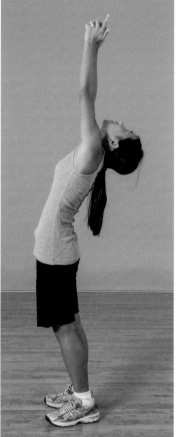
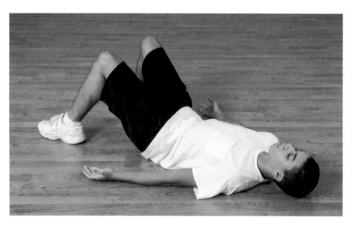

**Take action by managing your stress with relaxation exercises.**

# CHAPTER REVIEW

## Reviewing Concepts and Vocabulary

As directed by your teacher, answer items 1 through 5 by correctly completing each sentence with a word or phrase.

1. _____ is the body's reaction to a demanding situation.
2. The first phase of general adaptation syndrome is called the _____.
3. _____ is described as positive stress.
4. Coping that includes physical activity and reducing your breathing rate is called _____ coping.
5. Problem solving is a type of _____ coping.

For items 6 through 10, as directed by your teacher, match each term in column 1 with the appropriate phrase in column 2.

6. Stress Management Pyramid step 1
7. Stress Management Pyramid step 2
8. Stress Management Pyramid step 3
9. Stress Management Pyramid step 4
10. Stress Management Pyramid step 5

a. identify causes of stress
b. understand effects of stress
c. get help
d. identify signs of stress
e. learn coping skills

For items 11 through 15, as directed by your teacher, respond to each statement or question.

11. What is the difference between eustress and distress?
12. What are some guidelines for helping a friend who is depressed?
13. How can physical activity help you deal effectively with stress?
14. What is cyberbullying, and why is it a problem?
15. Describe some negative effects of competitive stress and explain how to manage it in a positive manner.

## Thinking Critically

Write a paragraph to answer the following questions.

You've been asked to give a speech to your class. You're concerned that if you refuse the opportunity, you may feel disappointed in yourself. However, you're also afraid that you'll be too nervous to speak in front of a large group. What are the positive and negative consequences of each choice? What decision would you make? How could you manage the stress associated with whichever decision you made?

## Project

Keep a journal for one week that documents incidents of stress in your life and observed stress in the lives of friends. Record incidents of bullying and cyberbullying. Use the information from your journal to create a brochure to help teens manage stress or prevent bullying and cyberbullying.

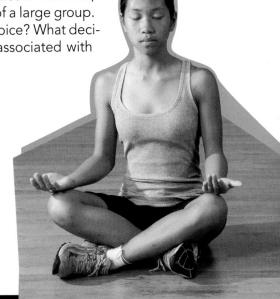

# 18

# Making Choices and Planning for Health and Wellness

## In This Chapter

 **Student Web Resources**
www.fitnessforlife.org/student

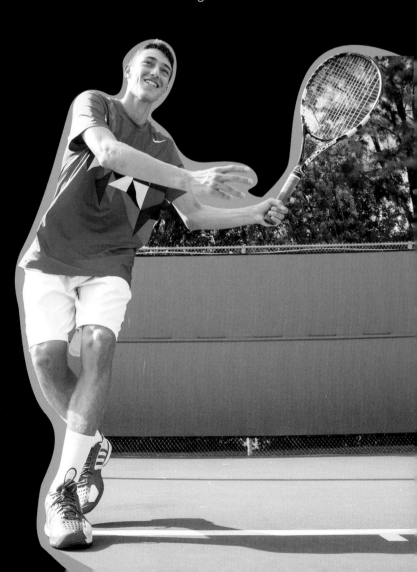

# Lesson 18.1

# Lifestyle Choices for Fitness, Health, and Wellness

## Lesson Objectives

After reading this lesson, you should be able to

1. describe several lifestyle choices—other than priority healthy lifestyle choices—that contribute to fitness, health, and wellness;
2. describe factors associated with the physical environment that affect fitness, health, and wellness; and
3. describe factors associated with the social environment that affect fitness, health, and wellness.

## Lesson Vocabulary

accelerometer, built environment, controllable risk factor, lifestyle, sleep apnea, uncontrollable risk factor

**If** you asked everyone you know, you would probably find that they would all like to have good health and wellness. But how many are aware of all the things they can do to achieve it? In this lesson, you'll learn about healthy lifestyle choices and how they can help you achieve good fitness, health, and wellness. You'll also learn about environmental and social factors that can influence your fitness, health, and wellness.

As you can see in figure 18.1, four major factors contribute to early death. Most early deaths result from unhealthy lifestyle choices. This means that these problems could be prevented if people changed the way they live. Making healthy lifestyle choices not only reduces the risk of disease and death from disease but also enhances wellness. For example, not smoking greatly reduces your risk of heart disease and cancer and also increases your quality of life. You can breathe better, you have a keener sense of smell, and you save the money you would have spent on tobacco and medical care.

## Healthy Lifestyle Choices and Risk Factors

You know by now that the word **lifestyle** refers to the way you live. A healthy lifestyle is a way of living that helps you prevent illness and enhance wellness. Healthy lifestyle choices are ways that you can reduce **controllable risk factors**—the risk factors that you can act upon to change. Healthy lifestyle choices are in your control, and if you choose well you reduce your risk of many major health problems. For example, one controllable risk factor is sedentary living; simply by being active, you can reduce your health risks.

Other risk factors—such as age and sex—are not in your control and thus are called **uncontrollable risk factors**. Because you cannot do anything about these risk factors, focus instead on those that you can control. This chapter describes several healthy lifestyle choices over which you do have some control.

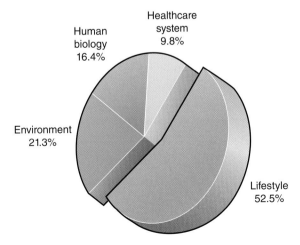

**FIGURE 18.1** Four main factors contributing to early death.

# Making Healthy Lifestyle Choices

This book focuses on three priority lifestyle choices: regular physical activity, healthy eating, and stress management. These lifestyle choices are considered to be most important because they can improve the fitness, health, and wellness of virtually all people. However, they are not the only lifestyle choices you can make to promote fitness, health, and wellness. This lesson describes other lifestyle choices you can make to maximize your fitness, health, and wellness.

## FIT FACT

Even though the dangers of tobacco use are well known, 17 percent of 12th graders, 11 percent of 10th graders, and 5 percent of 8th graders smoke. The good news is that smoking is less common than it used to be in all of these grades. Why? For one thing, social norms have changed, and smoking is less fashionable. In addition, public policies now often limit or prohibit smoking in public places, limit tobacco advertisements, and tax tobacco purchases.

## Adopt Good Personal Health Habits

In elementary school, you most likely learned about personal health habits, such as regular tooth brushing and flossing, good grooming (for example, hair and fingernail care), hand washing before meals and after bathroom use, and a healthy amount of sleep. But how many of these habits have you adopted? Practicing good health habits is one way you can prevent illness and promote optimal quality of life.

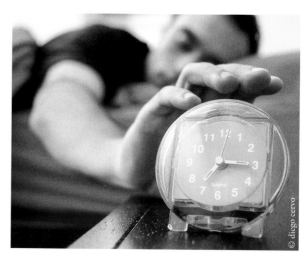

Getting enough sleep and practicing other simple personal health habits enhance health and wellness.

## ♥ FITNESS TECHNOLOGY: Sleep Tracking

Considerable evidence indicates that insufficient sleep can lead to health problems. Teens need about nine hours of sleep each night, but 9 out of 10 teens report getting less than that, and 10 percent get less than six hours. But the number of sleep hours is not the only issue; your sleep patterns are also important. People who wake up numerous times, or toss and turn frequently during the night, are not getting restful sleep.

For years, scientists have used sophisticated machines to detect **sleep apnea** and other serious sleep disturbances. Now, **accelerometers** (such as those worn to count steps) called *sleep trackers* can be used to determine movement patterns during the night. Experts caution against overgeneralizing the results from a sleep tracker because it is possible that a person sleeps well most of the

time but still has periodic restless nights. They also point out that sleep trackers do not sense different levels of sleep (light versus deep sleep). While sleep-tracking devices cannot directly determine the quality of sleep that a person gets, they can be used to screen for sleep problems in people who frequently feel tired or suspect that they have a problem.

### Using Technology

Investigate sleep-tracking devices and evaluate the pros and cons of using one. Check to see if activity-tracking devices cost more when they also include sleep-tracking functionality.

For example, if you have an illness that could have been prevented by means of proper health habits, you'll feel bad and will have at least a temporary reduction in your quality of living. Adopting good personal health habits is important throughout your life, and it can help you look and feel your best.

## Avoid Destructive Habits

Just as adopting healthy habits contributes to good health, practicing destructive habits detracts from your fitness, health, and wellness. Examples include, among many others, smoking and other tobacco use, legal and illegal drug abuse, and alcohol abuse. These destructive habits can impair your fitness, detract from your performance of physical activities, and result in various diseases, lowered feelings of well-being, and reduced quality of life.

## FIT FACT

Texting while driving is a major source of automobile accidents. In fact, doing so makes you 23 times more likely to crash. More generally, driver distraction is the cause of one out of every five fatal accidents in the United States (killing more than 3,000 people each year).

## Adopt Good Safety Practices

Reports of injuries and deaths caused by motor vehicle accidents fill the news each day. Other common causes of death and injury include falls, poisonings, drownings, fires, bicycle accidents, and accidents in and around the home. Many of these injuries and deaths could have been prevented if simple safety rules had been followed. Therefore, one national health goal in the United States is to reduce the number of deaths and injuries resulting from accidents. For your part, you can make a number of healthy lifestyle choices to reduce your risk of accidents, including wearing a seat belt, wearing a helmet when riding a bike or doing in-line skating, making sure that poisons are properly labeled, installing and maintaining smoke detectors, practicing water safety, and keeping your

home in good repair. And remember—being physically fit can also help you prevent accidents.

## Learn Cardiopulmonary Resuscitation (CPR)

Cardiopulmonary resuscitation (CPR) is a first aid procedure that is performed when the heart or breathing has stopped, and it saves many lives each year. The procedure uses chest compressions to keep blood flowing, preventing brain damage and death until expert medical help arrives. CPR training is strongly recommended, and many schools and several national organizations offer CPR classes and certification. According to the National Institutes of Health, "Even if you haven't had training you can do 'hands-only' CPR for a teen or an adult whose heart has stopped." Hands-only CPR is *not* recommended for use with children.

The American Heart Association recommends "two steps to staying alive": First, call 911 or direct someone else to call 911. Second, start chest compressions—push hard and fast at the center of the chest. The technique for chest compression is shown in figure 18.2. When two people are available, both mouth-to-mouth breathing and chest compression can be used.

CPR techniques and procedures are often revised based on new research and findings. For this reason, a regular check of the National Institutes of Health website for the latest information is recommended.

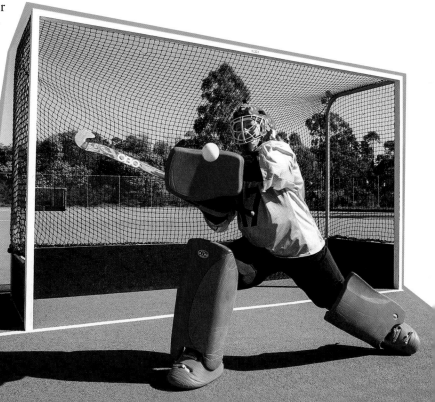

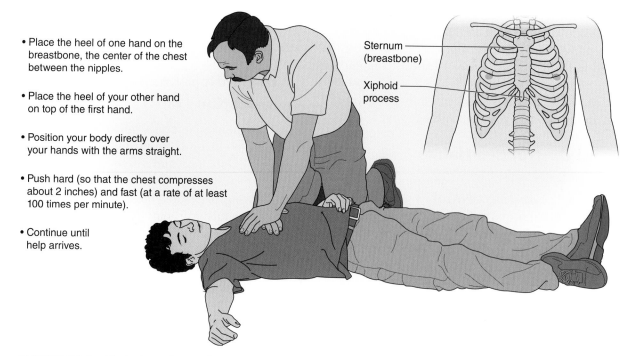

• Place the heel of one hand on the breastbone, the center of the chest between the nipples.

• Place the heel of your other hand on top of the first hand.

• Position your body directly over your hands with the arms straight.

• Push hard (so that the chest compresses about 2 inches) and fast (at a rate of at least 100 times per minute).

• Continue until help arrives.

Sternum (breastbone)

Xiphoid process

**FIGURE 18.2** Technique for performing hands-only CPR.

## Learn the Heimlich Maneuver (Abdominal Thrusts)

The Heimlich maneuver (also called abdominal thrusts) is performed when an object blocks a person's windpipe (air pathway). As shown in figure 18.3, the person administering the maneuver stands behind the person who is choking with his or her arms around the person's waist. The fist of one hand is placed just above the choking person's navel, with the thumb side of the fist against the body. The other hand is held over the fist. Pulling upward and inward causes pressure to force the object from the windpipe. As with all first aid procedures, training in the Heimlich maneuver is highly recommended.

## Learn Other First Aid Procedures

Even people who make healthy lifestyle choices and adopt good safety practices can have accidents. Because accidents can happen to anyone, all people should maintain a first aid kit and know how to administer first aid. In addition to learning how to perform CPR and the Heimlich maneuver, you should also learn how to apply pressure to prevent bleeding, how to clean and treat cuts and open wounds, how to use the RICE formula (rest, ice, compression, and elevation) to treat sprains and strains, and how to use other accepted first aid techniques.

## FIT FACT

Among adults, the most common reasons for not seeing a doctor include excuses such as, "I'm too busy," "It's only a minor problem that will go away on its own," "I can't afford it," and "I don't like to go to doctors." In reality, the best evidence suggests that putting off doctor visits for prevention and treatment can result in more time lost from work and more cost over the long run.

## Seek and Follow Appropriate Medical Advice

Even if you make healthy lifestyle choices, you may occasionally become ill. In those cases, seek and follow appropriate medical advice. In fact, for best results, get regular medical and dental checkups to help you prevent problems before they even start. Consult your physician and dentist to determine how often you should be seen. Some people avoid seeking medical help, but as noted in the Fit Fact, this practice can be dangerous because early detection of health problems is often important to an ultimate cure.

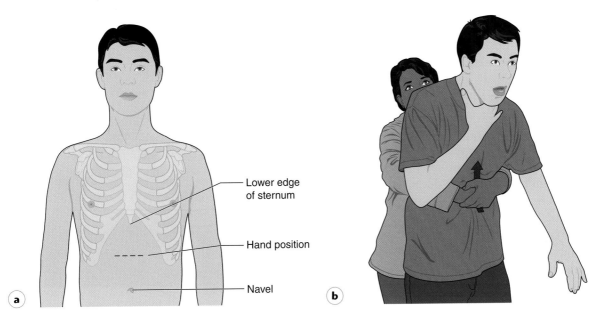

FIGURE 18.3 The Heimlich maneuver: *(a)* hand placement; *(b)* action—pull upward and inward.

# The Environment and Fitness, Health, and Wellness

The second leading contributor to early death (see figure 18.1) is an unhealthy environment. An environment is unhealthy if it causes health problems or detracts from personal wellness. Your physical and social environments are both important to your health and wellness.

## Physical Environment

The physical environment refers to the air, land, water, plants, and other physical things that exist around you. We know that certain physical environments can be very harmful to your health. For

## ⚛ SCIENCE IN ACTION: The Evolution of CPR

Over the past 50 years, new methods of CPR have been developed, resulting in thousands of saved lives. Mouth-to-mouth resuscitation was first used in France in the 1700s, and medical doctors used chest compression to revive people in the late 1800s.

Later, "artificial respiration" was modified to use a back-pressure arm-lift method, which in turn was replaced by chest compression and mouth-to-mouth breathing in the 1960s. Later,

one-person CPR alternated chest compression with mouth-to-mouth breathing. Doctors started using these procedures before they were recommended to the general public.

In recent years, CPR has changed considerably. As shown in figure 18.2, the hands-only method (chest compression) is now used for helping adults and teens in distress. This procedure is easier to do, and experts feel that it will be used more often as a result.

### Student Activity

Do a search to determine which local organizations offer CPR classes. If possible, take a class and get certified.

example, people who live in polluted cities are at greater risk than those who live in the countryside, where the air is often cleaner. Similarly, people who work in a coal mine or an area in which smoking is allowed have a higher risk of illness than those who work in less polluted areas. Your work environment is sometimes referred to as your vocational environment, and it can have serious consequences for your health. If your job requires you to sit all day and your work environment doesn't allow you to get up and move around frequently, you will have higher health risks.

You may not be able to change some physical environment factors, such as the place where you live. You can, however, take action to improve your environment. For example, you can avoid or minimize exposure to smoke-filled places, excessive exposure to the sun, and exposure to pollutants, such as weed killers and insecticides. To avoid excessive air pollution, exercise away from heavily traveled streets. You can also take certain steps to improve the physical environment—for example, recycling household materials and conserving water and electricity. You can also help people in your community who are making efforts to improve what is called the **built environment**—the physical characteristics of our neighborhoods. Improvements in the built environment—such as adding sidewalks and bike paths and improving street lighting and street crossings—have been shown to increase healthy physical activity such as walking and biking in neighborhoods.

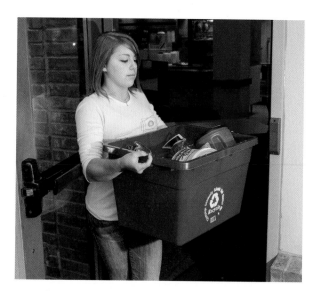

Recycling is something everyone can do to aid the environment.

> Earth provides enough to satisfy every [person's] need, but not every [person's] greed.

—Mahatma Gandhi, human rights leader

## Social Environment

Your social environment refers to the settings in which your social interactions take place. Social interactions refer to your contacts, conversations, and activities with friends, teachers, work colleagues, and others in leisure-time situations.

Researchers have shown that teens whose friends make unhealthy lifestyle choices are likely to try risky behavior such as abusing tobacco, drugs, or alcohol. In contrast, teens whose friends and family members make healthy lifestyle choices are more likely to practice healthy behaviors such as being physically active and eating well. With these two scenarios in mind, choosing supportive friends is important to your health and wellness.

Even if you make good choices, you, like most people, will probably be exposed to unhealthy social environments at some point in your life. If this does happen to you, consider using some of the self-management skills described in this book to help you make good choices in the heat of the moment. For example, learn to think critically, learn relapse prevention strategies, and practice ways to say no so that you can stick with your healthy behaviors. You do not need to be embarrassed or apologize for practicing healthy behaviors.

## Lesson Review

1. What are several lifestyle choices—other than priority lifestyle choices—that contribute to fitness, health, and wellness? How do they affect fitness, health, and wellness?
2. What factors associated with the physical environment affect fitness, health, and wellness?
3. What factors associated with the social environment affect fitness, health, and wellness?

Wellness is the positive component of good health. The five components of wellness include physical, emotional-mental, social, intellectual, and spiritual wellness. Complete the questionnaire to assess your current wellness. (Your teacher may give you a worksheet to use.) Remember that the information is personal and confidential. Don't share it with others without the permission of the person being assessed.

1. Read each wellness statement and decide whether you strongly agree, agree, disagree, or strongly disagree.

2. Record your results as directed by your teacher.

3. Calculate your score for each wellness component by adding your results for the three questions in that component.

4. Add all five component scores to get your overall wellness score.

5. Use table 18.1 to determine your rating for each component and your overall score.

### Healthy Lifestyle Questionnaire

| Wellness statement | Strongly agree | Agree | Disagree | Strongly disagree |
|---|---|---|---|---|
| 1. I am physically fit. | 4 | 3 | (2) | 1 |
| 2. I can do the physical tasks needed in my work. | 4 | (3) | 2 | 1 |
| 3. I have the energy to be active in my free time. | 4 | (3) | 2 | 1 |
| **Physical wellness score =** 8 | | | | |
| 4. I am happy most of the time. | 4 | (3) | 2 | 1 |
| 5. I do not get stressed often. | 4 | 3 | (2) | 1 |
| 6. I like myself the way I am. | 4 | 3 | 2 | (1) |
| **Emotional-mental wellness score =** 6 | | | | |
| 7. I have many friends. | 4 | (3) | 2 | 1 |
| 8. I am confident in social situations. | (4) | 3 | 2 | 1 |
| 9. I am close to my family. | (4) | 3 | 2 | 1 |
| **Social wellness score =** 11 | | | | |
| 10. I am an informed consumer. | 4 | (3) | 2 | 1 |
| 11. I check facts before making health decisions. | 4 | (3) | 2 | 1 |
| 12. I consult experts when I'm not sure of health facts. | 4 | 3 | (2) | 1 |
| **Intellectual wellness score =** 11 | | | | |
| 13. I feel a sense of purpose in my life. | (4) | 3 | 2 | 1 |
| 14. I feel fulfilled spiritually. | (4) | 3 | 2 | 1 |
| 15. I feel strong connections to the world around me. | 4 | (3) | 2 | 1 |
| **Spiritual wellness score =** | | | | |
| **Total wellness score =** | | | | |

Adapted from C. Corbin et al., 2013, *Concepts of fitness and wellness*, 10th ed. (St. Louis, MO: McGraw-Hill).

### TABLE 18.1 Rating Chart: Wellness

| Wellness rating | Three-item score | Total wellness score |
|---|---|---|
| Good | 10–12 | ≥50 |
| Marginal | 8 or 9 | 40–49 |
| Low | ≤7 | ≤39 |

# Lesson 18.2

# Healthy Lifestyle Planning and Career Opportunities

**Lesson Objectives**

After reading this lesson, you should be able to

1. describe the five steps involved in planning for health behavior change and
2. describe several career options in fitness, health, and wellness.

**Lesson Vocabulary**

consumer community, professional

In other chapters of this book, you've learned about healthy lifestyle planning and had the opportunity to prepare several types of physical activity plans. It's also important to plan for the healthy lifestyle choices discussed in this chapter.

## Healthy Lifestyle Planning

The same five steps you've used to plan physical activity can be used to prepare plans for eating better, reducing stress in your life, and adopting other behavior described in this chapter's first lesson. We'll use the example of Jeff, who was already implementing his physical activity plan but also wanted to make some other changes. To plan these changes, he used the five-step approach.

### Step 1: Determine Your Personal Needs

As part of learning about SMART goals, Jeff learned that it's important to make goals realistic. If he was going to be successful in adding to his current plan, he knew he shouldn't try to make too many changes at once. He reviewed some of the healthy lifestyle choices described in this chapter's first lesson, then decided to start by choosing one area in which he needed improvement. As indicated by the checkmark in the following list, he chose to eat better.

> " Don't dig your grave with your own knife and fork. "
>
> —English proverb

Check one or more areas of personal need in which you want to plan a change.

| | |
|---|---|
| ✔ Eat better | ___ Adopt safety habits |
| ___ Reduce stress | ___ Seek and follow medical advice |
| ___ Adopt personal health habits | ___ Learn first aid |
| ___ Avoid destructive behaviors | ___ Learn CPR |

When studying nutrition earlier, Jeff did a daily self-assessment of his eating habits and found that he could improve in several areas. Specifically, his diet included too much fat, he ate more calories than he should, and he didn't eat the recommended amount of fruits and vegetables.

### Step 2: Consider Your Program Options

Based on his needs and nutrition assessments, Jeff's options included changing his eating habits to be healthier.

- Cut the fat in his diet
- Eat more fruits
- Eat more vegetables
- Consume fewer calories

### Step 3: Set Goals

To help him eat better, Jeff set some SMART goals. That is, he set specific, measurable, attainable, realistic, and timely goals for changing his diet.

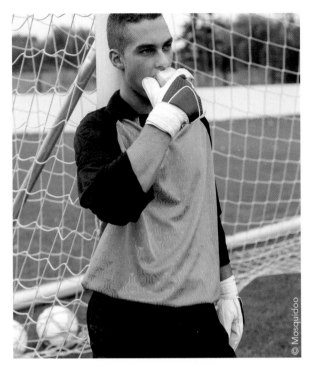

Dietary planning can help you eat more healthfully.

- Goal 1: Eat at least two servings of vegetables every day for two weeks.
- Goal 2: Eat at least two servings of fruits every day for two weeks.
- Goal 3: Eat at least five total servings of fruits and vegetables every day for two weeks.
- Goal 4: Drink two glasses of skim milk rather than whole milk each day.

## Step 4: Structure Your Program and Write It Down

Jeff prepared a written plan (see figure 18.4) that included each of his SMART goals and a calendar showing each day of the week. He posted the chart on the refrigerator (for the second week, he posted a clean copy of the same chart).

## Step 5: Keep a Log and Evaluate Your Program

Jeff used checkmarks on his written plan (see figure 18.4) to track whether he met each of his daily goals. His results? He did meet his goal for fruits and his goal for vegetables on all of the days, but on two days he did not eat five fruits and vegetables combined. He met his goal of drinking two glasses of skim milk on five of the seven days. During the second week, he was able to meet all of his goals on every day of the week.

When the two-week period ended, Jeff evaluated his results. He thought he had done pretty well. He was eating more fruits and veggies and had reduced the fat in his diet by drinking skim rather than whole milk. He decided to renew the plan for two more weeks just to be sure he kept on track. After that, he would consider making other healthy lifestyle changes based on the changes in his life. In the Taking Action feature, you'll have the opportunity to prepare your own healthy lifestyle plan using the same steps as Jeff. You can also use the planning steps to make changes later in life as circumstances change (for example, when you go to college, when you get a job).

# Careers in Fitness, Health, and Wellness

In this book, you've learned about various scientists who do research related to fitness, health, and wellness. Scientists do research to find new knowledge. In many ways, what they do is like finding pieces of a puzzle. But new information is not of much value

| Goal | Mon. | Tues. | Wed. | Thurs. | Fri. | Sat. | Sun. |
|---|---|---|---|---|---|---|---|
| Eat at least 2 daily servings of vegetables. | ✔ | ✔ | ✔ | ✔ | ✔ | ✔ | ✔ |
| Eat at least 2 daily servings of fruit. | ✔ | ✔ | ✔ | ✔ | ✔ | ✔ | ✔ |
| Eat at least 5 total daily servings of vegetables and fruit. | ✔ | ✔ | | ✔ | | ✔ | ✔ |
| Drink 2 daily glasses of skim milk rather than whole milk. | ✔ | ✔ | | ✔ | | ✔ | ✔ |

**FIGURE 18.4** Jeff's weekly plan and log.

## 👥 CONSUMER CORNER:  Consumer Communities

How do you get good consumer information? One way is to consult a book like *Fitness for Life*. You can also consult experts at your school or high-quality websites such as those described in this book. Another method is to establish a **consumer community** for finding and disseminating good information. Some schools have consumer communities that review scientific information and answer student questions related to fitness, health, and wellness. Some consumer communities provide a newsletter or contribute articles to the school newspaper. Others use the web or the school's intranet (local network) to provide information. Consumer communities with web access may also offer a website devoted to consumer issues. The site may feature articles

by students, provide sources of good consumer information, and answer questions from students. Some high school consumer communities have also used social media, such as Facebook.

Just as the work of scientists has to be reviewed by peers before it can be published, consumer communities must review the information that they provide to make sure that it is accurate and responsibly reported. They typically have older members who assume leadership roles and guide the review of information presented by the group. A consumer community provides a great opportunity to learn and serve for teens who are interested in a career in fitness, health, and wellness.

unless it is made available to the general public. This is where **professionals** come in. They deliver and apply the research knowledge developed by scientists; in other words, they put the pieces of the puzzle together so that the public can use the information. Professionals go through an extended education, typically a bachelor's degree or higher,

and often they must also be certified by a professional organization or governmental agency.

Now that you're nearing completion of this course, you may want to consider a career in fitness, health, and wellness. Table 18.2 lists various science and professional careers, as well as some examples (the table is not meant to be comprehensive).

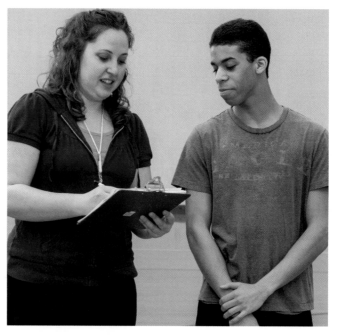

Qualified professionals are a good source of fitness, health, and wellness information.

**TABLE 18.2  Selected Careers in Fitness, Health, and Wellness**

| Science career | Description | Professional career | Description |
|---|---|---|---|
| Kinesiology | Biomechanics<br>Exercise anatomy<br>Exercise physiology<br>Exercise sociology<br>Motor learning/control<br>Sport/exercise psychology<br>Sport pedagogy | Physical education teacher<br>Coach<br>Fitness management<br><br>Fitness leader<br>Personal trainer<br><br>Sport management<br><br>Sport psychologist<br><br>Athletic trainer<br>Physical therapist<br><br><br>Occupational therapist<br><br><br>Strength coach<br><br>Dance teacher<br><br>Recreation leader/<br>therapist | Teaches physical education<br>Coaches sport teams<br>Manages corporate and commercial fitness<br>Leads exercises at clubs and worksites<br>Assesses and prescribes personal exercise<br>Applies business principles in sport settings<br>Helps athletes achieve optimal performance<br>Provides health care for athletes<br>Provides preventive and rehabilitative health care related to musculoskeletal problems<br>Provides rehabilitative health care related to musculoskeletal problems; helps people with tasks of daily life<br>Helps athletes and exercisers build muscle fitness<br>Teaches dance in schools, studios, other settings<br>Organizes programs and treats problems through recreation |
| Nutrition | Food science<br>Food services<br>Food technology<br>Sport nutrition | Clinical dietitian<br><br>Community dietitian<br>Management dietitian | Works in hospitals and nursing facilities<br>Works with organizations<br>Works in schools, health care facilities, and institutions such as prisons |
| Health | Environmental health<br>Epidemiology<br>Health statistics<br>Public health | Health educator<br>School health<br>Public health<br>Worksite wellness | Teaches health concepts in schools<br>Provides healthy school environment<br>Works in public health agency<br>Conducts programs in businesses |
| Medical and life sciences | Genetics<br>Immunology<br>Medical technology<br>Microbiology<br>Pathology<br>Virology | Medical doctor<br><br>Nurse<br><br>Dentist<br>Veterinarian<br>Medical technician<br>Physician's assistant<br>Chiropractor | Provides health care (diagnoses and treats)<br>Provides health care as part of health care team<br>Provides dental health care<br>Provides animal health care<br>Performs laboratory analysis<br>Helps physicians provide health care<br>Provides health care focused on musculoskeletal system |

**Lesson Review**

1. What are the five steps involved in planning for health behavior change?
2. What are several career options in fitness, health, and wellness?

An optimist is a person who expects a good or favorable outcome. This positive thinking is an example of thinking success. The optimist thinks that he or she can succeed at a specific activity. A person who thinks success, or has positive thoughts, will succeed more often than a person who has negative thoughts. Here's an example.

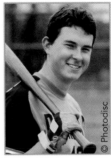

Aaron loves baseball. For two years, he played on a team that won most of its regular season games. The team even played in the league's championship game. During that time, Aaron played well at second base and hit a few home runs.

This year, Aaron moved up to a new team. Most of the players at the new level were older, bigger, and stronger than Aaron. During the first game, he was hit by a pitch once and struck out in his other at bats. In fact, he didn't get the bat on the ball even one time.

Aaron's coach noticed that he was no longer swinging with confidence. Luckily, he also knew that Aaron had the physical strength and skills needed to hit the ball. He knew Aaron just needed to change the way he was thinking. He wouldn't hit the ball until he thought he could. The coach had Aaron do some practice drills that he could successfully complete. He taught Aaron to visualize himself hitting the ball and to say and believe "yes, yes, yes" as he stood waiting for the pitch.

The coach also taught Aaron not to think obsessively about the times he'd struck out or failed to make a play. "After all," the coach said, "even the best professionals only get a hit about one out of every three tries. The next play is the one to think about." As Aaron regained his confidence, he improved his hitting.

## For Discussion

How did Aaron's negative feelings affect the way he played baseball with the new team? How was he able to change his attitude to think about success? What are some other ways in which a person can change negative thoughts into positive ones? Consider the guidelines presented in the Self-Management feature when answering the discussion questions.

# SELF-MANAGEMENT: Skills for Thinking Success

One reason that some people fail to stick with a healthy lifestyle program is that they don't believe in themselves. Many people make New Year's resolutions, but not all accomplish their goals. Use the following guidelines to help you succeed.

- Assess your feelings about success. Complete the worksheet provided by your teacher, and then use your answers to see where you might change in order to improve your chances of being successful.

- Set realistic, attainable goals and use self-monitoring to reinforce your successes.

- Use self-assessments to help you set goals and evaluate your progress.

- Choose activities that you enjoy and that match your abilities.

- Practice to improve your performance skills.

- Find friends with similar interests who support you.

- Take steps to avoid relapse and say no to things you don't want to do.

- Learn how to overcome the barriers to success.

- Work to build healthy self-perceptions and self-confidence.

- Practice relaxation techniques that can help you overcome competitive stress.

- Learn the steps in planning for healthy lifestyle change.

- Become an informed consumer.

- Avoid unhealthy physical and social environments.

- Use other self-management techniques that you have studied in this book.

In the second lesson of this chapter, you read about Jeff's plan for adopting a healthy lifestyle. Use the same five steps that Jeff used and **take action** by selecting at least one of the healthy lifestyle choices presented at the beginning of this lesson and preparing a plan to make a positive change in this area. You won't be able to take this action in class; it will be something that you do on your own.

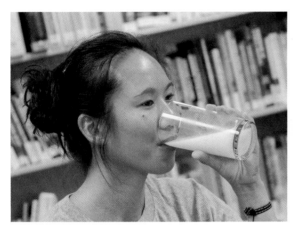

Take action by making a positive change to a lifestyle, such as eating more healthfully.

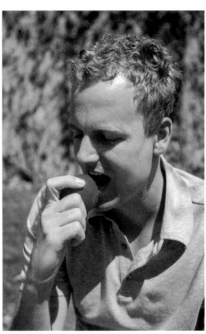

# CHAPTER REVIEW

## Reviewing Concepts and Vocabulary

As directed by your teacher, answer items 1 through 5 by correctly completing each sentence with a word or phrase.

1. Risk factors that you can change are referred to as _____ risk factors.
2. _____ is another name for mouth-to-mouth breathing and chest compression.
3. A technique to prevent choking is called _____.
4. Changing the physical environment to make it easier to walk or ride a bicycle is referred to as changing the _____ environment.
5. A _____ helps athletes achieve optimal performance.

For items 6 through 10, as directed by your teacher, match each term in column 1 with the appropriate word or phrase in column 2.

6. career in kinesiology
7. career in nutrition
8. career in health
9. career in medical or life science
10. texting

a. veterinarian
b. athletic trainer
c. frequent cause of accidents
d. dietitian
e. epidemiologist

For items 11 through 15, as directed by your teacher, respond to each statement or question.

11. Describe several healthy lifestyle changes that can be made to improve a person's fitness, health, and wellness.
12. Explain the difference between controllable and uncontrollable risk factors. Give examples.
13. Identify one healthy lifestyle choice and describe how it contributes to fitness, health, and wellness.
14. Explain how a person's environment relates to personal wellness.
15. Discuss career options in one of the areas of science identified in this chapter.

## Thinking Critically

Interview several people who are currently active in careers described in this chapter. Ask how their time is spent in a typical day and what roles and responsibilities they enjoy or struggle with. Keep a journal of their comments. Based on the information in this chapter and your journal, identify a career that interests you. In one to three paragraphs, describe why this career might be a good option for you.

## Project

Many schools have a wellness committee that includes students, teachers, parents, and other school staff. Wellness committees often schedule special events such as wellness weeks, during which a schoolwide effort is made to promote fitness, health, and wellness. If your school has a committee, attend a meeting and prepare a report of its activities. Indicate how students can become involved. If your school doesn't have a committee, explore ways to create one.

# UNIT VII
# Moving Through Life

## Healthy People 2020 Goals
- Increase the percentage of teens who meet physical activity guidelines for teens.
- Reduce time spent watching television and playing computer games.
- Increase biking to school.
- Improve community facilities to promote activity.
- Increase physical education in schools.
- Increase education to promote health-enhancing behaviors and reduce health risks.
- Increase education designed to prevent inactivity.
- Reduce overweight and obesity among teens.
- Improve teens' comprehension of health promotion and disease prevention concepts.
- Increase the number of people who achieve high-quality, longer lives by reducing preventable disease, injury, and early death.
- Create environments that promote health, fitness, and wellness for all.

## Self-Assessment Features in This Unit
- Assessing Game Strategy and Tactics
- Analyzing Basic Skills
- Modifying Rules in Games

## Taking Charge Features in This Unit
- Developing Tactics
- Positive Self-Talk
- Conflict Resolution

## Self-Management Features in This Unit
- Skills for Developing Tactics
- Skills for Positive Self-Talk
- Skills for Conflict Resolution

## Taking Action Features in This Unit
- Cooperative Games
- Applying Principles
- Team Building

# 19

# Strategies for Active Living

## In This Chapter

 **Student Web Resources**
www.fitnessforlife.org/student

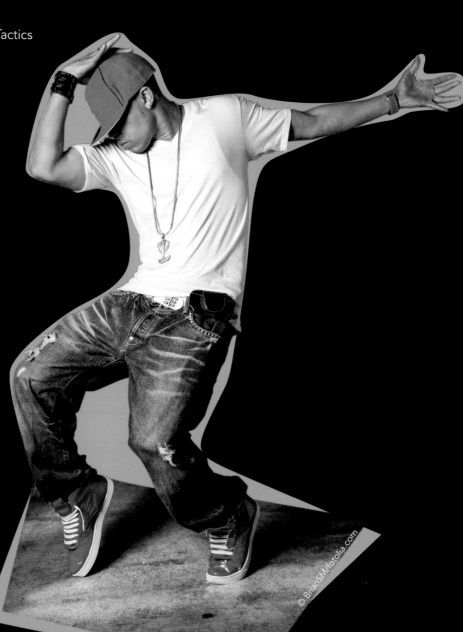

© BrianSM/fotolia.com

# Lesson 19.1

# Opportunities in Physical Education

## Lesson Objectives

After reading this lesson, you should be able to

1. name the five characteristics of a physically educated person,
2. describe the top 10 reasons that high-quality physical education is needed, and
3. describe several approaches to physical education.

## Lesson Vocabulary

adventure education, cooperative game, dance education, fitness education, outdoor education, physical literacy, sport education

**Are** you physically literate? Do you know what **physical literacy** is? Physical literacy refers to being physically educated. A physically literate (or physically educated) person has the knowledge, skills, and confidence to enjoy a lifetime of healthful physical activity. According to the Society of Health and Physical Educators (SHAPE America), a person who achieves these five goals is considered to be a physically literate or physically educated person. Specifically, a physically literate person

- participates regularly in physical activity,
- is physically fit,
- has learned skills necessary to perform a variety of physical activities,
- values physical activity and its contribution to healthy living, and
- knows the implications and benefits of being involved in physical activities.

Adapted from SHAPE America.

## FIT FACT

Literacy refers to being educated or "cultured." Early definitions of literacy referred only to the ability to read and write (prose and document literacy). Literacy has been expanded to include other skills, such as oral, quantitative, computer and technical, problem-solving, and physical. The types of literacy apply to all subject matter areas, including the sciences, the humanities, the arts, math, health, and physical education (physical literacy).

## Physical Education Units

Virtually all schools conduct physical education classes that help teens learn to perform a variety of physical activities included in the Physical Activity Pyramid. Classes are normally organized in units, each of which typically focuses on one type of activity from the pyramid. A unit can last a few weeks or as long as a full semester. It isn't possible to show all of the activities that can be included in the units, but some examples are illustrated in figure 19.1. Learning more about different programs and units within physical education can help you to make choices both in future physical education classes and about participation in physical activity programs after you graduate.

## Physical Education Program Approaches

Within physical education, several approaches have gained popularity in high schools in recent years. All of these are part of the regular physical education program, but each focuses on achieving certain physical education objectives in certain ways. Some examples are described in the following discussion.

### Fitness Education

**Fitness education** refers to physical education classes or units that focus on teaching fitness and activity concepts and learning self-management skills that can help you be active for a lifetime. Fitness education classes often use a text such as *Fitness*

## FIT FACT

A survey from the Harvard School of Public Health found that more than 90 percent of parents believe schools should provide physical education, particularly for fighting obesity.

*for Life* and include some classroom study and some participation in activities either in the gym or on the playing field. Fitness education can be mixed in a variety of units or taught as an independent class. One key feature of fitness education is to help students learn to be independent thinkers capable of solving problems and making informed decisions. One example of a desired outcome of fitness education is for students to plan personal programs based on self-assessment and sound personal goals. Teens who complete a fitness education class are more likely to be active several years after they graduate from high school than those who don't.

## Sport Education

**Sport education** is an approach to teaching physical education that is designed to make playing sport fun, interesting, and authentic. In sport education, as in the sporting world itself, the year is divided into several "seasons" (for example, baseball season or soccer season). During a season in sport education, several different activities are performed, including sport, recreational, and fitness activities. Early in each season, three to five teams are formed within the class, and members remain with the same team throughout the season. Teams practice together to learn skills and compete against other teams in the class. An effort is made to balance teams to make competition fair. Games are modified to accommodate team size, equipment, and rules.

In sport education, team members develop a sense of belonging (or team affiliation). During a season, members play different roles such as coach, fitness trainer, statistician, publicist, equipment

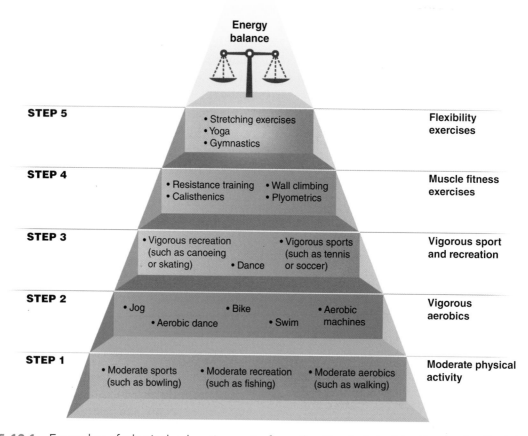

**FIGURE 19.1** Examples of physical education units from the Physical Activity Pyramid. All of the units shown contribute to energy expenditure and aid in energy balance.

# SCIENCE IN ACTION: Top 10 Reasons for High-Quality Physical Education

Scientists from several areas of kinesiology have identified 10 research-based reasons that high-quality physical education (HQPE) is important. HQPE programs offer the opportunity for *all* students to learn, provide meaningful content, provide quality instruction by trained teachers, and offer student and program assessments.

1. **Regular physical activity helps prevent disease.** Regular physical activity reduces risk of hypokinetic diseases, including heart disease, cancer, diabetes, and osteoporosis.

2. **Regular physical activity promotes lifetime wellness.** Health involves more than freedom from disease. Being regularly active improves wellness (quality of life, sense of well-being).

3. **HQPE provides unique opportunities for activity.** Physical education, including dance education, is the primary subject that provides an opportunity to be active during school hours. Teens who do physical education meet national activity goals more often than those who do not.

4. **HQPE helps fight obesity.** About one-third of youth and two-thirds of adults are overweight or obese. Being active in physical education classes and at other times during the school day helps expend calories to reduce the risk of overweight and obesity.

5. **HQPE helps promote lifelong physical fitness.** Regular physical activity using the FIT formula for each type of physical activity helps build all parts of health-related physical fitness. This enhances health and increases your ability to function effectively in work and play.

6. **HQPE teaches self-management and motor skills.** Teens who learn self-management skills are more likely to be active after they graduate from school. They know how to plan personal activity programs and avoid quackery. Students who learn a variety of motor skills are more active later in life.

7. **HQPE and regular physical activity promote learning in other academic areas.** Teens who are active and fit score better on academic tests than those who are inactive. Evidence shows that physical activity is necessary for the brain to function optimally. Active students are less likely to miss school or have discipline problems.

8. **HQPE and regular physical activity make good economic sense.** The annual cost of sedentary living in the United States exceeds $150 million. Worksite wellness programs enable many companies to save money, reduce absenteeism, and increase job satisfaction. High-quality physical education promotes the same benefits.

9. **HQPE is widely endorsed.** More than 50 organizations in the U.S. support the value of HQPE in schools, including the American Academy of Pediatrics (AAP); the American College of Sports Medicine (ACSM); the American Heart Association (AHA); the U.S. Centers for Disease Control and Prevention (CDC); and the President's Council on Fitness, Sports, and Nutrition.

10. **HQPE helps educate the total person.** As President John F. Kennedy said, "physical fitness is the basis of all the activities in our society. And if our bodies grow soft and inactive, if we fail to encourage physical development and prowess, we will undermine our capacity for thought, for work, and for the use of those skills vital to an expanding and complex America."

Adapted from Le Masurier and Corbin 2006.

---

### Student Activity

Interview at least one teacher who is not a physical education teacher. Ask questions to see if he or she is aware of the 10 reasons for high-quality physical education.

manager, scout, scorekeeper, or referee. Game results are posted, and standings are updated regularly. Each season concludes with postseason playoffs and an award ceremony. A key aspect of sport education is that team members provide leadership and assume responsibility for activities conducted during each season.

## Adventure Education

**Adventure education** typically focuses on challenging recreational activities such as rock climbing, orienteering, boating, rafting, and ropes courses. Adventure education units are sometimes taught as part of physical education and sometimes used in camp settings, recreational programs, and even programs designed to train business executives. Among the principal goals of adventure education are trust building, problem solving, and enhancement of self-confidence. This approach often uses teams, and it emphasizes placing trust in team members and working together to overcome risks. While adventure education is often conducted in outdoor and wilderness settings, it can also be conducted indoors using trust-building activities

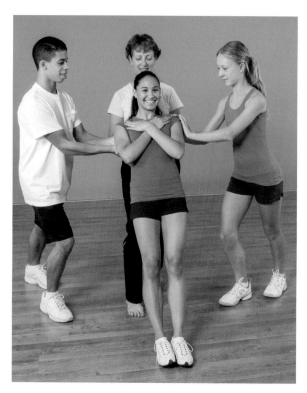

Trust-building activities can be part of the adventure education curriculum.

and cooperative games. Like fitness education and sport education, adventure education is really a way of teaching physical education.

## Outdoor Education

**Outdoor education** is education that occurs in an outdoor classroom. One type of outdoor education is adventure education that is conducted outside. Like adventure education, outdoor education uses activities such as camping, fishing, and hiking to develop physical literacy. Some schools conduct camps where students participate for several days and learn in outdoor settings.

## Cooperative Games

Like sport education, **cooperative games** use teams to help students learn cooperation, have fun, and overcome challenges. But cooperative games focus on working *together* in teams rather than competing or winning. Some physical education programs include units focused on cooperative games; as previously mentioned, cooperative games are also sometimes part of adventure education. Many books describe cooperative games that keep all people active and emphasize working together to solve problems. Cooperative games are sometimes used to help people get to know each other (through "icebreakers") and build trust. You can try some cooperative games in this chapter's Taking Action feature.

## Dance Education

**Dance education** can be part of a physical education program or a separate program that focuses on teaching various forms of dance both in and out of school. Dances are performed in many cultures and can be done individually, with a partner, or in a group. For example, ballet is a form of classical dance that is often performed by accomplished dancers as a form of art. Modern dance is a more contemporary form of dance. Dance education can include classes or units focused on these forms or others, ranging from social dances of moderate intensity to more vigorous options such as ballroom dance. Traditional types include ballroom dances such as the waltz, foxtrot, and quickstep. Latin dances include the samba, cha-cha, and rumba. Hip-hop is a vigorous type of dance popular among

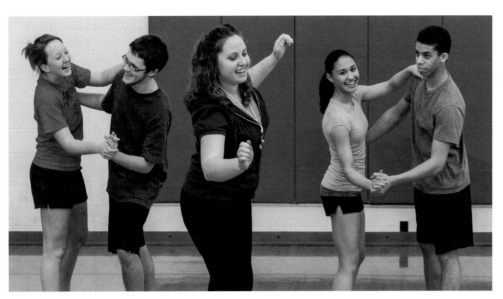

Dance in many forms can be included in physical education units or separate dance education classes.

youth. Other currently popular types include jazz, country and western, line dance, swing dance, and the jitterbug. Dance education classes often include various dances strongly associated with a particular culture, such as square dance, Irish dance, and African dance. Aerobic dance and other types of fitness dance such as Zumba may be included as part of dance education or fitness education units.

"
I do not try to dance better than anyone else. I only try to dance better than myself. "

—Mikhail Baryshnikov, professional dancer

## Lesson Review

1. What are the five characteristics of a physically literate (educated) person?
2. What are the top 10 reasons for conducting high-quality physical education?
3. Describe several approaches to conducting physical education.

In this chapter's second lesson, you'll learn several steps for developing strategy and tactics in various situations. In this self-assessment, you'll do an experiment to determine the effectiveness of different game strategies and tactics. As directed by your instructor, record your results and report on the effectiveness of the various options. Remember that self-assessment information is personal and considered confidential. It shouldn't be shared with others without the permission of the person being tested.

## Directions

1. Form teams of 2 to 4 players. Each team must have the same number of players.

2. Place four hoops on flat ground such as a gym floor or outdoor field. The hoops are placed at the following distances from a throwing line: 10 feet (3 meters), 20 feet (6 meters), 30 feet (9 meters), and 40 feet (12 meters). See figure 19.2.

3. Each team member throws three beanbags at each hoop target.

4. Record the number of beanbags that land inside each hoop for each team (more than half of the bag must be in the hoop). Score 1 point for every beanbag that lands inside the first target (the one that is 10 feet, or 3 meters, from the throwing line), 2 points for each bag in the second target, 3 points for each bag in the third target, and 4 points for each bag in the fourth target. Total your team's points and record your team score.

5. After completing step 4, each team decides on a short- or long-toss strategy for achieving the highest possible team score. In the short-toss strategy, only targets 1 and 2 can be used. In the long-toss strategy, only targets 3 and 4 can be used.

6. Each player on each team tosses three beanbags at the chosen targets (short or long toss). All players must throw only at the two targets chosen based on team strategy.

7. At least one player on each team must throw at each target. For example, if you have three players on a team, two can throw at the same target, but the third must choose the other target.

8. Decide tactics as a team. Who will throw at which target? How many players will throw at the shorter of the two targets?

9. After all players have completed their throws, calculate your team's score by adding the scores of all team members' throws (see step 4 for scoring). Record individual and team results.

10. Play again using the same procedures, but use the opposite strategy (if your team used the long-toss strategy the first time, use the short-toss strategy this time, or vice versa). As noted in item 7, at least one player on each team must throw at each target.

11. Using the same scoring procedure, calculate your team's score for the second strategy. Record your individual and team results.

12. Based on previous scores, determine which of the two strategies gives your team the better probability of success.

13. Prepare a brief report that includes the results of all trials. If more time was provided to practice the task, how might the probability of success change for each strategy? Comment on whether the group would use the same strategy after having time to practice.

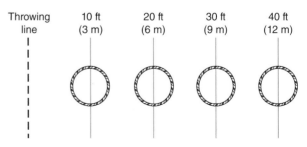

**Figure 19.2** Setup for the strategy and tactics assessment game.

# Strategy and Tactics

## Lesson Objectives

After reading this lesson, you should be able to

1. define *strategy* and provide examples that relate to physical activity and healthy lifestyle choices,
2. define *tactic* and explain its role in implementing a strategy, and
3. explain the five steps for planning strategy and tactics.

## Lesson Vocabulary

strategy, tactic

**Success** in sport and other physical activities requires certain physical abilities, including good fitness and good motor skills. People who train properly can achieve fitness and, with good practice, can master skills. But physical abilities are not the only requirements for success. You also need a good strategy and sound tactics.

## Strategy

A **strategy** is a master plan for achieving a goal. The word *strategy* comes from the Greek word *strategos*, which refers to the general or leader of an army. Consistent with its origin, many early uses of the word *strategy* were associated with military planning. Today, the word *strategy* is still often used in military contexts, as when referring to a war strategy. In modern times, however, it is also used in business and organizational contexts. Marketing, for example, is an aspect of business that helps companies develop strategies for selling their products. Strategies are also useful in sport and other physical activities. In sport, for example, coaches develop strategies or master plans for winning games, and players use strategies to be effective team members.

> " A strategy lays out a plan for reaching your goals; tactics help you carry out your strategy. "
>
> —Phil Abbadessa, teacher and coach

## Tactics

A **tactic** is a specific method for carrying out a strategy. The word *tactic* derives from the Greek *taktikos*, which refers to arranging forces in a battle formation. As with strategy, tactics were first used in the military, in this case to carry out a fighting strategy. Generals first developed a master plan or strategy, then developed specific tactics or procedures to carry out the strategy or battle plan.

Similarly, in marketing a product or service, companies first develop a strategy, then use specific

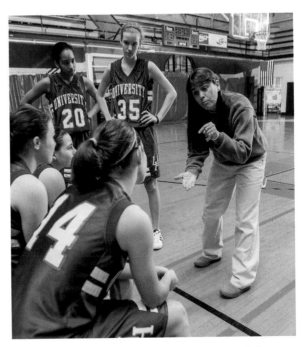

Strategies and tactics are used in sports, and they are also important in other areas of life.

tactics to carry it out. For example, a food manufacturer might adopt a strategy of selling cereals high in sugar and low in nutrients. In this example, the strategy is to convince children that they want the cereal. Even though adults buy the cereal, children have a big influence on what adults buy. Specific tactics might include placing ads for the cereal on Saturday morning TV shows aimed at children or placing toys in cereal boxes. Children see the ad or want the toy and beg a parent to buy the cereal.

In sports and games, a coach, team leader, or (in an individual sport or game) individual competitor develops the strategy. For example, a basketball team might decide to adopt a defensive strategy—that is, to emphasize defense in order to force the other team to make errors. Within this strategy, one specific tactic would be to use a full-court press, in which players guard their opponents at both ends of the court. Another defensive tactic might be to double-team the other team's best shooter (that is, to have two players guard one very good player on the other team).

You can also use strategy and tactics in other areas of your life. Some examples are provided in table 19.1.

## FIT FACT

The game of chess requires both strategy and specific tactics. In fact, many coaches and military leaders use the game to sharpen their ability to use tactics to carry out a strategy.

# Planning a Strategy and Developing Tactics

As shown in table 19.1, a strategy and accompanying tactics can be useful in many areas of your life. But how do you develop a strategy and tactics? You can use steps similar to those in the scientific method and those used in program planning. Since tactics are used to implement a strategy, the strategy is planned first.

## Step 1: Use Existing Information

Much is already known about strategies for various sports and activities. Therefore, a good first step is to read books and articles about the strategies that have been used successfully in your chosen sport

### TABLE 19.1  Examples of the Use of Strategies and Tactics

| Situation | Strategy example | Tactic examples |
|---|---|---|
| **Healthy eating** Person consumes more calories than expended each day. | Eat less food with empty calories. | Remove food with empty calories from house. Learn to say no. Eat healthy snacks. Avoid buying food from vending machines. |
| **Physical activity** Person does not meet national activity guidelines. | Prepare a written physical activity plan. | Follow the five steps for writing a plan. Log daily activity. |
| **Managing stress** Person has too many things to do and not enough time to do them. | Reduce commitments and spend more time on important things. | Self-assess current time use. Rank current commitments from high to low importance. Focus on high-importance commitments. Learn to say no to unimportant commitments. |
| **Playing a team sport** Person's intramural team wants to do well in the soccer league. | Focus on defense. | Assign more players to defense. Use zone defense because some players lack skills. Use long defensive kicks to clear ball and reduce shots on goal. |
| **Preventing back pain** Person wants to reduce risk of back pain. | Focus on good posture in standing, sitting, and moving. | Assess current posture and core fitness. Perform core exercises. Practice good posture. |

## 👥 CONSUMER CORNER: TV Tactics—Creating Needs

You've now learned about developing a strategy and using tactics to achieve a goal. Companies also develop strategies and tactics. Sometimes their strategies help them but are not good for you. For example, a company's strategy may be to get you to buy something you don't really want or need. To help them carry out their strategies, companies buy advertising in various media—such as television, the web (pop-up ads), magazines, radio, and newspapers. The money these companies pay for advertisements is what allows media outlets to survive. So both the companies that sell the products and the media outlets who sell the ads are trying to influence your consumer behavior in order to make money. In fact, marketers create media messages that flood our senses every day. Of course, not all advertisements are deceptive, but many are. It takes a very critical eye to detect the messages being conveyed in ads and to distinguish between good and bad information.

As you're exposed to media advertisement, try to determine the strategy and tactics being used. Ask the following questions: What is this ad trying to get me to do? Is the product they're selling something I really need? Is the product likely to work as advertised? In this chapter, you learn how to develop a strategy and identify tactics to carry out that strategy. You can use this knowledge to help you analyze marketing strategies and become an informed consumer.

or activity. You can also consult with experts and others who have succeeded in the sport or activity. For example, if you're playing tennis, you can learn about successful tennis strategies used by others—or by yourself in past matches. Keeping notes about successful strategies can help you carry out steps 2 through 5.

### Step 2: Collect New Information

One way to decide which available strategy will work best for you is to conduct a self-assessment of your strengths and weaknesses (for planning a sport performance) or of your personal needs (for planning a lifestyle change). If you're planning to play a sport, let's say tennis, it would also be helpful to assess your opponent's strengths and weaknesses. Coaches do this by means of "scouting reports" that describe other teams' strengths and weaknesses and identify strategies and tactics they have been known to use. To help you plan, write down what you learn about your own strengths and weaknesses and about the strengths and weaknesses of an opponent. Even the pros collect information. For example, professional basketball player LeBron James, who has excellent physical abilities and skills, also studies video of opponents and reads the full scouting report of other teams. He does this to implement a strategy and use tactics that keep him one step ahead of opponents.

### Step 3: Prepare a Plan

After considering available strategies and collecting information about yourself and your opponent, prepare a written plan. In competitive sport, you consider how you or your team can use your strengths and take advantages of your opponent's weaknesses. For example, if your strength in tennis is your serve and your opponent's weakness is return of serve, you might consider an offensive strategy. On the other hand, if you're quite fit and your opponent is not so fit, you might consider a strategy of trying to tire out your opponent so that you could take advantage later in the match.

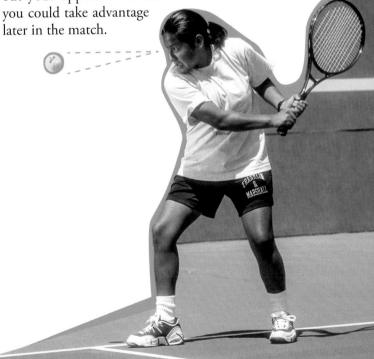

**FITNESS TECHNOLOGY: Computers Keep Getting Smarter**

New technology allows large amounts of information to be stored in the tiny chips that make up a computer's "brain." It has also allowed computers to process information much faster than in the past. In this light, perhaps it's no surprise that a computer (named Watson) used its "artificial intelligence" to beat two human competitors on the TV game show *Jeopardy*. Watson was developed by researchers at IBM and is named after the company's founder, Thomas Watson. The two human competitors were the biggest winners in the show's history, Ken Jennings and Brad Rutter. Watson won the million-dollar prize by using information stored in its computer memory. It was able to quickly retrieve and analyze information in ways similar to those of the human brain. Watson also performed some physical tasks in ways similar to or better than those of humans. For example, it had better reaction time and thus was able to respond to the buzzer more quickly than the human contestants. Watson was also immune to psychological strategies employed by some contestants. Watson did have some problems interpreting clues provided by the show's host.

**Using Technology**

Prepare a report to answer this question: How can computers be used to help people who have physical disabilities?

## FIT FACT

Preparing a written plan is a commitment to action. People who make a formal commitment are more likely to act than those who do not make a commitment.

## Step 4: Include Tactics in Your Plan

To carry out your strategy, plan to use specific tactics. For example, if you want to implement an offensive strategy in tennis, you might consider coming to the net after each of your serves to take advantage of your good serve and your opponent's poor service return. If your opponent is out of shape, you might use the tactic of making him or her move around a lot by hitting the ball first to one side of the court and then to the other.

When deciding on tactics, you can use the same steps as in planning a strategy. First, become familiar with existing information (study known tactics), then collect information, and then make a list of the tactics to consider. Rank the possible tactics and decide which ones are best for implementing your strategy.

## Step 5: Practice

When most people think of practice, they think of practicing skills to get better at performance. Doing that is indeed very important, but so is practicing your strategy and tactics. Once you've chosen a strategy and tactics, practice them. For the tennis player in our example, this practice would involve serving, coming to the net, and volleying. It would also include hitting the ball from side to side to make the opponent move.

As with any plan, you should also evaluate the success of the strategy and tactics you implement. What you learn will become part of step 1 when you plan your next strategy. The examples used here are for playing a sport, but you can use the same steps for making lifestyle changes as well (for examples, see table 19.1).

## Lesson Review

1. Define *strategy* and explain how it is relevant to physical activity and healthy lifestyle choices.
2. Define *tactic* and explain its role in implementing a strategy.
3. What are the five steps for planning strategy and tactics?

# TAKING CHARGE: Developing Tactics

Jason, Ali, Lucy, and Katie have been friends since elementary school. When Ali's mother was diagnosed with breast cancer, the friends wanted to do something to show Ali and his family how much they cared. Jason, Lucy, and Katie got together to plan a strategy. First, they considered what they already knew. They knew the dangers of breast cancer. They also knew that they were not qualified to help medically. After collecting information and considering all options, the group decided on a strategy. They would raise money for breast cancer by entering a Relay for Life event in their local community.

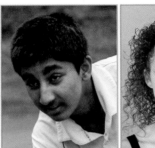

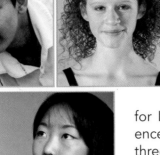

© Peter Mueller

© Photodisc

The Relay for Life is an annual event that takes place in communities throughout the world. This American Cancer Society event raises money for the fight against cancer. People from communities form relay teams that camp out overnight. Team members walk or run around a track or a predetermined course. Cancer survivors run or walk the first lap,

caregivers perform the second lap, and team members take turns walking or running additional laps over a predetermined amount of time, often 24 hours. Contributions are made for laps completed by team members. The funds raised from the Relay for Life are used to make a difference in the fight against cancer. The three friends needed to find other team members, ask supporters for pledges, and take care of other details such as arranging for an overnight stay.

## For Discussion

Is the friends' strategy a good one for people in their situation? What other strategies might they have considered? What tactics should they consider to carry out their strategy? How can they best recruit other team members, get the most pledges, and arrange for the details of the event? Consider the skills in the Self-Management feature when answering the discussion questions.

# SELF-MANAGEMENT: Skills for Developing Tactics

You will have opportunities to use strategies and tactics in the future. Use the following guidelines to help you succeed.

- **Plan your strategy.** Use the five steps described in this lesson. Plan tactics after you adopt a strategy.
- **Learn about and list available tactics.** Read, consult with others who have expertise, and observe. Make a list and rate tactics in terms of their likely effect on your strategy's success.
- **Collect information about yourself (or your team or group).** Choose tactics that emphasize your strengths and minimize your weaknesses.

- **Collect information about others who are involved.** If you're competing against another team or individual, collect information about your opponent. If you're planning an event, collect information from others who've been successful and find out as much as you can about the event (for example, Race for the Cure).
- **Choose the best tactics.** If you're working with others, consult with your group when making decisions about which tactics to use. If someone else decides the tactics (for example, a coach or team leader), provide input.
- **Commit.** Once you've decided, commit to your strategy and tactics.

You're more likely to be active and lead a healthy lifestyle if you have friends and family members who are also active. Sometimes it's fun to be active with friends without the competition that's typical in many sports and games. You can do this by playing cooperative games, such as footbagging, throwing a flying disc, and participating in a volleyball circle. Activities that enable everyone to participate and succeed are also great for social events such as cookouts, work parties, and group gatherings at a park or beach. Cooperative activities are relaxing because the emphasis isn't on winning. You can also have a lot of good laughs when people are encouraged to fool around while playing. **Take action** by trying several cooperative games.

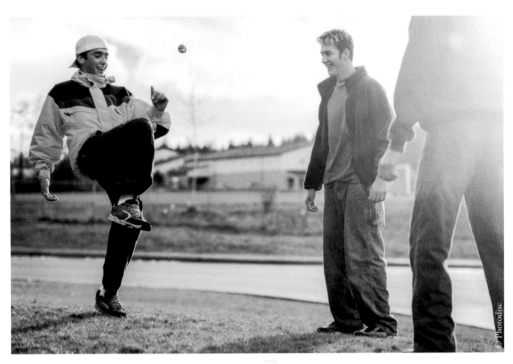

Take action by trying cooperative games.

## Reviewing Concepts and Vocabulary

As directed by your teacher, answer items 1 through 5 by correctly completing each sentence with a word or phrase.

1. A _____ person does regular activity, is fit, has skills, values activity, and knows the benefits of activity.
2. Activities that use teams to teach cooperation and overcome challenges are called _____.
3. A _____ is a master plan for achieving a goal.
4. _____ are specific methods for carrying out a strategy.
5. Watson is the name of a computer that uses _____ to solve problems and answer questions.

For items 6 through 10, as directed by your teacher, match each term in column 1 with the appropriate phrase in column 2.

6. sport education
7. adventure education
8. outdoor education
9. dance education
10. fitness education

a. uses challenging recreational activities
b. uses seasons and teams to educate
c. uses cultural movement activities
d. teaches concepts and self-management skills
e. may use camps to teach activities

For items 11 through 15, as directed by your teacher, respond to each statement or question.

11. Discuss 2 of the top 10 reasons for providing high-quality physical education in schools.
12. Describe adventure education. Why can it be an important part of physical education?
13. Describe dance education. Why can it be an important part of physical education?
14. Describe how the five steps for developing strategy and tactics can be used in a sport of your choice.
15. Describe several guidelines for developing tactics.

## Thinking Critically

Choose a member of your family that you would like to encourage to be more active or eat better. Write a paragraph to devise a strategy for helping that person change.

## Project

Media outlets—such as newspapers and radio and television networks—are major news and information sources. But in recent years, blogs and podcasts have become more prominent in providing information. Prepare a blog (a written article that could appear on a blog) or podcast (a recording that could appear on a podcast) describing reasons why high-quality physical education is important.

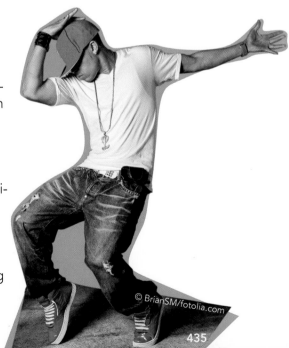

© BrianSM/fotolia.com

# 20

# The Science of
# Active Living

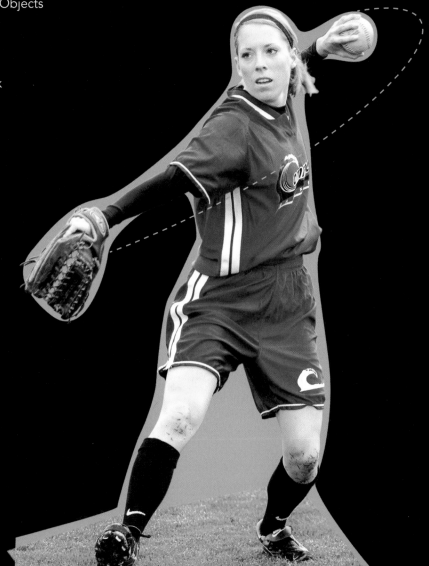

## In This Chapter

 **Student Web Resources**
www.fitnessforlife.org/student

# Lesson 20.1

# Moving Your Body

## Lesson Objectives

After reading this lesson, you should be able to

1. describe nine key biomechanical principles of motor skill learning,
2. describe the two stances commonly used in physical activity,
3. describe several forms of locomotion, and
4. explain the meaning of the term *biomechanical analysis*, and describe how it is used to aid motor skill performance.

## Lesson Vocabulary

acceleration, aerodynamics, biomechanical principles, center of gravity, deceleration, force, hydrodynamics, locomotion, stance, velocity

**Why** do some people let themselves go and become out of shape and unhealthy as they move into adulthood while others continue to be active? For example, when Gretchen was a teen she played softball and basketball. During her 20s and 30s, her job and home responsibilities kept her from playing these team sports, but she stayed active by doing aerobic dance and muscle fitness and flexibility exercises at the local fitness club. During her 40s, Gretchen had more time to get back into sports, so she joined a slow-pitch softball league with some friends at work. She also kept up her aerobic dance and other exercises at the gym. In her 50s, she decided to try tennis at the urging of a friend who needed a doubles partner. Today, at 74, she walks, does her muscle fitness and flexibility exercises, and plays doubles tennis in a local league. Thus, while her activities have changed, she's never been inactive, and along the way she's developed some great friendships and had a lot of fun.

Early in life, Gretchen was fortunate to have a physical education teacher and coach who taught her the principles of movement. As her life changed, her activities also changed, but she could apply those principles of movement to them. In addition, knowing some movement basics enabled her to have fun participating in activities with friends.

Throughout this book, you've learned various principles and how you can apply them in various situations. In this chapter, you'll review some of these principles and learn about others that can help you move efficiently throughout your life.

When performing activities from the Physical Activity Pyramid, you use motor skills, which range from simple to complex. Successful performance of motor skills requires you to apply principles of human movement. Experts in biomechanics study human movement and help us understand and apply the principles in all types of activity.

> Excellence is the gradual result of always striving to do better.
>
> —Pat Riley, basketball coach

## Biomechanical Principles

The principles of biomechanics are based on the basic laws of physics and are complex enough to be the subject of college courses and even college degrees. Physical education teachers and other exercise professionals typically take at least one class in biomechanics, and the **biomechanical principles** summarized here are only a few of the many. Those that were chosen for this discussion relate directly to the motor skills described in this chapter.

### 1. Stability

Stability of the body, at rest or in movement, is related to the location of the body's **center of gravity** and the base of the body's support. Stability while standing is increased by a wide base of support and a low center of gravity.

## 2. Force

To get a body or object moving, or to make a moving body or object stop, **force** must be applied. Many forces are involved, but the contraction of muscles provides the primary force that moves the body (or an object such as a thrown ball). External forces such as gravity and air resistance slow a body in motion. Applying force in one direction results in the production of force in the opposite direction (for every action there is an equal and opposite reaction).

## 3. Acceleration, Deceleration, and Velocity

**Velocity** is speed of movement. **Acceleration** (increase in velocity) occurs when a force is applied to a body or object. The bigger the object's mass, the more force must be applied to cause acceleration. **Deceleration** (a decrease in velocity) occurs when resistance is applied to an object.

## 4. Accumulation of Forces

Greater force can be applied to an object or body if each new force is added sequentially. For example, when a person throws a ball effectively, the lower body moves first, the trunk moves second, the upper body moves third, and then finally the arm and hand move (see the Self-Assessment later in this chapter). Force production is greatest if each movement is added after the previous movement has reached its greatest acceleration.

## 5. Resistance

Resistance is opposition to a force or movement. One source of resistance is friction. Friction is a force caused by one surface rubbing against another. Factors such as the air (including wind) and water offer resistance. Gravity is a source of resistance in motions such as jumping and throwing an object for distance. Resistance can also be applied by an opposing force such as another player pushing you in football or by a weight on a barbell in progressive resistance training.

## 6. Levers

A lever is a very basic machine—a bar or stiff, straight object that can be used to lift weight or increase force. Levers can be used to increase force for producing movement. The body has three types of lever: first, second, and third class. Third-class levers are the most common. Bones act as levers, and muscle contractions create the force that moves the levers.

## 7. Angles

An angle is defined as a figure formed by two lines originating in the same place. Angles are important for successful physical performance. For example, when you throw a ball, the angle of release affects the distance it travels. The ground is one line in the angle, and the trajectory of the ball is the other line. The size of an angle is measured in degrees—for example, a right angle is a 90-degree angle.

## 8. Aerodynamics

In physics, the study of dynamics addresses the causes of motion, including factors that cause changes in motion. **Aerodynamics** includes the study of motion in the air (represented in the term by *aero*). Performance is influenced by various factors associated with motion in the air; examples include spin (on a ball, for example), wind (air resistance in running, for example), and other factors (such as turbulence, humidity, and altitude).

## 9. Hydrodynamics

**Hydrodynamics** refers to the study of motion in fluids. Factors that affect movement in water include water resistance, turbulence (water movement patterns), and temperature.

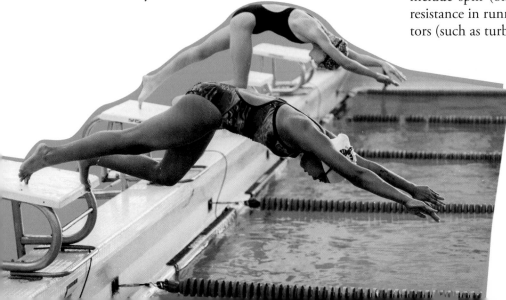

# Fundamental Skills: Stance and Locomotor Skills

Fundamental skills are those that are common to many activities. If you understand and learn to apply the principles of biomechanics when performing fundamental skills, you can use them to help you learn new skills. Virtually all skills are affected in some way by every one of the nine biomechanical principles.

## Balanced (Athletic) Stance

**Stance** is a way of standing, and the most basic stance is standing with good posture and stability. When performing in sport and other physical activities, you need to use a stance that prepares you for action. For this reason, the balanced stance is basic to many sport and other physical activities. The balanced stance, sometimes called the ready stance or athletic stance, allows you to be stable when standing and prepares you to move in any direction. Figure 20.1 shows the balanced stance. Some of its characteristics include a wide base (feet shoulder-width apart or slightly more), lowered center of gravity (knees bent), and center of gravity located within the body (body is not leaning backward, forward, or to either side).

Variations of the balanced stance are used, for example, by baseball and softball players when playing in the field, basketball players when playing defense, tennis players when getting ready to receive a serve, and many other participants in a wide variety of physical activity situations. Balance and stability are needed in these cases because the performer doesn't know in which direction he or she will need to move—forward, backward, right, or left.

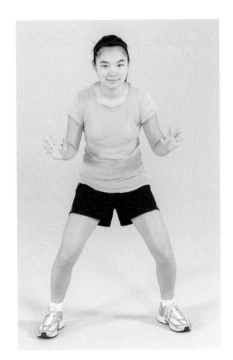

**FIGURE 20.1** The balanced stance.

## Unbalanced Stance

The unbalanced stance (figure 20.2) is used when a performer anticipates moving in a certain direction. This stance is used, for example, by sprinters and swimmers at the start of a race and by football players lined up for the start of a play. Rather than being stable, a performer using an unbalanced stance leans in the direction of anticipated movement, thus allowing the body to get moving more quickly.

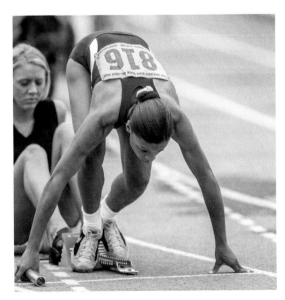

**FIGURE 20.2** The unbalanced stance.

##  SCIENCE IN ACTION: Biomechanical Analysis

Before the invention of motion pictures or video recording, scientists depended on live observation of sport and occupational skill performance to determine the most efficient and effective ways for people to perform motor skills. The first motion pictures were developed by the Frenchman Louis Lumière in the late 1800s. The American Thomas Edison invented the first movie projector that was a commercial success. This invention allowed motion pictures to be used for analyzing work skills during the early 1900s. As sport became more popular in the United States after World War II, moving pictures were also used to analyze the performance of sport skills by baseball players to improve their mechanics in batting and pitching. Researchers such as John Cooper at Indiana University and Richard Nelson at Pennsylvania State University used special high-speed cameras to perform slow-motion analysis of very fast movements recorded on film.

In the early 1950s, the magnetic video tape recorder replaced film as the most popular method of recording and analyzing movements in physical activity. Digital photography was used by the U.S. National Aeronautics and Space Administration for space exploration in the 1960s but did not become commercially available until 1981, when Sony introduced the first mass-produced digital (filmless) camera. In 1995, Sony introduced the first digital video camera. Now, digital cameras are used with computers to analyze movement. The software was originally developed for use in research laboratories and by sport teams but is now available for use by people who participate in leisure-time sport and recreational activities. For example, many golf stores use special cameras and software to offer motion analysis of a person's golf swing. Programs are also available to help individuals use a home computer to analyze their own sport performance.

### Student Activity

Investigate motion analysis systems. If your school has one for student athletes, ask for a demonstration. If not, check with a local golf or tennis store to get a demonstration, or investigate the motion analysis systems found in the student section of the Fitness for Life website. Write a brief report summarizing your investigation.

## FIT FACT

It takes 30 times as much force to lift an object as to push it. Pushing is also more efficient than pulling.

## Lifting

Lifting is a motor skill used in resistance training and in sports such as weightlifting, powerlifting, and wrestling. Principles 1 through 7 as described earlier are particularly relevant in lifting.

## Locomotion (Walking, Running, and Sprinting)

**Locomotion** refers to moving the body from place to place. The most basic forms of locomotion (that is, using locomotor skills) are walking and running. In walking, one foot or the other is in contact with the ground at all times. In running (or jogging), both feet are off the ground for a short time during each stride. Biomechanical principles 1 through 8 are especially important to apply when performing walking, running, and other locomotor skills. Sprinting, or fast running, is used in track and field for events such as the 100-meter dash and the run-up to a long jump and in sports such as soccer (for example, sprinting to get to a loose ball).

## Locomotion (Jumping and Leaping)

Two other common forms of locomotion in sport and other physical activities are jumping and leaping. In jumping, a person leaves the ground with both feet and lands on both feet (see figure 20.3). For example, in the standing jump you push against the ground with both feet and land on both feet. The standing jump can be forward, as in the standing long jump, or upward, as in the vertical jump (figure 20.3). Both the standing long jump and the vertical jump are used as tests of leg power. In leaping, a person leaves the ground on one foot and lands on the opposite foot (see figure 20.4). Leaps are common in ballet and gymnastics. Leaping is different from hopping. In hopping, one foot leaves the ground and the landing is on the same foot. Elements of jumping and leaping are often combined in physical activities. For example, in the running long jump, the performer leaves the ground on one foot and lands on two feet (see figure 20.5). Although this type of movement is a combined movement, it is commonly referred to as a jump. Plyometrics uses jumping and leaping to build power and muscle fitness.

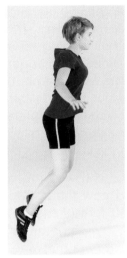
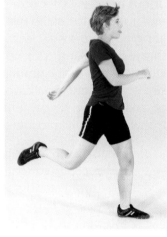

**FIGURE 20.3**
Vertical jump.

**FIGURE 20.4**  Leap.

## Other Locomotor Movements

Space constraints do not allow for discussion here of all forms of locomotor movement. Some examples of other forms are skipping, hopping, galloping, and skating. Shuffle and crossover running are also common in many sports, and there are many variations of moving in water.

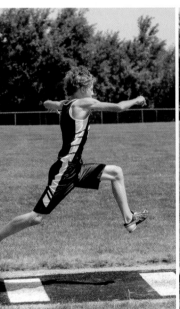
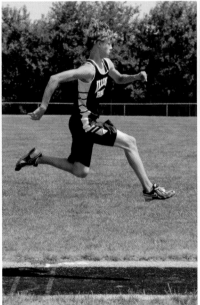
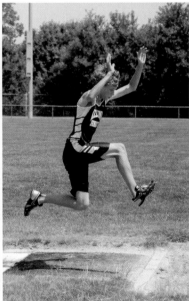
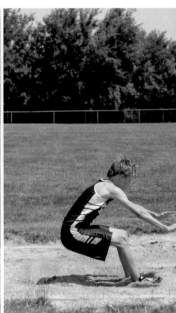

**FIGURE 20.5**  Running jump.

### Lesson Review

1. What are nine biomechanical principles? How are they important to learning motor skills?
2. What are the two basic stances, and when should each be used?
3. What are some examples of locomotor skills? Describe them.
4. What is biomechanical analysis, and how can it be used to improve motor skills?

In the first lesson of this chapter, you learned about a variety of motor skills, including several locomotor skills (walking, running, and jumping). In the next lesson, you'll learn about throwing, striking, striking with an implement, kicking, and other fundamental skills. In this self-assessment, you'll work with two partners to analyze the fundamental skill of overhand throwing. Use the following steps.

1. Perform an overhand throw using a baseball or softball. Throw the ball to a partner standing 30 feet (9 meters) away. Your target is the glove or mitt of the person to whom you are throwing. Repeat the throw several times.

2. Have a second partner watch your throws and rate them using table 20.1. This partner should record the results.

For each element of the throw listed in table 20.1, indicate whether you used good mechanics or need improvement in that area. Figure 20.6 in the next lesson may be useful as you make your assessment.

3. Rotate your duties so that each member of your team gets a chance to throw and rate.

4. When your ratings are done, use the information you gained to practice throwing properly. You can use peer teaching to help each other improve where needed.

Remember that self-assessment information is personal and considered confidential. It shouldn't be shared with others without the permission of the person being tested.

## TABLE 20.1  Rating Chart: Overhand Throwing

| Throwing mechanics | Needs improvement | Good mechanics |
|---|---|---|
| Preparation phase: Stands with the side pointing in the direction of the throw. | | |
| Force production phase 1: Reaches backward with the throwing arm and hand, and the elbow is at or above shoulder height. | | |
| Force production phase 2: Makes a long step forward with the foot opposite of the throwing arm. | | |
| Force production phase 3: Turns the lower body toward the target, and the upper body lags behind. | | |
| Force production phase 4: The shoulders turn toward the target, and the upper arm lags behind. | | |
| Force production phase 5: The upper arm moves forward, and the elbow remains high. | | |
| Force production phase 6: Flexes the wrist prior to follow through. | | |
| Critical instant: Releases the ball at an angle that is appropriate for reaching the target. | | |
| Recovery phase: Follows through across the body with the throwing arm after ball release. | | |

# Lesson 20.2

# Moving Implements and Objects

## Lesson Objectives

After reading this lesson, you should be able to

1. describe three methods (and the related principles) of moving objects with body parts;
2. describe how striking with an implement (and the related principles) can be used in physical activity;
3. define *aerodynamics*, *hydrodynamics*, and *complex skills*, and explain how each is important to human movement; and
4. define *motor learning* and describe some factors that help you learn motor skills.

## Lesson Vocabulary

complex skill, implement, jai alai, object, pelota, tracking

**Do** you ever think about the large number of physical skills you use every day? It's amazing to consider how many actions we perform without even thinking about them. In many things we do, whether work or play, we use an **implement**—a device or tool that helps us perform a task. For example, we use a rake to clean up leaves in the yard, a shovel to dig holes, brushes and rollers to apply paint, and hammers to pound nails. We also use implements in sport—for example, bats, rackets, clubs, and paddles to hit balls and birdies; paddles and oars to propel boats and canoes; sticks to play pool; and mallets to play croquet and polo. Of course, we can also use the body alone (most often a hand, arm, foot, or leg) to move an **object** without the aid of an implement. For example, we kick footballs and soccer balls, throw baseballs and softballs, and strike volleyballs. In all of these examples—those using an implement and those using only body parts—we are producing force to move an object.

## Skills That Move Objects

Too many skills involve moving implements and objects for us to consider them all here. However, the sections that follow describe some of the more basic skills that use body parts to move objects (for example, throwing and kicking). The descriptions also identify the principles related to performing each skill.

## Throwing

The word *throw* means to propel an object through the air using a forward motion of the arm and hand. A throw can be underhand (as in bowling and softball pitching), sidearm (as in some baseball pitches), or overhand (as in most baseball pitches). The focus in throwing is sometimes on accuracy and sometimes on speed or velocity (how hard or fast you throw).

When learning a skill such as throwing, you go through three stages. In the first (cognitive) stage, you have to think about what you're doing, which slows you down. In this stage, you may have to sacrifice speed for accuracy (this is sometimes called the speed–accuracy trade-off). As you move through the second (associative) stage, you get better as you automatically associate your knowledge about throwing with the physical skill itself. You can now move more quickly and still be accurate. In the final

### FIT FACT

The angle of a thrown object's release differs depending on the purpose of the throw. To throw a ball as far as possible, use a release angle of about 45 degrees. For hitting a target, especially one close to you, use a much lower angle of release (see principle 7 in lesson 1).

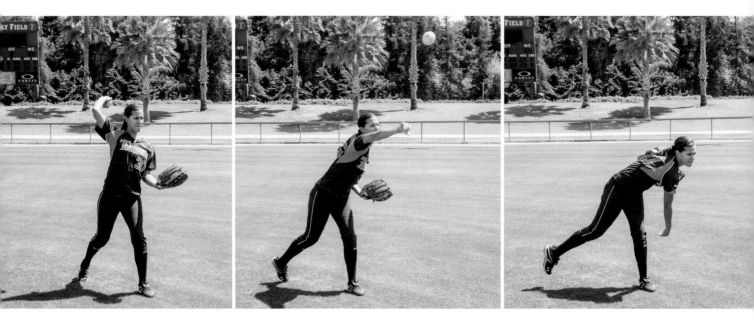

**FIGURE 20.6** Overhand throwing.

(autonomous) stage, your performance becomes automatic. You can perform the skill, in this case throwing, with both speed and accuracy.

All types of throwing are used in a variety of settings, but only overhand throwing is described here (see figure 20.6). The photos show (1) force production (levers moved by muscles to produce force in proper sequence), (2) ball release (at the critical instant and at the appropriate angle), and (3) follow through (during the recovery phase).

## Striking (With a Body Part)

Striking involves delivering a blow or making contact forcefully. It can be done with a body part, as in using a hand to spike a volleyball or deliver a karate blow. Like throwing, striking can be done at many arm angles, and contact can be made with the hand (open hand or fist), the heel of the hand, the forearms (as in a volleyball dig), or the elbows. Figure 20.7 shows one form of striking—the

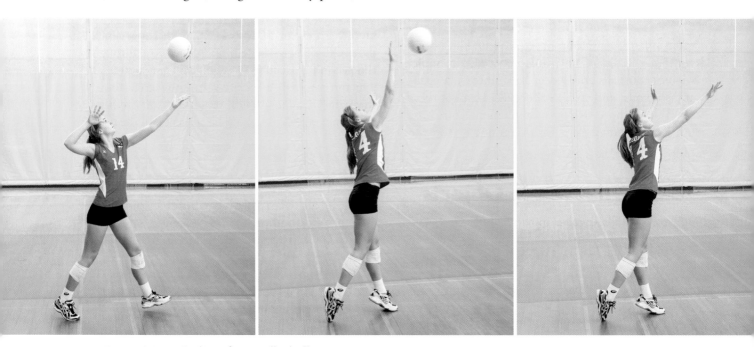

**FIGURE 20.7** Striking for a volleyball serve.

volleyball serve—which uses a motion very similar to the standard throwing motion. The photos show (1) force production (levers moved by muscles to produce force in proper sequence), (2) ball strike (at the critical instant and at the appropriate angle), and (3) follow through (during the recovery phase). The strike can be done from a standing jump or a running jump. In this example, the focus is on the mechanics of striking the ball with the arm and hand, but, as discussed in a later section, striking can also be done with an implement.

## Kicking (Striking With a Foot or Leg)

Kicking, which involves striking with a foot or leg, is used in various sports, including football (in punting and place-kicking), rugby, and soccer, and in games such as footbagging. Various kicks are also used in martial arts such as judo and karate. Kicking often involves contact, as when a foot hits the ball in soccer or strikes an object in karate, but some kicks do not make contact. In dance, for example, many types of kick are performed without striking. Kicked objects may be still at the time of contact (as in a soccer corner kick) or moving (as when the ball is rolling toward you in soccer). Kicking is often preceded by running, as in a football kickoff, and the performer sometimes alternates kicking and running (as in soccer dribbling). Figure 20.8 shows a soccer kick.

## Catching

The skills described in this section allow you to receive objects that have been thrown, kicked, or propelled by an implement, such as a bat. For each skill, the discussion also identifies the related biomechanical principles.

The word *catch* carries many meanings. In sport and other physical activities, it means to grasp and hold onto an object, such as a ball. You can catch with one hand, two hands, or an implement. Several kinds of catching are shown in figure 20.9.

Both one-hand and two-hand catches can be performed either bare-handed (as when catching a bouncing tennis ball or a soccer shot on goal) or with the assistance of a glove (as in baseball and softball). Sometimes a two-hand catch also requires the use of the arms; for example, a football player catching a punt or kickoff might use arms as well as hands.

Some sports require you to use an implement to catch an object. For example, a lacrosse stick is used to catch and throw a ball. In **jai alai** (pronounced hi' lie), a wicker basket glove is used to catch and throw the **pelota** (ball; pronounced puh low' tuh).

Certain steps in catching are typical regardless of the type of catching. Specifically, you need to track the object, receive it, and absorb its force. Before you can catch an object, you must locate it and track it. **Tracking** involves keeping track of the object to be caught from the time it is thrown or projected (for example, kicked) until it gets close enough to

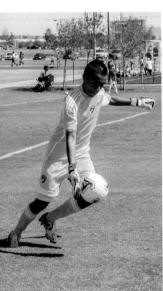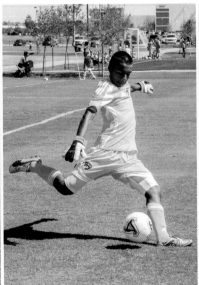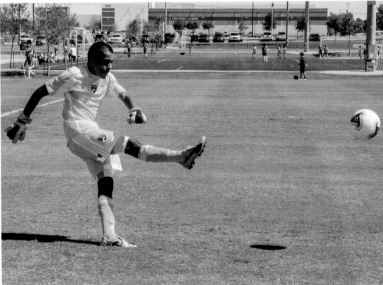

**FIGURE 20.8** Kicking.

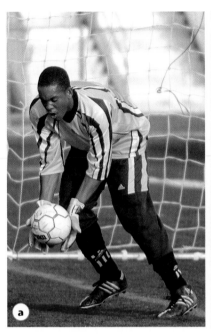
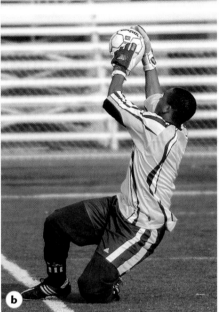
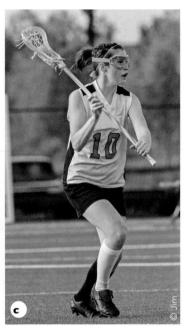

**FIGURE 20.9** Examples of different kinds of catching: *(a)* two hands, below the waist; *(b)* two hands, above the waist; *(c)* with an implement.

catch. One key to catching, then, is expressed in the adage "keep your eye on the ball."

In football, players who catch passes are called receivers because catching really is a form of receiving an object. After tracking the ball, you must move your hands, arms, glove, or other catching implement to a location that makes the object easy to receive. The exact positioning depends on where you will receive the object. For example, when catching a ball below your waist, your palms should face away from your body, but your thumbs should face away from each other (figure 20.9*a*). For

a catch above your waist, the palms of your hands should face away from your body with your thumbs together (figure 20.9*b*). When making an over-the-shoulder catch in football, your palms should face up with your thumbs facing away from each other.

In many types of catching, the object is moving very fast. As a result, once the object hits your hands, glove, or other implement, you should "give" with the blow to absorb the force by allowing the object to continue moving a bit before totally stopping it (figure 20.9*c*). For this reason, people who are good at catching are said to have "soft" hands.

 **FITNESS TECHNOLOGY: Movement Analysis Apps**

In this chapter's Science in Action feature, you learned about motion analysis systems that use special cameras and software to analyze physical performance. Coaches and athletes use these systems to study sport skill performance and identify areas for improvement. For example, softball pitchers study their pitching mechanics to see if changes are needed. Similarly, a batter can make a video when performing well and compare it with a video of his or her performance when not hitting well. Specialized apps even allow you

to record and analyze your performance with a computer tablet or smartphone.

**Using Technology**

Visit the Fitness for Life website and read about sport performance apps. If possible download a free app and use a tablet or smartphone to analyze a sport performance. If a download is not possible, read about the app. Prepare a brief report.

**FIT FACT**

Some sport and work skills require both hands to control an implement—for example, swinging an ax, digging with a shovel, hitting a two-hand tennis backhand, and swinging a baseball bat.

# Striking (With an Implement)

As you may recall, an implement is a tool or piece of equipment used to accomplish a specific task. Examples of using an implement to apply force in sport include serving a tennis ball and hitting a baseball. Implements are typically used as levers to create a force greater than could be created by the body alone. For example, the most powerful major league pitchers can throw a baseball about 100 miles (160 kilometers) per hour, whereas the most powerful tennis players can serve a ball more than 150 miles (240 kilometers) per hour. Because a tennis racket provides greater leverage (longer lever), it creates greater ball speed.

The process of striking is typically referred to as the swing (as in swinging a hammer or a softball bat). Some implements are used to strike a moving object, as in tennis, whereas others are used to strike a still object, as in golf and croquet. Both kinds of striking are complex skills, but striking a moving object requires the ability to track it (figure 20.10)—and, in some cases, to toss it so that it can be struck properly, as in a tennis serve. Objects are struck at different angles depending on the sport. For example, a tennis serve goes from high to low, a golf swing from low to high, and a softball swing from front to back at about waist height.

# Complex Skills

Walking and running are examples of basic motor locomotor skills. The basic skills described in this chapter are the most often used in sport and physical activity. Many activities, however, require **complex skills**. Some complex skills require the use of several basic skills in sequence. For example, in softball an outfielder must run, catch, and quickly throw the ball. Dance involves a wide range of intricate sequential steps, including ballet movements, Latin dance moves, and complex hip-hop maneuvers. Other complex skills require the coordination of several different movements. For example, swimming uses virtually all body parts at the same time, and the levers of the upper and lower body must be used in the proper sequence. Even the trunk must move to produce optimal movement through the water.

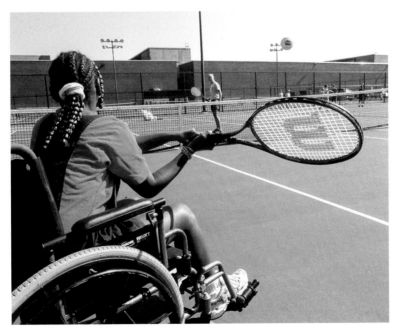

**FIGURE 20.10** To strike a moving object with an implement, you must first track it visually.

# Aerodynamics and Hydrodynamics

Aerodynamics refers to the study of motion in the air. When you use skills at work or play, air can affect your performance. Spin, for example, affects the motion of an object that has been thrown or struck by an implement. Here are some examples from softball in which spin is imparted by the use of the body without an implement.

- Forward spin (topspin) causes the ball to drop faster than normal.
- Backward spin (backspin) creates lift so that the ball appears to rise (does not drop as fast as normal).
- Sidespin causes the ball to "break" or curve from its normal path.

Spin can also be imparted to an object by means of an implement. For example, tennis players swing from low to high to create topspin, which allows them to hit the ball hard and still keep it in bounds because the spin causes the ball to come down faster than normal. As with a pitched baseball, sidespin causes a tennis ball to curve. Spin on a football causes it to spiral and stay stable in the air. Spin on a pool or billiard ball causes it to curve or even jump.

Wind (a type of air movement) can cause resistance to movement; a headwind, for example, slows a runner. Wind can also exaggerate the effect of spin on a ball. For example, if a ball is curving because of spin, the wind may either cause more spin or cause resistance to the curving caused by the spin. In sailing, the wind is essential to the boat's movement, and skilled sailors can use it to move a boat in all directions.

Moving objects, including your body, can also be affected by humidity, temperature, and altitude. Dry air, for example, provides less resistance than humid air. Very cold air cools an object, which may limit the distance it travels when struck or kicked. The air at high altitude is thinner and therefore provides less resistance than air at lower altitudes.

Hydrodynamics refers to the study of motion in fluid. It's especially important to swimmers and people who do other water activities, such as surfers, boaters, kayakers, and rowers. Water causes resistance to movement and therefore affects the movement of swimmers and boaters. In fact,

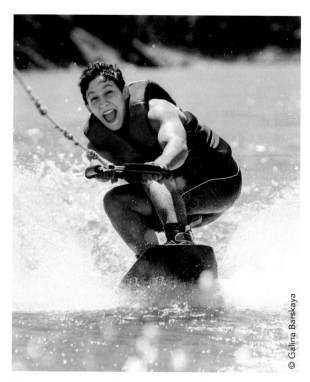

© Galina Barskaya

**Water resistance affects a variety of water activities.**

pushing against the resistance of water is what propels you forward when swimming or using an oar. Water itself moves because of various forces, including wind and gravitational pull, which can cause waves. Swimmers' movements also cause the water to move, as does splashing of water against the side of a pool. Waves and other water movements affect performance in water.

## Motor Learning

Motor learning involves practicing movements in order to improve motor skills. Some movements are voluntary; others are involuntary. Involuntary movements occur when a reflex initiates the movement. A reflex is an automatic movement that does not require your brain to directly stimulate your nerves to cause your muscles to contract. One example is the knee jerk reflex that occurs when a doctor taps your knee with a small hammer during a physical exam.

Most movements involved in motor skills are voluntary. When you perform a voluntary movement, such as throwing a ball, your brain signals your nerves, which signal your muscles to contract. The contraction of your muscles then moves your bones (in throwing, the bones or levers of your arm). The movement of the levers provides the force to throw the ball. Some principles of motor learning are described in this section.

## Practice

With good practice, you can improve your motor skills. You can get the most out of your practice by getting specific feedback from an instructor or using a video that teaches you about specific things to practice.

## Skill Transfer

Once you learn the basics of a motor skill, you can transfer it—that is, use it when learning a similar skill. For example, if you use practice to become good at throwing a baseball, it will be easier for you to learn to throw a football and even to strike a ball as in volleyball spiking.

## Skill Change

If you learn a skill very well and then try to change your technique, it will take some time before you see improvement. For example, if you practice for a long time to learn to bowl using a straight ball, then decide to change your delivery to a hook, you may not see immediate improvement. It took a lot of practice for you to learn the first delivery, and it will take time and practice to "forget" it and learn the new one. Allow yourself time to learn the new delivery before expecting improvement in your performance. It's also advisable to avoid making big changes in the way you perform a skill right before you compete or have a test of performance. Change when you have time to practice before performing.

> " Just keep going. Everybody gets better if they keep at it. "
> —Ted Williams, Hall of Fame baseball player

## Mental Practice

Mental practice involves rehearsing a skill in your mind without moving the relevant body parts. It is useful for rehearsing the biomechanics of a movement and has been shown to help people learn skills.

## Lesson Review

1. What are three methods (and the related principles) of moving objects with body parts?
2. How can striking with an implement (and the related principles) be used in physical activity?
3. What are aerodynamics, hydrodynamics, and complex skills? How is each important to human movement?
4. What is motor learning, and what factors help you learn motor skills?

Alexis was not on the school golf team, but she did like to play golf. She thought about trying out for the team, but she wasn't sure that she was good enough. When she played with her family, she did well, but when she played with people she didn't know, she didn't do as well. Sometimes she talked to herself while playing, saying things like, "Why did you do that, dummy?" or "Oh, no—I'm starting to play badly again." Sometimes she even talked to herself out loud, saying things like, "I got a 7 on that hole? Now I don't even have a chance for a good score!"

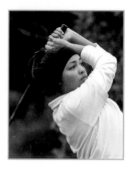

After one particular round in which she didn't play as well as she would have liked, Alexis asked her mother, "Why do things always go wrong when I play with people I don't know?" Her mother said that she had read a book by a sport psychologist who recommended avoiding negative self-talk (saying negative things to yourself, which affects your self-confidence and leads to poor play). The key is to replace the negative self-talk with positive self-talk. As Alexis' mom said, "If you expect bad things to happen, they probably will. Next time you play, try to cut the negative talk and focus on positives. If you have a bad hole, say to yourself, 'It's just one hole—I'm going to do better on the next one.'"

## For Discussion

What are some examples of negative self-talk common in sport and other activities? What are some examples of positive self-talk that can be used to replace negative self-talk? What other suggestions do you have for Alexis and other people who are in sporting situations? In crafting your advice, consider the guidelines presented in the Self-Management feature.

 **SELF-MANAGEMENT: Skills for Positive Self-Talk**

You know that some people are considered pessimists and others optimists. A pessimist thinks bad things are going to happen, and an optimist believes good things are sure to come. Experts in exercise and sport psychology have found that with practice, you can develop "learned optimism." Specifically, you can replace negative thoughts and negative self-talk with positive thoughts and positive self-talk. Follow these guidelines to use positivity to improve your performance.

- **Learn the ABCs.** A stands for adversity, which can lead to negative thoughts and negative self-talk. Learn to recognize when you're facing adversity. B stands for beliefs. If you believe that you're going to do poorly when you face adversity, you probably will. Learn to recognize negative beliefs when you face adversity. C is for consequences. Learn to recognize your feelings about the consequences of adversity. A pessimist might say, "If I do poorly on one hole in golf, I have no chance to get a

reasonable score." Learning to reassess consequences and be more realistic can help you become more optimistic.

- **Accept adversity as a challenge rather than a sure cause of failure.** Adversity causes negative self-talk only if you let it.

- **Alter your beliefs about adversity.** If you accept adversity as a challenge, you can tell yourself to avoid negative thoughts and replace them with positive ones. Experts suggest that replacing negative comments (such as "That was a dumb decision!") with positive ones (such as "I know I can do it!") leads to better performance. So when you're faced with adversity, respond with positive self-talk. Tell yourself, "I believe I can do this!"

- **Don't overdramatize the consequences of adversity.** Think realistically about adversity. Ask yourself if your view of the potential consequences is pessimistic. If so, replace it with a more realistic or even positive view.

- **Put the past behind you.** Failing at a task or doing less well than you'd like doesn't necessarily mean you'll fail next time. For example, in golf, don't let one bad hole get you down. You can't change the past—only the future. Worrying about the last hole leads to negative thoughts when you play the next one. Playing a hole badly creates adversity, but positive thinking and positive self-talk can turn the last bad hole into the next good one.

- **Practice creating a positive circle of success.** Pessimists think negatively when faced with adversity. Negative beliefs lead to poor performance, which contributes to more negative thoughts, thus creating a negative circle. Work instead to create a positive circle of success. Every time you face adversity, remember the ABCs (recall the first item in this list) and practice them. Recognize adversity when it arises and establish positive beliefs ("I know I can do this"). This can lead to positive consequences (improved performance).

- **Be realistic.** In learning about SMART goals, you've learned that being realistic is important to setting effective goals. Setting unrealistically high goals can lead to feelings of failure even when you're doing quite well. Remember that practice is necessary for success.

 **ACADEMIC CONNECTION: Multiple Meanings**

Meeting standards for English language arts requires an understanding of the multiple meanings of words. The word *force* has many meanings. For example, there is military force (troops and ships), violent force (a physical attack), and mechanical force (energy exerted). In this chapter, *force* refers to energy exerted by the muscles to cause tension or to cause the body or an object to move. Force can also be used to stop a body or object from moving (resistance force). The definition in the box is the one included in the glossary.

Identify other words used in this book that have multiple meanings. An example is the word *power*, which refers to a part of health-related

> **force**—In physical activity, it is energy exerted by the muscles to cause movement or resist movement; other uses include military force (ships and troops), violent force (a physical attack), or resistance force (stopping a moving body or object).

fitness (strength $\times$ speed) in this book. But *power* can also refer to possession of influence or control (political power) or a source of energy (electric or solar power). You may want to use the glossary to assist you.

In this chapter, you've learned nine biomechanical principles that are important for performing motor skills. These principles apply to skills used in a variety of work and play situations.

**Take action** by trying several different skills and describing the principles that apply to the performance of each one.

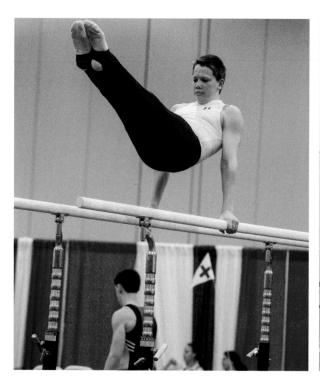 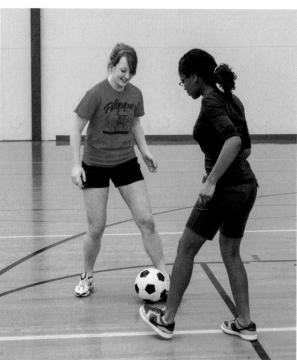

Take action by applying biomechanical principles as you perform different skills.

## Reviewing Concepts and Vocabulary

As directed by your teacher, answer items 1 through 5 by correctly completing each sentence with a word or phrase.

1. A _____ refers to a way of standing.
2. Moving your body from place to place is called _____.
3. _____ is the study of motion in fluids.
4. Delivering a blow or making contact forcefully is called _____.
5. When you perform the skill of _____, you must track the object before receiving it.

For items 6 through 10, as directed by your teacher, match each term in column 1 with the appropriate phrase in column 2.

6. transfer
7. mental practice
8. motor learning
9. aerodynamics
10. striking with an implement

a. study of motion in the air
b. using one skill to perform another
c. practicing to improve a skill
d. rehearsing a skill in your mind
e. tennis serve

For items 11 through 15, as directed by your teacher, respond to each statement or question.

11. Describe three different principles of biomechanics.
12. Describe biomechanical analysis and how it uses technology.
13. Give examples of striking a ball with an implement.
14. What are some aerodynamic factors that influence the flight of a ball?
15. What are some guidelines for eliminating negative self-talk?

## Thinking Critically

Write a paragraph to answer the following question.

A friend has been selected to kick a 15-yard field goal at your school's next home football game. If she succeeds, she wins a prize. When she was younger she played soccer, but she has not played in a while. Now she would like your help to improve her kicking. How would you help her win the prize?

## Project

To improve academic performance, many schools perform three- to five-minute exercise breaks in the classroom. The breaks include by-the-desk exercises that can be performed in a small space and often include dance steps (thus also involving motor skills). Plan an exercise break for one of your classes. You can use video or music or just lead the group in an exercise. Show it to one of your teachers and ask to present it to the class.

# 21

# Lifelong Activity

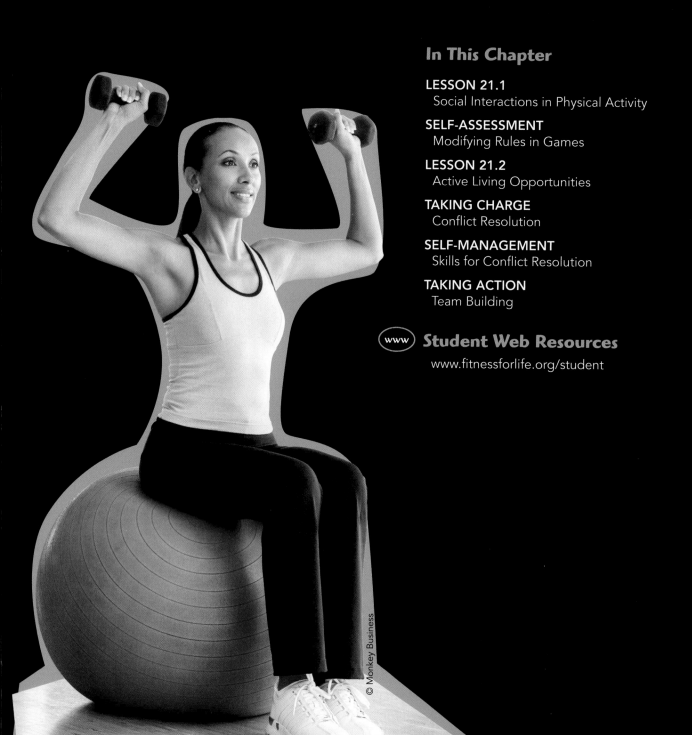

www **Student Web Resources**
www.fitnessforlife.org/student

© Monkey Business

# Social Interactions in Physical Activity

## Lesson Objectives

After reading this lesson, you should be able to

1. describe five leadership skills,
2. define *teamwork* and describe five guidelines for becoming an effective team member,
3. define *group cohesiveness* and factors that develop it,
4. define *rule* and *etiquette* and explain how they are important in sport and physical activity, and
5. describe *sportsmanship*, *diversity*, and *bullying* and explain how they are important in sport and physical activity.

## Lesson Vocabulary

etiquette, group cohesiveness, leadership, rule, sportsmanship, teamwork

---

**Have** you ever played on a sport team? Have you been part of a different kind of team? If you answered yes to either question, what role did you play on the team, and how comfortable were you in that role? Did the team have good chemistry, or were there issues that kept team members distant from each other?

One goal of this book is to help people move from dependence to independence, whether in working out to get fit or in making decisions about what to eat. This growth involves not only engaging in positive social interactions in school but also developing skills that will help you in the future. In school, teachers and coaches often appoint leaders, and rules are often made and enforced by others. This chapter provides guidelines for helping *you* make responsible choices, especially in physical activity settings.

> If your actions create a legacy that inspires others to dream more, learn more, do more, and become more, then you are an excellent leader.
>
> —Dolly Parton, singer and actor

## Leaders and Leadership

A leader guides or directs a group of people, such as a sport team or club. **Leadership** involves actively assuming the role of a leader. You can't be a leader just because you want to. Becoming a leader requires leadership skills that can be developed, and some of the most important are presented in table 21.1. Like all skills, leadership skills must be practiced in order to be mastered.

One way to get leadership experience is to play sports and games. Another way is to participate in physical education class; for example, in the physical education approach known as sport education, students are grouped into teams whose members serve as leaders, team members, and referees. In the workplace, companies often use cooperative games to train their leaders (in this case, managers and executives).

## Teams and Teamwork

A team is a group of people who band together or are assigned to work together. Ideally, team members work together to achieve a common goal. Sometimes, however, not all team members are committed to the team's goal; in fact, some members may even work to subvert the team's efforts. **Teamwork** is effective, combined work by all team members toward achieving the common goal. In order to experience teamwork, group members often have to sacrifice personal recognition in favor of team goals. For this reason, sport teams often use the slogan "There is no I in TEAM" to emphasize that individual goals are secondary to team goals (figure 21.1).

## TABLE 21.1 Leadership Skills

| Skill | Description | How to build |
|---|---|---|
| Integrity | Integrity means being fair; for a leader, it means directing while adhering to rules and standards of the group. Not all leaders have integrity, but good leaders do. | Integrity is built over time. You establish a reputation based on your actions. |
| Communication | Good leaders are good listeners. They listen in order to understand the group's needs, then speak clearly to be understood. Good leaders also inspire and persuade. | Practice listening even when you have much to say. Keep track of what others say. Ask whether what you think they said is what they meant. Ask what they heard you say to see if they got your message. Get the facts to help you make good arguments. |
| Strategy and planning | Creating a strategy requires creating a clear vision of your goals. It also involves developing tactics for carrying out the plan. | Practice using the steps for developing a strategy and carrying out a plan. Get the facts before planning. |
| Management | Leaders help group members work together to meet goals. Keys include building teamwork (group unity) and building trust based on integrity. Relevant skills that can be learned include directing and supervising others, resolving conflicts, and negotiating. | Study the information presented in this chapter about teamwork and conflict resolution. |
| Other | Other characteristics of a good leader include self-confidence, optimism, enthusiasm, decisiveness, and being proactive. Good leaders can also accept criticism and are willing to learn better ways to reach group goals. | Most of these characteristics are built through experience. It also helps to practice the self-management skills presented in this book. |

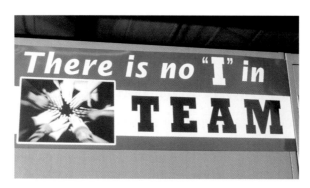

**FIGURE 21.1** Motivational slogans are sometimes used to promote teamwork.

Aristotle, the Greek philosopher, stated, "the whole is greater than the sum of its parts." The implication is that if people work together, they can accomplish things that they could not accomplish working independently. Consider the following guidelines about teamwork. They can be useful in helping groups to function effectively.

- **Learning your role.** What tasks are you best able to perform that will help the team? A team has a few common goals but many different roles. While some roles are more prominent (for example, pitcher on a softball team), all roles must be performed well for the team to succeed.

- **Accepting your role.** The role you want may not be the role you get. A person who accepts an assigned role is more likely to help the team than one who does not. In addition, carrying out a role that you don't prefer can lead to more desirable roles in the future. As illustrated in this chapter's Science in Action feature, teams can function effectively even if a member does not like his or her role—and even when team members don't get along well—as long as members *accept* their roles. Of course, being on a team is more fun if team members like each other and work well together.

- **Practicing your role.** As with being a leader, being an effective team member requires practice. Every role requires specific skills. For example, the pitcher on a softball team must have motor skills suited to that position but may not be an especially good hitter. For this reason, the pitcher may be called on to perform a sacrifice bunt to move a runner into scoring position. This pitcher will practice bunting more than other players because this is an assigned role. Of course, roles are often assigned by leaders on the basis of special skills that individuals possess. In an example from a school setting, one sophomore class president, named Hideko, sought artists to make posters, computer specialists to prepare websites, and other people with special skills for special roles.

- **Carrying out your role.** It's one thing to practice your role but another to carry it out effectively.

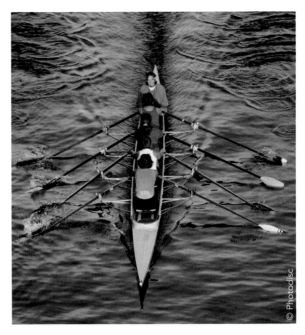

Group cohesiveness occurs when team members work together toward a common goal.

## ⚛ SCIENCE IN ACTION: Group Cohesiveness

Cohesion means sticking together tightly. In chemistry, it means uniting particles to form a single mass. When applied to groups of people, cohesion is referred to as **group cohesiveness**, which occurs when group or team members stick together in working toward common goals. Scientists have studied group cohesiveness in a variety of sports and found that several factors help groups stick together; they include small group size, friendship among members, commitment to the group's goals, group success or failure, and competitiveness of group members.

It's easier to achieve group cohesiveness in small groups because fewer people have to coordinate their efforts. For example, it's easier for 5 people on a basketball team to work together than for 11 people on a football team to do so. It's also easier for small groups to agree on goals.

In addition, if team members know and like each other, it's easier for them to agree on goals and work together. However, studies also show that some teams win championships despite dissension among their members because team members are strongly committed to the group's goals. Several studies of rowers, for example, show that personal feelings can be overcome if team members want strongly enough to win. Thus competitiveness is also a factor that creates desire among team members to work together, though it can cut both ways: Winning a competition can help members get along, but losing sometimes leads to disagreements between team members (see this chapter's Taking Charge feature).

Research also shows that it's important for group members to recognize that everyone makes mistakes sometimes. This acknowledgment reduces blaming when the team does poorly and increases the chances for achieving group cohesiveness in the future. It's crucial to support fellow team members when they're down.

### Student Activity

Search websites, magazines, or newspapers to find a true story about group cohesiveness. Describe how the group members worked together to achieve a common goal.

Even when everyone does his or her job as practiced, success may not follow. For example, the opposing team may use a tactic that overcomes your team's tactic. Or the other team may simply have players who are very good. Thus, carrying out your role may not always get the desired result, but it does give your team the best chance for success. For this reason, it's important not to get discouraged if you and your team are not successful every time that you perform your role well.

• **Adapting as necessary.** Again, even if all team members work hard and perform their roles well, success may not follow. If the team's strategy and tactics are not working, adjustments need to be made, and those adjustments could mean a change in some team members' role.

# Making and Enforcing Rules

A **rule** is a guideline or regulation for conduct or action. Rules help bring order and fairness to sports and games. They can be very formal—for

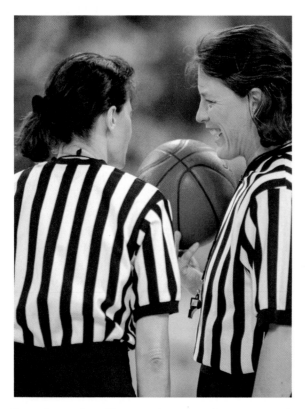

For rules to be effective, they must be consistently enforced.

example, the official rules of baseball. They can also be informal, as is the case for conduct of friends in an informal group.

There are many kinds of rules, ranging from societal laws (for example, the rules of the road for driving) to math and science laws and principles. Classrooms have rules, as do business meetings. Sport teams have rules for remaining in good standing with the team, and religions have rules of moral conduct. Violating a rule typically results in some sort of punishment, whereas regular adherence to rules is usually rewarded. Rules are enforced in a variety of ways; for example, police officers enforce laws, referees enforce sport rules, and coaches and team leaders enforce team rules.

## FIT FACT

A recent national survey found that nearly 85 percent of American adults agree that bending or breaking the rules in sport is cheating and should not be tolerated. A similar percentage agree that bending or breaking the rules is cheating even if no one notices. Despite the high number of people who feel that cheating is wrong and makes games less fun and fair, one in five admits to breaking rules in sports, and nearly half say they know someone who has bent or broken rules.

Experts agree that for rules to be effective, they must be consistently enforced. They should also be appropriate for the situation, and punishment should be consistent with the violation. Rules must be fair to all members of the group.

In some cases, not much can be done to change rules, at least not quickly. In sport, for example, teams are bound by existing rules as they are enforced by officials. Team and school rules, however, can be changed more quickly if they are not serving their intended purpose. Teams and team members can modify bad rules by using a version of the scientific method. After identifying the rules that seem to need changing, the group can collect information, then use it to articulate clear reasons (evidence) for changing the rules. Group members should consult with each other and debate the evidence, after which either the group as a whole or its leaders can make a decision. Once the decision is made, the group's effectiveness depends on whether group members comply with the new rules. A group member who finds the rules unacceptable can opt out; that is, he or she doesn't have to continue to be a member.

## Etiquette in Physical Activity

**Etiquette** involves acting in a way that is consistent with the typical or expected behavior of a social group. In Western society, for example, etiquette for eating indicates when to use a knife, a fork, or a spoon. In Eastern culture, however, etiquette for eating often calls for using chopsticks in particular ways. Sport also involves social situations subject to a code of etiquette. The code may not be written, but it is present nevertheless.

Some rules of sport etiquette are informal. In golf, for example, it is considered poor etiquette to talk while another player is swinging. Other rules of etiquette are more formal and may even be written. For example, tennis often involves a dress code, and many clubs and tournaments used to consider any color other than white to be inappropriate. In addition, for many years, female tennis players were expected to wear skirts rather than shorts. Over time, however, etiquette can change, and today it is common for women to wear shorts on the court. Clothing colors other than white are also now common.

Most people agree that following rules of etiquette, whether formal or informal, generally helps make

social situations more fun and enjoyable. Knowing the etiquette of a particular sport or social group can also help you feel more comfortable in the group, whereas not knowing it can make you quite uncomfortable.

## Diversity: Respect for Others

The word *society* refers to a large group of people who have a history of working and living together. It can refer to a neighborhood, a community, a nation, or an even larger group (for example, Western society). Characteristics of a society include traditions, organized laws and rules, and standards for living and conduct (social etiquette).

Societies provide for the common interests of their members and protect them from outside threats. One common interest in a society is that of providing for all members of the group, not just the biggest and strongest. Diversity in a society refers to the inclusion of different types of people, and the great diversity in many modern societies makes social sensitivity and responsibility necessary. Specifically, it requires sensitivity to others regardless of race, ethnicity, age, disability, culture, socioeconomic status, sex, or gender identity. To achieve the goal of treating all members equally and fairly, it is helpful to consider all people when selecting

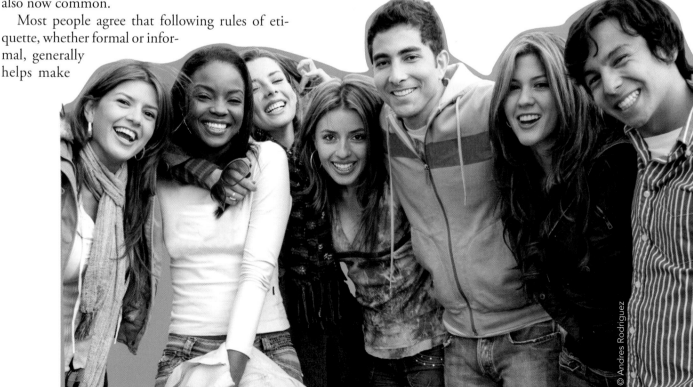

leaders; to follow the rules of the social group (such as a team or school); and to practice good etiquette in daily activities.

## FIT FACT

Two-thirds of American adults believe that winning is overemphasized, and more than half believe that unethical behavior is common in certain sports, particularly football, hockey, wrestling, and baseball.

# Sportsmanship

**Sportsmanship** is a term used to describe respect for opponents and grace in winning or losing when participating in a game or sport. A good sport exhibits good ethical conduct and plays by the rules. An overemphasis on winning can sometimes result in acts of poor sportsmanship, such as attempting to hurt an opponent or intentionally violating the rules to gain an advantage. You'll find that if you participate in games and sports for fun, health benefits, stress reduction, and social interaction you'll enjoy yourself much more than if you focus only on winning.

# Sensitivity, Trust, and Respect

Sensitivity refers to paying attention to the feelings and concerns of others. Ways to build sensitivity include listening (for example, hearing what others have to say rather than only telling others what to do) and communicating in nonthreatening language (for example, giving positive comments rather than harsh criticism). Trust refers to the belief that others are honest and reliable. Demonstrating honesty and reliability in your actions helps others learn to trust you. Trustworthy people keep their promises and are sensitive to the needs of others. People who are trustworthy and sensitive (including leaders) typically have the respect of others.

# Bullying

Bullying is a serious problem among teens. Experts in sport sociology indicate that half of all teens say they have been bullied, and nearly as many say they have bullied someone else. A U.S. government website (StopBullying.gov) describes several types of bullying, including verbal (name calling, teasing), social (spreading rumors, leaving people out, breaking friendships), physical (hitting, punching, shoving), and cyber (using the web and tech devices to do harm). Bullying shows disrespect for individual people and for the rules of the social group.

**Lesson Review**

1. What are the five leadership skills?
2. What is teamwork, and what are the five guidelines for becoming an effective team member?
3. What is group cohesiveness, and what are some factors that develop it?
4. What are rules and etiquette, and how are they important in sport and physical activity?
5. How are *sportsmanship*, *diversity*, and *bullying* defined, and how they are important in sport and physical activity?

This self-assessment will give you insight into the importance of fair rules when playing games. Perform the activity as described, then, as directed by your instructor, record information concerning the activity. Remember that self-assessment information is personal and considered confidential. It shouldn't be shared with others without the permission of the person being tested.

1. Each person in the class writes his or her name on a small piece of paper. Place the names in a box or bag. One member of the class draws the names of six people.

2. The people whose names are drawn come to the front of the class. Two teams are formed—the first three drawn are on one team, and the second three are on the other. Members of each team spread out in a defined game area in front of the class. They may stand wherever they want within the game area, but once their location is determined they cannot move from that spot (the right foot may not move).

3. The name of an additional person is drawn. This person is the referee. He or she tosses a small ball into the air within the playing area. When a player on either team touches the ball, the referee awards a point to one team. The referee decides which team gets the point and does not have to explain why the point was given. Points do not have to be awarded for the same reason for each throw. The referee retrieves the ball and continues to throw it and award points arbitrarily until the ball is thrown 10 times. The team with the most points is the winner. If the score is tied, the team that scores the next point wins.

4. Ask team members to explain how they felt about the game and its rules.

5. After the discussion, draw names for additional teams and referees, so that several games are played at the same time (all members of the class are involved). Before each group plays the game, both teams must agree on two or three rules for awarding points. The referee writes down the rules and uses them when throwing the ball and awarding points.

6. After all teams have finished playing their game, each group comes up with ideas for improving the game.

7. Each group then presents and justifies its list of rules to the rest of the class.

8. If time allows, play the game using rules created by one of the groups.

Adapted from an activity developed by the College of Education at the University of North Carolina.

# Lesson 21.2

# Active Living Opportunities

## Lesson Objectives

After reading this lesson, you should be able to

1. define *autonomy* and explain how it relates to decision making about healthy lifestyles,
2. describe five or more sources of information about opportunities for physical activity,
3. explain three guidelines for organizing for participation in physical activity, and
4. define *extrinsic motivation* and *intrinsic motivation* and explain the difference between them.

## Lesson Vocabulary

autonomy, extrinsic motivation, intrinsic motivation, optimal challenge, self-reward system

**Do** you feel like you have the power to make your own decisions in life? How do you feel when you have a choice compared with when you don't? Consider the following scenario.

Two years after graduating from high school, a group of friends gathered at a social. Hal hosted the party at his house. He was now married and worked full-time. He'd gained a few pounds since high school and wasn't as active as he had been when he played football in school. His wife, Fatima, had been a cheerleader in school but was also less active now because she also had a full-time job. Hal and Fatima stayed in touch with their friends, but some were off at college, and others were busy working.

Other people attending the social event included Kris, who had also played on the football team. He was now attending a local community college and working part-time. Like Hal, he knew he was less active than he should be. Jennifer was attending the local university, where she played on the soccer team. She was very active but missed interacting with her friends. Will was also attending the university, where he played some intramurals and worked out at the campus recreation center. Coretta and Josh had not gone to school with the others but were now neighbors of Hal and Fatima. Josh played slow-pitch softball, and Coretta used some home exercise videos. They had a four-year-old daughter named Clara.

The seven friends decided that it would be good if they could all be more active (except, of course, for Jennifer, the soccer player). They also wanted to spend more time together socially. They decided to do some type of physical activity together to help

them be more active and have fun at the same time. The rest of this lesson describes some of the steps that the friends used to investigate opportunities for their group.

## FIT FACT

Self-determination theory is one theory of human motivation. It places high importance on autonomy and intrinsic motivation. It is often used in the study of sport and physical activity. Students report that physical education classes are more enjoyable when they are given an opportunity to choose (to have autonomy in) some of the activities in their classes.

## Autonomy

**Autonomy** refers to self-direction or the ability to make decisions for yourself. One goal of this book is to help teens move from having others make decisions for them (dependence) to making decision for themselves (independence). Hal, Fatima, and their friends are at a stage of life where they make their own decisions. In elementary school, and even in middle school, many decisions had been made for them. Even in high school, they were somewhat dependent on others (such as parents, teachers, and coaches) for many things. Now, however, they have the autonomy to make their own decisions.

The friends applied some of the self-management skills they had learned in high school to their search for active living opportunities in their community.

For example, they had learned about the self-management skill of finding social support from friends, but they did have some barriers to overcome. For one thing, to be active together they would have to find activities that they were all interested in and find times when they would all be available. To solve this and other problems, they used elements of the scientific method and critical thinking skills. Like Hal, Fatima, and their friends, you can practice self-management skills and use the scientific method to become more autonomous in making decisions about healthy lifestyles.

# Finding Opportunities to Participate

One of the first steps in finding ways to be active is to find out what's available. Options in most communities include government agencies, community organizations, worksite programs, commercial options, and places of worship. Table 21.2 summarizes multiple types of opportunity for being active in your local area.

**TABLE 21.2  Finding Opportunities for Physical Activity in the Community**

| Type | Examples | How to contact |
| --- | --- | --- |
| • Government agencies<br>• Youth programs<br>• Sport leagues<br>• Facilities (tennis courts, bike trails, golf courses, hiking trails, parks)<br>• Community centers<br>• Zoos and cultural centers<br>• Museums | • Local parks and recreation department<br>• State parks and recreation department<br>• Local public school programs | Use a phone book or do a web search to locate the agency. Search for a specific department or facility. |
| National sport organizations | • U.S. Olympic Committee (TeamUSA)<br>• United States Tennis Association<br>• Amateur Softball Association of America<br>• National Senior Games Association<br>• Special Olympics<br>• U.S. Paralympics | Do a web search to locate the organization. For sites such as TeamUSA.org, use the pull-down menu to find specific sport pages. |
| Community organizations | • YMCA and YWCA<br>• Boys & Girls Clubs of America<br>• Activity-specific clubs (for example, walking, jogging, and tennis clubs)<br>• Sport organizations (for example, Little League baseball) | Do a web search for the organization name and your town or city name (for example, YMCA and Los Angeles). Contact the organization by phone or in person. |
| Worksite programs | • Company wellness programs<br>• Company fitness centers<br>• Company sport leagues and teams | Check with the human resources office at your worksite to see what's available. |
| Commercial options | • Health and fitness clubs and spas<br>• Private sport facilities (sport fields, ice rinks, skating rinks or parks, golf courses, leagues)<br>• Dance and yoga studios<br>• Martial arts studios<br>• Youth activity centers<br>• Physical therapy centers | Do a web search for the activity and your town or city name (for example, yoga and Detroit). Contact the facility by phone or in person. |
| Places of worship (for example, church, synagogue, mosque) | • Sport leagues<br>• Exercise groups<br>• Social groups | Check with your religious organization's office or look for listings in the bulletin or newsletter. |

# Organizing for Participation

After investigating opportunities, Hal and his friends decided to join a co-rec volleyball league sponsored by their community's parks and recreation department. They needed at least 10 people because a team requires 6 people every time it plays and they knew that not everyone would be able to make every game due to their busy schedules. They also needed their group to be evenly split between men and women because three of each had to be on the court during every game. The group elected Hal as captain and coach and recruited another couple (Nancy and Cole) who lived nearby. Jennifer also asked her friend Jasmine to join, which brought their total 10—5 women and 5 men.

Not all people have such a ready-made social group. Here are some good guidelines for finding or forming a group for physical activity participation.

- **Consider nonleague participation as a start.** Joining a club or league can be quite intimidating for some people. If you're just learning an activity, you may first want to join in recreational sessions or take a class at a local club before joining a league. For example, Coretta had not played much volleyball, so she joined with others in the group to practice at the park before the league started. Will went to the rec center at his university and played in some pick-up volleyball games to get some practice.

- **Check with friends at school or work.** Start with a few people, then each can recruit others with similar interests to participate. You might want to start with noncompetitive games before moving on to league play.

- **Check out your work wellness program or school recreation center.** See if there's a list of people interested in the same activity that you can recruit to join you. There might even be an existing club or exercise group that you can join. Club members often get to know each other and then form teams for leagues after starting with recreational play.

- **Check with the organizations listed in table 21.2.** See if they have opportunities for individuals or small groups to join larger teams.

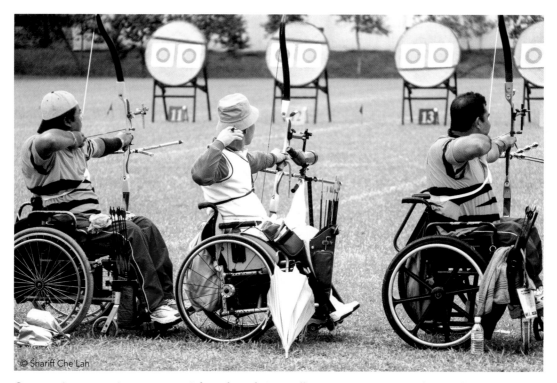
© Shariff Che'Lah

Community recreation, commercial, and worksite wellness programs provide good opportunities for lifelong participation.

# Daring to Try

Sometimes one of the hardest things to do is simply to dare to try. This can be especially true when you're starting something new and don't have others to do it with. Coretta had friends to support her, so joining them on a volleyball team was not as threatening as it might have been. Still, she lacked confidence, so before the volleyball league began she joined with others to practice. She was initially motivated by her desire to please her friends in the group; she didn't want to let them down.

Coretta's initial motivation for playing is called **extrinsic motivation**. Extrinsic motivation is motivation that comes from outside the individual (for example, pressure from others, external rewards). In this case, Coretta wanted to be on the team not because she particularly enjoyed volleyball but because the team needed another player. Even after trying recreational volleyball, she felt very nervous when she first played on the competitive team. As she practiced, however, she found success in serving

and digging, which encouraged her to keep trying. As she got better, she started to look forward to the games. She was not playing to please someone else (extrinsic motivation); she was now playing because she enjoyed it (**intrinsic motivation**). Intrinsic motivation comes from within the individual; the rewards for participation are personal and internal (for example, fun, joy of participation).

In school, Coretta had learned about **optimal challenge** (see figure 21.2). In her practice group, she tried to do things that were neither too easy nor too hard. Because the challenge was reasonable, she found success rather than failure. In turn, this success encouraged her to keep trying. Gradually, she started to enjoy herself, and that made her want to keep participating.

Coretta also learned to reward herself for her performance rather than rely on praise from others. If she had gone right into the volleyball league without practicing first, she might have become frustrated and quit trying.

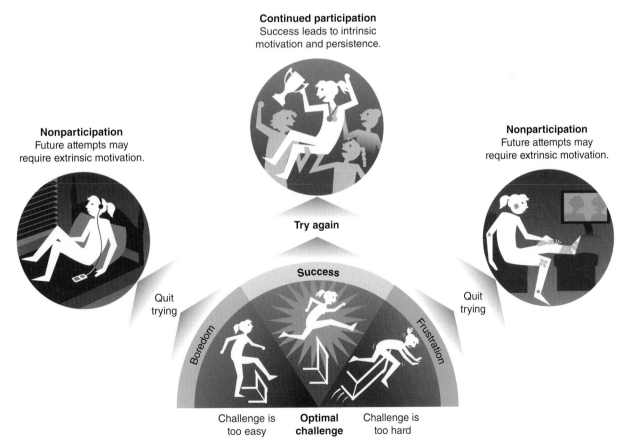

**FIGURE 21.2** Finding an optimal challenge helps you achieve success and intrinsic motivation.

## FIT FACT

Video game creators use the concept of optimal challenge. To ensure success, they design games that start players at a low level. This success creates intrinsic motivation that keeps players' interest high and encourages them to keep participating. Indeed, evidence shows that gamers play for hours with no extrinsic rewards.

Kris had a very different experience. He became bored with the volleyball team. Although he liked being with his friends, his volleyball skills were better than his friends' skills, and he lost interest in the games. It took encouragement and even pleading from his friends (extrinsic motivation) to keep him coming to the games. Ultimately, he dropped out of the league, and the team finished with nine players.

Sometimes you need a little extrinsic or external motivation to get you going. But researchers have shown that long-term participation requires intrinsic motivation. People who have intrinsic motivation (such as Coretta) are more likely to stick with participation than people who are extrinsically motivated (such as Kris). Being able to gradually build your skills and find success and ultimately intrinsic motivation is called having a **self-reward system**. You reward yourself rather than expecting others to reward you for your efforts.

##  FITNESS TECHNOLOGY: Social Support

Social support is important in helping people adopt and stick with healthy lifestyle changes. Weight Watchers is an organization that uses social support to help people maintain a healthy weight throughout life. Meetings allow group members to support each other and receive support from program leaders. Weight Watchers also uses the web to provide social support through interactive tools that help members self-monitor their eating and activity habits. Optimal challenges are provided to encourage success and intrinsic motivation. Even people who are intrinsically motivated benefit from the support of others, and Weight Watchers messages are sent periodically to provide support and encouragement. Some doctors now also provide messages to encourage patients.

You can use the web and social media to encourage others and help them be successful in making healthy lifestyle choices. You can do this through e-mail messages and tweets to support group members with similar goals. For example, Hal and his friends could use e-mails, text messages, phone calls, or tweets to encourage each other to come to practice and games.

Messages from others can also be harmful if not done properly. You've learned that autonomy is important and that we all want to make decisions for ourselves. Messages that encourage a person to stick with his or her plan encourage autonomy. On the other hand, messages or comments that treat a person as if you're trying to control his or her behavior do not encourage autonomy and may be ignored. For example, if a person misses a practice, a good message of support might be, "Missed you at practice—hope to see you next time." A not-so-good message might be, "If you keep missing, you will never get better." This message suggests that the person should attend to please someone else.

Appropriately supportive personal messages delivered via phone or the web have been shown to help people who are trying to stop smoking, maintain a healthy weight, or be active for health and fitness.

### Using Technology

Work with a group of friends to form a support network. Outline ways in which the group will use social support technology to help members meet their goals.

# Helping Others in Physical Activity

In this book, you've learned many self-management skills designed to help you be active for the rest of your life. In the years ahead, you'll find that having active people around you helps you be more active. You'll also have the opportunity to help others be physically active. A few of these opportunities are described in the following list.

- **Family activities.** A popular slogan says, "Families that play together stay together." You can use the skills you've learned in this class to help family members be active. Examples include family outings (such as camping, fishing, and biking trips), family exercise sessions (such as walks and hikes), and family activity nights (such as bowling or skating night). Since not all family members will always like the same activities, you can also support each other's activities.

Family support is a type of social support that can help family members stick with their exercise—for example, watching a family member's team play or praising the jogger in the family for sticking with it over time.

- **Coaching.** When you were younger, you may have played a sport such as soccer or tee ball. If so, someone coached your team. You can give back by volunteering to coach children in your neighborhood or your own children. Training for volunteer coaches is provided by many organizations.

> " You can motivate by fear, and you can motivate by reward. But both those methods are only temporary. The only lasting thing is self-motivation. "
>
> —Homer Rice, football coach

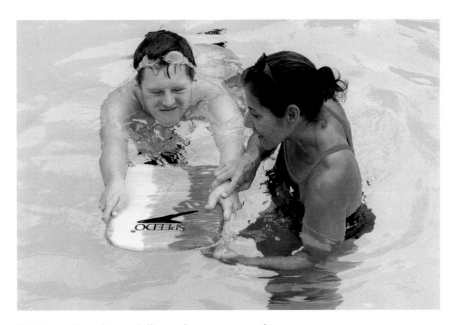

Helping others learn skills can be very rewarding.

## Lesson Review

1. What is autonomy, and how does it relate to decision making about healthy lifestyles?
2. What are some sources of information about opportunities for physical activity?
3. What are some guidelines for organizing for participation in physical activity?
4. What are extrinsic and intrinsic motivation, and how do they differ?

Conflict can be a barrier to participation; it can be the reason that a person doesn't stick to a physical activity plan. Here's an example. Monica and Juana developed a plan to walk to school five days a week for one month. Unfortunately, their friend Miguel kept offering them a ride to school. The third time Miguel offered, Monica accepted and left Juana to walk alone. Juana did not accept because she wanted to walk as planned. Juana then felt mad at both Monica and Miguel and didn't speak to them at school. The next day, Monica didn't

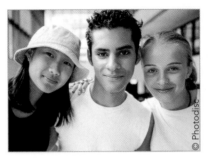
© Photodisc

stop by to walk with Juana—she just rode with Miguel. The friends did not speak at school. In fact, Monica said something to other friends about Juana that upset her.

## For Discussion

What could the friends have done to avoid the conflict? What steps should they take to resolve it? List possible solutions. Consider the skills in the Self-Management feature when answering the discussion questions.

 **SELF-MANAGEMENT:** *Skills for Conflict Resolution*

At times, all of us have disagreements with our friends. The disagreements are usually over small things and can be easily resolved. A conflict is typically bigger than a disagreement. When a conflict occurs, one or more of the people involved come to feel threatened, whether physically or emotionally. In sport, for example, one player may get angry with another, and strong emotions may lead to angry words. In extreme cases, the anger can result in fighting. Whether the conflict occurs in sport or daily life, the following steps can help you resolve it.

- **Consider the three Bs.** When working with others to resolve conflict, remember to *be calm*, *be patient*, and *be respectful*. Keeping emotions under control is essential.

- **Communicate.** To resolve a conflict, you need good communication. Be willing to listen to what the other person has to say. Watch what you say. Words can hurt, and it's crucial not to make the conflict worse.

- **Recognize that there is a conflict.** Don't ignore it. Avoiding a conflict can cause it to get worse.

- **Consider a meeting.** While a conflict can sometimes be resolved on the phone, by e-mail, through social media, or in other ways, it's often best to meet face to face. Meeting in person makes harsh

words less likely. The meeting should be held in a neutral and safe setting for all involved.

- **Set the scene.** Define the problem, and restate it if necessary. Using the three Bs, each person should describe the problem without interruption. After each person has done so, the parties can try to find a statement of the problem that all can agree to.

- **List possible solutions.** Make a list of possible solutions based on ideas from people on all sides of the conflict.

- **Consider the options.** Once options have been proposed, communicate respectfully to find the options that best meet the needs of all parties concerned.

- **Compromise.** If the people involved have very different ideas about the conflict, it may be necessary for each person to give up something in order to find a resolution.

- **Seek help.** Another way to resolve a conflict is through arbitration. If the parties involved cannot resolve the conflict on their own, an independent arbitrator may be used. In sport, a coach or referee can resolve some conflicts, and others may be resolved with the help of a common friend, but difficult conflicts may call for a professional arbitrator.

The TEAM concept (Together Everyone Achieves More) can help you succeed in all aspects of your life. It's an exciting challenge to build a team of individuals who work well together in pursuit of a common goal. **Take action** by performing a team-building activity in your physical education class.

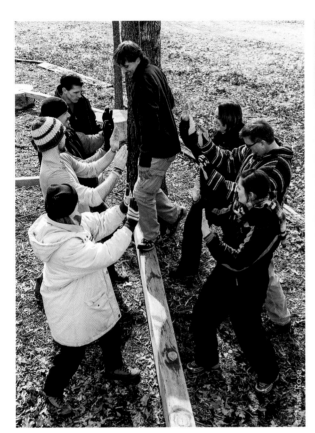

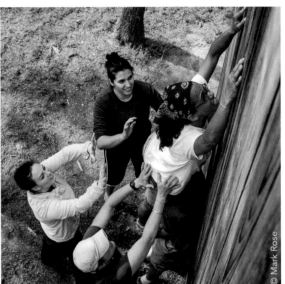

**Take action by trying team-building activities.**

## Reviewing Concepts and Vocabulary

As directed by your teacher, answer items 1 through 5 by correctly completing each sentence with a word or phrase.

1. _____ involves being fair and following the rules.
2. Sticking together when working toward a common goal is called _____.
3. _____ involves acting in a way that is consistent with expected behavior in a group.
4. People who have _____ are self-directed and make their own decisions.
5. People who need an external reward to do a behavior have _____ motivation.

For items 6 through 10, as directed by your teacher, match each term in column 1 with the appropriate phrase in column 2.

6. self-determination theory        a. places importance on autonomy
7. diversity                        b. respect for others
8. optimal challenge                c. person who guides or directs
9. leader                           d. comes from within
10. intrinsic motivation            e. neither too hard nor too easy

For items 11 through 15, as directed by your teacher, respond to each statement or question.

11. List and describe several leadership skills.
12. Explain some factors that contribute to good teamwork.
13. Discuss rules and their importance.
14. Describe groups that provide opportunities for physical activity in a community.
15. Describe the guidelines for resolving conflict.

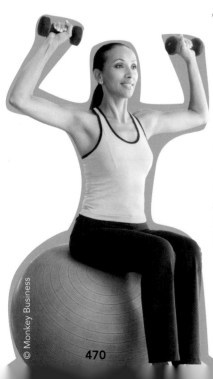

## Thinking Critically

You've been asked to form an intramural team for a school league. Write a paragraph to describe the steps you would take to get a team organized.

## Project

Work with a group to develop a directory of physical activity for your community. Include a list of agencies and businesses offering various kinds of physical activity. Consider the following categories and list the activities they provide: local government agencies, community sport organizations, worksite activity programs, commercial options (local businesses), places of worship, and other types. Use table 21.2 for ideas.

# Glossary

**absolute strength**—Strength measured by how much weight or resistance you can overcome regardless of your body size.

**acceleration**—Increase in velocity.

**accelerometer**—Device that measures movement; frequently used to measure steps, intensity of movement, and duration of physical activity.

**acronym**—Specific kind of mnemonic in which the first letters of each word in a phrase are combined to form an easy-to-remember word (for example, SMART—specific, measurable, attainable, realistic, and timely).

**active stretch**—Stretch caused by contraction of your own antagonist muscles.

**activity neurosis**—Condition in which a person feels overly concerned about getting enough exercise and upset if he or she misses a regular workout.

**Adequate Intake (AI)**—Dietary reference intake (DRI) used when there is insufficient evidence to establish a recommended dietary allowance (RDA).

**adventure education**—Physical education approach focused on challenging recreational activities, such as rock climbing, orienteering, and rafting.

**aerobic**—Term often used to describe moderate to vigorous physical activity that can be sustained for a long time because the body can supply adequate oxygen to continue activity; means "with oxygen."

**aerobic activity**—Activity that is steady enough to allow your heart to supply all the oxygen your muscles need.

**aerobic capacity**—The ability of the cardiorespiratory system to provide and use oxygen during very hard exertion over a specific amount of time. The maximal oxygen uptake test measures aerobic capacity.

**aerodynamics**—Study of motion in the air.

**agility**—Ability to change your body position quickly and control your body's movements.

**air quality index**—Scale used to rate pollution levels ranging from good air quality to very unhealthful.

**alarm reaction**—First stage of general adaptation syndrome; occurs when your body reacts to a stressor.

**amino acid**—Building block of protein.

**anabolic steroid**—Synthetic drug that resembles the male hormone testosterone but that has health risks. It produces lean body mass, weight gain, and bone maturation.

**anaerobic activity**—Activity so intense that your body cannot supply adequate oxygen to sustain it for a long time.

**anaerobic capacity**—The ability of the body to perform all-out exercise using the body's high energy fuel sources (ATP-PC and glycolytic systems); commonly measured using the Wingate Test.

**androstenedione**—Substance considered to be a steroid precursor because it is converted into anabolic steroids such as testosterone (male hormone) after it enters the body; also called andro.

**anorexia athletica**—Eating disorder with symptoms similar to anorexia nervosa; most common among athletes involved in sports in which low body weight is desirable (such as gymnastics and wrestling).

**anorexia nervosa**—Eating disorder in which a person severely restricts the amount of food eaten in an attempt to be exceptionally low in body fat.

**antagonist**—Muscle or muscle group having the opposite function of another muscle or muscle group.

**artery**—Vessel that carries blood from your heart to another part of your body.

**atherosclerosis**—Clogging of the arteries.

**attitude**—Your feelings about something.

**autonomy**—Self-direction; ability to make decisions for yourself.

**balance**—Ability to maintain an upright posture while standing still or moving.

**ballistic stretch**—Series of gentle bouncing or bobbing motions that are not held for a long time.

**basal metabolism**—Amount of energy your body uses just to keep you living.

**biomechanical principles**—Basic laws of physics that are used to help people perform physical tasks efficiently and effectively.

**biomechanics**—Branch of kinesiology that uses principles of physics to help us understand the human body in motion.

**blood pressure**—Force of blood against your artery walls.

**bodybuilding**—A competitive sport in which participants are judged primarily on the appearance of their muscles rather than how much they can lift.

**body composition**—The proportional amounts of body tissues, including muscle, bone, body fat, and other tissues that make up your body.

**body dysmorphia**—Condition in which a person is obsessed with building muscle.

**body fat level**—Percentage of body weight that is made up of fat.

**built environment**—Physical characteristics of a neighborhood.

**bulimia**—Eating disorder in which a person binges, or eats very large amounts of food within a short time, followed by purging.

**calisthenics**—Exercises done using all or part of the body weight as resistance.

**calorie**—Unit of energy or heat that describes the amount of energy in a food (the true term is *kilocalorie*).

**calorie expenditure**—Calories (energy) used in physical activity.

**calorie intake**—Calories (energy) ingested.

**calorimeter**—Apparatus used to determine the amount of heat generated by a chemical reaction; also can determine the number of calories in food.

**carbohydrate**—Type of nutrient that provides you with your main source of energy.

**cardiorespiratory endurance**—Ability to exercise your entire body for a long time without stopping.

**cardiovascular disease (CVD)**—A physical illness that affects the heart, blood vessels, or blood. Examples include heart attack and stroke. It's the leading cause of death in the United States.

**cardiovascular system**—Body system that includes your heart, blood vessels, and blood; provides oxygen and nutrients to the body.

**center of gravity**—The location of the center or midpoint of the total body weight.

**cholesterol**—Waxy, fatlike substance found in meat, dairy products, and egg yolk; a high amount in the blood is implicated in various types of heart disease.

**circuit training**—Performance of different exercises one after another, separated only by brief breaks, with the goal of keeping your heart rate in your target zone and building various components of health-related fitness.

**cognitive skills**—Abilities that help you gain knowledge from information; examples include being able to concentrate and focusing your attention.

**compendium**—List of physical activity that tells you the intensity of various activities.

**competitive stress**—The body's reaction to participation in a sport or other activity in which people or teams attempt to outperform an opponent; a stress condition that may be eustressful.

**complete protein**—Protein containing all nine essential amino acids; derived from animal sources, such as meat, milk products, and fish.

**complex skill**—Task that involves complicated movement sequences (for example, serving a tennis ball, hip-hop dancing) or integrating several movements at the same time (for example, stroking, kicking, and breathing in swimming).

**con artist**—Person who practices fraud.

**concentric**—A shortening isotonic muscle contraction.

**consumer community**—A school group or club that reviews scientific information and answers student questions related to fitness, health, and wellness.

**controllable risk factor**—Risk factor that you can act upon to change.

**cool-down**—Activity performed after a workout to help you recover.

**cooperative game**—Game in which teams work together rather than compete.

**coordination**—Ability to use your senses together with your body parts or to use two or more body parts together.

**coping**—Dealing with or attempting to overcome a problem.

**coping skill**—Technique that you can use to manage stress or deal with a problem.

**coronary artery disease (CAD)**—Specific kind of cardiovascular disease in which the arteries in the heart become clogged.

**CRAC**—Contract-relax-antagonist-contract; a type of PNF stretch that first requires the muscle or muscles to contract and then relax before being stretched by the contraction of the opposing muscle or muscles.

**creatine**—Natural substance manufactured in the body by meat-eating animals including humans and needed in order for the body to perform anaerobic exercise, including many types of progressive resistance exercise.

**creeping obesity**—Slow, gradual weight gain typically caused by consuming empty calories.

**criterion-referenced health standards**—Fitness ratings used to determine how much fitness is needed to prevent health problems and to achieve wellness.

**dance education**—An approach to physical education (or a separate program) that focuses on teaching various forms of dance, both in and out of school.

**deceleration**—Decrease in velocity.

**determinant**—Factor affecting your fitness, health, and wellness.

**diabetes**—Disease in which a person's body is unable to regulate sugar levels, leading to an excessively high blood sugar level.

**diastolic blood pressure**—Pressure in your arteries just before the next beat of your heart.

**Dietary Reference Intake (DRI)**—Amount of a given micronutrient that you should consume daily.

**dietitian**—Expert in nutrition who helps people apply principles of nutrition in daily life; has a college degree and certification by a reputable national organization.

**distress**—Negative stress from situations that cause worry, sorrow, anger, or pain.

**double progressive system**—The most-used method of applying the principle of progression for improving muscle fitness—first by increasing repetitions (reps) and second by increasing resistance or weight.

**dynamic movement exercises**—Exercises such as jumping, skipping, and calisthenics that are often used in a warm-up for activities requiring strength, power, and speed. They move the joints beyond normal resting ROM and cause the muscles and tendons to stretch. The stretch caused by dynamic movement exercise is followed by a contraction of the stretched muscle.

**dynamic stretch**—Slow movement exercises designed to lengthen the muscles.

**dynamic warm-up**—Dynamic movement exercises that increase body temperature and get muscles ready for more vigorous exercise; can serve as all or part of the general warm-up.

**dynamometer**—Device that measures the amount of force produced by a muscle or group of muscles.

**eating disorder**—Condition that involves dangerous eating habits and often excessive activity to expend calories for fat loss.

**eccentric**—A lengthening isotonic muscle contraction.

**electrolytes**—Minerals in your blood and body fluids that are important for normal body functioning and prevention of water loss during exercise.

**empty calories**—Calories that provide energy but contain few if any other nutrients.

**energy balance**—Balance between calorie intake and calorie expenditure.

**ergogenic aid**—Anything done to help you generate work or to increase your ability to do work, including performing vigorous exercise.

**ergolytic**—Term referring to substances that negatively affect performance (*ergo* meaning work, and *lytic* meaning destruction).

**essential body fat**—The minimum amount of body fat that a person needs to maintain health.

**etiquette**—Typical or expected behavior of a social group.

**eustress**—Positive stress.

**exercise**—Form of physical activity specifically designed to improve your fitness.

**exercise anatomy**—Study of how muscles work together with bones, ligaments, and tendons to produce human movement.

**exercise physiology**—Branch of kinesiology focused on how physical activity affects body systems.

**exercise psychology**—Study of human behavior in all types of physical activity, including exercise for fitness and sport.

**exercise sociology**—Study of social relationships and interactions in physical activity, including sport.

**extension**—A movement that increases the angle between the bones at a joint.

**extrinsic motivation**—Reason for doing something that comes from an outside source (for example, prizes, approval, or acceptance).

**fast-twitch muscle fiber**—Fiber that contracts quickly, is white because it receives less blood flow delivering oxygen, and generates more force than slow-twitch muscle fiber when it contracts (thus, muscles with many fast-twitch fibers are important for strength activities).

**fat**—Nutrient that provides energy, helps growth and repair of cells, and dissolves and carries certain vitamins to cells.

**feedback**—Information you receive about your performance, including suggestions for making changes in order to perform better.

**fiber**—Type of complex carbohydrate that your body cannot digest.

**fibrin**—Substance involved in blood clotting.

**fitness education**—Classes or units in physical education focused on learning fitness and activity concepts and self-management skills that can help you be active throughout your life.

**fitness profile**—Brief summary of your fitness self-assessment results.

**fitness target zone**—Optimal range of physical activity for promoting fitness and achieving health and wellness.

**FITT formula**—Prescription or recipe (based on the ingredients of frequency, intensity, time, and type) for appropriate physical activity.

**flexibility**—Ability to use your joints fully through a wide range of motion without injury.

**flexion**—A movement that reduces the angle between the bones at a joint.

**food label**—Nutritional information that appears on food packaging.

**food supplement**—Product taken by mouth as an addition to a person's basic diet (for example, vitamins, minerals, and herbs); also called a dietary supplement.

**force**—In physical activity, it is energy exerted by the muscles to cause movement or resist movement; other uses include military force (ships and troops), violent force (a physical attack), or resistance force (stopping a moving body or object).

**fraud**—Intentional use of deception to get you to buy products or services known to be ineffective or harmful.

**frequency**—How often a task is performed; in the FITT formula, it refers to how often physical activity is performed.

**functional fitness**—Capacity to function effectively when performing normal daily tasks.

**general adaptation syndrome**—Body's reaction to stress in three phases: alarm reaction, stage of resistance, and stage of exhaustion.

**goal setting**—Process of establishing objectives to accomplish; the objectives for lifetime fitness are to achieve good fitness, health, and wellness and to adopt a healthy lifestyle.

**graded exercise test**—Test used to detect potential heart problems by having you exercise on a treadmill while your heart is monitored by an electrocardiogram.

**group cohesiveness**—Sticking together in working toward a common goal.

**habituate**—To get used to something because of repeated exposure to it.

**health**—Freedom from disease and a state of optimal physical, emotional-mental, social, intellectual, and spiritual well-being (wellness).

**health and medical science**—Area of study that focuses on preventing and treating illness and promoting wellness.

**health-related physical fitness**—Parts of physical fitness that help a person stay healthy; includes cardio-respiratory endurance, flexibility, muscular endurance, strength, power, and body composition.

**heart attack**—Condition in which the blood supply within the heart is severely reduced or cut off, which can cause an area of the heart muscle to die.

**heart rate reserve (HRR)**—Difference between the number of times that your heart beats per minute at rest and during maximal exercise.

**heat index**—Scale that rates the safety of the environment for exercise based on temperature and humidity.

**high-density lipoprotein (HDL)**—Lipoprotein often referred to as good cholesterol because it carries excess cholesterol out of your bloodstream and into your liver for elimination from your body.

**human growth hormone (HGH)**—Illegal drug that is exceptionally dangerous, especially for teens; causes premature closure of bones and can have deforming and even life-threatening effects.

**humidity**—Relative amount of moisture in the air.

**hydrodynamics**—Study of motion in fluids.

**hyperkinetic condition**—Health problem caused by doing too much physical activity.

**hypermobility**—Unusually large range of motion in the joints; sometimes referred to as double-jointedness.

**hypertension**—Condition in which blood pressure is consistently higher than normal.

**hyperthermia**—Exceptionally high body temperature often associated with exposure to hot or humid environments.

**hypertrophy**—Increase in muscle fiber size.

**hypokinetic condition**—Health problem caused partly by lack of physical activity.

**hypothermia**—Abnormally low body temperature often associated with exposure to cold and windy environments.

**implement**—Device or tool used to perform a task.

**incomplete protein**—Protein that contains some, but not all, essential amino acids.

**intensity**—Magnitude or vigorousness of a task; in the FITT formula, it refers to how hard you perform a physical activity.

**intermediate muscle fiber**—Fiber with characteristics of both slow- and fast-twitch fibers.

**interval training**—Type of training that uses bouts of high-intensity exercise followed by rest periods.

**intrinsic motivation**—Reason for doing something that comes from within (for example, enjoyment, desire to be more fit).

**isokinetic exercise**—Type of isotonic exercise in which movement velocity is kept constant through the full range of motion.

**isometric contraction**—Contraction in which muscles exert force but do not cause movement at a joint.

**isometric exercise**—Exercise involving isometric contractions in which body parts do not move.

**isotonic contraction**—Muscle contraction that pulls on bone and produces movement of a body part.

**isotonic exercise**—Exercise involving isotonic contractions in which body parts move.

**jai alai**—Sport played on a large enclosed court similar to handball but using a wicker basket glove and a pelota (ball).

**kinesiology**—Study of human movement.

**kyphosis**—Posture problem characterized by rounded back and shoulders.

**laws of motion**—Rules of physics that help us understand human movements.

**leadership**—Ability to motivate and help people in a group work toward a common goal.

**lean body tissue**—All tissue in the body other than fat.

**leisure time**—Time free from work and other commitments; also called discretionary time.

**lifestyle**—The way you live.

**lifestyle physical activity**—Activity done as part of daily life (such as walking to school or doing yardwork).

**lifetime sport**—Sport in which you're likely to participate throughout your life.

**ligament**—Tough tissue that holds bones together.

**lipoprotein**—Protein that carries lipids and cholesterol through your bloodstream.

**locomotion**—Movement of the body from place to place.

**long-term goal**—Goal that takes months or even years to accomplish.

**lordosis**—Posture problem characterized by too much arch in the lower back; also called swayback.

**low-density lipoprotein (LDL)**—Type of lipoprotein often referred to as bad cholesterol because it carries cholesterol that is most likely to stay in your body and contribute to atherosclerosis.

**macronutrient**—Nutrient that supplies the energy your body needs to perform daily tasks; comes in three types—carbohydrate, protein, and fat.

**maturation**—Process of becoming fully grown and developed.

**maximal heart rate**—Number of times your heart beats per minute during very vigorous activity; the highest your heart rate can go.

**maximal oxygen uptake**—Lab measure considered to be the best for assessing fitness of the cardiovascular and respiratory systems; see also *aerobic capacity*.

**metabolic equivalent (MET)**—Measure that refers to metabolism (the use of energy to sustain life), with 1 MET representing the energy you expend while resting; multiples are used to describe the intensity of all types of physical activity.

**metabolic syndrome**—Condition in which a person has high body fat, large girth, and other health risks, such as high blood pressure, high blood fat, and high blood sugar.

**micronutrient**—Nutrient (vitamin or mineral) that your body needs in smaller amounts than it needs carbohydrate, protein, and fat.

**microtrauma**—Invisible injury, caused by repeated use or misuse of a body part, that may not result in immediate pain, soreness, or symptoms.

**mnemonic**—A term that is useful in remembering specific information, such as an acronym (for example, SMART).

**moderate physical activity**—Activity that requires energy expenditure four to seven times greater than that required by being sedentary (that is, 4 to 7 METs).

**motor learning**—Process of acquiring a motor skill; also an area of study within kinesiology that relates to acquiring motor skills.

**motor skill**—The learned ability to use the muscles and nerves together to perform a physical task (for example, throwing, running).

**motor unit**—A group of nerves and muscle fibers working together to cause movement. The nerves cause the muscle fibers to contract.

**muscle bound**—Having tight, bulky muscles that inhibit free movement.

**muscle-tendon unit (MTU)**—Skeletal muscles and the tendons that attach them to bones.

**muscular endurance**—Ability to use your muscles many times without tiring.

**nutrition science**—Study of the processes by which a plant or animal uses food to grow and sustain life.

**obesity**—Condition of being especially overweight or high in body fat.

**object**—An item used in sport and physical activity (for example, a ball or hockey puck).

**1-repetition maximum (1RM)**—Test of muscle strength in which you determine how much weight you can lift (or how much resistance you can overcome) in one repetition.

**optimal challenge**—Activity that is neither too hard nor too easy; activity that isn't too distressful compared to the competitive situation.

**osteoporosis**—Condition in which bone structure deteriorates and bones become weak.

**outdoor education**—An approach to physical education that occurs in an outdoor classroom.

**over-exercising**—Doing so much exercise that you increase your risk of injury or soreness.

**overuse injury**—Injury resulting from repeated movement that causes wear and tear in your body.

**overweight**—Condition of weighing more than the healthy range.

**passive exercise**—Use of a machine or device that moves your body for you. Programs using passive exercise are ineffective.

**passive stretch**—Stretch requiring an assist from an external source (gravity, a partner, or some other source).

**peak bone mass**—Highest bone density achieved during life; typically occurs in late adolescence or early adulthood.

**pedometer**—Small battery-powered device that can be worn on your belt to count your steps.

**pelota**—Ball used in jai alai.

**periodization**—Way of scheduling muscle fitness exercise in which you perform a given plan for a while, then alter it to perform different exercises or change the way you do your exercises.

**personal lifestyle plan**—Written schedule of activities designed to improve fitness, health, and wellness.

**personal needs profile**—Chart listing self-assessment scores and corresponding ratings.

**personal program**—Written individualized plan designed to change behavior (the way you live) to improve fitness, health, and wellness.

**physical activity**—Movement using the large muscles; includes sport, dance, recreational activity, and activities of daily living.

**Physical Activity Pyramid**—Diagram or model that describes the various types of physical activity that produce good fitness, health, and wellness.

**Physical Activity Readiness Questionnaire (PAR-Q)**—Seven-question assessment of medical and physical readiness that should be taken before beginning a regular physical activity program for health and wellness.

**physical fitness**—Capacity of your body systems to work together efficiently to allow you to be healthy and effectively perform activities of daily living.

**physical literacy**—Being physically educated; a physically literate person does regular activity, is fit, has skills, values activity, and knows the implications and benefits of physical activity.

**Pilates**—Form of training, quite popular in recent years, designed to build core muscle fitness; named for Joseph Pilates, who described core exercises and developed special exercise machines for building core muscles.

**plyometrics**—Type of training designed to increase athletic performance using jumping, hopping, and other exercises to cause lengthening of a muscle followed by a shortening contraction.

**PNF stretching**—Flexibility exercise using proprioceptive neuromuscular facilitation; a variation of static stretching that involves contracting a muscle before stretching it.

**power**—Capacity to use strength quickly; involves both strength and speed.

**powerlifting**—Competitive sport using free weights and involving only three exercises: bench press, squat, and deadlift.

**principle of overload**—The most basic law of physical activity, which states that the only way to produce fitness and health benefits through physical activity is to require your body to do more than it normally does.

**principle of progression**—Principle stating that the amount and intensity of your exercise should be increased gradually.

**principle of rest and recovery**—Principle stating that you need to give your muscles time to rest and recover after a workout.

**principle of specificity**—Principle stating that the type of exercise you perform determines the type of benefit you receive.

**priority healthy lifestyle choice**—One of the key lifestyle choices (regular physical activity, sound nutrition, and stress management) that help you prevent disease, get and stay fit, and enjoy a good quality of life.

**process goal**—Goal relating to what you do rather than the product resulting from what you do.

**product goal**—Goal relating to what you get as a result of what you do.

**professional**—Highly educated person who delivers information and helps people apply it to improve their lives.

**progressive resistance exercise (PRE)**—Exercise that increases resistance (overload) until you have the amount of muscle fitness you want; also called progressive resistance training (PRT).

**protein**—Group of nutrients used for building, repairing, and maintaining your body cells.

**ptosis**—Posture problem characterized by protruding abdomen.

**public health scientist**—Expert who studies disease prevention and wellness promotion in communities.

**quack**—Person who practices quackery.

**quackery**—Method of advertising or selling that uses false claims to lure people into buying products that are worthless or even harmful.

**range of motion (ROM)**—The amount of movement in a specific joint that is considered to be healthy (neither too much nor too little).

**range-of-motion (ROM) exercise**—Exercise that requires a joint to move through a full range of motion by using either your own muscles or the assistance of a partner or therapist.

**reaction time**—Amount of time it takes to move once you recognize the need to act.

**Recommended Dietary Allowance (RDA)**—Minimum amount of a nutrient necessary to meet the health need of most people.

**recreation**—Something you do during your free time.

**relative strength**—Strength adjusted for your body size.

**reps**—Short for *repetitions* (the number of consecutive times you do an exercise).

**respiratory system**—Body system made up of your lungs and the passages that bring air, including oxygen, from outside of your body into your lungs.

**resting metabolism**—Number of calories expended by your body for basic functions and typical light activities done during the day.

**rhabdomyolysis**—Condition in which muscle fibers break down and the bloodstream absorbs muscle fiber elements.

**RICE**—Formula in which each letter represents a step in the treatment of a minor injury: R = rest; I = ice; C = compression; E = elevation.

**risk factor**—Any action or condition that increases your chances of developing a disease or health condition.

**rule**—Guideline or requirement for conduct or action.

**runner's high**—The eustress people feel when they run or do exercise that they enjoy.

**saturated fat**—Fat that is solid at room temperature and is derived mostly from animal products, such as lard, butter, milk, and meat.

**sedentary**—Not engaging in regular physical activity from any of the steps of the Physical Activity Pyramid.

**self-management skill**—Skill that helps you adopt a healthy lifestyle now and throughout your life.

**self-reward system**—System for gradually building skills and finding success and, ultimately, intrinsic motivation; involves rewarding yourself rather than expecting others to reward you for your efforts.

**set**—One group of repetitions.

**short-term goal**—Goal that can be reached in a short time, such as a few days or weeks.

**side stitch**—Pain in the side of the lower abdomen that people often experience during sport activity, especially running.

**skill**—Ability to perform a specific task effectively that results from knowledge and practice.

**skill-related physical fitness**—Parts of fitness that help a person perform well in sports and activities requiring certain skills; the parts include agility, balance, coordination, reaction time, and speed.

**skinfold**—Fold of fat and skin used to estimate total body fat level.

**sleep apnea**—Disorder that results in poor sleep or inability to sleep, characterized by pauses in breathing or shallow breathing during sleep.

**slow-twitch muscle fiber**—Muscle fiber that contracts at a slow rate, is usually red because it has a lot of blood vessels delivering oxygen, and generates less force than fast-twitch muscle fiber but is able to resist fatigue.

**SMART goal**—Goal that is specific, measurable, attainable, realistic, and timely.

**spa**—Facility offering saunas, whirlpool baths, and other services such as massage and hair or skin care.

**speed**—Ability to perform a movement or cover a distance in a short time.

**sport**—Physical activity that is competitive (has winners and losers) and has well-established rules.

**sport education**—Approach that seeks to make physical education both fun and interesting by dividing the year into seasons similar to those found in the sport world.

**sport pedagogy**—Art and science of teaching physical activity; includes applying motor learning principles to help people learn motor skills and studying the best ways to teach and learn the principles of physical activity derived from the sciences.

**sportsmanship**—Having respect for people on opposing teams; being a good winner and not being a poor loser.

**sprain**—Injury to a ligament.

**stage of exhaustion**—Third stage of general adaptation syndrome; occurs when the body is not able to resist a stressor well enough.

**stage of resistance**—Second stage of general adaptation syndrome; occurs when the immune system starts to resist or fight the stressor.

**stance**—Way of standing.

**state of being**—Overall condition of a person.

**static stretch**—Stretch performed slowly as far as you can without pain, until you feel a sense of pulling or tension.

**strain**—Injury to a tendon or muscle.

**strategy**—Master plan for achieving a goal or set of goals.

**strength**—Maximal amount of force your muscles can produce.

**stress**—Body's reaction to a demanding situation.

**stressor**—Something that causes or contributes to stress.

**stretching warm-up**—A way of preparing for physical activity using flexibility exercises performed after several minutes of general exercise.

**stroke**—Condition in which the supply of oxygen to the brain is severely reduced or cut off.

**systolic blood pressure**—Pressure in your arteries immediately after your heart beats.

**tactic**—Specific method for carrying out a strategy.

**tai chi**—Ancient form of exercise that originated in China and whose basic movements have been shown to increase flexibility and reduce symptoms of arthritis in some people.

**target ceiling**—Your upper recommended limit of activity for optimally promoting fitness and achieving health and wellness.

**teamwork**—Cooperative effort of all team members to strive for a common goal in the most effective way.

**tendon**—Tissue that connects muscle to bone.

**threshold of training**—Minimum amount of overload you need in order to build physical fitness.

**time**—Length of a task; in the FITT formula (first *T*), it refers to the optimal length of an activity session designed to improve fitness and promote health and wellness.

**Tolerable Upper Intake Level (UL)**—Maximum amount of a vitamin or mineral that can be consumed without posing a health risk.

**tracking**—Using vision to follow the path of an object (for example, watching the path of a thrown ball).

**trans-fatty acid**—Product made from unsaturated fat, such as can be found in vegetable oil, by means of a process that renders it solid at room temperature (for example, solid margarine); also known as trans fat. It has been banned from food by the FDA.

**type**—The specific kind of task; in the FITT formula (second *T*), it refers to the specific kind of physical activity that is performed.

**uncontrollable risk factor**—Risk factor that you cannot do anything to change.

**underweight**—Condition of weighing less than the healthy range.

**unsaturated fat**—Fat that is liquid at room temperature; derived mostly from plants, such as sunflower, corn, soybean, olive, almond, and peanut.

**vein**—Vessel that carries blood filled with waste products from your muscle cells back to your heart.

**velocity**—Speed of movement.

**vigorous aerobics**—Aerobic activities intense enough to elevate your heart rate above your threshold of training and into your target zone for cardiorespiratory endurance.

**vigorous recreation**—Activity done during your free time that is fun and typically noncompetitive but intense enough to elevate your heart rate above your threshold of training and into your target zone for cardiorespiratory endurance.

**vigorous sport**—Sport activity that elevates your heart rate above your threshold of training and into your target zone for cardiorespiratory endurance.

**warm-up**—A series of activities that prepares the body for more vigorous exercise.

**web extension**—Ending of a web address, such as .gov, .org, and .com.

**weightlifting**—Olympic sport involving free weights in which athletes try to lift a maximum load; includes two lifts—the snatch and the clean and jerk.

**wellness**—Positive component of health that involves having a good quality of life and a good sense of well-being as exhibited by a positive outlook.

**wind-chill factor**—Index used to determine when dangerously low temperatures and unsafe wind conditions exist.

**workout**—The part of the physical activity program during which a person does activities to improve fitness.

**yoga**—Activity that originated in India and that in its traditional forms includes meditation as well as the exercises and breathing techniques common to modern forms; involves poses called asanas that are similar to many flexibility exercises and can offer improved flexibility and other health benefits.

# Index